W9-CKR-701

Learning and Individual Differences

Learning and Individual Differences

PROCESS, TRAIT, AND CONTENT DETERMINANTS

Edited by
Phillip L. Ackerman
Patrick C. Kyllonen
Richard D. Roberts

AMERICAN PSYCHOLOGICAL ASSOCIATION • WASHINGTON, DC

LIBRARY
COLBY-SAWYER COLLEGE
NEW LONDON, NH 03257

BF
318
.L3853
1999
c.1

39812319

Copyright © 1999 by the American Psychological Association. All rights reserved. Except as permitted under the United States Copyright Act of 1976, no part of this publication may be reproduced or distributed in any form or by any means, or stored in a database or retrieval system, without the prior written permission of the publisher.

Published by
American Psychological Association
750 First Street, NE
Washington, DC 20002

Copies may be ordered from
APA Order Department
P.O. Box 92984
Washington, DC 20090-2984

In the U.K., Europe, Africa, and the Middle East, copies may be ordered from
American Psychological Association
3 Henrietta Street
Covent Garden, London
WC2E 8LU England

Typeset in Electra by EPS Group Inc., Easton, MD
Printer: Data Reproductions Corporation, Auburn Hills, MI
Cover Designer: Berg Design, Albany, NY
Technical/Production Editors: Marianne Maggini and Anne Woodworth

Library of Congress Cataloging-in-Publication Data
Learning and individual differences : process, trait, and content
    determinants / edited by Phillip L. Ackerman, Patrick C. Kyllonen,
    and Richard D. Roberts.
        p.   cm.
    Includes indexes.
    ISBN 1-55798-536-7 (casebound : alk. paper)
    1. Learning, Psychology of.   2. Individual differences.
    I. Ackerman, Phillip Lawrence. 1957–   II. Kyllonen, Patrick C.
    III. Roberts, Richard D.
    BF318.L3853   1998
    153.1′5–dc21   98-31084
                                                                                            CIP

British Library Cataloguing-in-Publication Data
A CIP record is available from the British Library.

Printed in the United States of America
First Edition

*This book is dedicated to the memory of
Richard E. Snow (1936–1997).
A pioneer in learning and individual-differences research
and a scholar, teacher, and friend.*

Contents

Contributors

PHILLIP L. ACKERMAN   School of Psychology, Georgia Institute of Technology

PATRICIA A. ALEXANDER   Department of Human Development, University of Maryland, College Park

ALAN BADDELEY   Center for the Study of Memory and Learning, Department of Psychology, University of Bristol, England

MARK L. DAVISON   Department of Educational Psychology, University of Minnesota, Twin Cities

IAN J. DEARY   Department of Psychology, University of Edinburgh, Scotland

IAN DENNIS   School of Mathematics and Statistics, University of Plymouth, England

SUSAN GATHERCOLE   Center for the Study of Memory and Learning, Department of Psychology, University of Bristol, Bristol, England

GINGER NELSON GOFF   Metrica, Inc., San Antonio, Texas

JAN-ERIC GUSTAFSSON   Department of Education, University of Göteborg, Mölndal, Sweden

ERIC D. HEGGESTAD   U.S. Air Force Armstrong Laboratory, Brooks Air Force Base, Texas

EARL HUNT   Department of Psychology, University of Washington

MANUEL JUAN-ESPINOSA*   Universidad Autononma de Madrid, Spain

RUTH KANFER   School of Psychology, Georgia Institute of Technology

SE-KANG KIM   Department of Educational Psychology, University of Minnesota, Twin Cities

---

*Indicates additional discussion participant, although not a chapter contributor.

HAIJIANG KUANG   *Department of Educational Psychology, University of Minnesota, Twin Cities*

DAVID F. LOHMAN   *Division of Psychological and Quantitative Foundations, College of Education, University of Iowa*

GERALD MATTHEWS   *Department of Psychology, University of Dundee, Scotland*

P. KAREN MURPHY   *Department of Human Development, University of Maryland, College Park*

EDWARD NĘCKA   *Psychology Institute, Jagiellonian University, Kraków, Poland*

GERRY PALLIER   *University of Sydney, Australia*

DAVID B. PISONI*   *Department of Psychology, Indiana University*

RICHARD D. ROBERTS   *U.S. Air Force Armstrong Laboratory, Brooks Air Force Base, Texas*

LAZAR STANKOV   *Department of Psychology, University of Sydney, Australia*

KEITH E. STANOVICH   *Department of Human Development and Applied Psychology, Ontario Institute for Studies in Education, University of Ontario, Canada*

HEINZ-MARTIN SÜß   *Department of Psychology, Universität Mannheim, Germany*

RICHARD K. WAGNER   *Department of Psychology, Florida State University*

RICHARD F. WEST, *Department of Psychology, James Madison University*

KEITH F. WIDAMAN   *Department of Psychology, University of California, Riverside*

WERNER W. WITTMANN   *Department of Psychology, Universität Mannheim, Germany*

DAN J. WOLTZ   *Department of Educational Psychology, University of Utah*

DAVID E. WRIGHT   *School of Mathematics and Statistics, University of Plymouth, England*

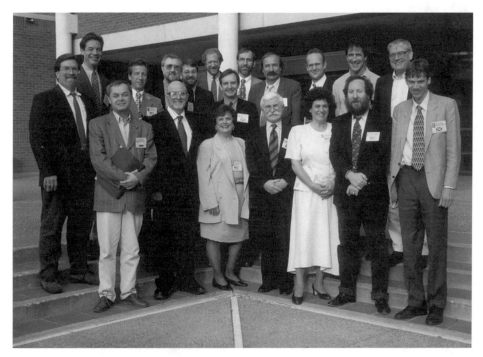

Conference Participants

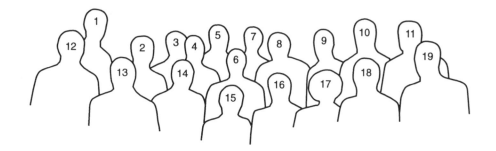

1. Patrick C. Kyllonen
2. Richard K. Wagner
3. Keith E. Stanovich
4. Dan J. Woltz
5. Jan-Eric Gustafsson
6. Ian J. Deary
7. David F. Lohman
8. Werner W. Wittmann
9. David E. Wright
10. Richard D. Roberts
11. Alan Baddeley

12. Keith F. Widaman
13. Edward Nęcka
14. Earl Hunt
15. Patricia A. Alexander
16. Lazar Stankov
17. Ruth Kanfer
18. Phillip L. Ackerman
19. Gerald Matthews

Not pictured:
Mark L. Davison

Foreword

In late 1996, when Phil Ackerman first suggested to Bill Howell, then Executive Director for Science, that the APA should publish the volume expected to result from a planned conference on the future of learning and individual differences research, Bill responded with an enthusiastic "absolutely!" Those of us in the Science Directorate and in the APA Books department knew that Phillip L. Ackerman, Patrick C. Kyllonen, and Richard D. Roberts would put on a first-rate conference and that the volume coming from it would maintain that level of excellence.

Indeed, this volume includes the research results and commentary of some of the most distinguished scientists who work in the area. We believe you will find it a stimulating collection of perspectives on a subject that is at the core of psychological science.

This volume continues a long-standing tradition of the APA publishing books that represent the best of psychological science. We are committed to the further development of this science series and we invite your suggestions for topics for future volumes.

RICHARD C. MCCARTY, PHD
Executive Director for Science

VIRGINIA E. HOLT
Assistant Executive Director for Science

Preface

Research into learning and individual differences has traditionally included laboratory, school, and job learning and learning in children and adults. In many ways, the growth of this field has paralleled that of modern psychology through this century. In 1908, E. L. Thorndike posed the question of whether individuals become more similar or more different with practice on mental tasks. In nearly every subsequent decade of this century, there have been significant contributions in both theory and practice associated with this topic, such as E. L. Thorndike's work in the 1910s and 1920s, A. Anastasi's work in the 1930s, H. Woodrow's work in the 1940s, and E. L. Fleishman's work in the 1950s. None of these research programs, though, have had the immense impact on the field as have the contributions by L. J. Cronbach, in his 1957 *American Psychologist* article in which he put forth a challenge for unification of experimental and correlational scientific psychologies, and later by Cronbach and R. E. Snow, in their 1977 book *Aptitudes and Instructional Methods*. Such developments are spelled out in three previously published collections.[1]

Because much of the research reported in this book is truly multidisciplinary — crossing methodology, process, trait, and content approaches to learning and individual differences — categorization of the chapters was a difficult task. Nonetheless, we have divided the book into five parts that make a rough delineation of the major themes of the chapters. The first part, General Background and Perspectives, contains perspectives from cognitive psychology, neuropsychology, instructional psychology, and ecological psychology. Hunt's chapter reviews a broad array of issues and findings from cognitive psychology as applied to individual differences in intelligence, especially in the domain of work and employment. The chapter by Bad-

---

[1]Ackerman, P. L., Sternberg, R. J., & Glaser, R. (1989). *Learning and individual differences: Advances in theory and research.* New York: Freeman. Gagné, R. M. (Ed.). (1967). *Learning and individual differences.* Columbus, OH: Charles E. Merrill. Kanfer, R., Ackerman, P. L., & Cudeck, R. (1989). *Abilities, Motivation, and Methodology: The Minnesota Symposium on Learning and Individual Differences.* Hillsdale, NJ: Erlbaum.

deley and Gathercole takes a micro-oriented approach to individual differences in learning and memory by focusing on evidence from experimental clinical and neuropsychological research. Lohman reviews issues of learning and intelligence from an instructional and educational attainment perspective. The last chapter in this section, by Wittmann and Süß, presents an approach to several issues of learning and individual differences, such as working memory and complex problem solving, with a perspective that is based on Egon Brunswik's concept of symmetry.

The second part of the book, Processes, concentrates on the basic process determinants of learning and individual differences, namely, visual and auditory processing, priming, and automaticity. Deary's chapter is organized around a critical review of extant research and current developments in the area of individual differences in visual and auditory information processing, including a discussion of inspection time issues. The chapter by Woltz discusses theoretical and empirical work concerning individual differences in reactions to stimulus priming, which is viewed as a particularly useful window in evaluating how individuals differentially process and accumulate information. Next, Nęcka reviews a series of experiments on individual differences in the development and expression of information-processing automaticity and discusses how these differences relate to extant measures of intellectual abilities.

The third part of the book, Methodological Strategies, concentrates on new developments in quantitative methodology for assessing learning and individual differences, namely, profile analysis, path analysis and structural equation modeling, and speed–accuracy trade-off analysis. The chapter by Davison, Kuang, and Kim presents a new approach to evaluating the interrelations among individuals and tests within a test battery. This approach uses multidimensional scaling techniques to establish test and participant profiles that can be used to derive groupings of similar individuals. Widaman returns to enduring issues of changes in abilities over time, with new developments in structural equation modeling techniques. In the Wright and Dennis chapter, tests are specially constructed to allow for modification of presentation time to evaluate individual differences and to determine whether these techniques can be used to improve old tests and develop new computer-based tests.

The fourth part of the book, Traits, focuses on cross-comparisons between individual differences in traits and learning, including personality traits, general intelligence, motivational traits, and sensory abilities. In his chapter, Matthews reviews relations among personality traits such as introversion–extroversion and anxiety, task information-processing demands, and individual differences in cognitive performance within a larger cognitive–adaptive framework. Gustafsson provides a perspective of general intelligence that is founded on the integration of experimental and correlational research. In their chapter, Kanfer and Heggestad discuss how motivational traits (such as anxiety and achievement orientation) and skills affect individual differences in learning and performance. Stankov's chapter reviews evidence relating personality traits with intellectual abilities and includes work on emotional intelligence. In the chapter by Roberts, Pallier, and Goff, the authors review a domain of abilities that has received little attention in recent years — sensory abilities — and they discuss how such abilities relate to broader indexes of intellectual ability.

The fifth and final part of the book, Content, concerns larger-scale issues in learning and individual differences, including expertise, heuristic reasoning, classroom learning, and adult intellectual development. Wagner discusses individual differences in performance at the upper reaches of attainment by focusing on the determinants of expertise. In their chapter, Stanovich and West consider higher-level cognitive problem solving, including the use of heuristic strategies, and discuss how abilities relate to individual differences in strategies and biases in problem solving. The chapter by Alexander and Murphy considers learning in college and university domains, and they describe the implications of profiles that are common to clusters of learners. The final chapter, by Ackerman, describes a perspective on adult intelligence that concentrates on knowledge and the ability, personality, and interest determinants of individual differences in knowledge attainment.

The reader will find both historical and current theory and research described in this book. He or she will find discussions and citations to work from around the world, some of which appear for the first time in an English-language publication. The discussions among chapter authors provide the reader with a rare view of the theoretical and empirical tensions that permeate this multidisciplinary field. We hope that the reader will get a sense of the issues of consensus and contention in this area. We also hope that the reader will get an unvarnished representation of how paradigms can be set in opposition to one another, or fused together, to reveal new opportunities for future research and theory. These chapters show the "lay of the land" in the field of learning and individual differences, and describe the uncharted territory for future investigations.

PHILLIP L. ACKERMAN
Atlanta, Georgia

PATRICK C. KYLLONEN
Brooks Air Force Base, Texas

RICHARD D. ROBERTS
Brooks Air Force Base, Texas

Acknowledgments

This book is based on a conference held at the University of Minnesota, Twin Cities, in October 1997. In addition to the 20 invited chapter authors who represent eight countries, the meeting was attended by 50 local, national, and international observers, including poster presentations from 20 attendees. The invited speakers had previously distributed draft copies of their chapters, and each presentation was followed by a discussion that was recorded and later edited for this volume.

The completion of this project is due to the efforts and contributions of many individuals and organizations. We are grateful for the financial support that allowed the meeting and this book to come to fruition. An early commitment of support from John Tangney at the U.S. Air Force Office of Scientific Research (AFOSR) allowed us to pursue both domestic and internationally distinguished researchers for the meeting and this book. Funding for the meeting was provided by the AFOSR, the University of Minnesota, Twin Cities, and the APA. We especially wish to acknowledge the enthusiastic support of John F. Tangney, Program Manager for Perception and Cognition at AFOSR, Robert H. Bruininks, Executive Vice President and Provost at the University of Minnesota, Twin Cities, and Gary R. VandenBos, Executive Director of Publications and Communications at the APA. Local support was provided by students in the Kanfer/Ackerman Cognitive Ability, Motivation, and Learning Laboratories and by the Herculean organizational efforts of Michelle Adamiak. Support for the time and effort for preparation of this book was generously provided by the School of Psychology at the Georgia Institute of Technology. Most of all, we wish to thank the authors and meeting participants for their cutting-edge papers and penetrating and critical discussion of the papers, much of which we have recorded in this book. The future for the study of learning and individual differences, as demonstrated by these chapters, is bright. As we enter modern psychology's second century, these innovative inquiries suggest many new areas for fruitful investigation and promise to bring greater order to the field.

When we started planning for the book and meetings in late 1996, Dick Snow was one of the first individuals we had invited, and he cordially accepted our invitation. However, he became ill in the spring of 1997 and was unable to complete his chapter for this book or to attend the conference. His presence was genuinely missed at the conference, but many of the chapters of this book serve as a salient reminder of his contributions to this field.

I

GENERAL BACKGROUND AND PERSPECTIVES

1

Intelligence and Human Resources: Past, Present, and Future

EARL HUNT

How many intelligences are there? How can I count the ways? A Harvard professor has shown that there are multiple intelligences (Gardner, 1983; Gardner, Kornhaber, & Wake, 1996). Disconcertingly, in the widely read *The Bell Curve,* another Harvard professor has told us that there is a single general intelligence (Herrnstein & Murray, 1994). Cattell and Horn assured us that there are two intelligences: fluid and crystallized (Cattell, 1971; Horn, 1985; Horn & Noll, 1994). Eysenck (1986) said that there are three: Intelligences A, B, and C. Generalizing on Eysenck in both number and content, R. J. Sternberg (1990) and several other publications have said that there are 3^k intelligences, where $k > 1$. To top it all off, Guilford (1967) offered us over 100 intellectual abilities. Just to show that psychometricians are not the only ones who are confused, a recent rebuttal of *The Bell Curve* insists that a proper analysis will show that intelligence is not general, is not important, and probably is not hereditary (Fischer et al., 1996).

Cognitive psychology is neither better nor worse. Psychologists have production system models, schema theory, connectionism, cognitive neurosciences, and situated cognition. What is the way to truth? A disinterested observer, or maybe even a funding agent, might decide to just turn away. This, of course, is intolerable!

I believe that much of this noise is just that, noise. Newton regarded his predecessors as giants, and said he stood on their shoulders. Twentieth-century psychologists have had a discouraging tendency to regard their predecessors as dwarfs and to stand on their faces. Newton's way is better, and not just because it is more polite. The production, nurturing, and use of cognitive abilities are important national

The preparation of this chapter was partially supported by a grant to the University of Washington by the James S. McDonnell Foundation.

issues. If scientists fail to state clearly what is known, people with political axes to grind will invent the facts they want to have. Scientific debate should never minimize differences between researchers, but magnifying them will lessen the chance that established findings have the social impact that they ought to have.

The purpose of this chapter is to highlight commonalities in psychologists' views of human cognition and then to use those commonalities to point the way to future research. I hope that I will not be seen as developing my own theory, for that is neither my intention nor, to be frank, do I think that it is a particularly desirable outcome. What I want to do is to show that various approaches to cognition are complementary rather than opposed. I will attempt a unification of some diverse findings in order to point toward some of the major questions about individual differences in human cognition that face us as we enter the 21st century. As my opening remarks suggest, I do not think that determining the number of intelligences is one of those questions.

The Psychometric View of Intelligence

Most tests of intelligence are actually batteries of subtests. The subtests evaluate narrow cognitive skills, such as paragraph comprehension or arithmetical reasoning. The Wechsler Adult Intelligence Scale (WAIS), the Armed Services Vocational Aptitude Battery, and the Scholastic Assessment Test (SAT) are good examples. The correlations between different subtests are high enough to support a strong case for general intelligence (g). Unfortunately, the correlations are also low enough to support a case for correlated multiple intelligences. What cannot be denied, however, is that a few broad dimensions of individual differences can account for the measurements that are obtained with test batteries. Also, when serious attempts are made to construct tests of pure reasoning, notably by Cattell (Institute for Personality and Ability Testing, 1973) and Raven (1965), these tests define statistical markers for g.

The history of debates about general versus multiple dimensions underlying the psychometric data is well-known, so I do not attempt to repeat it here. (Interested readers should consult Brody, 1992, Gardner et al., 1996, and R. J. Sternberg, 1990.) What is not well-known is that the issue has been pretty well settled. Carroll (1993) has written a superb, detailed statistical analysis of virtually all the major data sets.[1] He concluded that intellectual abilities form a hierarchy. A graphic summary of part of his argument (modified from Carroll, 1997) is shown in Figure 1.1. At the bottom level (*stratum*, in Carroll's terms), there are a variety of specific abilities, such as the speed of accessing a word or the ability to recite a small number of words, letters, or digits in a memory span experiment. The correlations between these microabilities indicate that they are specialized expressions of several broad-ranging abilities. These form Carroll's middle, or *second-order*, stratum. The most important of the second-order abilities is a general reasoning factor, the ability to use cultural knowledge, visual–spatial reasoning, and the ability to reason quickly.

---

[1] Although Carroll's (1993) analysis is well-known to specialists in the field, it is relatively inaccessible to a layperson because of its highly technical nature. Therefore, it has had little influence on many of the current public debates on intelligence. Carroll (1997) has since provided a much less technical discussion of his conclusions.

4

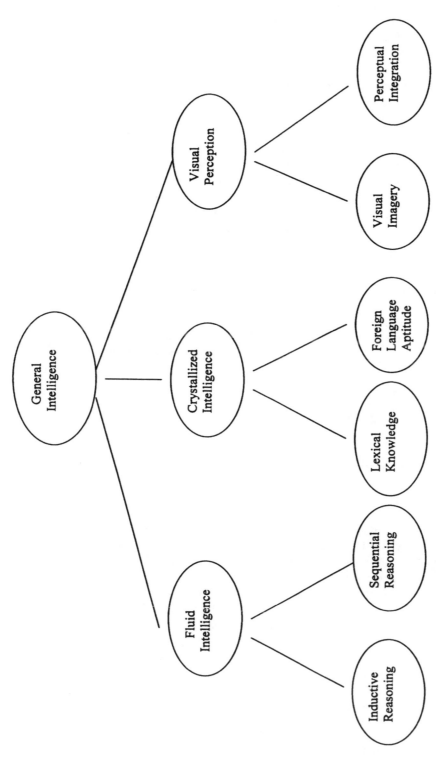

Figure 1.1. A schematic of Carroll's (1993) hierarchical model of intelligence, as defined by performance on psychometric tests. The items shown are intended to illustrate the nature of Carroll's model (see Carroll, 1993, Figure 15.1, for a much more complete diagram).

As Carroll acknowledged, his hierarchical analysis is closely related to the fluid intelligence–crystallized intelligence model put forward by Cattell (1971) and Horn (1985; Horn & Noll, 1994). I adopt their terminology and concentrate first on *fluid intelligence* (Gf), defined loosely as the ability to represent and reason about novel problems, and *crystallized intelligence* (Gc), defined as the ability to apply previously acquired, culturally defined definitions or problem-solving methods to a current situation. I offer a few remarks about *visual–spatial reasoning*, but only to provide some specific illustrations.

In most data sets, the correlations between the Gf and Gc factors are in the .5–.7 range. This would be consistent with thinking of a third-order general intelligence factor, g, either as a statistical combination of Gc and Gf or as a causal agent that precedes both of them. Although these are much different conceptual explanations for the data, they make no difference for the use of intelligence tests. When subtests are moderately or highly correlated with other, general factor scores are useful statistical indicators for personnel screening regardless of why the factor itself exists.

Although the psychometric data cannot discriminate between the two interpretations of g, other data can. When this is done, conceptualizations of g as a causal factor run into difficulties. The clearest example is gerontology, wherein the influence of age on cognition has been studied extensively. Gf decreases over the adult life span, whereas Gc increases slightly (Horn & Noll, 1994). In the terminology of experimental psychology, age acts as an independent variable that has different effects on two measures. This is sufficient to show that the measures are measures of different underlying processes. That point is going to be important when I move from discussing what causes intelligence to a discussion of what intelligence causes.

Cognitive Psychology: Information Processing and the Neurosciences

Correlational analyses are useful ways of defining the dimensions of human intellectual variation, but they do not define the process of thought. That is the province of cognitive psychology. Cognitive psychology has to be related to psychometrics, but the purpose of this relation is not, and never has been, to produce a better test. The purpose is to assist in understanding why the dimensions of human cognition are what they are. There are both scientific and practical reasons for doing this. The scientific reason is that analyses based on cognitive psychology are an important step in the reductionist goal of relating psychometric findings to biological measures. The practical reason is that if we wish to gain acceptance for the use of intelligence testing in school and in the workplace, we must explain why the tests work the way they do. People who question policies that are based on psychometric results are not interested in correlational analyses. They want causal models, and with justification (Hunt, 1996).

Cognitive psychology consists of two quite different subdisciplines. One is the study of human information processing. This is my first concern. The second subdiscipline is a loosely defined field that I will refer to as the *organization of knowledge*. This subdiscipline will be of concern when I discuss the uses of intelligence.

The goal of information-processing studies is to understand those aspects of human cognition that depend only minimally on the meaning of information a person is processing. Perhaps one of the best examples of this approach is Sternberg's (1975) famous work on short-term memory scanning. S. Sternberg wanted to determine how people scan information held in short-term memory. The stimuli chosen for memorization were arbitrary sets of words or alphanumeric characters. Symbol strings that made up a sentence were avoided. This was reasonable to do, for the goal was to reveal the architecture and operating characteristics of the human information processor. For this purpose, the use of meaningful sentences would simply have confused the issue. On the other hand, in everyday life people spend more time understanding sentences than they do memorizing telephone numbers. This point should be kept in mind.

Although the information-processing approach often uses terminology borrowed from computer science, the approach itself does not imply a commitment to the use of modern computers as metaphors for the brain. Both symbol processing (Simon & Kaplan, 1988) and connectionist architectures (Rumelhart, 1988) lie within the information-processing framework. The key point is that what is being examined are the information-processing characteristics of humans. Although those who build information-processing models of thought do not study how meaning and understanding influence thought, they certainly do not deny these influences.

Information-processing approaches to thought are closely linked to the neurosciences. A major goal of cognitive neuroscience is to locate those brain structures and neurochemical processes that support cognitive actions. Therefore, information-processing models are essential to relate neuroscience observations to behavior. It would not be terribly useful to look at a positron–emission tomography (PET) scan or a functional magnetic resonance imaging picture of a person reading a newspaper. You would simply discover that there was lots of activity all over the brain. It is instructive to contrast the brain images obtained when an individual is (a) looking at lines that do not form letter or words, (b) looking at words, and (c) looking at words and thinking of a word that semantically related to the word in view. Task A requires vision alone, Task B requires vision and the retrieval of lexical information, and Task C requires controlled processing of that lexical information. Knowing the difference between the information-processing demands of any two tasks informs researchers when they look at the difference between levels of brain activity during each task (Posner & Raichle, 1994; Smith & Jonides, 1997).

More generally, both neuroscientific and psychometric data have to be examined in the context of a theory of cognition. What information-processing psychology provides is a theory that can unite the two. What does that theory look like?

Information-processing studies have resulted in a consistent functional (not biological) model of the mind. This is shown in Figure 1.2. It consists of two major systems, each with their own subdivisions.

The major division between systems is between working memory and long-term memory. *Working memory*, a term first introduced by Baddeley (1986), refers to people's functional ability to construct, hold over time, and manipulate an internal representation of objects that conceivably could be perceived by their sensory apparatus. The second subdivision, *long-term memory*, refers collectively to people's stored representations (engrams) of facts and procedures. A pattern recognition process recognizes data structures in working memory and activates related engrams. The actions associated with the engrams may in turn produce new data structures

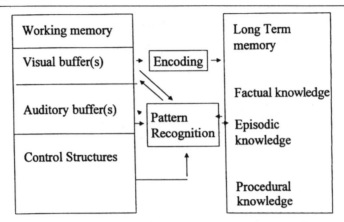

Figure 1.2. The standard information-processing theory of mental architecture. Memory is divided into working memory and long-term memory. Within working memory there are buffer memories for auditory and visual representations and a central control section. An encoding process moves information from working to long-term memory. A pattern matching process connects the information in working memory to previously acquired information in long-term memory.

in working memory, leading to a new cycle of action of representation construction, pattern recognition, and manipulation.

This is an extremely long-winded way of saying "When you see 2 + 2 on a sheet of paper, think 4" and "When you see a red traffic light, stop." The principles behind these rules can be used to construct a detailed theory of human thought (Anderson, 1993; Newell, 1990).

Baddeley (1986) proposed that working memory consists of three structures. Two of them, the iconic and echoic buffers, are devices for holding sensory-coded messages. These can be received either from the environment or from long-term memory, such as when one images a memorized picture or explicitly recalls the rules for solving a particular type or problem. In addition to the iconic and echoic buffers, working memory contains control structures that enable people to fix attention on one or another item in memory. The control structures also ensure an orderly flow of information into working memory, both from the external world and from memory itself, either by blocking extraneous information or by dropping out those pieces of information that do not appear to be being used in the problem-solving process. The phrases "Paying attention to all relevant variables" and "Holding the relevant variables in working memory" are virtually synonymous.

It is one thing to say that attention must be paid and quite another to say how it is paid. One of the major theoretical problems facing cognitive neuroscientists today is to find a description of what "paying attention" means in terms of more primitive functions. This problem has to be attacked at the information-processing level, without appealing to some sort of homunculus that has access to information about the meaning of brain activities in terms of the external world. Researchers do have some hints about the solution of this theoretical problem. I mention a few shortly. For the moment, I accept "paying attention" as a primitive concept and continue looking at how thought proceeds at the functional level.

Because people do learn, there must be an encoding system that uses information in working memory to create new productions in long-term memory. Again, as a matter of logic, this has to be an entirely automatic process that is contingent only on information structures being in working memory in appropriate temporal contiguity. To repeat, an information-processing model deals with internal configurations of the brain–mind system, not with the external meanings of those configurations.

The standard information-processing model does not include a commitment to there being unique physical locations for working memory and long-term memory, akin to a stage and a set of actors waiting for their cue lines. On the other hand, there must be anatomical locations for the functions that collectively produce the working memory/long-term memory distinction. These brain structures may also be used for other cognitive functions, notably perception. I argue that the anatomical distribution of functionality in the brain has implications for the study of intelligence. Second, the model, as presented, contains no role for what has been called *unconscious processing* or *implicit memory*. It is possible to expand the model to include these features of human thought, but this is not the place to do so. Finally, nothing here is new. Elements of these ideas can be found in many publications (Anderson, 1983, 1993; Hunt & Lansman, 1986; Newell, 1990; Thibadeau, Just, & Carpenter, 1982). My contribution is to try to summarize a quarter century of research relating these concepts to the psychometric definition of intelligence.

Any psychometric task that depends on the development and manipulation of a complex, multivariable problem representation should tax working memory. Two such tasks come immediately to mind: matrix tests (Raven, 1965) and the analysis of complex sentences.

Matrix tests are particularly interesting because, as already noted, they are good markers for Gf. Task analyses of the individual steps required to solve matrix problems have shown that, as a matter of logic alone, these tasks cause considerable strain on working memory. Different patterns have to be abstracted from an examination of different parts of the matrix, and then these patterns must be combined (Carpenter, Just, & Shell, 1990; Hunt, 1974). This is illustrated by the problem shown in Figure 1.3. Similar remarks can be made about logic problems, in which people have to restrict their attention to relevant elements and combine statements about them. Another example is the analysis of electronic circuits, in which it is necessary to keep in mind the implications of combinations of multiple states of circuit elements. The results of several studies have shown that measures of working memory capacity do indeed correlate strongly with performance on matrix problems, logic problems, and circuit analysis problems (Carpenter et al., 1990; Kyllonen & Christal, 1990; Kyllonen & Stephens, 1990).

Language comprehension is an interesting task because it is obviously a crucial cognitive skill, clearly shows individual differences, and yet is usually considered separately from reasoning ability. Nevertheless, the two share a common dependence on working memory. Language comprehension depends on being able to extract information from words and on being able to hold that information in abeyance until there is something to attach it to. In the extreme, the receiver's initial representation of the meaning of a sentence may have to be redeveloped (i.e., a data structure in working memory may have to be rebuilt) when new information is received. This is shown in the classic "garden path" sentence: "The horse raced past the barn fell."

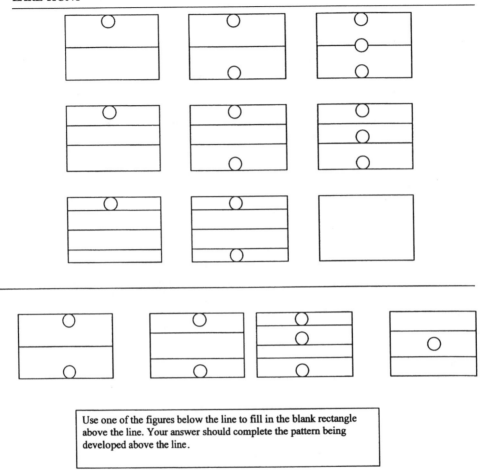

Figure 1.3. An example matrix problem constructed to illustrate the general principles behind such problems. The problem shown is relatively easy. Much harder problems can be constructed.

In other cases, the meaning of the entire sentence can be determined only by selecting a meaning that makes sense in context. A recent radio announcement by the Washington State Department of Transportation informed me that "The Seattle to Bainbridge ferry is not running on time as usual." This was said in the context of a story about a fire on the Bainbridge loading dock rather than in an expose of poor service by Washington State's Ferry system. Using more prosaic examples, Just and Carpenter (1992) have shown that the ability perform such linguistic tasks is related closely to performance on a short-term memory task involving linguistic stimuli.

These examples have only touched the surface of the literature. There is now a substantial body of evidence showing that, in Kyllonen and Christal's (1990) apt title, "Reasoning Ability Is (Little More Than) Working Memory Capacity." This opens thinking about intelligence to some of the recent findings in the neurosciences.

Working memory is a function, not a place. Modern neuroscientific findings (Gazzaniga, 1995; Posner & Raichle, 1994) strongly indicate that the brain does not have centers that produce grand intellectual themes, such as love, thought, or patriotism. Rather, the brain is more like a toolkit that provides low-order primitive functions from which the mind constructs its general themes. Baddeley's (1986) concept of working memory depends on three separate functions: auditory and visual sensory coding areas, in which internal and external images may be maintained and rehearsed, and a control element. These functions are produced in three separate areas of the brain, and these areas can be broken down further into noncontiguous regions that are involved in still more primitive functions. Individual differences in the brain's capacities to execute the primitive functions will place limits on a person's ability to develop representations of the world.

Tasks that require auditory or visual "images," such as thinking of a word or imaging a scene, involve regions that are associated with (although not exactly identical to) those regions involved in direct perception. Some relevant regions are the temporal cortex for audition and widely distributed but specific regions of the brain for vision, imaging, and spatial reasoning (Jonides et al., 1993; Kosslyn, 1994; Logie, 1995; Posner & Raichle, 1994). The frontal cortex seems to be involved in a wide variety of intellectual functions, as I discuss in more detail. Pathological damage to these regions can result in major dysfunction in perception and imagery. It is unlikely in the extreme that these regions just do or do not work. As neural imaging and other biological tools become more widespread, researchers can certainly hope for a better understanding of how auditory and visual imaging abilities relate to individual differences in representation manipulation and, at a grosser level, the statistical abstraction that psychologists call *fluid intelligence*. However, I do not think that that is going to be the whole story.

By definition, difficult problems unfold over time. To solve them, people have to keep their internal (imaged?) representations focused on the problem at hand. It is now clear that the frontal cortex performs this function. This was illustrated in one of the earliest reports of clinical neuropsychology on record, the case of Phineas Gage. Gage, a nineteenth century railroad foreman, suffered a freak accident in which a railroad spike was driven through his forehead. Gage went from being a well-respected worker to being an aggressive, impulsive social misfit. When Gage died, his brain was preserved. A century later, an analysis using modern imaging techniques showed that Gage had suffered severe damage to his prefrontal cortex (Damasio et al., 1994). The finding was not unexpected. Since Gage's day, numerous studies of injuries to the frontal cortex have confirmed the early report. Damage to the prefrontal cortex is associated with a reduced ability to focus attention and a failure to inhibit actions that are inappropriate in context (Shimamura, 1995).

The effects of frontal cortical injuries are dramatic when the injury is severe enough to intrude on social behaviors, as Gage's was. They are less dramatic, but consistent with the social observations, in situations that call for "pure thought." Patients with frontal injuries are handicapped whenever the situation requires that they selectively attend to one aspect of a situation while ignoring others. This is especially true if the aspect to be ignored is usually salient or when it is necessary to suppress previously learned responses to acquire new associations. Computer simulations in which it is assumed that the difference between people is the extent to which they can control attention can mimic the contrasts between patients with

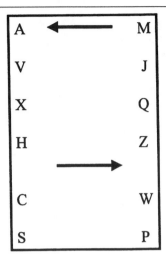

Figure 1.4. A schematic of the monitoring task used by Duncan, Emslie, Williams, and Johnson (1996).

frontal lobe injuries and a control group in tasks that require these sorts of control of attention, such as the Stroop task and the Wisconsin Card Sorting Test (Kimberg & Farah, 1993).

Neuropsychological studies show what happens when a brain structure suffers major damage. Because brain tissue does not turn off and on, it seems reasonable to expect that studies of normal individuals will show some relationship between performance on tests designed to evaluate damage to specific brain regions, such as microscopic tasks involving the control of attention, and more global Gf tasks. An important article by Duncan, Emslie, Williams, and Johnson (1996) has linked these observations to intelligence, as defined by conventional intelligence tests. Participants were shown two streams of letters and told to monitor, aloud, letters appearing in either the right- or left-hand stream (see Figure 1.4). Aperiodically, they were told either to continue monitoring the same side or to switch to the other side. Thus, the task requires both selective attention and an ability to switch attention from one part of a stimulus complex to another. Duncan et al. found that patients with frontal lobe lesions performed exceptionally poorly on this task compared with control participants or patients with posterior lesions. As further evidence of the validity of the task, the performance of uninjured participants on the monitoring task was positively related to scores on Cattell's Culture-Fair Intelligence Test, a good marker of Gf.

The Duncan et al. (1996) experiment is a nice demonstration of the continuity from neuropsychological to normal data because different populations, including patients and carefully matched controls, were tested on the same task with exactly the same procedures. Das and his colleagues have been making the same point for a number of years, relying on data from less tightly controlled situations. Das and his associates used adaptations of neuropsychological tests for frontal lobe damage to evaluate goal-directed planning abilities in normal participants, including schoolchildren. They have found that test performance shows a clear-cut developmental trend that parallels the development of planning and purposeful behavior before adolescence. These are also individual differences in the performance of normal adults who have to deal with planning situations. In one experiment, there was a correlation of .53 between bank financial officers' performance on tests of frontal lobe functioning and ratings of their performance by bank managers (Das, Kar, & Parrila, 1996).

To complete the picture, neuroimaging studies have shown that when people attack matrix problems, metabolic activity increases in the forebrain. Furthermore, precisely where in the forebrain the activity increases depends on the type of problem. Problems that involve perceptual analysis primarily activate regions in the right frontal and parietal regions. Problems that require analytical strategies activate other areas that are known to be associated with verbal working memory and domain-independent control processes (Prabhakaran, Smith, Desmond, Glover, & Gabrieli, 1997).

Summing these findings up, I can make certain major assertions. There is a psychometric dimension of Gf, performance along this dimension is closely associated with working memory capacity and the ability to control attention, and these functions are largely mediated by forebrain structures. Those who feel that psychology simply recycles old issues should rethink their position. None of these propositions could be made with so much confidence 50 years ago.

I now shift the discussion of information-processing functions away from working memory toward long-term memory to examine pattern recognition, because this is the way in which long-term memories are aroused, in situations in which people can safely assume that the relevant memories are indeed present. During the 1970s and 1980s, several studies by my colleagues and me, as well as by others (reviewed by Hunt, 1987), showed that there are differences in the speed with which people can access their memories of common words, such as on the California Achievement Tests. These differences are positively related to measures of verbal intelligence. Of course, it can be argued that lexical access is not all there is to verbal intelligence. For that matter, my colleagues and I never said that it was. However, verbal performance will not go forward without lexical access. More generally, the ability to use previously acquired problem-solving procedures depends on the ability to recognize that the previously acquired problem is relevant to the current problem. The lexical access studies showed that even when it is clear what the appropriate pattern is (a visual word form), there are still differences in access to the engram.

Another important long-term memory function is the encoding function. To acquire Gc, people have to be able to store information in memory. Neuropsychology provides some of the most dramatic examples of loss of this function. Patients with severe damage to the hippocampus and associated areas of the medial temporal lobes may develop almost complete anterograde amnesia; that is, they are unable to develop permanent memories for events that occur to them after their injury (Cohen & Eichenbaum, 1993; Squire & Knowlton, 1995). Such people are sometimes said to have normal intelligence because they pass all but the short-term memory tests on the WAIS. I dissent. I cannot see how anyone can possibly be said to have normal intelligence, in any meaningful sense of the word, if they have to be hospitalized for life because of deficiencies in cognitive functioning. I am not disputing the finding about unimpaired WAIS scores. I am disputing the identification of a useful but imperfect indicator, the WAIS, with the concept of intelligence.

There is still no direct evidence that individual differences in medial temporal lobe functioning influence normal memory. Although I am hopeful that subsequent studies may establish this link, psychologists have to realize that the neurological and neuroanatomical processes involved in long-term memory and retention are complicated. Although the hippocampus and its related structures are clearly necessary for encoding, they are not sufficient. One can see this by looking at a much more common form of memory disorder, Korsakoff's syndrome.[2]

Korsakoff's syndrome is a disorder of memory that, in prototypical cases, includes profound anterograde amnesia. Because the amnesia can be as complete as seen in the (much rarer) cases of hippocampal removal, many discussions of Korsakoff's syndrome in the cognitive psychology literature leave the impression that the two syndromes represent the same sorts of memory loss, with different etiologies. This is not so. There are important behavioral and neurological differences between the two syndromes, and these differences point to some of the complexities researchers deal with in uncovering the biological basis of intelligence. To explain why, I must briefly describe the clinical and neurological aspects of Korsakoff's syndrome, as presented by an authoritative monograph in the field (Victor, Adams, & Collins, 1989).

Most patients with Korsakoff's syndrome have a history of prolonged alcoholism accompanied by dietary deficiencies. In the typical case, the patient presents in a severe and disabling state of confusion, characterized by apathy and characteristic nervous tics, especially in the eyes. This condition is called *Wernicke's syndrome*. After the Wernicke's syndrome signs have subsided enough so that the patient can be tested, the severe anterograde amnesia is noted. Researchers do not know whether nonpathological anterograde amnesia was present before the onset of the Wernicke's syndrome attack. It is hard to see how this information could be obtained because the investigator would have to identify Wernicke–Korsakoff cases in advance of the display of symptoms.

The memory disorders of patients with Korsakoff's syndrome and hippocampal injuries are not identical. Both display anterograde amnesia. Patients with Korsakoff's syndrome, but not hippocampal injuries, may also display retrograde amnesia. Also, the former patients vary greatly in the degree of the anterograde amnesia. In some cases, they may recover a degree of memory function after treatment with improved, thiamin-rich diets.

Brain imaging and pathological examinations show a much different pattern between the two syndromes. Patients with Korsakoff's syndrome show extensive damage to the dioncephalon, particularly to the mammallary bodies. However, the degree of this damage does not correlate with behavioral indications of memory loss. Furthermore, patients with Korsakoff's syndrome do not show damage to the hippocampi. This, together with the data from patients with hippocampal injuries, indicates that hippocampal functioning is a necessary but not sufficient part of the encoding process.

A recent study by Paller et al. (1997) suggested what may be occurring in Korsakoff's syndrome and established a tenuous but perhaps important link to individual

---

[2]These comments on Korsakoff's syndrome represent additions to my thinking following comments by Baddeley at the conference. (See Baddeley's, 1986, comments in the discussion of this chapter.) I thank Arthur Shimamura for his assistance in pointing out some of the recent literature on the topic.

differences in normal memory function. Paller et al. used PET scanning to examine brain metabolism in Korsakoff's syndrome and control patients while the subjects were performing a variety of memory tasks. They found correlations in the .5 range between behavioral measures of memory and measures of hypometabolism in several areas of the brain. The highest correlations were found for the frontal cortex, the area that is also heavily involved in working memory functions. Paller et al. suggested that damage to the dioncephalon produces the hypometabolism in the frontal cortex. Although further research is certainly necessary, I shall speculate a bit on why this finding may help in clarifying findings from studies of normal memory.

First, there are clearly individual differences in normal long-term memory functioning. This has been shown by both psychometric and experimental studies of cognition. The experimental studies are clearest because they can control for exposure to the information being tested in a way that psychometric studies cannot. In one of the early studies of individual differences in information processing, Underwood, Boruch, and Malmi (1978) found that university students varied in their ability to memorize information and that this ability was general across a wide variety of tasks. Underwood et al. were disappointed in the result because they had hoped to use individual differences to test a multifaceted theory of memory. In hindsight, what they may have observed was the widespread effect of individual differences in the ability to organize and store information in general. The organization point is crucial.

The organization of information is central both to encoding and to controlled recall. To organize information, it is necessary to process it in depth, abstracting key elements and making associations that will be useful in later recall. In fact, this point generalizes beyond memory studies to studies of thinking in general. The brain, like any other computer, is only as good as its cabling. Therefore, several attempts have been made to relate brain functioning to general neural functioning rather than to the functioning of particular centers.

Most of these studies have used gross measures, varying from conduction velocity in the arm to electroencephalographic measures of responsiveness, and even size of the brain (Vernon, 1993). There is a consistent finding of modest but reliable relationships to gross measures of Gf. Probably, the most interesting of these measures is the inspection time task, in which the correlations with test performance are somewhat higher (.3−.4; Deary & Stough, 1996). In this task, all the observer does is make a simple perceptual comparison (e.g., between line lengths), so there is no argument that the untimed task tests anything that one normally would call *intelligence*. In addition, neuroimaging studies of brain metabolism during the performance of simple perceptual comparisons and of complex reasoning have shown that the latter problems draw on brain regions that are not heavily involved in tasks similar to the inspection time task. Compare, for instance, the brain regions involved in simple and complex tasks that have been identified by Posner and Raichle (1994) and by Prabhakaran et al. (1997). Therefore, the biological link between inspection time and psychometric measures of intelligence is probably attributable to individual differences in general brain processes rather than to the efficiency of particular structures required by both tasks.

These biological observations fit well with another well-known fact about intelligence, the influence of aging. It is well-known that aging results in a decline in scores on Gf measures (Salthouse, 1990). There is also a concomitant loss in the speed of elementary cognitive functioning. This can be explained by a surprisingly simple model in which the key assumption is that as people lose neural elements, their brain has to do more rechecking to protect against unreliable transmissions from center to center (Myerson, Hale, Wagstaff, Poon, & Smith, 1990). A considerable amount of decline in Gf in the later years of the life span can be accounted for by measures related to cognitive slowing (Salthouse, 1996).

The final point I would like to make about the relation between neuroscientific evidence and the brain concerns an old argument: the relation of nature and nurture to intelligence. Psychometric test scores, and especially scores on g and reasoning factors, show that in Western industrial society there is heavy genetic involvement in intelligence. Heritability estimates are between .4 and .7, and there is no reason (that I can think of) to want to tie them down more accurately. There has been more than enough debate in the scientific literature about the fact of genetic intelligence (Hunt, 1997a). It is still true, however, that many people hesitate to accept what seems, to a naive behavioral scientist, to be an obvious conclusion. There is a genetic component to human mental competence. How can anyone who is even marginally familiar with the evidence debate this?

Fortunately, a not-so-naive social scientist with extensive experience in policy analysis has explained why there are objections. Jencks (1992) observed that nonscientists dislike the argument that genetics causes intelligence for two reasons. First, no mechanism has been offered. Obviously one does not inherit an SAT score from one's parents in the same sense that one inherits eye color from them. So what does a child inherit? Second, the general public, and not a few social scientists (Fischer et al., 1996), seems to believe that high heritability of intelligence implies immutability of cognitive functioning. Although geneticists deny this, the way that the denial is stated can often be easily interpreted as their saying, "In principle, the mean could rise without affecting the variance, but in practice it probably will not." Herrnstein and Murray (1994) provided some particularly good examples of this sort of remark. Suggestions of immutability are not acceptable because modern Western traditions are far from fatalistic. Some people think they can reform the world, and someone who tells them that they cannot must be wrong. That is not good logic, but it is understandable psychologic. Furthermore, there is something to the argument.

The request for a mechanism behind the genetic correlations is a reasonable one. In fact, this issue is being pursued by teams of geneticists, neuroscientists, and molecular biologists (Plomin, 1995). The results so far have not been startling, but, to take a historical analogy, Columbus did not bring back much gold from his voyages. The conquistadors who followed him did. There is every reason to be optimistic that in the near future, researchers will be able to trace the mechanisms behind the heritability coefficients. Although the resulting discoveries could conceivably raise some issues that will require deep thought from society, a far more likely result is that researchers will be able to treat several currently disabling conditions. It seems unlikely that researchers will develop a pill to make people smart because, as I argue, smartness is probably specialized and largely dependent on hard work. It is reasonable to hope that research in the neurosciences will lead to therapy for major deficiencies associated with genetic and in utero damage.

The Relation to Intelligence: A Résumé of the Argument So Far

Claims that intelligence resides in a specific place in the brain belong to the nineteenth century, not the twentieth and certainly not the twenty-first centuries. The brain is the toolkit for the mind. Different information-processing tasks draw on particular tools to different degrees, and one tool may appear in many processes. The idea is shown in broad outline in Figure 1.5, in which Carroll's (1993) tree structure has been replaced by an alternative structure, a lattice. Each of Carroll's first-order, specific factors, such as lexical identification, depends on certain elementary information-processing functions, and these are associated both with general neural functioning and the efficiency of mechanisms in specific regions of the brain. This model can be used to address important issues about the distribution of test scores in the population.

When we teach students the statistical theory behind mental tests, we typically begin with a statement about assuming multivariate normality. This is a lie; intellectual skills are not normally distributed. At the bottom of the distribution, scores on cognitive tests are grouped tightly together, implying a strong general factor. Test scores at the top of the distribution are much more independent of each other, supporting the idea of specific intelligences. This fact has long been suspected but was verified only recently, first in an important article by Detterman and Daniel (1989) and then in several confirmatory studies (Deary et al., 1996; Hunt, 1997b; Legree, Pifer, & Grafton, 1996).

This finding becomes reasonable if one assumes, as I do, that having a good brain permits intelligent performance but does not dictate it. In the next section I argue that in our society, and in probably every society that depends on specialization of the roles of its members (i.e., every society that moves beyond the tribal level, as defined by Diamond, 1997), exceptional performance is almost always specialized. Therefore, high-level performance depends heavily on how efficiently people use their brain rather than what the brain's information-processing capacities are. On the other hand, if the brain has not provided the mind with adequate computing capacities in one or more areas (e.g., memorization, control of attention), there are going to be relatively few things that people can learn to do. This is essentially an anti-Mensa argument; there are no generally intelligent people, but there are some generally stupid ones.

To make the argument somewhat more scientific, I suggest that there is a nonlinear relation between brain functioning and intelligence, in which the latter is defined as a general ability to advance in society. When brain functioning falls below an acceptable level, as is certainly the case in Korsakoff's syndrome and Alzheimer's dementia, and marginally the case in cases of closed head injury (Sunderland, Harris, & Baddeley, 1983), and normal aging, the ability to perform elementary cognitive functions becomes inadequate. In particular, the weakened brain is not able to perform those functions associated with memory and control of attention. Below the point at which these functions become critical the biological functioning of the brain centrally determines a person's ability to be part of human society. Above the critical level, however, biological functions still count, but they count for much less. The issue becomes the content of the information that a person has to process more than the person's content-free ability to process information.

17

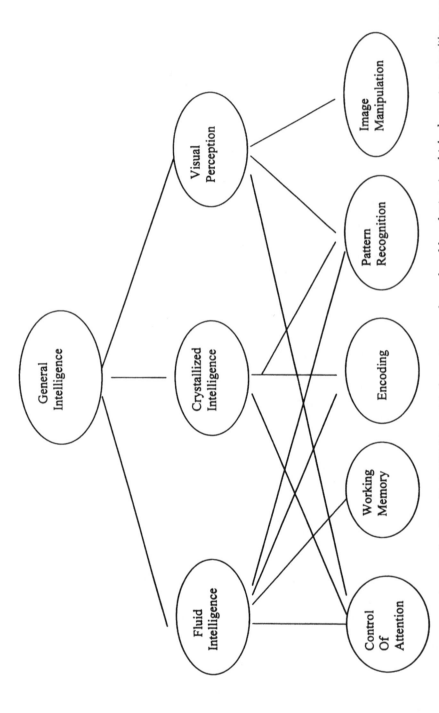

Figure 1.5. A schematic showing that Carroll's (1992) hierarchical structure can be replaced by a lattice, in which elementary cognitive processes contribute to more than one higher order ability. These abilities, in turn, are statistically related to observable complex behaviors. The underlying abilities are related to brain areas that support this function. The example is intended for illustration only, not as a theory of intelligence.

Nonreductionist Issues: Contention About What Intelligence Is Worth

I now move from discussions of reductionist approaches to intelligence to a discussion of issues surrounding the use of intelligence in both academics and the workplace. Again, I first present some facts and then use cognitive psychology to expand on them. This time, however, instead of being concerned with information processing, I am going to be concerned with the organization of knowledge.

There has been a great deal of contention over the use of psychometric scores to make personnel decisions in both education and the workforce. Contention is likely to continue because we are dealing with a sensitive issue. Although every society has disparities in wealth, the disparities in the United States are greater than the disparities in other comparable nations (Fischer et al., 1996). The disparity has fluctuated markedly over time. During the Great Depression, wealth was distributed much more unequally than it is today. Disparities declined until about 1970, at which point inequalities in income and wealth began to increase. That trend has continued steadily. The United States will go into the twenty-first century with one of the largest disparities in income among the industrial nations. I believe, along with former Labor Secretary Robert Reich, that most of the trend is attributable to the increasing importance of people who deal with symbols and a concomitant lessening of the role of those who deal with things and even with other people (Hunt, 1995; Reich, 1991). Whatever the reason, the finding itself is sufficient to make reasonable people curious about any correlate of social success in our country.

A second fact is that the probability of receiving negative social sanctions, such as being in prison or on welfare, is related to psychometric intelligence scores (Gordon, 1997; Herrnstein & Murray, 1994). The third, and most explosive, fact is that ethnic differences in both the rewards and punishments received from society are closely mirrored by ethnic group differences in intelligence test scores. (Gordon's, 1997, analyses are particularly cogent here.) Although alternative explanations are possible, this statistical finding, combined with the undoubted involvement of genes and intelligence, permits but does not demand an explanation of ethnic group differences that, to put it mildly, is socially explosive. Therefore, it is advisable to proceed carefully. One has to look at the social situation first and then decide just how intelligence might be used. This will dictate both the scientific methodologies that one wants to use and the perspectives that have to be taken to deal with a complicated problem.

A high IQ score, in itself, is worth nothing at all. Employers do, and should, pay for specific cognitive skills required in the workplace. These are sometimes vaguely defined, such as the frequently cited "knowing how to learn." In other situations, the skills required are specified precisely. Mental test scores can assess how close a person is to having the requisite skills and to estimate how much training will be required before an acceptable skill level is reached. Note that this covers the two extreme positions. If the people involved cannot be trained, the costs are infinite; if the applicant already has the needed skills, the cost of training is zero.

An important methodological point follows from this. The percentage of variance, a statistical concept that is useful in some scientific analyses, is of less interest in workplace applications. Another statistic, the percentage of people with a given skill who can perform acceptably on the criterion task (the Brogden–Taylor approach), is somewhat more interesting but is ultimately unsatisfactory because performance is seldom either acceptable or unacceptable. What is most interesting is the expected performance of a workforce given that its members have been selected on the basis of passing some criterion score (the cut score) on the selector variable.

In an employer's ideal world, the cut score would be established solely by the number of positions to be filled; if an employer wants 100 employees (or 100 graduate students), the employer can offer jobs to the 100 with the highest scores. However, as any personnel or admissions officer knows, people do not always accept the offer. The situation can vary drastically over relatively short time periods. In the late 1980s the United States was in the midst of a serious recession. While doing research for a book on the workforce, I encountered several incidents in which companies had 10–15 times the number of applicants as they had open jobs. Ten years later, unemployment was under 5% and "help wanted" signs were all over my local shopping mall. At the same time, German unemployment was above 10%.

The employment situation determines the worth of personnel selection because of the interaction between the validity coefficient and the cut score. Research psychologists are well familiar with the validity coefficient; it is the correlation between a test score and some measure of criterion performance. The cut score is the fraction of applicants who are to be accepted. The relation between the validity coefficient, the cut score, and the mean utility of performance are shown in Figure 1.6. The relation is shown for two levels of validity correlation, .25 and .5. These were chosen because they represent low and high estimates of performance–test relationships in academia and the workplace (Hunt, 1995). Also shown are the effects of test and cut scores in two different settings. One is the selection of managers in the communications industry ($r = .38$, with a cut score estimated at about .15; Howard & Bray, 1988). The other is acceptance of first-year students at the University of Washington ($r = .36$, cut score at .67; data supplied by the university).

One might conclude from this analysis that one should test only in recessions, and therefore personnel selection is a countercyclic industry. That is not correct. There are always more than enough applicants for the really good jobs, as the managerial example shows. In cases in which a high percentage of applicants have to be offered jobs, test scores can still be useful to estimate the costs of training after selection. Cognitive tests are good for this purpose. Figure 1.7 shows data from studies of enlisted performance in the military (Wigdor & Green, 1991). Hands-on tests of job qualifications were related to time on the job, which could be more than 3 years, and the enlistee's scores on the Armed Forces Qualification Test. Test performance was best for people with the highest Armed Forces Qualification Test scores at all levels of experience, but the differences were greatest early in training. Also, and of considerable importance, the highest scoring soldiers required less experience to reach their maximum level of performance.

A Second Look at Cognitive Psychology: The Organization of Knowledge

It has been observed, and unfortunately I have lost the citation, that if one looks only at information-processing measures, he or she will conclude that everyone older than 25 years of age is deteriorating and that by 35 everyone is slow moving, error

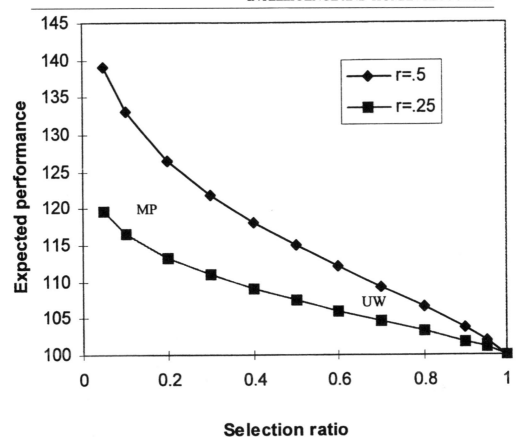

Figure 1.6. The relation between the utility of using a personnel screening test, the predictive validity of the test, and the cut score used to select applicants. Utility is expressed in standard score units, and the cut score is expressed as the ratio (number of jobs)/(number of applicants). Two points are shown, for management personnel selection (MP) and for the selection of freshman applicants to the University of Washington (UW).

prone, and distractible. If one combines this assertion with the recent finding that men have more neurons than women, one could be forced into admitting that the smartest person in the world is a 17-year-old male. Since this is the demographic group whose members are most likely to be involved in automobile accidents, the conclusion is suspect. Fortunately, cognitive psychology offers hope, with a bit of help from anthropology.

Although researchers can make people perform as information-processing machines in the laboratory, outside of the laboratory people's performance is largely determined by what they already know. Experience results in organized methods of problem solving called *schemas*. Schemas are used to focus attention on the relevant variables in frequently experienced problems and to guide the information processing required to handle these problems efficiently. Individual differences in recurring, extralaboratory problem solving may be much more determined by individual differences in the schematic organization of knowledge than individual differences in information-processing power. This idea can be demonstrated for highly intellectual problem solving,

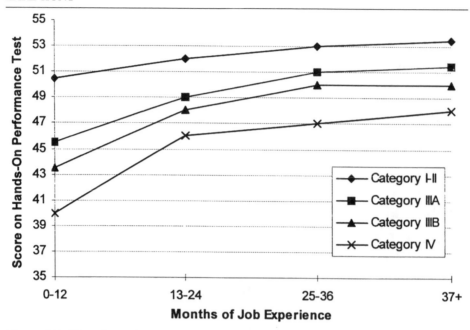

Figure 1.7. The relation between performance on a hands-on test of job competence, years of experience, and category of score on the Armed Services Vocational Aptitude Battery. The data are shown for a variety of enlisted military occupational specialities in the military. From *Performance Assessment in the Workplace* (p. 164), by A. K. Wigdor and B. F. Green, 1991, Washington, DC: National Academy Press. Copyright 1991 by the National Academy of Sciences. Courtesy of the Joseph Henry Press, Washington, DC. Adapted with permission.

such as solving problems in physics (Larkin, 1983). The same principle applies to the problem of organizing the motor actions required to operate a piece of machinery. In fact, in this case neuroimaging has been used to show that when a person learns a motor action, the memory migrates away from forebrain involvement to involve the motor cortex (Shadmehr & Holcomb, 1997). This would hardly surprise Bartlett (1958), the originator of the term *schema*, for in his later work he emphasized the application of schemas to both motor movements and problem solving.

Given this, one would expect that as people gain experience, their performance would be less predictable from intelligence measures than it would be early in training. This effect is clearly demonstrated in Figure 1.7. It has also been shown in extensive studies of expert performance (Ericsson, 1996; Ericsson & Smith, 1991). People who do well in jobs simply learn a great deal about their field. This can vary from simple examples such as learning how to visualize the way to pack a truck with standard-size boxes (Scribner, 1984) to learning how to apply the complicated concepts of medicine, law, or physics. The same point can also be studied in the laboratory, where it has been shown that extensive training on a task typically reduces interindividual variability as people approach their individual asymptotes and also reduces the correlation between task performance and intelligence measures (Ackerman, 1987).[3]

---

[3]Paradoxically, in certain situations interindividual variations will first increase and then decrease (Ackerman & Woltz, 1994). This happens if people differ markedly in the rate at which they discover and apply the most efficient strategies for the task at hand. This does not invalidate the main point of the argument.

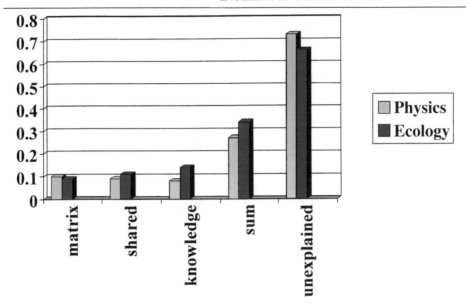

Figure 1.8. Percentage of variance on a high school science final examinations (ordinate) predicted by a progressive matrix test and by knowledge of the topic before taking the test. Data are from Levidow (1994) and Barnes (1997).

Although it is possible to invent tasks for which people have no cultural experience, in the ordinary world people move from a familiar task to a less familiar one, so that knowledge builds on knowledge. This does not mean that Gf is unimportant, but it does mean that knowledge also counts. To illustrate this, I offer two pieces of data from research projects that my colleagues and I have been conducting on the improvement of science instruction (Hunt & Minstrell, 1994).

Instructors using our procedures begin a course by giving students a pretest that evaluates their knowledge before instruction. This is used to select further instruction. In some of our research studies, the students were also given a matrix reasoning test as a content-free evaluation of their problem-solving skill. After instruction, they were, naturally enough, given a postinstruction test to see what they have learned.

Figure 1.8 shows the percentage of variance in the final test that could be predicted by the pretest, the problem-solving test, and the interaction between the two. Results are shown for two different courses: a high school course in introductory physics (Levidow, 1994) and a junior high school course in ecology (Barnes, 1997). The results are highly similar for each course. Predicting the problem-solving skills and knowledge that the students had coming out of the course required knowledge of both abstract problem-solving skills (intelligence, if you will) and knowledge of what the students already knew about the topic. Most importantly, more than half the variance could not be predicted by any of the measures we took. What do these results indicate about intelligence?

Cattell (1971) and Horn (1985) referred to Gc as the application of acquired problem-solving methods to current problems. Operationally, and probably because they wished to apply the concept to the population in general, Cattell and Horn evaluated Gc by using tests of knowledge that one would expect to be generally acquired by all participants in a culture. This is a reasonable thing to do if the examinees are from a culturally homogeneous background. However, the concept of Gc is a broader one. From the cognitive psychology viewpoint, a person's capability to solve a problem depends on (a) possession of a schema that applies to the problem at hand and (b) having the information-processing capabilities required to execute that schema. People's capabilities are dictated by what they know, not what somebody else knows. Physicists' concepts of "balance of forces" and psychometricians' concepts of "hierarchical factor analysis" are parts of Gc for specialists in those fields. Of course, it makes no sense to evaluate the Gc of a physicist by asking questions about factor analysis. That is just the point. In our highly specialized society, Gc is not a unitary thing, especially in at its higher levels.

This lets me close my review on an upbeat note. Today there is a great deal of talk about "learning how to learn" but little discussion about precisely how teachers are supposed to teach people to learn. Teachers certainly can teach specific skills, Gc in its broadest framework. Students who complete a course in psychological statistics will be able to solve problems that baffled Gauss and Pascal. Does this mean that today's students are more intelligent than Blaise Pascal? In a sense, no, but who cares? They are better statisticians.

And on to the Future

Intelligence test scores have been shown to be influenced by heritability and to be important predictors in education and the workplace. The first finding is so common that I coined the term *vuja de* (meaning, the uncanny feeling that I do not want to be caught here again) to express my feelings about the continued revolving debate about nature and nurture (Hunt, 1997a). The second finding is now so well established that if I am asked to comment on a meta-analysis of the validity of intelligence, I shall title my paper "Vuja de" All Over Again. That does not mean that research on intelligence should end just yet. But the end is near!

People do clearly vary in that statistical abstraction, Gf. They also vary in visual–spatial reasoning and in a number of other important aspects of intellectual competence. Some of this variation is clearly tied to information-processing capacity, differentiated along the lines mentioned in the first part of this chapter. We need to know the biological mechanisms by which this is achieved. This is partly because we want to understand the gene–performance relationships. In part, and equally important, it is because we want to understand what other physical factors can affect mental competence and how we can avoid or ameliorate them. The persistence of recreational drugs, including alcohol, stands high on the list of danger factors to be investigated, but they are by no means alone. We need a better understanding of nutritional effects and deterioration of intellectual competence associated with aging and disease. We do not need to know the value of the heritability coefficient to the third decimal place, or even the second.

Cognitive competence, as indexed by intelligence tests, is clearly an important factor in the workplace. It may even be the most important single factor in terms of prediction. However, in virtually every study I have read, in either academics or the workplace, half the variance or more remains unexplained. Intelligence is a can-do concept for both workforce and school. It indicates what a person could do if he or she chooses to work hard and is afforded the opportunity to do so. We need a much better understanding of how present intellectual competence interacts with personality and social variables to produce future intellectual competence. Studies such as Ackerman's (1996) recent approach are a step in the right direction. However, researchers are going to have to expand their methods because this is not an issue that is likely to be determined by gazing at correlations. Laboratory and field studies will be required. Psychometricians may even have to talk to anthropologists. The issues are too complex to be studied from the perspective of just one discipline.

Understanding the interactions among intelligence, personality, and situational variables is also an important social goal. Numerous researchers have documented the fact that Americans think of mental power as fixed. (Citizens of other countries do not.) The way in which psychologists have talked about intelligence has not dictated this conclusion, but I think it may inadvertently have reinforced it. The correct statement is that some aspects of mental competence are either fixed or, if they are not, we do not know how to change them. Other aspects are not fixed. Instead, they depend on the individual's interacting with situations in a way that ensures that appropriate knowledge is acquired. Steinberg (1996) has argued that intellectual disengagement, a sort of fatalistic belief that a person either is smart or is not, is one of the biggest detriments to education in the United States. Gc counts, and in the workplace it counts a great deal. The social science goal of understanding how to foster it is every bit as important as the biological goal of finding the power of the mind in the brain.

REFERENCES

Ackerman, P. L. (1987). Individual differences in skill learning: An integration of psychometric and information processing perspectives. *Psychological Bulletin, 102*, 3–27.

Ackerman, P. L. (1996). A theory of adult intellectual development: Personality, interests, and knowledge. *Intelligence, 22*, 227–257.

Ackerman, P. L., & Woltz, D. J. (1994). Determinants of learning and performance in a memory/substitution task: Task constraints, differences, volition, and motivation. *Journal of Educational Psychology, 86*, 487–515.

Anderson, J. R. (1983). *The architecture of cognition*. Cambridge, MA: Harvard University Press.

Anderson, J. R. (1993). *Rules of the mind*. Hillsdale, NJ: Erlbaum.

Baddeley, A. D. (1986). *Working memory*. Oxford, England: Oxford University Press.

Barnes, A. (1997). *A field study of school computer use: Examination of the effects of student learning and perceptions of learning*. Unpublished doctoral dissertation, University of Washington, Seattle.

Bartlett, F. C. (1958). *Thinking*. London: Allen & Unwin.

Brody, N. (1992). *Intelligence* (2nd ed.). New York: Academic Press.

Carpenter, P. A., Just, M. A., & Shell, P. (1990). What one intelligence test measures: A theoretical account of processing in the Raven Progressive Matrix Test. *Psychological Review, 97*, 404–431.

Carroll, J. B. (1993). *Human cognitive abilities*. Cambridge, England: Cambridge University Press.

Carroll, J. B. (1997). Psychometrics, intelligence, and public policy. *Intelligence, 24*, 25–52.

Cattell, R. B. (1971). *Abilities: Their structure, growth, and action*. Boston: Houghton Mifflin.

Cohen, N. J., & Eichenbaum, H. (1993). *Memory, amnesia, and the hippocampal system*. Cambridge, MA: MIT Press.

Damasio, H., Grabowski, T., Randall, F., Galaburda, A. M., & Damasio, A. R. (1994). The return of Phineas Gage: Clues about the brain from the skull of a famous patient. *Science, 264*, 1102–1104.

Das, J. P., Kar, B. C., & Parrila, R. K. (1996). *Planning: The psychological basis of intelligent behavior*. Thousand Oaks, CA: Sage.

Deary, I. J., Egan, V., Gibson, G. J., Austin, E. J., Brand, C. R., & Kellaghan, T. (1996). Intelligence and the differentiation hypothesis. *Intelligence, 23*, 105–132.

Deary, I. J., & Stough, C. (1996). Intelligence and inspection time: Achievements, prospects, and problems. *American Psychologist, 51,* 599–608.

Detterman, D. K., & Daniel, M. H. (1989). Correlations of mental tests with each other and with cognitive variables are highest in low IQ groups. *Intelligence, 13,* 349–360.

Diamond, J. (1997). *Guns, germs and steel: The fates of human societies.* New York: Norton.

Duncan, J., Emslie, H., Williams, P., & Johnson, R. (1996). Intelligence and the frontal lobe: The organization of goal directed behavior. *Cognitive Psychology, 30,* 257–303.

Ericsson, K. A. (Ed.). (1996). *The road to excellence: The acquisition of expert performance in the arts and sciences, sports, and games.* Mahwah, NJ: Erlbaum.

Ericsson, K. A., & Smith, J. (1991). *Towards a general theory of expertise.* New York: Cambridge University Press.

Eysenck, H. (1986). The theory of intelligence and the psychophysiology of cognition. In R. J. Sternberg (Ed.), *Advances in the psychology of human intelligence* (Vol. 3, pp. 1–34). Hillsdale, NJ: Erlbaum.

Fischer, C. S., Hout, M., Jankowski, M. S., Lucas, S. R., Swidler, A., & Voss, K. (1996). *Inequality by design.* Princeton, NJ: Princeton University Press.

Gardner, H. (1983). *Frames of mind: The theory of multiple intelligences.* New York: Basic Books.

Gardner, H., Kornhaber, M. L., & Wake, W. K. (1996). *Intelligence: Multiple perspectives.* New York: Harcourt Brace.

Gazzaniga, M. S. (Ed.). (1995). *The cognitive neurosciences.* Cambridge, MA: MIT Press.

Gordon, R. A. (1997). Everyday life as an intelligence test: Effects of intelligence, and intelligence context. *Intelligence, 24,* 203–230.

Guilford, J. P. (1967). *The nature of human intelligence.* New York: McGraw-Hill.

Herrnstein, R. J., & Murray, C. (1994). *The bell curve: Intelligence and class structure in American life.* New York: Free Press.

Horn, J. L. (1985). Remodeling old models of intelligence. In B. B. Wolman (Ed.), *Handbook of intelligence: Theories, measurements, and applications* (pp. 267–300). New York: Wiley.

Horn, J. L., & Noll, J. (1994). A system for understanding cognitive capabilities: A theory and the evidence on which it is based. In D. Detterman (Ed.), *Current topics in human intelligence: Vol. 4. Theories of intelligence* (pp. 151–204). Norwood, NJ: Ablex.

Howard, A., & Bray, D. W. (1988). *Managerial lives in transition: Advancing age and changing times.* New York: Guilford Press.

Hunt, E. (1974). Quote the raven? Nevermore! In L. W. Gregg (Ed.), *Knowledge and cognition* (pp. 129–158). Potomac, MD: Erlbaum.

Hunt, E. (1987). The next word on verbal ability. In P. A. Vernon (Ed.), *Speed of information processing and intelligence* (pp. 349–392). Norwood, NJ: Ablex.

Hunt, E. (1995). *Will we be smart enough? A cognitive analysis of the coming workforce.* New York: Russell Sage Foundation.

Hunt, E. (1996). When should we shoot the messenger? Issues involving cognitive testing, public policy, and the law. *Psychology and Public Policy, 2,* 486–505.

Hunt, E. (1997a). Nature versus nurture: The feeling of vuja de. In R. J. Sternberg & E. Grigorenko (Eds.), *Intelligence, heredity, and the environment* (pp. 531–551). Cambridge, England: Cambridge University Press.

Hunt, E. (1997b). The concept and utility of intelligence. In B. Devlin, S. Feinberg, D. Resnick, & K. Roeder (Eds.), *Intelligence and success: Is it all in the genes? Scientists respond to The Bell Curve* (pp. 171–190). New York: Springer.

Hunt, E., & Lansman, M. (1986). A unified model of attention and problem solving. *Psychological Review, 93,* 446–461.

Hunt, E., & Minstrell, J. (1994). A collaborative classroom for teaching conceptual physics. In K. McGilly (Ed.), *Classroom lessons: Integrating cognitive theory and the classroom.* Cambridge, MA: MIT Press.

Institute for Personality and Ability Testing. (1973). *Measuring intelligence with the culture-fair tests.* Champaign, IL: Author.

Jencks, C. (1992). *Rethinking social policy: Race, poverty, and the underclass.* Cambridge, MA: Harvard University Press.

Jonides, J. E., Smith, E. E., Koepe, R. A., Awh, E., Minoshim, S., & Mintun, M. A. (1993). Spatial working memory in humans as revealed by PET. *Nature, 363,* 623–625.

Just, M. A., & Carpenter, P. A. (1992). A capacity theory of comprehension: Individual differences in working memory. *Psychological Review, 99,* 122–149.

Kimberg, D. Y., & Farah, M. J. (1993). A unified account of cognitive impairments following frontal lobe damage: The role of working memory in complex organized behavior. *Journal of Experimental Psychology: General, 122,* 411–428.

Kosslyn, S. M. (1994). *Image and brain.* Cambridge, MA: MIT Press.

Kyllonen, P. C., & Christal, R. E. (1990). Reasoning ability is (little more than) working memory capacity?! *Intelligence, 14,* 389–433.

Kyllonen, P. C., & Stephens, D. L. (1990). Cognitive abilities as determinants of success in acquiring logic skills. *Learning and Individual Differences, 2,* 129–160.

Larkin, J. (1983). Problem representation in physics. In D. Gentner & A. Stevens (Eds.), *Mental models.* Hillsdale, NJ: Erlbaum.

Legree, P. J., Pifer, M. E., & Grafton, F. C. (1996). Correlations among cognitive abilities are lower for higher ability groups. *Intelligence, 23,* 45–58.

Levidow, B. (1994). *The effect of high school physics instruction on measures of general knowledge and reasoning ability.* Unpublished doctoral dissertation, University of Washington, Seattle.

Logie, R. H. (1995). *Visuo-spatial working memory.* Hillsdale, NJ: Erlbaum.

Myerson, J., Hale, S., Wagstaff, D., Poon, L. W., & Smith, G. A. (1990). The information-loss model: A mathematical theory of age-related cognitive slowing. *Psychological Review, 97,* 475–487.

Newell, A. (1990). Unified theories of cognition. Cambridge, MA: Harvard University Press.

Paller, K. A., Acharya, A., Richardson, B. C., Plaisant, O., Shimamura, A. P., Reed, B. R., & Jagust, W. J. (1997). Functional neuroimaging of cortical dysfunction in alcoholic Korsakoff's syndrome. *Journal of Cognitive Neuroscience, 9,* 277–293.

Plomin, R. (1995). Molecular genetics and psychology. *Current Directions in Psychological Science, 4,* 114–117.

Posner, M. I., & Raichle, M. E. (1994). *Images of mind.* New York: Freeman.

Prabhakaran, V., Smith, J. A. L., Desmond, J. E., Glover, G. H., & Gabrieli, J. D. E. (1997). Neural substances of fluid reasoning: An fMRI study of neocortical activation during performance of the Raven's Progressive Matrices test. *Cognitive Psychology, 33,* 43–63.

Raven, J. C. (1965). *Advanced Progressive Matrices: Sets I and II.* London: H. K. Lewis.

Reich, R. (1991). *The work of nations: Preparing ourselves for 21st century capitalism.* New York: Knopf.

Rumelhart, D. E. (1988). The architecture of mind: A connectionist approach. In M. I. Posner (Ed.), *The foundations of cognitive science* (pp. 133–160). Cambridge, MA: MIT Press.

Salthouse, T. A. (1990). *Theoretical perspectives on cognitive aging.* Hillsdale, NJ: Erlbaum.

Salthouse, T. A. (1996). The processing-speed theory of adult age differences in cognition. *Psychological Review, 103,* 403–428.

Scribner, S. (1984). Studying working intelligence. In B. Rogoff & J. Lave (Eds.), *Everyday cognition: Its development in social context.* Cambridge, MA: Harvard University Press.

Shadmehr, R., & Holcomb, H. H. (1997). Neural correlates of motor memory consolidation. *Science, 277,* 821–824.

Shimamura, A. P. (1995). Memory and frontal lobe functioning. In M. S. Gazzaniga (Ed.), *The cognitive neurosciences* (pp. 803–812). Cambridge, MA: MIT Press.

Simon, H. A., & Kaplan, C. A. (1988). Foundations of cognitive science. In M. I. Posner (Ed.), *The foundations of cognitive science* (pp. 1–48). Cambridge, MA: MIT Press.

Smith, E. E., & Jonides, J. (1997). Working memory: A view from neuroimaging. *Cognitive Psychology, 33,* 5–42.

Squire, L. R., & Knowlton, B. J. (1995). Memory, hippocampus, and brain systems. In M. S. Gazzaniga (Ed.), *The cognitive neurosciences.* Cambridge, MA: MIT Press.

Steinberg, L. (1996). *Beyond the classroom: Why school reform has failed and what parents need to do.* New York: Simon & Schuster.

Sternberg, R. J. (1990). *Metaphors of mind.* Cambridge, England: Cambridge University Press.

Sternberg, S. (1975). Memory scanning: New findings and current controversies. *Quarterly Journal of Experimental Psychology, 27,* 1–32.

Stoddard, G. D. (1943). *The meaning of intelligence.* New York: Macmillan.

Sunderland, A., Harris, J. E., & Baddeley, A. D. (1983). Do laboratory tests predict everyday memory? A neuropsychological study. *Journal of Verbal Learning and Verbal Behavior, 22,* 341–357.

Thibadeau, R., Just, M. A., & Carpenter, P. A. (1982). A model of the time course and content of reading. *Cognitive Science, 6,* 157–203.

Underwood, B. J., Boruch, B. F., & Malmi, R. A. (1978). Composition of episodic memory. *Journal of Experimental Psychology: General, 107,* 393–419.

Vernon, P. A. (Ed.). (1993). *Biological approaches to the study of human intelligence*. Norwood, NJ: Ablex.

Victor, M., Adams, R. D., & Collins, G. H. (1989). *The Wernicke–Korsakoff syndrome and related neurologic disorders due to alcoholism and malnutrition*. Philadelphia: F. A. Davis.

Wigdor, A. K., & Green, B. F., Jr. (1991). *Performance assessment in the workplace*. Washington, DC: National Academy Press.

Discussion

Discussion following Hunt's paper focused on general issues about the continued role of intelligence during an individual's career and about the controversial issue of the relationship between intelligence and individual earnings.

Unidentified: Buz, you show the prediction of performance over time for high and low groups — and you show that there's a decrease. I think that seriously underestimates the effectiveness of IQ. Because in fact, one of the real features of the modern complex world is that people move from job to job. And if you get that big spread at the beginning every time you step to a new job, that picture underestimates the long-term effect with intelligence on any given individual's career.

Dr. Hunt: The question is, do they do it? The average American, in fact is estimated to move six times in his or her job, to change his or her employer six times. He or she does not change jobs six times. Let's take one that's a good example is aircraft mechanics. Aircraft mechanics or engineers working on aircraft may work for Boeing, but they may work for Boeing in different states. But the fact seems to be that there is relatively little movement completely across jobs. You change employers and chase jobs. Now, that may change. We don't really know. And how much training will come in? You then have just guesses as to whether it will be easier for employers to provide on-the-job training or to simply go chasing around after better or new work forces, which would cause a lot of thrashing. And that gets us into issues of socioeconomic policies that are far beyond this conference.

Dr. Wittmann: I have two points. I do not believe that the correction for unreliability will not make a big difference because I have data where I can demonstrate that the variance portion of 30% goes up to 70% if you do make the correction, but we should look at the data to solve that. Your other example, your income figure, that spread, very interesting. What about the credibility of that explanation where you pointed to technology, but what about alternative explanations like politics or other explanatory constructs?

Dr. Hunt: Well, it appears to be happening in every industrial country. The United States is the second highest of the industrial countries in the spread in income between the top and bottom. But there is not that big of a difference. Ireland is the highest for some reason. I don't know quite why. But this has been happening overall in every country. What seems to happen is if you do forced political things, like very progressive income taxes and such, then people who make a lot of money simply move out.

Dr. Ackerman: Well, let me ask the general question. Who mandated that intelligence and income should be related to one another?

Dr. Hunt: Empirically they are.

Dr. Ackerman: But they're not, as you showed, they're not very highly related to one another. Who said they should be highly related to one another? I don't understand the philosophy or the construct that says that intelligence and income should be highly related to one another.

Dr. Hunt: Well, intelligence and income are not necessarily linked, but intelligence and trained ability. . . . In a highly technical society, there is a tremendous payoff for education. We as professors, lamentably paid, tend to be kind of frustrated and say we're as smart as those Microsoft programmers, how come they're making so damn much money? But the real payoff is not there. There's a huge penalty for not completing high school in this country. There is a substantial penalty for not having some college, and there's benefits all the way through. And that is definitely linked.

Dr. Ackerman: But that addresses a point that George Stoddard (1943) made in his book *The Meaning of Intelligence*, which is that the credential is the important thing, and realistically there is almost as much variance in intelligence at school entry as school leaving, and that includes college and graduate school as well. So it's the credential that drives the income, not intelligence. Although intelligence is related indirectly by getting you into school.

Dr. Hunt: I guess the way I would put that is slightly different. The income variance across occupations is increasing now. We see at the universities where there is a greater variance in pay across departments than there used to be because of industrial competition for some fields and not others. I don't know how you would answer that. I don't think anybody knows how you'd answer the credentialing versus knowledge acquisition thing. And I think the answer is probably not the same for different areas. In medicine, for instance, you can only fake it so far. You just have the same thing for computer programming and engineering, aeronautical engineering. Other fields . . . generalized social skills may carry you further. So I think that's an answer that's going to be very specific to the particular occupation. But you still got to get the credential.

2

Individual Differences in Learning and Memory: Psychometrics and the Single Case

ALAN BADDELEY and SUSAN GATHERCOLE

Over the past 50 years, it could be argued that the greatest impact of psychology on society has come from psychometrics, the attempt to study and measure individual differences. At a practical level, the use of psychometric measurements in the selection, training, and the assessment and treatment of patients represents a substantial and growing international industry. Public discussion and dissent on the nature of intelligence, particularly on issues of nature and nurture, race, and gender, have had a continuing major impact on the public's perception and evaluation of psychology. Although that discussion has not always been informed or informative, there is no doubt that the underlying issues are of great practical and conceptual significance. Yet, despite this impressive history of public impact, psychometrics has had relatively little influence on the development of related areas of psychology, and, although the area is certainly continuing to develop in statistical sophistication, it could be argued that there has been much less evidence of genuine theoretical progress.

Psychometric Conservatism

This personal view may, of course, simply reflect ignorance, but the theoretical issues that appear to concern researchers in the field tend to have a traditional feel to them. The preoccupation with the concept of intelligence, and the extent to which it may be reflected in basic cognitive functions such as reaction time or

We acknowledge the support of Medical Research Council Grant G9423916 with thanks.

31

LIBRARY
COLBY-SAWYER COLLEGE
NEW LONDON. NH 03257

inspection time, reflects some of the concerns of James McKeen Cattell in the last century, whereas the issue of whether it is better to consider intelligence as a unitary or multiple process reflects the Spearman versus Thurstone controversies of more than 50 years ago. The role of cultural and educational factors in performance is another important issue, and the fear that the general intelligence of the population is declining because the less able tend to have larger families caused a major uproar when Herrnstein and Murray published their book *The Bell Curve* in 1994. Exactly the same idea was proposed by the Reverend Malthus in the nineteenth century. Although it would be wrong to say that the field is not progressing, to the outsider at least, psychometrics appears to be one of the more conservative fields of psychology.

We suggest that the very success that psychometrics has had in tackling important practical problems may tend to bring with it entirely appropriate constraints that have the tendency to limit theoretical innovation. What might these be?

Practical Constraints

At a practical level, the success of psychometrics is reflected in the existence of standardized tests that are used widely within and beyond the profession. Tests are easy to invent but hard to develop. For a test to be useful, it must be both reliable and valid. There are now sophisticated ways of increasing the reliability of a test, but to do so still requires skill, persistence, and a good deal of hard work. The same applies to a greater extent to obtaining adequate validity for a test, a point we return to later. Having achieved a reliable and valid test, it is then necessary to collect adequate norms, which involves substantial expense and considerable difficulty if one is to sample the population adequately. Finally, having developed a new test, it is necessary to persuade one's colleagues to use it.

"If a man can invent a better mousetrap, then the world will beat a path to his door" must be one of the most misguided gems of folk wisdom. In the case of tests, there are good reasons for sticking with what one knows. First, familiar tests allow a comparison of one's current results with one's past experience in a straightforward, meaningful way. If the assessment is open to question, or even challenged in a court of law, it is much safer to rely on measures that are tried and trusted and used by everyone in the field rather than trusting new measures however attractive they may sound.

This situation is less true for tests that attempt to measure newly investigated psychological functions when older, more familiar instruments are not available. In this case, however, the practitioner needs to be convinced of the desirability of such new measures, which can raise problems for the test developer because such novel tests are by definition not assumed to correlate highly with existing measures, so evaluating their validity can be difficult.

One might expect that it is in the interest of test manufacturers to sell the user other new tests. Up to a point this is certainly true, although there is no reason to seek novelty for its own sake. Scientists usually want to do something different. However, manufacturers' profit comes from doing the same thing many, many times to minimize new problems and development costs. A sensible strategy would therefore appear to be incremental evolution rather than a search for radical new solutions.

Suppose, however, that the innovative, tireless, meticulous, and persuasive psychometric scientist does succeed in developing an ingenious new measurement instrument and that he or she persuades the publisher to fund and promote this new test. How is this event likely to be seen by his or her colleagues? In cognitive psychology at least, test development is likely to be viewed at best as a tedious and slightly odd hobby, like building cathedrals out of matchsticks, and at worst as a form of academic prostitution driven by the urge for easy money. There are therefore some good practical reasons, and some not so professional considerations, why one might expect practical psychometrics to remain a somewhat conservative discipline.

Theoretical Limitations

We suggest, however, that there is an even more fundamental reason for the apparent conservatism of psychometrics that stems from the methods it has traditionally used. The field began to tackle important practical problems in the 1930s and 1940s, a time when the development of theory within mainstream psychology was such that it was likely to offer psychometrics relatively little help. It was therefore important to find a method that would allow a test to be progressively refined regardless of whether the underlying concepts were theoretically productive. This was made possible by choosing a criterion, such as success in a particular job, and statistically selecting those tests that were the most successful in achieving that criterion, a form of natural selection among test items. This was and continues to be an enormously powerful technique, but it has a major limitation. The success of the test is constrained by the adequacy of the items that are initially fed into the test. At base, therefore, test development remains an art coupled to a powerful technology rather than a science. There have, of course, been enormous developments in statistical analysis that allow the development of ever more ingenious models of the data. These are typically based on correlation, that is, on the association between two variables, leading the modeler to collapse them into a single variable. Although this may provide simple ways of describing complex data patterns, we argue that *dissociation* is a more powerful method of analyzing a complex system such as the human mind. Although nature occasionally performs good experiments (see the next section), these are rare and we are yet to be convinced that even the most ingenious statistical analysis can cut through the patterns of associated variables that constitute a representative sample of participants given a broad cognitive test battery.

Neuropsychology and the Single Case

We now consider an alternative way of studying individual differences that is complementary to the psychometric approach, and does indeed rely heavily on psychometric measures, but that attempts to use dissociations rather than associations to analyze cognitive deficits. The area in question is sometimes known as "cognitive neuropsychology," and over the past 20 years it has reflected a fruitful alliance between the clinician attempting to understand the cognitive deficit shown by a patient with brain damage, and the cognitive psychologist attempting to produce general theories of cognition. Whereas psychometrics is principally concerned with the range of functioning in the normal population, neuropsychology is principally concerned with deficits. Furthermore, whereas mainstream psychometrics has the practical aim of measuring the range of normality, and as such must deal with large numbers of representatively selected individuals, the neuropsychologist is typically concerned with the assessment of a single patient and in teasing apart the nature of any cognitive deficits from which the patient might suffer.

From a practical viewpoint, neuropsychology relies heavily on psychometrics, and, in terms of its impact, it influences far fewer lives, probably to a much less dramatic extent than does the psychometric testing industry. In terms of theoretical impact, however, we suggest that the alliance between neuropsychology and cognitive psychology has been and is continuing to be extremely productive. Researchers now know much more about human memory, language, perception, and reading than they did 10 years ago; although this has not yet had a major impact on the capacity to remediate the cognitive effects of brain damage, the flow of information does occur in both directions, with neuropsychology enriching cognitive theory, which in turn helps the neuropsychologist understand the nature of the patient's deficit, and, in some cases at least, begin to develop better treatment methods (Baddeley, Wilson, & Watts, 1995; Wilson & Moffat, 1992).

If, as we suggest, it has proved easier to form an alliance between cognitive theory and neuropsychology than it has with classical psychometrics, why should this be? Suppose we return to our claim of two major sources of conservatism: practical and methodological. Neuropsychologists who have been most actively involved in the development of cognitive neuropsychology, clinicians such as Elizabeth Warrington, for example, tend to have been involved in extensive face-to-face interaction with patients, developing and using a range of different tests in order to analyze the nature of the dysfunction. At this level of dealing intensively with a small number of patients, a test can be developed and, if successful, passed on relatively easily. Because the initial studies typically concentrated on patients with clear and dramatic deficits, the need for extensive norms was much less, allowing a large range of novel tests to be developed relatively quickly.

Once an attempt is made to make such tests more widely available, of course the same constraints begin to apply as were described earlier. However, between the classic psychometric tests that appear to be dominated by large established companies and the informal borrowing of new techniques has grown up, in Britain at least and we suspect in the United States as well, a range of small companies with relatively low overheads able to deal with the much smaller neuropsychological test market in a more flexible, innovative way. Examples include the Test for the Reception of Grammar, which Dorothy Bishop, the scientist who invented the test, decided to market herself, and the Thames Valley Test Company, which started as a one-man business to publish a single test, the Rivermead Behavioural Memory Test (RBMT), and is now a three- to four-person business publishing more than a dozen tests. Another example is Psychology Press, which branched out from publishing psychological and neuropsychological books and journals to test publishing. In each case, the relatively modest size of the operation has allowed the flexibility to innovate in a way that seems difficult for large publishing corporations.

At a methodological level, cognitive neuropsychology has tended to use dissociations to analyze, rather than using statistical techniques to synthesize, as often happens with the large data sets required by classical psychometrics. The classic analytical tool in neuropsychology is the double dissociation, in which two types of patient, often in the first instance individual patients, are shown to have contrasting deficits. For example, the patient with classical amnesia will have grossly impaired performance on a range of tasks that are assumed by cognitive psychologists to measure episodic long-term memory (LTM) while having preserved immediate memory tested for example by digit span or by the recency effect in free recall (Baddeley & Warrington, 1970), whereas, patients with short-term memory (STM) deficits may show apparently normal LTM and grossly impaired immediate memory span and recency (Shallice & Warrington, 1970).

Although double dissociation does not prove the existence of two separate systems, it provides strong evidence for such a dissociation, particularly when the dissociation is supported by other evidence. This was the case with the evidence for LTM and STM; indeed, the reason for identifying and testing such patients came from earlier evidence for a dichotomy in normal people. It is, of course, highly desirable to replicate such findings before reaching firm conclusions, something that proved possible for both types of patients (Shallice, 1988). The two memory systems have in turn proved fractionable into a multicomponent working memory (Baddeley & Hitch, 1974) and an LTM system that involves both implicit and explicit memory systems, together with a somewhat more controversial distinction between semantic and episodic memory systems (Squire, 1992).

However, although single cases with pure and specific cognitive deficits may be extremely productive, they are very rare, representing experiments of nature that just happen to be well controlled. Furthermore, neuropsychologists with the skills to identify such patients, coupled with the necessary flow of suitable patients, are few and far between. Hence, although neuropsychology will continue to be a fruitful source of progress in cognitive psychology, it is not a substitute for the capacity to use individual differences within the normal population as a scientific resource. Researchers clearly need to take advantage of both; a brief account of our own attempts to do so follows.

Individual Differences in Learning and Memory

There are several advantages to studying the psychometrics of learning and memory as opposed to the more extensively explored area of individual differences in intelligence. The comparative lack of earlier work means that there has been less development of strongly entrenched positions. Furthermore, measuring memory performance appears to be perceived as less threatening than measuring intelligence; people readily admit to having a terrible memory but rarely claim to be stupid. The general acceptability of poor learning and memory is indeed reflected in the use of the term *memory clinic* to refer to what is in reality investigation for dementia in older people, whereas in Britain at least the term *learning disability* is perceived as less demeaning than *mental handicap*, which in turn replaced *mental deficiency*, which itself supplanted terms such as *idiocy* and *imbecility*. Partly because of the more neutral nature of the capacity to learn and remember, the area seems to have avoided some of the more heated controversies that have beset the study of intelligence.

Despite a call to arms by Underwood (1975), psychometric approaches to learning and memory have been less prominent than those concerned with intelligence. There is, of course, a long tradition of testing in this area, particularly as applied to neuropsychology, where the Wechsler Memory Scale (WMS) continues to be used extremely widely. The WMS was developed by Wechsler (1945) to use alongside the Wechsler Adult Intelligence Scale (WAIS; Wechsler, 1955), with performance being assessed as a memory quotient that indicates the ratio of the patient's memory performance to his or her intelligence. The fact that the WMS is still used, albeit in a somewhat modified form after 40 years, is a tribute to its usefulness. However, it reflected the state of cognitive psychology at that time and consequently has a number of major shortcomings. Probably the most serious of these in the original scale was the combination into a single score of tests, which represented a mixture of tasks reflecting long-term episodic memory, together with working memory and attentional measures. Because these represent quite different systems, it is possible to have a patient who is clearly densely amnesic when tested on episodic measures but who does sufficiently well on the attentional and working memory tasks to bring him or her within the normal range when the measures are combined (e.g., Patient K.J. studied by Wilson & Baddeley, 1988). The revised WMS (Wechsler, 1987) abandoned the ideal of combining scores into a single figure, but it then leaves the issue of interpreting each of the subscores to the clinician. Because the tests were not based on any clear theoretical basis in the first place, this remains problematic.[1]

If one regards the WMS as being representative of the psychometric approach to the measurement of learning and memory deficits, what can recent developments in cognitive psychology offer that might be of further value to the clinician? We present two contrasting developments that represent aspects of recent research in cognitive psychology. The first of these represents the everyday cognition movement, which has been concerned with mapping the study of cognitive function in the laboratory onto its operation in everyday life, that is, to check the ecological validity of laboratory findings. Questions about the ecological validity of intelligence testing have, of course, been raised for many years (e.g., McClelland, 1973), but in the field of memory the movement is more recent. Probably its most outspoken recent advocate has been Neisser (1978), resulting in a much discussed attack on this view (Banaji & Crowder, 1989), followed by an attempt to agree on some middle ground (see discussions in *American Psychologist*, 1991, Vol. 46, pp. 19–48).

Within clinical psychology, there is a legitimate concern about whether the standard clinical measures based on laboratory paradigms such as paired-associate learning and the free recall of meaningless figures provides a good assessment of the nature and type of problem encountered by patients going about their everyday business. Although there is no doubt that patients who suffer from brain damage tend to both perform badly on such tasks, and to complain of memory problems, an attempt to find detailed association between the two using a range of standard tasks, together with diaries and ratings from patients and caregivers, suggested that although such tasks were sensitive to head injury, they were poor predictors of com-

---

[1] A third edition of the Wechsler Memory Scale has now been developed, but we have not yet had the opportunity to study it.

plaints from patients and caregivers of everyday memory problems (Sunderland, Harris, & Baddeley, 1983).

This led a clinical neuropsychologist, Barbara Wilson, to develop a new kind of memory test based on her observation of the memory lapses and problems encountered by her patients with brain damage. She developed the RBMT, which has 12 subtests, each based on an everyday memory problem. They measure tasks such as remembering someone's name, recognizing faces and objects that have just been seen, learning a simple route, orientation to time and place, memory for a brief prose passage, and measuring *prospective memory*, the capacity to remember to do something. The test was initially validated by comparing the mean performance on each of the subtests of patients rated by their therapists as having memory problems severe enough to interfere with treatment and those who did not. All of the subtests proved to discriminate reasonably well. The test was further validated by correlating performance with the likelihood of memory lapses, as measured by therapists working with each patient over a period of many hours. The association was approximately .75, higher than earlier tasks used by earlier measures such as paired-associates learning ($r = .40$). In a subsequent study, Wilson (1991) followed-up a group of memory patients she had seen some 5–10 years earlier, giving them both the RBMT and the WMS. She recorded the extent to which the patient had managed to become independent, as measured by returning to work, living independently, or both. Her results are shown in Figure 2.1, from which it is clear that performance on the RBMT did a reasonably good job of predicting capacity for independent living, whereas the WMS was much less successful.

The original RBMT was designed as a screening test, aimed at identifying patients who are likely to have significant everyday problems. Consequently, in its original form it was useless for testing normal participants because they all performed at ceiling. However, an extended form of the test has now been developed by taking the four parallel forms and combining them to make two more difficult tests. Although the test is relatively new, preliminary data appear promising (de Wall, Wilson, & Baddeley, 1994).

Other examples of ecologically based tests include the Behavioural Assessment of the Dysexecutive Syndrome (Wilson, Alderman, Burgess, Emslie, & Evans, 1996), which is a test of executive dysfunction, and the Autobiographical Memory Inventory (Kopelman, Wilson, & Baddeley, 1989, 1990), which measures the patient's capacity to recollect autobiographical information of both an episodic and a personal semantic nature. Both tests are designed to measure aspects of cognition that are of theoretical concern, executive processing (see the section on working memory), and autobiographical aspects of episodic memory. However, they attempt to investigate real-world problems rather than to provide a pure measure of some hypothetical underlying memory system. As such, their usefulness does not depend on the validity of the underlying theory.

The concern for ecological validity has introduced a new dimension to the more classical approach to psychometrics; however, it does tend to be relatively atheoretical, attempting to adapt the test to the everyday environment of the patient, rather than to investigate the nature of the underlying deficit. A test that attempts to be more analytical in nature, while also retaining a degree of face validity, is the Doors and People test (Baddeley, Emslie, & Nimmo-Smith, 1994).

Although most existing clinical memory tests load heavily on episodic memory,

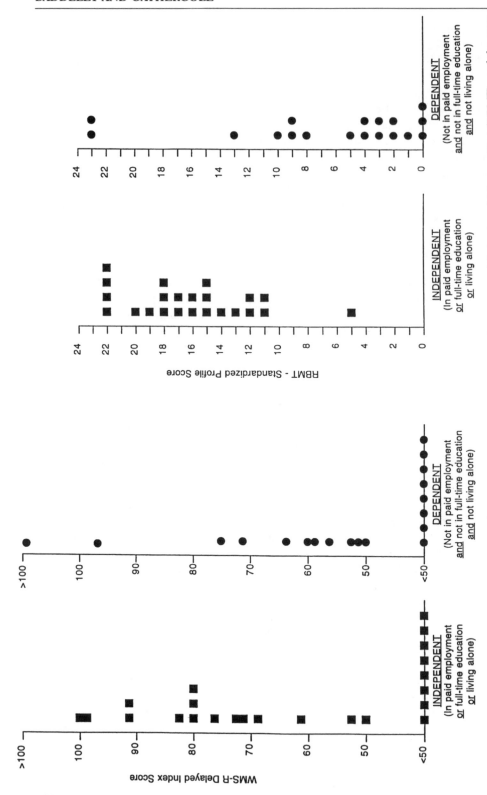

Figure 2.1. Performance of patients who had previously been diagnosed as amnesic on the Rivermead Behavioural Memory Test (RBMT); and the most discriminating of the Wechsler Memory Scale—Revised (WMS–R). Patients capable of living independently are shown in the left panels and dependent patients on the right. Although the Wechsler Memory Scale is capable of detecting amnesia, it is less good at predicting everyday functioning.

as we discussed earlier in the case of the WMS, they also tend to involve other variables. A good example of this is the Consortium for Experimental Research on Alzheimer's Disease (CERAD) verbal learning test, developed by a U.S. consortium of departments studying Alzheimer's disease. The test contains a list of words to be presented and tested on three occasions, followed by a delayed recall and recognition test. It is sensitive to the effects of Alzheimer's disease, as is the case with virtually any measure involving the learning of word lists. In addition, however, it suggests that patients with Alzheimer's disease forget more rapidly than older control participants, a less well-established finding. Careful examination of the data, however, suggests that patients and control participants show evidence of using different strategies, with patients relying on recency across the three successive trials to boost their performance, whereas control participants appear to use the more standard procedure in this context, of clustering on the basis of other variables such as semantic associations, leading to a much more marked recency effect in the patient group (see Figure 2.2). The recency effect is, of course, highly subject to even brief delay, leading to a more marked tendency for forgetting in the patient group (Greene, Baddeley, & Hodges, 1996).

The Doors and People test was in some ways relatively traditional, measuring recall and recognition for visual and verbal materials and including simple measures of learning and forgetting after a brief delay. It differed from many existing tests in that it had two measures of each function to minimize the possibility of drawing false conclusions from a temporary lapse of concentration during one subtest. The material was also chosen to be realistic and attractive while attempting to ensure that even densely amnesic patients could feel that they were performing reasonably well and stretching the capacity of young, bright normal participants. For each subtest, scaled scores were used to allow scores to be combined, hence providing separate measures of recall and recognition, visual and verbal memory, learning, and forgetting. A carefully selected and stratified sample of normal participants was tested to allow the scaling.

One problem in attempting to test visual and verbal memory is that participants readily recode, naming even meaningless figures, and forming images of meaningful words. We attempted to avoid this in the case of visual coding by making a verbal label readily available but unhelpful. The material we selected for visual recognition comprised a series of color photographs of doors, each of which subsequently had to be recognized from a set of four. On first presentation, the item would be accompanied by an appropriate label, such as, *church door* or *door of a French barn*. The items would then be tested by recognizing that item from a set of four, for all of which the given label would be appropriate. The visual recall and learning test involved four versions of the cross differing in overall shape, the nature of the crux, and the presence of elaboration at the four points. They were readily drawn, and the features were easily scored. In the case of verbal recall and recognition, we opted to use people's names because these are typically not readily semantically codable, and, even when they are, people tend to ignore that fact as being irrelevant. Mr. Black and Mr. Brown, for example, are unlikely to differ in predictable ways in hair or skin color. Finally, possible deficits in perception or production can be checked by using the initial copy of the crosses, the capacity to read the names, and, if necessary, to discriminate among the doors.

Validity was checked using a number of selected patient groups. As mentioned

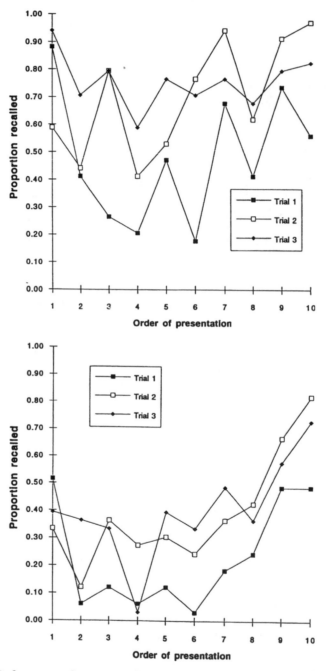

Figure 2.2. Performance of patients suffering from probable Alzheimer's disease (bottom panel) and control patients on three successive learning trials of the Consortium for Experimental Research on Alzheimer's Disease List Learning test. The patients show a greater reliance on the recency effect, which is known to be vulnerable to a brief filled delay. This is reflected in the greater forgetting shown by patients on this test, but not on the Doors and People test, which avoids this short-term component.

earlier, normal older participants tend to have a deficit that is greater for the verbal than the visual test; this does not simply reflect the greater difficulty of that component because patients with schizophrenia tend to show the opposite pattern (Baddeley, 1996a). A study of patients with temporal lobectomies (Morris, Abrahams, Baddeley, & Polkey, 1995) demonstrated a clear crossover interaction, with patients with left hemispherectomies being more impaired on the verbal subtests and the opposite being true for patients with right hemispherectomies. The effects were equivalent for recall and recognition, as is usually the case.

Recall–recognition differences can occur, however, as shown in the case of J.F., a patient who showed grossly reduced hippocampal development, probably as a result of anoxia at birth, but who nevertheless showed normal intelligence and semantic memory (Vargha-Khadem et al., 1997). On recall measures he showed clear evidence of impairment, with a scaled score of 1 for visual and 3 for verbal memory. When tested by recognition, however, his performance was entirely normal, with scale scores of 11 and 10 for visual and verbal recognition, respectively, a pattern that also emerged on a range of other recall and recognition tests (Baddeley et al., 1998).

Finally, the value of the forgetting measure was shown in a study of patients suffering from the early stages of Alzheimer's disease. On both the previously described CERAD test of verbal learning and recall and on immediate and delayed recall of a short story, they showed significantly more forgetting than an older control group. A detailed analysis of their CERAD scores, as described earlier, indicated that the effect stemmed from the use of a recency strategy and suggested that a similar mechanism may operate within prose recall, a hypothesis that has been subsequently pursued with some success (Baddeley, 1998).

The Doors and People test is conceptually traditional; the distinction between recall and recognition, verbal and visual memory, learning, and forgetting have all been around for more than 50 years. It is innovative in its methods of minimizing the role of other aspects of memory, in its basing of all estimates on at least two measures, its use of scaled scores to allow a combination of measures, and in its choice of material.

Theory has played a more important role in the development of measures for semantic memory, a concept that had not been developed when the Wechsler tests were first produced. This is an area in which tests are still being developed, but examples for use with patients with semantic memory deficits include the Pyramids and Palm Trees Test (Howard & Patterson, 1992), on which respondents attempt to match pairs of pictured objects in terms of their semantic associations; hence, given a picture of a pyramid, a pine tree with a broadly triangular outline, and a camel, the respondent is assumed to link the pyramid and the camel. Other tests of semantic processing have been developed to examine the breakdown of semantic coding in Alzheimer's disease, showing as it does a tendency for patients to occasionally lose whole categories and more generally to lose the capacity to make detailed assignments, such as failing to recognize a rabbit but being able to classify it as an "animal." Hodges has developed a set of materials specifically for this purpose and used them to study the deterioration of semantic memory in patients with dementia (see Patterson & Hodges, 1995).

Such tests do, however, tend to be aimed at identifying patients with semantic processing deficits and are typically performed perfectly by normal adults. Some aspects of semantic memory do tend to be well preserved even in older patients or those with brain damage, something that has been capitalized on in the Spot-the-Word Test, on which respondents are given pairs of items, one a real word and one a pseudoword, and required to mark the word. The words range from simple ones such as *kitchen* or *oasis*, to obscure words like *trireme* and *shako*. The test correlates with verbal intelligence as measured on the WAIS, is resistant to aging, and is comparatively resistant to the effect of dementia, although in the later stages of Alzheimer's disease virtually all tasks show an impairment. It can be combined with another semantic memory test that, by contrast, is highly sensitive to the respondent's current state. This is a speeded test on which the respondent must verify a series of statements about the world as rapidly as possible. These are selected to be within the respondent's knowledge base. Half are true (e.g., *nuns have a religious vocation, shoes are sold in pairs*), and half are false, comprising a re-pairing of true items (e.g., *nuns are sold in pairs, shoes have a religious vocation*). Because the information is within the knowledge base of virtually all respondents, it is essentially a measure of the speed of processing, with errors tending to be minimal. Spot-the-Word and the Sentence Verification Task, which is nicknamed "Silly Sentences," can be used together, with one giving an estimate of premorbid verbal intelligence and the other providing an indication of the respondent's current state of functioning. Norms for these two and for their combination are published as part of the Speed of Comprehension and Language Processing Test (Baddeley, Emslie, & Nimmo-Smith, 1992). The Silly Sentences component of SCOLP is also a useful measure of current stressors such as alcohol (Baddeley, 1981), or concurrent information processing load (Baddeley, Eldridge, Lewis, & Thomson, 1984), and has been adapted for use with Third World children (Baddeley, Gardner, & Grantham-McGregor, 1995), where it proved to correlate highly with educational achievement.

Working Memory

The term *working memory* is typically applied to a system that is assumed to be responsible for the temporary holding and manipulating of information in the performance of such complex cognitive tasks as reasoning, learning, and comprehension. Although the term is used in a somewhat different way in animal learning (Olton, Walker, & Gage, 1978) and artificial intelligence (Newell & Simon, 1972), these uses are not considered here. Although the origin of the term is uncertain, it was used by Miller, Galanter, and Pribram (1960) and subsequently applied by Baddeley and Hitch (1974) to their model, which proposed the replacement of the earlier concept of a unitary STM system, such as that proposed by Atkinson and Shiffrin (1968), with a multicomponent system. Baddeley and Hitch specifically proposed three subsystems: (a) an attentional controller that they termed the *central executive*, supported by two subsidiary active memory systems; (b) the *articulatory*, or *phonological*, *loop*, which maintains speech-based information; and (c) the *visuo-spatial sketchpad*, which performs a similar function for visual and spatially coded stimuli. The two slave systems enable the active maintenance of information using stores that are multimodal in input. Hence, the visuospatial sketchpad can be accessed through touch or vision, or indeed may be fed from LTM, such as when participants are asked to describe the layout of their home or to give directions on how to get from one part of town to another. The capacity for spatial visualization is, of course, one that is already familiar to psychometricians and that forms part of selection tests for jobs such as an architect or civil engineer, in which the capacity to imagine complex spatial arrangements plays an important role. For our purposes, we concentrate on the other subsystems.

Central Executive

The central executive component of working memory has sometimes been associated with general intelligence (Duncan, 1993; Kyllonen & Christal, 1990), making this of considerable relevance to the development and refinement of psychometric measures of cognition. As will be clear from other presentations, there has been good progress made by using an operational definition of working memory in terms of tasks that demand the simultaneous storage and manipulation of information (e.g., Daneman & Carpenter, 1980; Kyllonen & Christal, 1990). There has, however, been less concern with the analysis of the system or systems underlying performance, leading to a danger of possible theoretical sterility. This may result in some practically useful new tasks being absorbed into the existing psychometric framework, with no attempt at deeper analysis. A notable exception to this has been the work of Engle and his colleagues, who attempted to analyze a range of working memory span measures in terms of potential underlying variables with some success (e.g., Engle, 1996, for a review).

Our own, more piecemeal approach to the problem of the central executive has been to postulate a number of possible executive subprocesses such as the capacity to focus, switch, and divide attention (Baddeley, 1996b) and then to attempt to measure these using several converging experimental paradigms. We hope eventually to be able to answer questions about the interrelationship between these various subprocesses of the central executive, allowing us to decide whether they are a series of semiautonomous but interactive processes, analogous to an executive committee, or whether the system is more hierarchical, a committee run by a strong executive. Our research so far has concentrated on the capacity to divide attention, which we have found to be particularly impaired in Alzheimer's disease (Baddeley, Bressi, Della Sala, Logie, & Spinnler, 1991). We have made encouraging experimental progress and are now attempting to increase reliability to be able to produce a clinical tool with adequate psychometric reliability.

Phonological Loop

The task associated most closely with the phonological loop is digit span, developed by a London schoolmaster to measure the capacity of his pupils (Jacobs, 1887). Although it tends not to cluster with other measures of general intelligence, over the years it has continued to be included in tests such as the WAIS and to be valued by clinicians as providing another less central but nevertheless important feature of cognitive performance. For example, it tends to be impaired in children with dyslexia (Miles, 1993) and in certain patients with left hemisphere damage (Shallice, 1988).

Verbal memory span has also proved to be a convenient task for use within the cognitive psychology laboratory, showing evidence of the importance of phonological similarity among the items to be recalled, with a sequence such as *B, C, P, G,*

T being harder than *F, W, K, M, Y* (Conrad & Hull, 1964), suggesting some kind of acoustic or phonological code. When unrelated words were used, phonological similarity was again important, with a sequence such as *man, cat, map, cap, mad* being harder than *pit, day, cow, pen, hot* and the similarity of meaning, *huge, big, long, wide, tall* having little effect (Baddeley, 1966a). With an LTM task, involving the delayed recall of longer lists of items, however, semantic similarity becomes the important variable, with acoustic similarity losing its importance (Baddeley, 1966b). The STM storage system appears to be fed and maintained by an articulatory rehearsal system, which appears to operate in real time, with the result that a sequence of long words such as *refrigerator, tuberculosis, university, opportunity, telephonist* leads to poorer performance than an equivalent set of shorter words (Baddeley, Thomson, & Buchanan, 1975). This probably results from both the slowed rate of rehearsal of long words and from delayed recall output they produce if spoken response is required (Cowan et al., 1992). Baddeley and Hitch (1974) proposed to interpret this pattern of data as reflecting a phonological store, within which memory traces would fade over a period of about 2 s, together with an articulatory rehearsal process capable of recoding nameable visual items and of maintaining items in store by continued rehearsal. The patients with impaired STM, described earlier, were assumed to have a deficit in this system, a hypothesis that was broadly supported by the detailed analysis of a pure STM patient, S.R. (Vallar & Baddeley, 1984). Such patients typically have damage to the perisylvian region of the left hemisphere (Vallar & Shallice, 1990). Recent neuroradiological studies have indicated the importance of two separate areas within the left hemisphere (Brodman areas 40 and 44), with one associated with storage and the other rehearsal (see Smith & Jonides, 1995, for a review).

One major puzzle remains, however. Patients such as S.R., despite having a major disruption to their immediate phonological memory performance, nevertheless appear to have few difficulties in their everyday cognition, raising the question of what the functional significance of such a system might be. One classical suggestion is that the STM system is necessary for comprehending speech, possibly holding on to each sentence until parsing and semantic processing is complete (Clark & Clark, 1977).

This hypothesis has now been extensively investigated. Although an occasional patient is found who shows a major disruption of comprehension apparently associated with STM deficit, and an occasional patient who appears to show no impairment whatsoever, the typical pattern is that of an impaired comprehension of complex sentences, in which it is necessary to hold the surface structure throughout the sentence, but otherwise of comparatively normal comprehension capacity. Speech production also appears to be normal, both in content and prosody (Shallice & Butterworth, 1977). In general, then, apart from a minor role in backing up speech perception, there is little evidence for the major significance of the phonological loop in language perception or production (Vallar & Shallice, 1990).

An alternative hypothesis proposed that the system had evolved to facilitate new phonological learning, something that would be important during the acquisition of language but much less so for a mature adult. This was tested by attempting to teach Patient P.V. the vocabulary of an unfamiliar language, Russian. Although she was normal in her capacity to associate pairs of words in her native language of Italian, something that typically depends on semantic coding, her Russian vocabulary acquisition was grossly impaired (Baddeley, Papagno, & Vallar, 1988). We were able to further implicate the phonological loop by demonstrating a similar dissociation between the acquisition of foreign language vocabulary and meaningful paired-associates learning in normal participants under conditions that disrupted the operation of the phonological loop (Papagno, Valentine, & Baddeley, 1991; Papagno & Vallar, 1992).

At this point, we had reached the following conclusion: We had a reasonable account of the system that underpinned the traditional psychometric measure of digit span. The neuropsychological evidence suggested that the system may have evolved to facilitate language acquisition (Baddeley, Gathercole, & Papagno, 1998). If so, then one might expect the system to be associated with capacity for second-language learning and to be of particular significance in children acquiring language.

Evidence for an association between phonological memory and second-language learning comes from several sources. Service (1992) studied the acquisition of English by young Finnish schoolchildren, finding that a nonword repetition task was the best predictor of their success at language learning some 2 years later, whereas in the case of adults, Atkins and Baddeley (in press), using a distributive method of teaching Finnish vocabulary, found that performance was well predicted by a series of short-term phonological memory span measures but not by their visuospatial equivalent. There is clearly a need to relate this approach to language learning to earlier work on second-language acquisition within the psychometric tradition, such as that of Carroll (1962, 1993).

We began our own investigation of language acquisition with a group of children who were identified as having specific language impairment; they were 8 years of age and of normal nonverbal intelligence, but they were 2 years behind in their language development. We began by testing them on a standardized test: Goldman–Fristoe–Woodcock's Test of Auditory Discrimination (Goldman, Fristoe, & Woodcock, 1974). One particular component of performance was especially impaired, namely sound mimicry, in which the child had to echo back an unfamiliar item, typically a single nonsense syllable. On this test, the children were approximately 4 years behind their age norms. We were unhappy with a number of features of the sound mimicry test and developed a task that we called *nonword repetition*, in which the child repeats back pseudowords ranging in length from one to five syllables, all selected to be phonotactically acceptable and hence pronounceable by English speakers. We replicated the major deficit and ruled out any obvious problems of speech perception or production (Gathercole & Baddeley, 1990).

Our next step was to apply the nonword repetition test to a sample of more than 100 4- to 5-year-olds who were starting school (Gathercole & Baddeley, 1989). They were also given the sound mimicry test, the Raven's Progressive Matrices test of nonverbal intelligence, and a vocabulary test. This involved presenting the child with four pictures and speaking the name of one of them. The child then responded by pointing to the appropriate picture. If the phonological loop is necessary for acquiring language, then one might predict that the nonword repetition test, which depends on the temporary storage of novel phonological information, would predict vocabulary. This proved to be the case, with nonword repetition predicting vocabulary ($r = .525$, $p < .01$) better than sound mimicry ($r = .295$, $p < .01$) or indeed general intelligence ($r = .388$, $p < .01$).

An association between vocabulary and nonword repetition could imply that a common phonological store underlies both, but it could also suggest that having a good vocabulary helps one perform the nonword repetition task. It is certainly the case that nonword repetition performance increases with age and that performance tends to be better for items that are more wordlike (Gathercole, 1995). However, two factors tend to suggest the primacy of the phonological loop in language acquisition. The first of these comes from a cross-lagged correlation in which children's nonword repetition and vocabulary were measured at ages 4 and 5. If good vocabulary produces good nonword repetition, then one might expect vocabulary at age 4 to predict nonword repetition 1 year later, whereas if phonological loop capacity is primary, then one would expect the opposite pattern. This proved to be the case, with nonword repetition at age 4 predicting vocabulary 1 year later significantly better than the reverse (Gathercole, Willis, Emslie, & Baddeley, 1992). A second source of evidence for a link of this kind comes from the observation by Gathercole (1995) that, although high wordlike items are easier, items that are low in word likeness are better predictors of subsequent vocabulary acquisition.

Therefore, we propose that the task of nonword repetition is one that is influenced both by phonological loop capacity and the existing state of phonological development. Children with good phonological STM are able to acquire new words more rapidly. As children get older, however, their phonological representations become richer, allowing them to repeat longer and more complex nonwords. The result is that the association between nonword repetition and vocabulary becomes gradually more interactive as the child develops more words that can serve as a basis for pronouncing new items.

What is the relationship between nonword repetition and digit span? Our hypothesis should predict that the two will be correlated and that digit span should also be a predictor of vocabulary development. That is indeed the case, although digit span typically underperforms nonword repetition. Why should that be? If one assumes that the phonological loop has evolved as a mechanism for acquiring new vocabulary, then one might expect that the best way of testing its success is to present it with a task analogous to new vocabulary learning, namely the repetition of an unfamiliar sequence of phonemes. It is assumed that the more durable the short-term trace, the better the opportunity of long-term learning. In the case of digit span, participants are given a sequence of separate familiar words. The task resembles learning a novel word in demanding the holding of a phonological sequence but differs prosodically from the presentation of a single novel sound sequence. We therefore would argue that nonword repetition is a better task than digit span for predicting the capacity for language development.

The nonword repetition test has been standardized and published only recently (Gathercole & Baddeley, 1996; Gathercole, Willis, Baddeley, & Emslie, 1994), but it is already proving useful. For example, Bishop, North, and Donlan (1996) included nonword repetition, and several other possible predictors of language development, in a study involving pairs of twins selected because one of the pair had evidence of specific language impairment. The purpose of the study was to assess the extent to which this particular form of language impairment was heritable and hence involved contrasting identical and nonidentical twin pairs. The children were given the nonword repetition test and a range of other measures, including Raven's Progressive Matrices, a test involving the repetition of sentences increasing in syntactic complexity, and two measures of comprehension, the Test for the Reception of Grammar, and the Comprehension subtest of the Wechsler Intelligence Scale for Children — Revised. Nonword repetition proved to be the best indicator of inheritability of language deficit, showing significant impairment even in children whose problems had largely resolved, suggesting that it provides a valuable marker of the phenotype of heritable forms of developmental language impairment.

We suggest that the development of the nonword repetition test offers a good example of the way in which cognitive psychology, neuropsychology, and psychometrics can interact. Jacobs's (1887) original psychometric measure developed for use with children, digit span, led to a relatively detailed model of the system used by normal adults to perform the task. Data from adult neuropsychological patients broadly confirmed this picture but raised the question of the functional significance of such a memory system, in turn allowing a hypothesis to be tested and supported. The hypothesis in question, namely that the phonological loop serves as a language acquisition mechanism, then required the detailed study of children's memory and the development of appropriate psychometric methods. The result is a new measure to use alongside the traditional test of digit span, whose underpinnings are relatively well understood in theoretical terms and whose practical value has been established. We see this as one example of the way it which the three disciplines of cognitive psychology, neuropsychology, and psychometrics can effectively interact to provide measures that are well-standardized, broadly based, and valid indicators of important cognitive processes.

REFERENCES

Atkins, P. W. B., & Baddeley, A. D. (in press). Working memory and distributed vocabulary learning. *Applied Psycholinguistics.*

Atkinson, R. C., & Shiffrin, R. M. (1968). Human memory: A proposed system and its control processes. In K. W. Spence (Ed.), *The psychology of learning and motivation* (Vol. 2, pp. 89–195). New York: Academic Press.

Baddeley, A. D. (1966a). Short-term memory for word sequences as a function of acoustic, semantic and formal similarity. *Quarterly Journal of Experimental Psychology, 18,* 362–365.

Baddeley, A. D. (1966b). The influence of acoustic and semantic similarity on long-term memory for word sequences. *Quarterly Journal of Experimental Psychology, 18,* 302–309.

Baddeley, A. D. (1981). The cognitive psychology of everyday life. *British Journal of Psychology, 72,* 257–269.

Baddeley, A. D. (1996a). Applying the psychology of memory to clinical problems. In D. Herrmann, C. McEvoy, C. Hertzog, P. Hertel, & M. K. Johnson (Eds.), *Basic and applied memory research* (Vol. 1, pp. 195–220). Hillsdale, NJ: Erlbaum.

Baddeley, A. D. (1996b). Exploring the central executive. *Quarterly Journal of Experimental Psychology, 49A,* 5–28.

Baddeley, A. D. (1998, June). *Is STM simply the activated portion of LTM?* Paper presented at the Quebec STM Conference, Quebec, Canada.

Baddeley, A. D., Bressi, S., Della Sala, S., Logie, R., & Spinnler, H. (1991). The decline of working memory in Alzheimer's disease: A longitudinal study. *Brain, 114,* 2521–2542.

Baddeley, A. D., Eldridge, M., Lewis, V., & Thomson, N. (1984). Attention and retrieval from long-term memory. *Journal of Experimental Psychology: General, 113,* 518–540.

Baddeley, A. D., Emslie, H., & Nimmo-Smith, I. (1992). *Speed and Capacity of Language Processing Test (SCOLP).* Flemptonbury St. Edmunds, United Kingdom: Thames Valley Test Company.

Baddeley, A. D., Emslie, H., & Nimmo-Smith, I. (1994). *Doors and People: A test of visual and verbal recall and recognition.* Flempton, Bury St. Edmunds: Thames Valley Test Company.

Baddeley, A. D., Gathercole, S., & Papagno, C. (1998). The phonological loop as a language learning device. *Psychological Review, 105,* 158–173.

Baddeley, A. D., & Hitch, G. (1974). Working memory. In G. A. Bower (Ed.), *The psychology of learning and motivation* (pp. 47–89). New York: Academic Press.

Baddeley, A. D., Gardner, J. M., & Grantham-McGregor, S. (1995). Cross-cultural cognition: Developing tests for developing countries. *Applied Cognitive Psychology, 9,* 173–195.

Baddeley, A. D., Papagno, C., & Vallar, G. (1988). When long-term learning depends on short-term storage. *Journal of Memory and Language, 27,* 586–595.

Baddeley, A. D., Thomson, N., & Buchanan, M. (1975). Word length and the structure of short-term memory. *Journal of Verbal Learning and Verbal Behavior, 14,* 575–589.

Baddeley, A. D., & Warrington, E. K. (1970). Amnesia and the distinction between long- and short-term memory. *Journal of Verbal Learning and Verbal Behavior, 9,* 176–189.

Baddeley, A. D., Wilson, B. A., & Watts, F. N. (1995). *Handbook of memory disorders.* New York: Wiley.

Banaji, M. R., & Crowder, R. G. (1989). The bankruptcy of everyday memory. *American Psychologist, 44,* 1185–1193.

Bishop, D. V. M., North, T., & Donlan, C. (1996). Nonword repetition as a behavioral marker for inherited language impairment: Evidence from a twin study. *Journal of Psychology and Psychiatry, 37,* 391–403.

Carroll, J. B. (1962). The prediction of success in intensive language training. In R. Glazer (Ed.), *Training research and education* (pp. 87–136). Pittsburgh, PA: University of Pittsburgh Press.

Carroll, J. B. (1993). *Human cognitive abilities.* New York: Cambridge University Press.

Clark, H. H., & Clark, E. V. (1977). *Psychology and language.* New York: Harcourt Brace Jovanovich.

Conrad, R., & Hull, A. J. (1964). Information, acoustic confusion and memory span. *British Journal of Psychology, 55,* 429–432.

Cowan, N., Day, L., Saults, J. S., Keller, T. A., Johnson, T., & Flores, L. (1992). The role of verbal output time in the effects of word length on immediate memory. *Journal of Memory and Language, 31,* 1–17.

Daneman, M., & Carpenter, P. A. (1980). Individual differences in working memory and reading. *Journal of Verbal Learning and Verbal Behavior, 19,* 450–466.

de Wall, C., Wilson, B. A., & Baddeley, A. D. (1994). The Extended Rivermead Behavioral Memory Test: A measure of everyday memory performance in normal adults. *Memory, 2,* 149–166.

Duncan, J. (1993). Selection of input and goal in the control of behaviour. In A. D. Baddeley & L. Weiskrantz (Eds.), *Attention: Selection, awareness and control* (pp. 53–71). Oxford, England: Clarendon Press.

Engle, R. W. (1996). Working memory and retrieval: An inhibition-resource approach. In J. T. E. Richardson, R. W. Engle, L. Hasher, R. H. Logie, E. R. Stoltzfus, & R. T. Zacks (Eds.), *Working memory and human cognition* (pp. 89–119). New York: Oxford University Press.

Gathercole, S. E. (1995). Is nonword repetition a test of phonological memory or long-term knowledge? It all depends on the nonwords. *Memory & Cognition, 23,* 83–94.

Gathercole, S. E., & Baddeley, A. D. (1989). Evaluation of the role of phonological STM in the development of vocabulary in children: A longitudinal study. *Journal of Memory and Language, 28,* 200–213.

Gathercole, S. E., & Baddeley, A. D. (1990). Phonological memory deficit in language-disorder children: Is there a causal connection? *Journal of Memory and Language, 29,* 336–360.

Gathercole, S. E., & Baddeley, A. D. (1996). *The Childrens' Test of Nonword Repetition.* London: Psychological Corporation UK.

Gathercole, S. E., Willis, C. S., Baddeley, A. D., & Emslie, H. (1994). The Childrens' Test of Nonword Repetition: A test of phonological working memory. *Memory, 2,* 103–128.

Gathercole, S. E., Willis, C., Emslie, H., & Baddeley, A. D. (1992). Phonological memory and vocabulary development during the early school years: A longitudinal study. *Developmental Psychology, 28,* 887–898.

Goldman, R., Fristoe, E. M., & Woodcock, R. W. (1974). *Auditory Skills Test Battery.* Minneapolis, MN: American Guidance Service.

Greene, J. D. W., Baddeley, A. D., & Hodges, J. R. (1996). Analysis of the episodic memory deficit in early Alzheimer's disease: Evidence from the Doors and People test. *Neuropsychologia, 34,* 537–551.

Herrnstein, R. J., & Murray, C. (1994). *The bell curve: Intelligence and class structure in American life.* New York: Free Press.

Howard, D., & Patterson, K. (1992). Pyramids and palm trees. Flemptonbury St. Edmunds, United Kingdom: Thames Valley Test Company.

Jacobs, J. (1887). Experiments on "prehension." *Mind, 12,* 75–79.

Kopelman, M. D., Wilson, B. A., & Baddeley, A. D. (1989). The Autobiographical Memory Interview: A new assessment of autobiographical and personal semantic memory in amnesic patients. *Journal of Clinical and Experimental Neuropsychology, 11,* 724–744.

Kopelman, M. D., Wilson, B. A., & Baddeley, A. D. (1990). *Autobiographical Memory Interview.* Bury St. Edmunds, United Kingdom: Thames Valley Test Company.

Kyllonen, P. C., & Christal, R. E. (1990). Reasoning ability is (little more than) working memory capacity?! *Intelligence, 14,* 389–433.

McClelland, D. C. (1973). Testing for competence rather than intelligence. *American Psychologist, 28,* 1–14.

Miles, T. R. (1993). *Dyslexia: The pattern of difficulties* (2nd ed.). London: Whurr.

Miller, G. A., Galanter, E., & Pribram, K. H. (1960). *Plans and the structure of behavior.* New York: Holt, Rinehart & Winston.

Morris, R. G., Abrahams, S., Baddeley, A. D., & Polkey, C. E. (1995). Visual and verbal memory following unilateral temporal lobectomy. *Neuropsychology, 9,* 464–469.

Neisser, U. (1972). Changing conceptions of imagery. In P. W. Sheehan (Ed.), *The function and nature and imagery* (pp. 3–24). New York: Academic Press.

Neisser, U. (1978). Memory: What are the important questions? In M. M. Gruneberg, P. E. Morris, & R. N. Sykes (Eds.), *Practical aspects of memory.* London: Academic Press.

Newell, A., & Simon, H. A. (1972). *Human problem solving.* Englewood Cliffs, NJ: Prentice Hall.

Olton, D. S., Walker, J. A., & Gage, F. H. (1978). Hippocampal connections and spatial discrimination. *Brain Research, 139,* 295–308.

Papagno, C., Valentine, T., & Baddeley, A. D. (1991). Phonological short-term memory and foreign language vocabulary learning. *Journal of Memory and Language, 30,* 331–347.

Papagno, C., & Vallar, G. (1992). Phonological short-term memory and the learning of novel words: The effect of phonological similarity and item length. *Quarterly Journal of Experimental Psychology, 44A,* 47–67.

Patterson, A., & Hodges, J. R. (1995). Disorders of semantic memory. In A. D. Baddeley, B. A. Wilson, & F. N. Watts (Eds.), *Handbook of memory disorders* (pp. 167–186). New York: Wiley.

Service, E. (1992). Phonology, working memory and foreign language learning. *Quarterly Journal of Experimental Psychology, 45A,* 21–50.

Shallice, T. (1988). *From neuropsychology to mental structure.* Cambridge, England: Cambridge University Press.

Shallice, T., & Butterworth, B. (1977). Short-term memory impairment and spontaneous speech. *Neuropsychologia, 15,* 729–735.

Shallice, T., & Warrington, E. K. (1970). Independent functioning of verbal memory stores: A neuropsychological study. *Quarterly Journal of Experimental Psychology, 22,* 261–273.

Smith, E. E., & Jonides, J. (1995). Working memory in humans: Neuropsychological evidence. In M. Gazzaniga (Ed.), *The cognitive neurosciences* (pp. 1009–1020). Cambridge, MA: MIT Press.

Squire, L. R. (1992). Declarative and non-declarative memory: Multiple brain systems supporting learning and memory. *Journal of Cognitive Neuroscience, 4,* 232–243.

Sunderland, A., Harris, J. E., & Baddeley, A. D. (1983). Do laboratory tests predict everyday memory? *Journal of Verbal Learning and Verbal Behavior, 22,* 341–357.

Underwood, B. J. (1975). Individual differences as a crucible in theory construction. *American Psychologist, 30,* 128–134.

Vallar, G., & Baddeley, A. D. (1984). Fractionation of working memory: Neuropsychological evidence for a phonological short-term store. *Journal of Verbal Learning and Verbal Behavior, 23,* 151–161.

Vallar, G., & Shallice, T. (Eds.). (1990). *Neuropsychological impairments of short-term memory.* Cambridge, England: Cambridge University Press.

Vargha-Khadem, F., Gadian, D. G., Watkins, K. E., Connelly, A., Van Paesschen, W., & Mishkin, M. (1997). Differential effects of early hippocampal pathology on episodic and semantic memory. *Science, 277,* 376–380.

Wechsler, D. (1945). A standardized memory scale for clinical use. *Journal of Psychology, 19,* 87–95.

Wechsler, D. (1955). *Adult intelligence scale.* New York: Psychological Corporation.

Wechsler, D. (1987). *Wechsler Memory Scale–Revised.* San Antonio, TX: Psychological Corporation.

Wilson, B. A. (1991). Long-term prognosis of patients with severe memory disorders. *Neuropsychological Rehabilitation, 1*, 117–134.

Wilson, B. A., Alderman, N., Burgess, P., Emslie, H., & Evans, J. J. (1996). *Behavioural assessment of the dysexecutive syndrome*. Flemptonbury St. Edmunds, United Kingdom: Thames Valley Test Company.

Wilson, B. A., & Baddeley, A. D. (1988). Semantic, episodic and autobiographical memory in a post-meningitic amnesic patient. *Brain and Cognition, 8*, 31–46.

Wilson, B. A., & Moffat, N. (1992). *Clinical management of memory problems* (2nd ed.). London: Chapman & Hall.

Discussion

The open discussion following Baddeley's presentation concerned the usefulness of psychometric techniques like factor analysis in the investigation of experimental treatments and phenomena. Additional discussion focused on where information-processing investigations fit into a larger conceptualization of individual-differences theory and research.

Dr. Widaman: I don't know if these are questions or comments. But first of all, in other talks there's been a conflation I think of the notions of psychometrics and mental ability testing. And it was sometime after Thurstone — in the next generation of scholars after Thurstone that the two became widely separated, and psychometrists now — most psychometricians I know either never published anything on a substantive topic, or if they are involved with the collection of any data, it's in the context of big testing companies where they have some vested interest in trying to verify the scores on those tests. I think the conservatism you might be talking about is not in psychometrics but in the testing of memorabilities.

Secondly, I do think that — I wish people would go back and read Thurstone's work because he was really a substantive psychologist, and psychometrics was only an offshoot. And in the forward to *Multiple Factor Analysis* and in the first chapter or two, he said a couple of things that are extremely interesting. One is that techniques like factor analysis are only valuable at the forefront of science when you go into a domain and try to characterize it; and he hoped that people would use factor analysis to characterize different domains, find the important dimensions of individual differences, and he had made some movements clearly in the ability domain. Thurstone said, "I trust that the experimental psychologists" — nowadays we call them cognitive psychologists — "would go into the laboratory and do experiments to try to find out why it is that various tests loaded on the same factor."

Cognitive psychology finally started fulfilling that request about 30 years later. Psychometrics is a set of procedures and it's very useful. It is not content based. And one of the problems with working in cognitive psychology is that cognitive psychologists tend not to know very much about psychometrics. When they do experiments and they find differences in response times in different conditions or different rates of recognition memory and other conditions, frequently it's possible to write statistical models to estimate parameters. They don't do that. What they do is they find a significant difference, and if there's a significant difference in the direction they're interested in, they think this must be an important component that we could develop some test for. But if you go to any one of the testing companies with reliabilities of .7 or .8 — these might be good enough for government work. But when you're trying to develop tests that really tap individual differences, well, we're talking about needing reliabilities of .93, .94, something like that. Very highly reliable measures. And I do believe that it's likely the case, given the way in which many kinds of measures in cognitive psychology are obtained, that if you estimated the parameters associated with those models, the reliabilities would be abysmal even though you could reliably find mean differences across conditions. Those are parameters that could be estimated, and they never are estimated. And once they were estimated, you could do some psychometrics on those estimates to see whether they had any hope of being valid in any kind of predictive situation.

And then the final note on conservatism. I think once you find a final model then there's a reason to be conservative. There's been a hundred years of research on mental abilities. At this point the theory of fluid and crystallized intelligence, which is embedded to a certain extent in John Carroll's work but is represented best in the work of John Horn, has about seven major second- or third-order abilities, about seven different kinds of functions. Once you find a model, there should be other evidence to lead you to reject that model. I think we found in personality, for anyone interested in personality, that was a field that was rife with problems. Now they finally have the Big Five as an organizing framework. Thurstone hoped that those mental abilities would provide an organizing framework for experimental psychologists to then investigate. And I think that they should, and they should with proper psychometric techniques.

Dr. Baddeley: Well, there are a whole lot of points there. Just starting at the beginning, we have often used factor analysis to investigate a new area or an area we knew something about. On the whole, it's rarely been enormously informative. Now, you could argue that perhaps we weren't asking the right questions, but very often where we know, because of other neuropsychological evidence, that one can fractionate something, it doesn't fractionate in the general population. Now, if you're interested in fractionation, then finding that it doesn't fractionate in the general population isn't very helpful. If psychometrics can help us, I'm happy to have that help. But it certainly isn't, I think, the case that starting with factor analysis is a good way forward. Because that depends on what you put in there anyway which depends on what your hypotheses are.

Dr. Ackerman: It seems that a lot of the difficulty at the juncture between cognitive psychology and individual differences, differential psychology, or what some people here are calling psychometrics (which we'll not worry about slicing the small part of that), has to do with a problem in distinguishing between *reliable* effects (those that are replicable) from *large* effects. Now, what you're talking about is very illustrative of where in neuropsychological situations the effects are very large. I'm wondering if you could address your sense of the magnitude of these effects in the normal population as they might be encompassed in a larger individual-differences scheme.

Dr. Baddeley: I can address it in the sense that one can talk about the range, because one uses the normal range as a yardstick for assessing the impairment. To what extent these situations would be useful in asking questions about the normal range, well, I think clearly in the case of the nonword-repetition test, the answer is "yes, it would." Because there is a substantial minority of children who are likely to have difficulty in performing the task. For example in a twin study on heritability of language disability, this particular measure came out as being the best measure of the particular phenotype. So I think the answer varies according to the particular measure. I accept that in some ways working with abnormal populations is easier because you are getting larger effects. And if one is interested in using individual differences to understand the underlying system, then that's probably an easier population, a more fruitful population to work with. The question of "can one then turn it around and use it?" I agree is an open one. Certainly in terms of things like language learning there is evidence that memory span, for example, will predict who's going to be good and who's not so good at learning languages.

Dr. Wagner: Speaking of nonword repetition, you mentioned you'd be willing to say a few words about how you're trying to decompose it or understand what goes into performance of nonword repetition. What are you doing with that?

Dr. Baddeley: I think one particularly interesting finding that Sue Gathercole has recently come up with resulted from wanting to develop a nonword-recognition measure that wouldn't require output, so that you could use it with kids who had articulatory problems. If you do that, what you find is that the "wordlikeness effect" disappears. So items that are not at all wordlike are no harder than items that are wordlike. What that seems to point to in terms of the model is that the wordlikeness effect seems to be operating at the output, the articulatory level, that this suggests that there is a temporary storage system that is not influenced by that. Now, that has implications for the underlying model of what's going on. It clearly will have implications for developing measures and the extent to which one can use these measures in children who can or can't articulate.

Dr. Wittman: I find your work from a paradigm viewpoint very interesting and often ask myself what can be detected with your mainly experimental one which I prefer to call *mean-difference psychology* in contrast to a *differential–correlational* one, where all these means are removed in computing covariances and correlations. Theoretically it's possible that all your resources never will be detected in individual-differences research. All the three resource systems could be perfectly correlated within each person, and you will never detect it with individual-differences research after factoring the correlation matrix of the tasks mapping your different resources you'll only get a *g* factor. But with experimental research, you can detect the usefulness of the different resources by manipulating the memory load and content and find that performance deteriorates with certain manipulations directed to postulated resources. What I mean is, do you expect the same number of systems you found in experimental research also in individual-differences research?

Dr. Baddeley: If we take, for example, the nonword-repetition task that came from a single-subject experiment essentially, the hypothesis that this is a system for acquiring language was tested using individual-differences measures. Initially using an extreme group, subsequently using the general population. So I think there are certain circumstances that give you a way into a separate subsystem, a separate bit of what's going on, but it's very important to extend that to use correlational methods to understand the degree of generality. PET [positron–emission tomography] scanning actually can pull apart the different components so we know that the Wernike's area seems to be responsible for the storage part and Broca's area for the rehearsal part. Now, that's not a general verbal system. That's if you like, a microsystem. And I think we do need to use both experimental and psychometric methods.

3

Minding Our p's and q's: On Finding Relationships Between Learning and Intelligence

DAVID F. LOHMAN

In this chapter, I discuss conditions under which researchers might observe relationships between the constructs of learning and intelligence and, more important, reasons why they generally should not expect these relationships to be strong. The history of attempts to relate these two constructs is remarkable in several respects. If there is a theme, it is the triumph of belief over evidence: that is, *belief* that learning and intelligence ought to be strongly related versus the *evidence* that they are only weakly related.

The expectation of strong relationships between learning and intelligence is based on several logical, statistical, and conceptual confusions. The primary logical confusion is between learning and attainment; the primary statistical confusion is between row and column deviation scores in data matrices (or, more subtly, between the mean of a deviation score and its variance or covariance); and the primary conceptual confusion is among psychological constructs defined by different aspects of score variation.

Background

From the earliest days of testing, scores on intelligence tests have been interpreted primarily as measures of scholastic aptitude (i.e., as the measures of the ability to learn the knowledge and skills taught in schools in the manner in which such things have been taught in schools). When used in this way, there is a clear expectation of a relationship between scholastic aptitude and scholastic attainment and, to the extent that rank orders of students on measures of scholastic attainment vary over time, between scholastic aptitude and individual differences in scholastic learning.

55

Those who interpret measures of intelligence more broadly have expected intelligence tests to predict individual differences in learning in *any* context. Several contributors to the 1921 symposium on intelligence offered definitions of intelligence as simply the ability or capacity to learn (see, for example, E. L. Thorndike, 1921). It is this broader definition that has guided most research. In other words, most systematic efforts to explore relationships between learning and intelligence have sprung not from the school but from the laboratories of experimental psychologists and thus have focused on the learning of laboratory tasks rather than the learning of academic tasks. Woodrow's (1946) studies exemplify this tradition. The results of this effort are well-known. His conclusions not only summarized his work, but they also set the stage for subsequent efforts to relate learning and intelligence. The conclusions were as follows:

1. The ability to learn cannot be identified with the ability known as intelligence.
2. Individuals process no such thing as a unitary general learning ability.
3. Improvement with practice correlates importantly with group factors, that is, relatively narrow abilities, and also with specific factors.
4. Even the group actors involved in learning are not unique to learning but consist of abilities which can be measured by tests given but once. (Woodrow, 1946, pp. 148–149)

Reactions

Woodrow's (1946) first two conclusions ran so completely counter to beliefs about the relationship between learning and intelligence that they were simply ignored by most differential psychologists and psychometricians (Cronbach & Snow, 1977, p. 111). One of the few who seemed to notice was Gulliksen, who, with his students and colleagues (Allison, 1960; Bunderson, 1967; Stake, 1961), doggedly pursued the problem in a series of studies. Others joined the effort or initiated independent attacks on the problem (see Gulliksen, 1961, for an overview of the early work). Their responses to Woodrow's challenge fell mostly into one of six categories: (a) Intelligence is not unitary; (b) learning is not unitary; (c) Woodrow's learning tasks were inappropriate; (d) gain scores are bad; (e) learning should be represented by attainment rather than by gain; and (f) measurement scales are inadequate. I briefly summarize each of these suggested solutions to the problem and then offer my own.

1. *Intelligence is not unitary.* To those trained in the shadow of Thurstone (such as Gulliksen), the most obvious limitation of some of the early investigations was the failure to decompose intelligence into the proper sort of primary mental abilities. Although Woodrow (1946) had included group ability factors in his work (see Simrall, 1946), others believed his tests and methods of factor analysis were inadequate. Correlations between learning and ability were indeed higher when learning tasks and ability tests were more carefully matched, although it now appears that the Cattell–Horn ability theory is more useful than Thurstone's theory for teasing out ability–learning relations (Snow, Kyllonen, & Marshalek, 1984). Nonetheless, replacing g (i.e., general intelligence) with three broad group factors or with seven or more primary ability factors was at best a partial solution.

2. *Learning is not unitary.* In one of the earliest discussions of relationships

between intelligence and learning, E. L. Thorndike, Bregman, Cobb, and Woodyard (1926) noted that most theorists distinguished between lower order association processes and higher order generalization, abstraction, and reasoning processes. One might reasonably expect individual differences in these different cognitive functions to show different relationships with intelligence (although Thorndike actually argued otherwise). Jensen (1973) offered a similar distinction between Level 1 and Level 2 learning abilities and their expected ability correlates. An even more extreme splintering was suggested by experiments showing low correlations among learning rate measures on different tasks (Woodrow, 1946) or when learning rate was estimated from different dependent variables (Cronbach & Snow, 1977). Nevertheless, many investigators hoped that stronger, more consistent relations between learning and intelligence would be found if the proper measure (or measures) of learning were used.

Most significant in this respect were the attempts to define learning not by a simple gain score computed from two waves of data but by the parameters of a learning curve fitted to each participant's performance over many trials. The preferred measure of learning was typically the curvature of this function, or the point at which its first derivative was maximum (i.e., the slope was steepest), indicating the maximal rate of learning (Woodrow, 1946). A variant of this theme was to compute the slope at two points, one estimating early learning and the other late learning (Allison, 1960).

Curve fitting to individual data is a good idea for both theoretical and methodological reasons (Bock, 1991; Estes, 1956; Rogosa, Brandt, & Zimowski, 1982; Woodrow, 1946). It is also useful to distinguish among various aspects of learning (such as initial level of performance, rate of improvement, and final level of performance) and to do so for different aspects of learning, retention, and transfer (Ferguson, 1956). Such methods are not without their problems, however. For example, in any curve-fitting exercise, participants vary in the extent to which their data is well described by functions fitted to the data. Should parameters of the learning curve be used only for those participants well fit by the model? If so, how should this be defined? More important, learning rate measures not only have the same sort of reliability, ceiling, and floor problems as gain scores, but they also show extremely skewed distributions. Interpretation of correlations between rate measures and other variables is thus fraught with difficulties. Nonetheless, rate measures have sometimes shown interesting and interpretable patterns of relationships with ability variables (Snow et al., 1984).

3. *Learning tasks are inappropriate.* A common critique of Woodrow's (1946) studies is that the learning tasks he used were too simple or too short (Humphreys, 1979). Indeed, learning on more complex tasks (e.g., concept attainment tasks) often shows stronger correlations with ability. Taxonomies of learning tasks (e.g., Bloom, 1956; Gagné, 1965; Kyllonen & Shute, 1989) can help guide these efforts to discover ways in which task characteristics moderate ability–learning relationships. Nevertheless, even on complex tasks, correlations between learning and intelligence are usually modest unless scores on the pretest are uniformly low or distributed randomly. Then, correlations between the learning gain score and other variables will be attenuated versions of the correlations between postscores (or final attainment scores) and these variables, which brings me to the troublesome and confusing problem of gain scores.

4. *Gain scores are bad.* Probably the most common critique of Woodrow's (1946)

studies — and many that followed in his wake — is that gain scores are unreliable, thereby severely attenuating relationships with other variables. For some, this means that the unreliable gain score should somehow be made more reliable, usually through disattenuation of its correlations with other variables. For example, Cronbach and Snow (1977) showed how disattenuation could transform negative correlations between mental age and yearly gains in mental age to moderately positive correlations. Yet, in a summary discussion, Cronbach and Snow (1977) eschewed gain altogether and advise that "outcomes in learning . . . ought to be expressed in terms of level (i.e., attainment) scores collected at some terminal point (and perhaps at intermediate points also)" (p. 116).

However, in the very next sentence, the same authors advised treating initial status as a covariate, thereby bringing back a modified gain score. Clearly, there is some confusion about what to do. On the one hand, individual differences in gain scores are unreliable. On the other hand, learning is defined by a change in performance with practice. It is thus naturally operationalized by a gain score or, better, by a curve fitted to multiple waves of data, each representing performance at a particular point in time. In the simplest case in which the investigator has only two waves of data, the observed gain is an unbiased estimator or true gain. From a statistical point of view, then, raw gain scores are preferred over residualized gains as estimators of true gain (Rogosa et al., 1982). Furthermore, the precision of estimated gain must not be confused with the reliability of *individual differences* in gain. For example, in the case in which all participants show the same gain, one can say precisely what this gain is even though the reliability of individual differences in gain will be zero. The reliability coefficient indicates only the accuracy with which individuals can be ranked on the basis of the score. If there is little variability in gain, the reliability of individual differences in gains will be low even though the precision of each estimated gain is high. Conversely, if the variability in true gain is substantial, then reliability of gain scores can also be substantial.

The conditions under which this is likely to occur can be deduced from an examination of the formula for the reliability of gain scores, which is shown in Equation 3.1:

$$\rho_{gg}' = \frac{\rho_{11}'\sigma_1^2 + \rho_{22}'\sigma_2^2 - 2\rho_{12}\sigma_1\sigma_2}{\sigma_1^2 + \sigma_2^2 - 2\rho_{12}\sigma_1\sigma_2}. \tag{3.1}$$

The reliability of gains (ρ_{gg}') is a complex function of the reliability of the pretest (ρ_{11}'), the reliability of the posttest (ρ_{22}'), the variance of the pretest (σ_1^2) and of the posttest (σ_2^2), and the correlation between pretest and posttest (ρ_{12}). One way to understand complex equations is to make some simplifying assumptions. The most common simplifying assumptions here are (a) the pretest and posttest have approximately the same reliabilities and (b) the variance of scores is uniform across time. Under these assumptions, Equation 3.1 reduces to Equation 3.2:

$$\rho_{gg}' = \frac{\rho_{xx}' - \rho_{12}}{1 - \rho_{12}}, \tag{3.2}$$

where ρ_{xx}' is the common pretest–posttest reliability. This formula shows clearly that the reliability of the gains decreases as the correlation between the two scores increases. In fact, ρ_{gg}' drops to zero when $\rho_{12} = \rho_{xx}'$. Thus, it would seem desirable to reduce the pretest–posttest correlation to improve the reliability of the observed gains. However, some have argued that a high correlation between pretest and posttest (here, ρ_{12}) is a necessary condition for test validity. The assumption seems to be that a test that does not show good stability may not be measuring the same trait on both occasions. This is the so-called reliability–validity paradox of gain scores. It is a short step from Equation 3.2 to a general indictment of gain scores. However, one gets to this unhappy place in part by assuming that score variances should be equal and that stability of individual differences over time should be high. Neither assumption is particularly reasonable when significant learning is interposed between pretest and posttest. Indeed, the variability of scores often changes dramatically over time. For achievement test scores, variances tend to increase systematically over the grade school years. Figure 3.1 shows this graphically for the Reading Vocabulary subtest of the Iowa Tests of Basic Skills (ITBS). Kenny (1974) dubbed this pattern of increasing score variance the "fan spread effect." It occurs in large measure because true gains are weakly but significantly correlated with initial status.

What is the effect of unequal variances on reliability of gains? Table 3.1 shows how the reliability of gain scores increases as the ratio of posttest to pretest standard deviation increases and as the correlation between pretest and posttest declines from the average reliability of the pre- and posttests. The good news, then, is that gains can be reliable if there is significant variability in true gain. The bad news is that this does not happen quickly, at least for the sorts of broad abilities students acquire through formal schooling. Table 3.2 and Figure 3.2 show some of the correlations Martin (1985) obtained in his investigation of gains on the ITBS for a sample of 6,321 Iowa students retested every year from third through eighth grade. Table 3.2 shows correlations between gains in different aspects of school achievement and general ability. One-year gains showed small correlations with ability, especially for individual subtests of the ITBS, but 5-year gains showed substantial correlations with ability.[1]

Thus, there is some confusion about gain scores. Sometimes researchers are admonished to avoid them altogether, or better, to reformulate their questions in ways that do not require that they use such measures (Cronbach & Furby, 1970). At other times they are admonished to disattenuate or to examine relationships among latent rather than observed variables. Implicit in the first suggestion is the idea that learning could somehow be operationalized without contrasting initial and final performance; implicit in the second is the idea that the only thing separating constructs of learning and intelligence are errors of measurement. Both suggestions mislead. Although there are times when attainment scores are to be preferred over learning scores, there are also times when the learning score is needed. Similarly, although errors of measurement are a problem, they are not the only reason, or even the main reason, for the relative independence of the constructs of learning and intelligence. About which more later.

---

[1]The low correlations between 1-year gains and ability mean that a model that claimed that status on year n was the sum of status on year $n - 1$ and random growth (e.g., Anderson, 1939) would fit the year-to-year gains well. However, such a model would not predict that growth over a longer period would show higher correlations with ability. Rather, the model would need to incorporate a small correlation between true gain during any 1-year period and ability. These small advantages cumulate over the years.

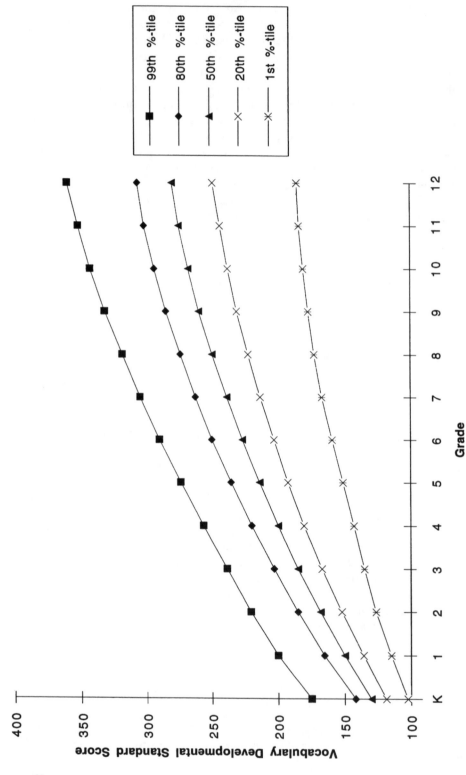

Figure 3.1. Developmental standard scores on the Reading Vocabulary subtest of the Iowa Tests of Basic Skills from kindergarten through Grade 12 for students scoring at the 1st, 20th, 50th, 80th, and 99th percentiles within each grade (spring norms; see Hoover, Hieronymous, Frisbie, & Dunbar, 1993).

TABLE 3.1 Reliability of Raw Gain Scores as a Function of the Ratio of the Pretest and Posttest True Score Standard Deviations

ρ_{12}	σ_1/σ_2			
	.40	.60	.80	1.00
.50	.70	.65	.61	.60
.60	.66	.58	.52	.50
.70	.61	.48	.37	.33
.80	.55	.33	.09	.00

Note. Assuming $\rho_{11}' = \rho_{22}' = .80$.

5. *Learning should be represented by attainment scores.* One response to the measurement difficulties posed by gain scores is to avoid them altogether. There are indeed many times when questions may be properly formulated in terms of attainment rather than learning. A common example is questions about individual differences in what individuals can do at a particular point in time. Although one may infer that doing has something to do with learning, individual differences in attainment scores may reflect primarily individual differences in initial status. Indeed, individual differences in learning may be small even though learning is substantial. In other words, although attainment invariably reflects learning, individual differences in attainment may better reflect individual differences in initial status than individual differences in learning.

A variant on this scheme is to record attainment scores at various stages of practice or learning and then to examine both the intercorrelations of the attainment scores

TABLE 3.2 Correlations Between Average One- to Five-Year Gains in Achievement and General Ability for 6,321 Iowa Students (see Martin, 1985)

Test	Years between pretest and posttest				
	1	2	3	4	5
Vocabulary	.167	.255	.334	.398	.437
Reading comprehension	.141	.270	.357	.441	.486
Spelling	.139	.281	.379	.452	.470
Capitalization	.126	.243	.342	.400	.453
Punctuation	.112	.216	.299	.361	.412
Language usage	.093	.179	.240	.314	.354
Language total	.183	.337	.441	.514	.554
Visual materials	.109	.218	.282	.378	.421
References	.134	.262	.354	.433	.480
Work study total	.154	.298	.386	.477	.519
Math concepts	.140	.260	.362	.440	.503
Math problems	.127	.238	.327	.393	.440
Math computation	.141	.244	.318	.392	.462
Math total	.193	.335	.435	.510	.567
Composite	.262	.445	.548	.625	.664

Note. Entries in column 1 are average correlations with ability for the five 1-year gains, in column 2 for the four 2-year gains, in column 3 for the three 3-year gains, in column 4 for the two 4-year gains, and in column 5 for the one 5-year gain.

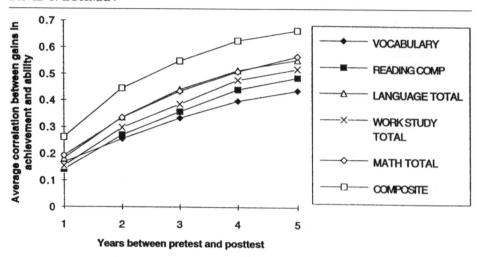

Figure 3.2. Average correlation between gains over periods of 1–5 years on subtests of the Iowa Tests of Basic Skills and an estimate of general ability for 6,321 Iowa students retested every year from third through eighth grade (see Martin, 1985). COMP = comprehension.

and their correlations with other variables. This is precisely the methodology adapted by many who have investigated changes in ability correlations during skill acquisition (Ackerman, 1989; Fleishman, 1972). Fleishman kept all variables in one matrix; Ackerman followed Humphreys's (1960) recommendation to analyze attainment scores from the learning task separately. Attainment scores do not directly compare final status with initial status. Therefore, such analyses reflect individual differences in learning only to the extent that they reveal changes over time in correlations between attainment scores and ability factors. This happens only if the matrix of learning scores is not of unit rank, which is generally the case. Analyses of the external correlates of attainment scores are not only informative in their own right, but they also avoid many of the difficult measurement problems that attend the use of learning scores. However, such analyses often show that the assumption that one is measuring the same thing early and late in learning may be unwarranted, which brings me to the scaling problem.

6. *The scales are inadequate.* One of the earliest criticisms of the Binet Scale was that it did not appear to be measuring the same thing for young children as for older children because there was little overlap in the tasks presented at different ages (Yerkes & Anderson, 1915). Yerkes and Anderson thus proposed that intelligence tests should contain subtests of relatively homogeneous items, such as series completion or vocabulary or analogies, that could be administered to all examinees. Yerkes's arguments and the tests he helped create (e.g., the Army Alpha and Beta, the National Intelligence Test) significantly altered testing in America. Later, investigators often worried about the purity of the scales defined by ability tests, and some even proposed methods for constructing equal-interval scales. Concerns about the scale move center stage, however, when one seeks to estimate learning or growth. Does a 10-point gain mean the same thing at all points along the score scale? If not, then, how can be gains be correlated meaningfully with other variables.

Recently, some have suggested that scales constructed by item–response theory (IRT) methods attenuate or even solve these problems (e.g., Embretson, 1991). Others, however, point to the fact that IRT-based ability estimates for high- or low-scoring examinees are highly unstable. For example, for the three-parameter logistic model, measurement error variance for extreme-scoring examinees can be 10 or even 100 times that for more typical examinees (Lord, 1980). Even more troubling is the fact that such methods can transform a raw score scale that shows a systematic increase in score variance with age into one that shows marked decrease in score variance with age (Hoover, 1984). Although score variance can reasonably remain steady or even decrease over time for closed-ended skills, there is little empirical or conceptual support for such effects in the complex, open-ended skills measured on school achievement tests. By the end of the grade school years, some low-scoring children are still struggling with elementary addition and subtraction, whereas their high-scoring peers are solving algebra problems. It makes little sense to say that somehow the variability in mathematics achievement or vocabulary knowledge has declined over the grade school years. Yet, this is precisely what happened when IRT methods were used to scale the California Achievement Tests (Hoover, 1984).[2]

The problem is not that IRT methods are flawed but that the model used may not really fit the data. Hoover's (1984) critique was aimed at attempts to fit a three-parameter logistic model to a heterogeneous achievement test. Furthermore, because no child takes the entire test, between-grades (or developmental) scales on such tests are often constructed by pasting together a chain of overlapping within-grade (or level) scales. Scaling problems at one level are compounded at the next. On the other hand, ability tests on which both person variance and item difficulty variance are unidimensional can be nicely scaled using the (much simpler) Rasch model, even when a multiage developmental scale is constructed from a series of overlapping within-age scales (see R. L. Thorndike & Hagen, 1997, for an example). Although researchers certainly need to devote more attention to the difficult issues of scale construction than they currently do, and even though IRT scales have many desirable properties and are known to work well when the underlying model fits the data, it is unlikely that IRT scales will resolve debates about the meaning of gain scores any more than improved methods of factor analysis have resolved debates about the number of ability factors and their organization (see also Cliff, 1991).

An even more difficult issue is the fact that scales are often bounded, and so gains are limited. For example, when latency is the dependent measure, those who respond faster in the initial task can improve less than those who respond more slowly. Transformations that linearize the scale provide some remedy and should probably be used more routinely than they are. At the least, it needs to be demonstrated that effects attributed to differential gains are not as easily explained by differences in initial response latencies.

---

[2]R. L. Thorndike (1966) leveled the same criticism at the use of IQ scores to study the relationship between intellectual status and intellectual growth: "By eliminating from the score scale the differences in standard deviation at different ages, that which is the essence of growth is eliminated — the greater variability of specimens as they mature. Imagine a group of adults whose heights and weights showed no greater standard deviations than those of newborn babies! . . . A statistical treatment that . . . excludes greater variability in intellect as we go from birth to maturity is equally absurd" (p. 126).

Summary

There was, and continues to be, an expectation that intelligence is related to learning. This assumption is particularly strong when intelligence is construed as scholastic aptitude and learning is assessed by complex educational tasks. Thus, claims by Woodrow (1946) that intelligence was unrelated to learning elicited either disbelief or a variety of repair strategies (cf. Brown & Burton, 1978). Some proposed that the problem lay in a conception of intelligence as unitary rather than as multiple. Others focused on the measures of learning and emphasized the construction of learning curves for extended, complex tasks. Others emphasized the unreliability of gain scores or the assumptions of interval scaling. Still others moved away from the measurement of learning per se and examined relations between ability tests and attainment scores at various stages of practice. Although each of these repair strategies has been shown to be effective to one degree or another, none has done so consistently and dramatically. As Cronbach and Snow (1977) put it, "the results have been mixed rather than obviously coherent" (p. 133).

A Resolution?

Every now and then, vigorous dispute about some experimental result can be quelled by the recognition of what (in retrospect at least) is an obvious statistical necessity. For example, Bloom (1964) was puzzled by negative correlations between initial IQ and gain in IQ. However, correlated errors will produce such a result. More important, IQ scores have fixed standard deviations, and so highs cannot (on average) improve their scores because that would increase the standard deviation. Rather, they must regress toward the mean, which contributes to the negative correlation. Thus, the negative correlation between gain in IQ and initial IQ is a statistical artifact, not a substantive finding.

Several years ago I experienced a similar dawning of the obvious as I puzzled over information-processing analyses of ability tests (Lohman, 1994). The goals of that research were to (a) understand the mental processes participants used when attempting to solve items on these tests and (b) explain overall individual differences on the tests in terms of individual differences on the component mental process. Although investigators have been generally successful in meeting the first goal, they have been less successful in achieving the second. In particular, although process-inspired models often showed good fits to the data, scores estimating the speed or efficiency with which participants performed particular mental processes showed inconsistent and often low correlations with reference ability constructs (Carroll, 1980). The reason component scores fail to decompose individual differences on tasks is the same reason individual differences in learning are at best weakly related to individual differences in intelligence.

Imagine a simple Person × Occasion data matrix whose entries X_{po} represent the scores of n_p persons on a task administered on n_o occasions. Figure 3.3 shows how the variability in scores may be partitioned into three sources: the person source, the occasion source, and the Person × Occasion/Residual source. The person source represents the variability in row means, that is, in the average attainment scores of persons on the tasks. The occasion source represents the variability in column

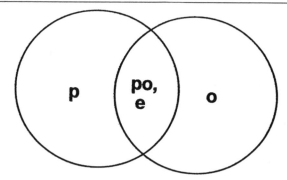

Figure 3.3. Venn diagram showing the partitioning of sources of variation in a Person × Occasion data matrix. The variation in row means ($\overline{X}_{p\cdot}$) captures differences among individuals in overall performance, whereas the variation in column means ($\overline{X}_{\cdot o}$) captures differences across occasions. Individual differences in learning scores capture neither of these sources of variation but instead reflect some portion of the $p \times o$ interaction.

means, that is, in average differences in performance on the tasks across time. The Person × Occasion interaction captures systematic differences in the way participants responded on each occasion that are not captured by the person or occasion sources. In the case of two occasions, it represents variability across persons in learning or gain scores. Changes in variability from pretest to posttest will also be reflected in the Person × Occasion component. Note, however, that average learning is captured by the occasion source and that individual differences that are consistent across time are captured by the person source.

Individual differences are represented by sources of variance that lie within the p circle in Figure 3.3. There are three claims here. First, if the goal is to understand individual differences on a task, then one is interested in *all* of the sources of variance in the p circle. Second, the p variance component is generally large when homogeneous ability tests or learning tasks are administered to samples that vary widely in ability. Third, learning or gain scores help explain variance in the o and po variance components, not the p variance component. The mean of these learning scores is reflected in the o component, their variance in the $p \times o$ component. In other words, the primary contribution of individual learning scores is to help explain individual differences that are independent of both overall individual differences on the task and average learning on the task. Individual differences in learning scores help capture systematic variance from the $p \times o$ component that is ignored when performance is represented by average attainment. However, the learning or gain scores do not decompose and therefore cannot help explain the typically much larger p variance component. This is why attainment scores (initial, final, or average) show correlations with ability variables when gains or rate parameters often do not.

When are individual learning scores most useful? Generally, such scores are most useful when the p variance component is relatively small and the $p \times o$ variance component is relatively large. In the extreme, this would be on a task on which everyone received the same total score ($\sigma^2_p = 0$) and on which individual differences were entirely reflected in differential pre- to posttest gains. In the language of interclass correlations, this means that the correlation between pre- and posttest would be small and the variability in true gains large.

A parallel scenario holds when the goal is to estimate scores for mental processes. Such scores will be most useful when the person variance component is relatively small and the Person × Item variance component is relatively large. For example, Ippel (1986) found that the Person × Item (or Person × Task) variance component was large when different embedded figures tasks were administered simultaneously. For any task (or combination of tasks), measures of internal consistency (e.g., co-efficient alpha) provide an estimate of the relative magnitudes of the person and Person × Facet interactions. When alpha is large, then $p \times i$ must be small. When alpha is small, then $p \times i$ may be large. Thus, if the goal is to measure individual differences in mental processes, then one should look for tasks that do not exhibit a high degree of internal consistency.

Like component scores for mental processes (e.g., Sternberg, 1977), learning is defined by some measure of within-person change. This can be a simple difference score or weighted difference score (such as a slope). (That slopes are difference scores is most readily seen in an analysis of variance model, in which a linear trend is estimated by multiplying cell means by coefficients such as -3, -1, 1, and 3. One is simply computing a non–unit-weighted difference score, but a difference score nonetheless.[3] The main conceptual difference is that whereas component mental processes estimated on one task are thought to explain performance on that same task (e.g., Sternberg, 1977), learning scores on one task are typically related to status or attainment scores on another task, at least when learning is correlated with intelligence. Furthermore, although within-subject deviation scores may be independent of between-subjects deviation scores on one task, these same within-subject deviation scores may indeed be related to between-subjects scores on another task. The key variable is the relationship between the between-subjects scores on the two tasks. The relationship between learning scores and ability test scores will be limited to the extent that attainment scores on the learning task are highly cor-related with status scores on the ability test. The limiting case occurs when the disattenuated correlation between attainment scores on the learning task and ability test is unity. In other words, from a statistical standpoint at least, learning scores on one task are more likely to relate to ability scores on another task when overall performance on the two tasks is *not* highly correlated. However, a psychological analysis would seem to lead to precisely the opposite conclusion. Perhaps this is the reliability–validity paradox written in still another form, or perhaps it is the reason why, for example, Martin (1985) observed small correlations between ability and differential gains in achievement over an entire school year, whereas Woltz (see chap. 6 in this book) finds relatively large correlations between repetition priming and academic achievement.

To recapitulate, then, the problem is not that measures of learning are unreliable (which they are), or that learning should be estimated from individual learning curves rather than simple gain scores (which is a good idea), or that learning needs to be measured on an interval scale (which is also a consummation devoutly to be wished). Nor is the problem that ability should be represented severally rather than singly. In short, my claim is that the primary problem lies not in the measurement of ability or learning but in a more fundamental conceptual confusion about the

---

[3]Kyllonen pointed out that an alternative way to think of this is that the slope is just the average of the difference scores between adjacent levels (e.g., the average of 5-4, 4-3, 3-2, and 2-1).

meaning of constructs defined by different, often highly independent aspects of score variation. Furthermore, the arguments apply with equal force to *any* measure of learning that is operationalized by subtracting one variable from another, whether the two variables are latencies, errors, or positron emissions tomography scan images; whether each is a simple sum of performance on several trials or the product of a more complex function; or whether the theory that guides the process is behavioral, cognitive, or even sociohistorical.

Critics of the arguments I have advanced here often point to cases in which measures of component mental processes or learning gain scores show moderate or even high correlations with other variables. (See, e.g., the correlations between 5-year gains in achievement and ability shown in Table 3.2.) This can happen in a variety of ways, some of which are artifactual and some which are not. First, it is important to emphasize that even relatively small amounts of variation in within-person scores can show substantial correlations with other variables, especially when correlations are disattenuated or reported as path coefficients among latent variables. Even in those cases in which such relationships are replicable, they may not mean what they seem to mean. A common problem — especially when latency is the dependent measure — is that the variability of scores is much greater in one condition than in another condition, and the difference in variability is not attributable to learning but to differences in task demands or scale restrictions. For example, on mental rotation problems (Shepard & Metzler, 1971), variance in response latencies increases dramatically with the amount of rotation required. A score estimating the rate of rotation is typically computed by regression response latency on angular separation between figures. This slope will show high correlations with time taken to solve problems requiring the most rotation. In such cases, correlations between individual slope scores and other measures may be little more than an attenuated version of the correlation between the time required to solve problems in the condition with the greater variance. The limiting case here occurs when the variance is zero in one condition (i.e., all participants have the same score). If scores in this condition are subtracted from scores in another condition, then the difference score will merely reflect the rank order of individuals in the condition with the nonzero variance. For example, if individuals are initially unable to perform a task but differ markedly in performance after practice, then gains will be highly correlated with final status. This is the model that seems to underlie many writers' expectations for strong relationships between learning and intelligence. What it fails to take into account is the fact that, on virtually any complex task, there will be substantial individual differences in initial performance and that these differences will be correlated both with final performance and with academic aptitude (see Woodrow, 1946, for discussion and illustration of this point).

A less extreme case occurs when the variance increases slightly across any two intervals, such as the year-to-year increases in score variance commonly observed on achievement tests (see Figure 3.1 and Table 3.1). It occurs because, although all children improve with education, high-scoring children tend to improve more. Over short intervals, however, differential gains are not large and are easily swamped by the doubly error-laden difference score. Over long periods, however, differential gains can be substantial. For example, Cronbach and Snow (1977) estimated that true mental age at age 6 correlated approximately .6 with true gain in mental age between ages 6 and 7 in Bayley (1949) data.

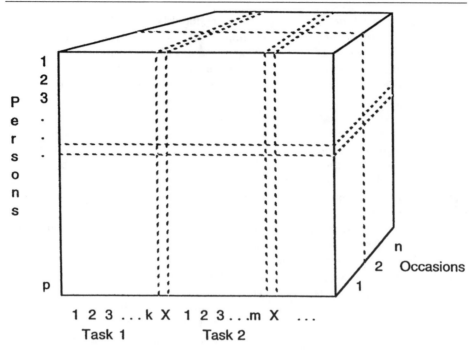

Figure 3.4. A Person × Task (with items nested within tasks) × Occasion data matrix. Note that constructs in psychology are often defined by much different, often independent aspects of score variation.

Construct Confusion

The difficulties in relating measures of learning and intelligence are only one example of a larger confusion in psychology. Many psychologists tend to think of all psychological constructs as belonging to the same conceptual category when in fact they may be conceptually and statistically independent. Although constructs in differential psychology are invariably defined by individual-differences variance, constructs in other domains may be defined by changes in performance across conditions, by rules that map scores onto content domains or absolute scales, and in other ways that reflect individual-differences variance incidentally rather than directly (and may even obscure it altogether).

A more systematic accounting for what sort of variability is represented by different constructs may help researchers keep track of their constructs and keep in line their expectations for relationships among them. Learning and ability scores are defined by different partionings of a simple Person × Occasion data matrix. Personality, developmental, and style variables complicate the picture. Figure 3.4 shows a modified version of Cattell's (1966) covariation chart: Persons × Items (nested within tasks) × Occasions (or situations). Differential psychologists typically worry about person main effects (or covariation of person main effects across several tasks). Experimental psychologists are less uniform. Those who follow an information-processing paradigm worry about variation over trials with a particular task. Situationalists, however, worry more about covariation of either task main effects (e.g., delay vs. no delay of reinforcement) or person main effects across occasions; they typically emphasize the magnitude of the former relative to the magnitude of the latter. Developmentalists do the opposite. Then there are those who worry about interactions. The point is that psychological constructs may be arrayed on several, not just two, dimensions and certainly not just one dimension. Person × Situation is not the same as Person × Items Within Task. When constructs are defined by individual-differences variance, then experimental analyses of tests may not indicate much about the source of these individual differences unless participants solve the tests in different ways and the experimental analyses can identify them. Similarly, when a construct is defined by condition or stimulus variance, then correlating individual scores on a task with other variables may not indicate much about it either.

Investigations of the generalizability of constructs show this confusion most clearly. The differential psychologist knows how to estimate the generalizability of individual differences across tasks, but that is not the aspect of generalizability that should most interest the experimentalist. In addition to the generalizability of individual differences across tasks, one can examine the consistency across tasks of treatment effects or even of score profiles (see Cronbach, 1957, for an example; see also Cattell, 1966). In other words, the experimentalist should be more interested in the covariation of response patterns between rows of the data matrix, not between columns, like the differential psychologist. Unfortunately, because the psychometrician is usually more adept at multivariate statistics, efforts to link experimental and differential psychology usually end up playing by differential rules. Entire research programs attempting to link experimental and differential psychology have risen and then collapsed on the basis of a few between-persons correlation coefficients. A better strategy would be to exploit the separate strengths of the experimental and differential traditions rather than trying to reduce them to a common enterprise. In other words, one might look to an experimental analysis to explain how participants solved tasks or learned from their exposure to them. Although such analyses can usefully inform understanding of individual differences when individuals differ in the parameters of a common model, they are most informative when qualitatively different models are needed to describe the performance of different individuals, and these differences show systematic relations with overall performance on the task or with other variables. Stage-theoretic models of cognitive development (such as the one advanced by Piaget) are an example. Baddeley's (see chap. 2 in this book) neuropsychological examples are another. In either case, logic and argumentation would seem to offer less hazardous avenues of commerce between the disciplines of psychology and their constructs than do between-persons correlation coefficients, no matter how carefully estimated and adjusted.

Conclusions

1. The fact that individual differences in measures of learning are generally weakly but positively related to measures of intelligence is an interesting fact of life, not a problem to be explained. Indeed, were the two not related at all, or more strongly related, then researchers would have more to explain. If learning and intelligence were not related, then differential maturation rates would

constitute the only explanation for imperfect relationships among true status scores on mental tests over time (assuming, of course, that the scales can be trusted). If learning and intelligence were more strongly related, then the differences between high- and low-ability learners would show a positively accelerated growth over time rather than the gentle fan that they seem to show.

2. The simple gain score is often the best measure of learning. If the data permit, then more sophisticated functions can be fitted to each participant's learning data and parameters of this function used to summarize the course of learning for each individual. (Aggregation of individuals comes later.) Gain scores should not be eschewed because of their low reliability. Indeed, ceiling effects (especially for accuracy) and floor effects (especially for latency) probably present more serious problems. Analyses that allow estimation of relations among latent variables can be performed and will often show patterns much unlike those observed among raw scores. When this happens, it would seem wise to report both.

3. Although gain scores are not to be eschewed, neither should they be used when questions more properly concern changes in relationships of attainment scores with other variables over time as, for example, in Ackerman's (1987, 1989) studies of skill acquisition.

4. The expectation of strong relationships between learning and intelligence is based on several logical, statistical, and conceptual confusions. The primary logical confusion is between learning and attainment. Indeed, although they are usually moderately correlated, individual differences in learning may be independent of individual differences in attainment. This illustrates the primary statistical confusion, which is between row and column deviation scores in data matrices or between within- and between-persons variation. More subtly, it is between the mean of a deviation score and its variance or covariance. Finally, the primary conceptual confusion is among psychological constructs defined by these (and other) different aspects of score variation.

In the old days, typesetters assembled words from individual letters, each stored alphabetically in small compartments; p's and q's were thus stored in adjacent bins and would appear reversed when arranged on the composing stick. It was easy to confuse them. Apprentices who disassembled type and re-stored the letters were thus admonished to "mind their p's and q's." A more colorful tale is that tabs in pubs once consisted of lists of p's (for pints) and q's (for quarts). Both the innkeeper and the drinker would have a stake in making sure p's were not confused with q's when the tally was reckoned. Like apprentice typesetters or wary pub sitters, researchers must attend carefully to the orientation of their data matrices. Constructs that explain much of the within-person variation on a task need not explain much of the between-persons variation either on that task or on other tasks.

REFERENCES

Ackerman, P. L. (1987). Individual differences in skill learning: An integration of psychometric and information processing perspectives. *Psychological Bulletin, 102*, 3–27.

Ackerman, P. L. (1989). Individual differences and skill acquisition. In P. L. Ackerman, R. J. Sternberg,

& R. Glaser (Eds.), *Learning and individual differences: Advances in theory and research* (pp. 164–217). New York: Freeman.

Allison, R. B. (1960). *Learning parameters and human abilities* (Rep. No. UM 60-4958). Princeton, NJ: Educational Testing Service.

Anderson, J. E. (1939). The limitation of infant and preschool tests in the measurement of intelligence. *Journal of Psychology, 8,* 351–379.

Bayley, N. (1949). Consistency and variability in the growth of intelligence from birth to eighteen years. *Journal of Genetic Psychology, 75,* 165–196.

Bloom, B. S. (1956). *Taxonomy of educational objectives: Handbook I. Cognitive domain.* New York: David McKay Co.

Bloom, B. S. (1964). *Stability and change in human characteristics.* New York: Wiley.

Bock, R. D. (1991). Prediction of growth: Implications of a multidimensional latent trait model for measuring change. In L. M. Collins & J. L. Horn (Eds.), *Best methods for the analysis of change: Recent advances, unanswered questions, future directions* (pp. 126–136). Washington, DC: American Psychological Association.

Brown, J. S., & Burton, R. R. (1978). Diagnostic models for procedural bugs in basic mathematical skills. *Cognitive Science, 2,* 155–192.

Bunderson, C. V. (1967). *Transfer of mental abilities at different stages of practice in the solution of concept problems* (Research Bulletin 67-20, Rep. No. UM 66-4986). Princeton, NJ: Educational Testing Service.

Carroll, J. B. (1980). *Individual differences in psychometric and experimental cognitive tasks* (ONR Final Rep. No. NU 150-406). Chapel Hill: University of North Carolina, L. L. Thurstone Psychometric Laboratory.

Cattell, R. B. (1966). *Handbook of multivariate psychology.* Chicago: Rand McNally.

Cliff, N. (1991). Comments on "Implications of a multidimensional latent trait model for measuring change" by S. E. Embretson. In L. M. Collins & J. L. Horn (Eds.), *Best methods for the analysis of change: Recent advances, unanswered questions, future directions* (pp. 198–201). Washington, DC: American Psychological Association.

Cronbach, L. J. (1957). The two disciplines of scientific psychology. *American Psychologist, 12,* 671–684.

Cronbach, L. J., & Furby, L. (1970). How we should measure "change" — Or should we? *Psychological Bulletin, 74,* 68–80.

Cronbach, L. J., & Snow, R. E. (1977). *Aptitudes and instructional methods: A handbook for research on interactions.* New York: Irvington.

Embretson, S. E. (1991). Implications of a multidimensional latent trait model for measuring change. In L. M. Collins & J. L. Horn (Eds.), *Best methods for the analysis of change: Recent advances, unanswered questions, future directions* (pp. 184–197). Washington, DC: American Psychological Association.

Estes, W. K. (1956). The problem of inference from curves based on group data. *Psychological Bulletin, 53,* 134–140.

Ferguson, G. A. (1956). On transfer and the abilities of man. *Canadian Journal of Psychology, 10,* 121–131.

Fleishman, E. A. (1972). On the relation between abilities, learning, and human performance. *American Psychologist, 11,* 1017–1032.

Gagné, R. M. (1965). Problem solving. In A. W. Melton (Ed.), *Categories of human learning.* New York: Academic Press.

Gulliksen, H. (1961). Measurement of learning and general abilities. *Psychometrika, 26,* 93–107.

Hoover, H. D. (1984). The most appropriate scores for measuring educational development in the elementary schools: GE's. *Educational Measurement: Issues and Practices, 3,* 8–14.

Hoover, H. D., Hieronymous, A. N., Frisbie, D. A., & Dunbar, S. B. (1993). *Iowa Test of Basic Skills: Norms and score conversions (Form K).* Chicago: Riverside.

Humphreys, L. G. (1960). Investigation of the simplex. *Psychometrika, 25,* 313–323.

Humphreys, L. G. (1979). The construct of general intelligence. *Intelligence, 3,* 105–120.

Ippel, M. J. (1986). *Component-testing.* Amsterdam: Free University Press.

Jensen, A. R. (1973). *Educability and group differences.* New York: Harper & Row.

Kenny, D. A. (1974). A quasi-experimental approach to assessing treatment effects in nonequivalent control group design. *Psychological Bulletin, 82,* 345–362.

Kyllonen, P. C., & Shute, V. J. (1989). A taxonomy of learning skills. In P. L. Ackerman, R. J. Sternberg,

& R. Glaser (Eds.), *Learning and individual differences: Advances in theory and research* (pp. 117–163). New York: Freeman.

Lohman, D. F. (1994). Component scores as residual variation (or why the intercept correlates best). *Intelligence, 19,* 1–12.

Lord, F. M. (1980). *Applications of item response theory to practical testing problems.* Hillsdale, NJ: Erlbaum.

Martin, D. J. (1985). *The measurement of growth in educational achievement.* Unpublished doctoral dissertation, University of Iowa, Iowa City.

Rogosa, D., Brandt, D., & Zimowski, M. (1982). A growth curve approach to the measurement of change. *Psychological Bulletin, 92,* 726–748.

Shepard, R., & Metzler, J. (1971). Mental rotation of three-dimensional objects. *Science, 171,* 701–703.

Simrall, D. V. (1946). *The effects of practice on the factorial equations for perceptual and visual-spatial tests.* Unpublished doctoral dissertation, University of Illinois, Urbana-Champaign.

Snow, R. E., Kyllonen, P. C., & Marshalek, B. (1984). The topography of ability and learning correlations. In R. J. Sternberg (Ed.), *Advances in the psychology of human intelligence* (Vol. 2, pp. 47–103). Hillsdale, NJ: Erlbaum.

Stake, R. E. (1961). Learning parameters, aptitudes, and achievement. *Psychometric Monographs,* No. 9.

Sternberg, R. J. (1977). *Intelligence, information processing, and analogical reasoning: The componential analysis of human abilities.* Hillsdale, NJ: Erlbaum.

Thorndike, E. L. (1921). Intelligence and its measurement: A symposium. *Journal of Educational Psychology, 12,* 124–127.

Thorndike, E. L., Bregman, E. O., Cobb, M. V., & Woodyard, E. (1926). *Measurement of intelligence.* New York: Teachers College Press.

Thorndike, R. L. (1966). Intellectual status and intellectual growth. *Journal of Educational Psychology, 57,* 121–127.

Thorndike, R. L., & Hagen, E. P. (1997). *Cognitive Abilities Test (Form 5) research handbook.* Itasca, IL: Riverside.

Woodrow, H. (1946). The ability to learn. *Psychological Review, 53,* 147–158.

Yerkes, R. M., & Anderson, H. M. (1915). The importance of social status as indicated by the results of the point-scale method of measuring mental capacity. *Journal of Educational Psychology, 6,* 137–150.

Discussion

The discussion of Lohman's paper started with a general question-and-answer exchange about situations in which learning and intelligence may not be related. Additional discussion focused on the measurement of "change." A final exchange between Lohman and Kyllonen illustrated that there is still substantial controversy about the relations between measures of intelligence on the one hand and measures of individual differences in learning on the other hand.

Dr. Baddeley: Thinking about it from a neuropsychological perspective, and it becomes very clear that there are certain cases like the classic amnesic syndrome where intelligence can be perfectly spared, certain types of learning can be unimpaired, and others dramatically impaired. I'm not quite so sure about the double dissociation of people with very low fluid intelligence and learning, but I think it's an interesting reflection on asking the same questions using different sources. And, I wonder, am I misconceptualizing, or do you feel that this is consistent. . . .

Dr. Lohman: Yes. That's a further complication. It was one I wanted to discuss but didn't really have the time to do here. I used the example of row and column deviation scores on a single matrix. But if you envision two matrices, one for the ability test and one for the learning task, then it is far less obvious how row deviation scores in one matrix may be constrained in their relationships with column deviation scores in the other matrix. One is now dealing with two different systems. The key is how strongly row deviation scores in Matrix 1 covary with row deviation scores in matrix 2 (i.e., the extent to which individual differences on the ability test are correlated with attainment scores on the learning task). If this correlation is high, then you may expect column deviation scores from Matrix 2 to be weakly correlated with row deviation scores in both matrices. But when the covariance between the two sets of row deviation scores is low, then there would be no such constraint. So yes, there are cases in which measures of learning and ability are not constrained in the ways that I have shown here. Furthermore, don't think I'm arguing against the specialized cases to which you refer.

Dr. Baddeley: Well, I'm not sure that it is separate. My assumption is that these are the same underlying neural systems that we're looking at in different ways.

Dr. Lohman: The measures you reported using differed importantly from the measures of learning I discussed in my talk. The measures that you used as indicators of a particular neurological deficit were generally total scores rather than difference scores. One score subtracted from another just doesn't work nearly as well as total or attainment scores for the analysis of individual differences.

Dr. Baddeley: I think with amnesic patients the two are virtually similar. If you're not learning anything, then you don't have any slump. So the subtleties almost drop out.

Dr. Wittmann: I want to comment on "change" — learning means change. Well, the first thing we have to answer how reliable is change. That means if it's unreliable it isn't worth the effort to be explained. I think somebody has to speak it out loud or talk straight about it. Lord and Cronbach are simply falsely interpreted on that postulate of the unreliability of change scores. What is wrong with the formula which you have demonstrated is that it contains basically no replication. You have the pretest, the posttest, and the correlation between both. Where is the replication of the difference scores? What you need is at each measurement point two parallel measures; that is, two parallel measures of the pretest and two parallel measures of the posttest. Then you can compute two difference scores, and then you can correlate that. I did that, and I'm able to demonstrate that these results are pretty much higher than applying the Lord or Cronbach formula.

Dr. Lohman: The key issue is the variability in true change. And when you have significant variability in true change — no matter how you compute it — then you will be more likely to find substantial correlations between gain and other measures. But in learning situations in which there is a complex task on which individuals differ meaningfully at pretest, and a short time for learning, you often don't obtain much variability in pretest to posttest gains. In the data I showed earlier, even after 1 year, the gains were not sufficiently variable among students to show much correlation with ability. But over longer periods — such as 3, 4, or even 5 years — these small advantages accumulated. In the reading literature, this is called the *Matthew effect*.

Dr. Wittmann: I completely agree. You got much more dosage in the treatment if you're going to aggregate over time. If you have only a short time, what's the dosage? What do we expect with such a weak treatment? Why should change result with weak treatments from a conceptual and theoretical standpoint?

Dr. Ackerman: I would like to ask a conceptual question. For example, when you talk about concept attainment tasks where everybody starts off at chance performance, then we can measure learning directly because everybody is essentially at zero or at chance performance. But maybe the problem that we have fundamentally and conceptually is thinking about learning as sort of an experimental treatment, whereas what we really deal with as correlational or differential psychologists is individual differences in transfer. Learning doesn't have a unitary meaning for people of low ability and high ability, for example. In contrast, in the aggregate, you get large correlations between intelligence and learning, like in your Iowa test.

Dr. Lohman: After 5 years.

Dr. Ackerman: After 5 years. But in the short term it's the low-ability people who learn the most because the high-ability people understand the instructions. And so the low-ability people have so much more to learn, so we would expect a negative correlation between ability and learning — even with true scores for gain.

Dr. Lohman: In certain cases, yes. But in many tasks — particularly in school-learning tasks that require more than the proceduralization of skills — individual differences at input are substantial, and at output are not constrained. The rich do indeed tend to get richer, although in fairly small increments over any short period of time; but over long periods these small advantages accumulate into a substantial advantage. So, for example, in the data for the Iowa tests that I showed, there were some eighth grade students who were scoring worse than the average first grader. And this is in Iowa where all the children are above average! The variability in performance is truly enormous at the end of grade school (and even more so by the end of high school) and these differences are built upon a much smaller variability at kindergarten.

Dr. Deary: This is just a reflection rather than a question, David [Lohman]. It seems that there's an application here for your criticism in the area of gerontology. One of the biggest interests at present is what determines people's differential decline in various abilities, especially fluid intelligence and memory. And much of it is designed along exactly the sort of design you're talking about which takes an initial ability level or social class or education and looks at to what degree that determines the decline over time. Although here we're talking largely about children and learning, it can be equally well applied to the change in ability with age; there exist the same inherent problems.

Dr. Lohman: I believe that Richard Wagner is going to talk about this in his presentation and will use methods that are actually much better suited for modeling growth. Basically, growth models in which you actually fit a model to the data are much better suited for the analysis of multiwave data than the sort of simple correlational analyses that I've presented here.

Dr. Kyllonen: In lots of studies we find an extremely high relationship, close to a perfect relationship, between learning and working memory capacity. The kind of learning that we're talking about is the acquisition of simple rules to classify stimuli. Given that high relationship, I'm confused about why this continues to be an issue.

Dr. Lohman: It is an issue when we measure learning by subtracting posttest from pretest, and there are significant individual differences on the pretest that are strongly correlated with individual differences on the posttest.

Dr. Kyllonen: Well, that's the case with, for example, the complex learning studies that we do to a certain extent, but with the simple learning studies where people are simply learning to classify stimuli according to some arbitrary rules . . . .

Dr. Lohman: Right. So people are at chance to begin with in which case . . . . in which case the learning score would be perfectly correlated with attainment or a final score.

Dr. Kyllonen: We find essentially, correlations that are indistinguishable from 1.0.

Dr. Lohman: Yes, that makes good sense. This will happen if either the variance of the initial scores is zero (everyone has the same score) or the initial scores are at a chance level. In the latter case, when you subtract one from the other, you're basically taking your final score and subtracting some noise. And that's a case where probably the attainment score would make more sense than the learning score, because the learning score is just adding noise.

Dr. Kyllonen: Given that's the case, I'm not sure why you're so quick to dismiss the argument that it's a scaling problem.

Dr. Lohman: I would certainly agree that scaling is an important issue — perhaps even the most important issue in modeling change scores. Although IRT [item–response theory]-based scales have many desirable properties, the procedures used to produce them sometimes do not work as expected. I cited one example in which this happened. In that case, the normal fan was actually reversed. And so I'm somewhat leery of such methods, especially attempts to apply the three-parameter model to scores from heterogeneous ability tests. There are many people actually who do these sorts of scaling on operational tests who are not at all convinced that IRT methods are going to be our salvation, primarily because you have to make many assumptions in order to use them. They're model-based procedures rather than data-based procedures. And if your model doesn't actually describe what's going on, you can be in great difficulty.

Dr. Kyllonen: Well, a scaling artifact would be more convincing if, in fact on that fan spread graph you showed, the fan went outward in both directions, but that doesn't happen. It's always the case that both the lowest end is moving up and the highest end is moving up.

Dr. Lohman: In fact, something like that did happen some years ago when the California Achievement Tests were scaled using a three-parameter logistic model. The variance of scores actually decreased across grades — which is bizarre.

Dr. Kyllonen: Well, I don't know why you can say that.

Dr. Lohman: Because by the time kids are in eighth grade, there is considerably more variability in what they can do in mathematics or in the number of words they can define than there is in first grade. Variables such as height and weight show the same sort of fan effect. It just doesn't make sense to me to envision a scale on which variability for such variables decreases with age.

Dr. Kyllonen: But it can. That could be a scaling artifact.

Dr. Lohman: In this case, I would have to disagree.

Dr. Ackerman: Can you tell that these two guys went to graduate school together?

4

Investigating the Paths Between Working Memory, Intelligence, Knowledge, and Complex Problem-Solving Performances via Brunswik Symmetry

WERNER W. WITTMANN and HEINZ-MARTIN SÜß

The future of interindividual-differences research as a scientific branch of psychology depends, as every science, on its ability to predict and explain criteria. What are those criteria? Psychology is the science of human behavior, that is, what psychologists try to predict and explain. Psychologists know that humans differ in performance whether in school, business, or other areas of life.

Cronbach (1957, 1975) distinguished between two scientific disciplines of psychology. Experimental psychology concentrates on the explanatory power of situational variables that are manipulated and analyzed for their effects on human behavior. Correlational psychology focuses on dispositional constructs within individuals to maximize prediction of behavior. We choose in our research program an emphasis on dispositional constructs even when borrowing constructs from experimental psychology. The criteria we use are individual differences in performance on computer-based games that are thought to be ecologically valid for real-life performance but have the advantage to be researched in our lab. The dispositional constructs we use are working memory capacity (WMC) psychometric intelligence, personality, biodata, and knowledge. The reasons for choosing these constructs are derived from the state of the art in modern personnel selection research (Hunter, 1986; Hunter & Hunter, 1984; Rumsey, Walker, & Harris, 1994; Schmidt, Ones, & Hunter, 1992). Meta-analysis has shown that intelligence, biodata, and task knowledge are among the most valid predictors. Personality is also often discussed and considered but does not demonstrate the same amount of predictive validity. This can be seen in the most comprehensive meta-analysis of personality's role conducted by Ackerman and Heggestad (1996). WMC was borrowed from experimental research on learning, memory, and cognition. Experimental researchers tried to isolate process components that were assumed to be centrally related to psychometric intelligence and able to explain interindividual differences as a function of manipulated task characteristics. Memory load in dual-task paradigms, information-processing speed, and capacity to process information are the most prominent ones. For example, Baddeley (1986) found evidence for a phonological loop and a visuospatial sketchpad. Verbal information is processed in the phonological loop and figural in the visuospatial sketchpad. Both are called *slave systems*. He also postulated a central executive system that is assumed to control, distribute, or supervise the information flow in the brain. Evidence for the separation of the two slave systems as two different resources is good compared with the one for the central executive. Baddeley's model is derived from experimental research that traditionally concentrated on mean reaction time and mean differences as a function of task characteristics. It is unclear whether the same structure will appear in correlational research, factoring the correlational pattern between different working memory tasks. Kyllonen and Christal (1990) were among the first to attempt this goal. Their main result was that WMC, defined as an aggregation of the working memory tasks used, was little more than reasoning (and thus closely related to *g*). The only drawback of their study was that some of their working memory tasks were conceptually highly similar to tasks used in psychometric intelligence research. Thus, the almost-perfect correlation between WMC and *g* could have been biased. In our research program, we have tried to assess WMC as broadly as possible by simply searching for the most typical and divergent tasks used by WMC researchers, and then we adapted the tasks to measures of interindividual differences and included them in our assessment battery.

In intelligence research many investigators have turned to Spearman's *g* and regard it as the most important explanatory construct in predicting human performance and other socially important criteria. Although *The Bell Curve* (Herrnstein & Murray, 1994) has attracted much controversy, it demonstrates for many people some unexpected relationships of a *g*-type intelligence measure to a variety of criteria. Only some (e.g., Ackerman, 1997, p. 172) are aware of the historical facts in pointing to Thorndike (1940), who stated this very fact. Discussions about the ubiquity of *g* are on the top of the agenda in learning ability and interindividual-differences research. A large-scale assessment program conducted by the U.S. Air Force using the Armed Forces Vocational Assessment Battery found only the battery's *g* to be the most important predictor, not specific abilities or aptitudes (Ree & Earles, 1994). Discussions and consequences of the results relate to the possible diminishing returns in further investments in researching other dimensions of ability (Alderton & Larson, 1994).

Reviewing personnel selection research, Schmidt et al. (1992) found little evidence for the incremental validity of specific aptitudes over the effect related to *g*. Schmidt (1994) believed that the small increments found were overestimates caused by statistical problems. A whole special issue of the leading journal *Intelligence*, edited by Gottfredson (1997), is devoted to intelligence and social policy. Many arguments about the importance of *g* can be found there. Although *g* is derived from theoretical conceptualization and encouraged through empirical results, we are concerned that concentrating only on *g* will turn out to be one of the greatest fallacies in intelligence research. At least in our German research we have found evidence that school grades at the gymnasium are not to be best predicted from g (Wittmann & Süß, 1996). To provide more evidence on that topic, we used in all our research a comprehensive intelligence battery related to the Berlin model of intelligence (Jäger, 1984; Jäger, Süß, & Beauducel, 1997; Süß, 1996; Wittmann, 1988), which measures g and specific ability factors at the same time. But first we turn to theoretical and methodological concepts that we think are at the heart of the future of learning and individual-differences research.

Some Basic Theoretical Assumptions and Methodological Principles

Success in prediction and explanation varies among different scientific disciplines. Psychology and the social sciences are at a considerable disadvantage compared with the natural sciences such as physics. There one finds powerful theories leading to strong and courageous predictions that experimenters try to falsify. An example is Gell-Mann's quark theory in particle physics. Recently at Fermi Laboratory they found the very existence of the last particle, the top quark. What a powerful and strong theory! Psychologists dedicated to science are deeply impressed by theories of that type. They can only dream about such types of theories in psychology. To get rid of the depression caused by comparing one's own research with topnotch science, we started guessing about the secrets behind questions to which nature gives clear answers. In doing so, we found in psychology and the social sciences explanations of failure related to cross-level fallacy, a theme emerging repeatedly every couple of decades (e.g., Alker, 1969; Robinson, 1950; Thorndike, 1939). Yet, explanations of success in science are related to the magic concept of *symmetry*. All the smart and successful researchers such as Richard Feynman, Murray Gell-Mann, Emmy Noether, Michael Faraday, to name a few, used principles of symmetry (see Zee, 1989). Guessing about secrets and finding symmetry, it was only a short step to find that principles of symmetry have been around for many years in Egon Brunswik's psychology, especially in his lens model (Brunswik, 1952, 1955, 1956). Predictors and criteria have to be symmetrical to one another to obtain maximum predictability. Predictors used in differential correlational psychology, such as intelligence, personality, and knowledge, have been extensively researched over the past century, and the best synthesis turns out to be in hierarchical models of intelligence (e.g., Carroll, 1993). Placing hierarchical models at the predictor side of the lens, gestalt principles force researchers to look at the criterion side for symmetrical hierarchical models as well. We comply with Karl Popper's recommendations to be courageous in proposing falsifiable series, so we postulate that the true latent structures of psychological constructs have to be symmetrical. We coined this axiom *Brunswik symmetry*. Figure 4.1 depicts what we mean by constructs that are symmetrical. Every level of generality at the predictor model has its symmetrical level of generality at the criterion side, and vice versa. If we could only know and adequately assess the respective components, all correlations in pairs between symmetrical levels would be perfect (i.e., one).

Our failures as cross-level fallacy can be seen in Figure 4.1. Looking at how we try to assess the true latent dimensions and structure with manifest variables, Type

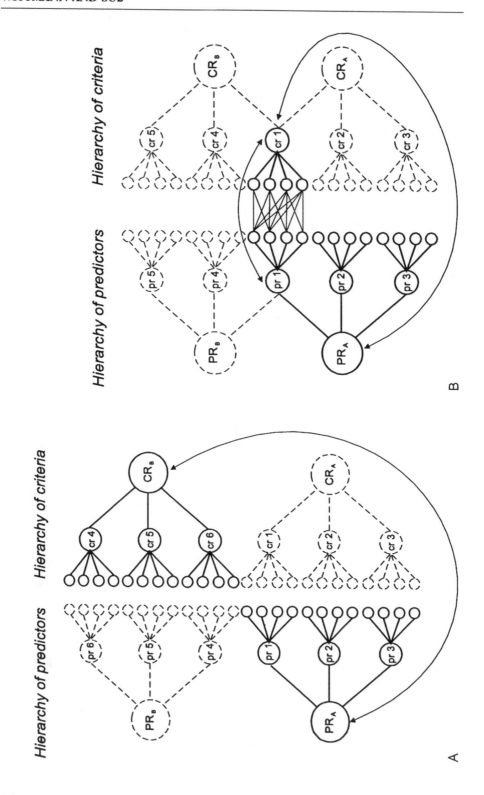

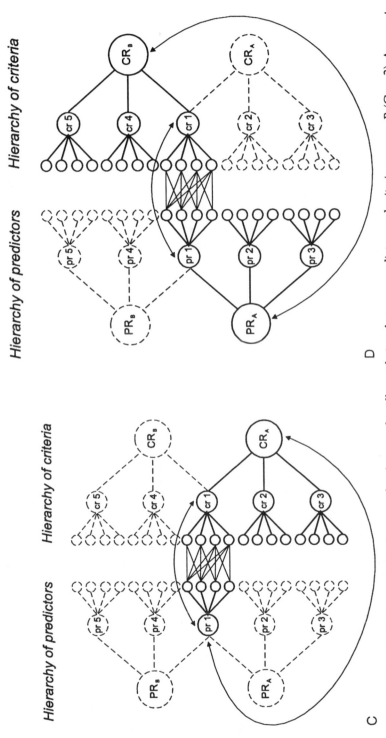

Figure 4.1. A (Case 1): Full asymmetry, the case of nothing works. A (Case 1): Full asymmetry, the case of nothing works. All correlations between predictors and criteria are zero. B (Case 2): Asymmetry that is due to a broad, higher level predictor and a narrower, lower level criterion. C (Case 3): Asymmetry that is due to a narrower, lower level predictor and a broad, higher level criterion. D (Case 4): The hybrid case of asymmetry, mismatch at the same level of generality. PR/pr = predictor; CR/cr = criterion.

III error (P. Cohen, 1982) comes into mind (i.e., measuring the wrong construct). We distinguish among four kinds of asymmetry that are shown in Figure 4.1 as Cases 1–4. Nesselroade and McArdle (1997) also have taken up these ideas in discussing mismatch in causal structural equation modeling.

Case 1 in Figure 4.1 denotes complete asymmetry, where we either measured the wrong criterion or the wrong predictor. Yet, this case suggests an important methodological principle given by Campbell and Fiske (1959) known as *convergent validation* and *discriminant validation*. What might be regarded as a complete mess here can be turned into helpful knowledge as discriminant validity. The missing link here is related to convergent validity. Cases 2 and 3 are one-sided asymmetries. In Case 2 the predictor model is far more general than the criterion model, and in Case 3 the criterion model is more general. Case 2 can be described as a prominent controversy in personality research related to the debate between Epstein and Mischel, or a similar one in attitude research (see Ajzen & Fishbein, 1980; Fishbein & Ajzen, 1975). Mischel (1968) reanalyzed studies that tried to predict behavior from broad dispositional personality constructs, resulting the overall mean correlation of .30. These coefficients challenge the utility of dispositional personality theories in predicting and explaining human behavior. However, Epstein (1979, 1980) pointed out that one of the fallacies in such an interpretation is related to the inevitable low reliability of single-act behavioral criteria in the majority of studies reviewed by Mischel and others. Aggregating repeated single acts leads to higher reliability, and aggregating repeated multiple acts leads to more general and broader nomothetic criteria. In terms of Brunswik symmetry, these broader and more reliable criteria can be better predicted from broad dispositional constructs. This does not imply that the problem of predicting single acts is solved, but it leads to a new type of criterion that we regard as more important than single-act ones.

Single acts often attract much public interest (e.g., Why do some highly intelligent people make bad mistakes?). Sternberg (e.g., 1994) often used examples of the single-act type to illustrate the limits of traditional dispositional intelligence constructs. But what about other types of criteria (e.g., What do people accomplish over at least one year aggregated over many single acts that are all functionally equivalent with respect to problem solving?). Criteria in business, such as a balance of wins and losses over a whole year, might be more appropriate for evaluating performance. Shouldn't it be interesting for psychologists to also use multiple-act criteria?

What does the concept of a disposition mean and imply? In a dictionary we found *disposition* defined as a tendency to act in a certain direction. Does this imply a certain direction in every single act according to the disposition? Clearly, no. Therefore, by conceptual analysis, we learn that dispositional constructs can be fairly validated only via repeated single acts or repeated multiple acts depending on the breadth of the disposition used. After using a multiple-act criterion of religious behaviors, Fishbein and Ajzen (1975) were able to demonstrate the predictive validity of a broad attitude scale against religion, whereas the majority of attitude researchers using only single acts did not get much higher than the infamous .30 correlation hurdle. Consequently, they proposed a principle of correspondence of attitude measures in terms of action, target, time, and context that could guide the attitude researcher in constructing either predictors or criteria at the same level of generality. In conceptualizing Brunswik symmetry, we acknowledge their influence. Principles of correspondence and Brunswik symmetry are basically the same. Yet, the lens model has the virtue of a mathematical equation derived and proposed by Tucker (1964), which explains asymmetry in the variants of the four cases shown in Figure 4.1. It describes the observed correlation of a predictor (PR) and a criterion (CR) model in analogy to Wiggins's (1973) notation as follows:

$$r_{PR,CR}^{observed} = G_{PR,CR} \cdot R_{PR} \cdot R_{CR} + C_{PR,CR} \sqrt{(1 - R_{PR}^2) \cdot (1 - R_{CR}^2)} \qquad (4.1)$$

where $G_{PR,CR}$ is the relationship between the linear model of the predictor and the linear model of the criterion; $C_{PR,CR}$ is the same for the incremental nonlinear models, respectively; and R_{PR} and R_{CR} are multiple linear correlation coefficients mapping the linear predictability of predictors and criteria, respectively, from the cues used. The parameters $(1 - R_{PR}^2)$ and $(1 - R_{CR}^2)$ map the nonlinear model confounded by error variance. The term *cue utilization* refers to the main use of the lens model in decision research, in which a decision researcher's model is compared with a true or an expert model of known ecological validity in the sense meant by Hammond (1966). Here, we use it for prediction and validation research in general. The cues in terms of structural equation modeling are the measurement (manifest) model of a latent structural model. From psychometric theory, psychologists know that observed empirical correlations are attenuated either by unreliability or restriction of range. Enhancement of range leads to overestimation if psychologists try to generalize from the sample to the population. Therefore, we incorporated psychometric theory into the lens-model equation for the linear and nonlinear part separately.

The observed correlation in Equation 4.1 is not a linear correlation but a nonlinear correlation coefficient of the eta type from analysis of variance designs (J. Cohen & Cohen, 1983; Hays, 1994). Because of the robust beauty of linear models in psychology (Dawes & Corrigan, 1974), we concentrate only on the linear part of the lens model (Equation 4.1). Equation 4.2 gives our variant of the lens model only as a linear model, in relegating possible nonlinearity to the error term *e*. Comparing that equation with those used in meta-analytic validity generalization developed by Hunter and Schmidt (1990), we will discover their basic identity. Equation 4.2 shows the many ways psychologists use sometimes dramatically attenuated correlations, whereas a powerful test of a theory should be based only on the corrected true correlations:

$$r_{PR,CR}^{observed} = S \sqrt{r_{tt}^{PR} \cdot r_{tt}^{CR}} \cdot G_{PR,CR}^{true} \cdot R_{PR} \cdot R_{CR} + e \qquad (4.2)$$

Psychometric reliabilities r_{tt}^{PR} and r_{tt}^{CR} and construct reliabilities R_{PR} and R_{CR} are always less than one. Parameter S in the case of restriction of range is also less than one; only in enhancement of range it is larger than one. The error term may be negative in some cases and positive in others. Therefore, one has six possibilities in which a true correlation is underestimated and only two in which it may be overestimated by the observed correlation. We call R_{PR} and R_{CR} the construct reliability of predictors and criteria, respectively, although most prefer to call them construct validity, as Hunter and Schmidt (1990) did. However, we insist on using the term *construct reliability* because these parameters map the degree of overlap of manifest indicators to the true wanted latent constructs. Wittmann (1988) distinguished among three types of variances: wanted, unwanted, and error variance. Wanted and unwanted systematic variance always make up psychometric theory's true variance. Unfortunately, psychometrics in emphasizing reliability is completely uninformed about theory. Profiting from the Spearman–Brown prophecy formula, we know that aggregation of parallel tests or indicators always leads to higher reliability at the composite level, whether the true scores of the parallel test are composed of wanted variance, unwanted variance, or both. Aggregation does not automatically lead to higher construct reliability, however. Only theory-derived aggregation leads to higher psychometric and construct reliability at the same time. Therefore, understanding aggregation and disaggregation is important and has been demonstrated in a multivariate reliability theory (Wittmann, 1988) that uses systematic suppressor principles and ideas proposed by Cattell and Tsujioka (1964). In our terms, construct validity is related, visible, and testable only in the amount of overlap between the wanted parts of predictor and criterion. The amount of overlap of all four variants of asymmetry determines the amount of correlation, holding all other attenuating factors constant. In Case 2 we should be precise at what level of generality our theory is directed. In removing or suppressing the unwanted variance in the predictor, we are interested in the lower level construct of the criterion. However, we could also search for the missing links in the criterion, looking for wanted variance missing in the criterion, thus demonstrating our interest in a higher level construct. If we are successful in both cases, the correlation goes up. To distinguish between both, we need a strategy we have already described as convergent and discriminant validation (Campbell & Fiske, 1959). We return to Case 1 again. We should always be precise about what construct A_{CR} is and is not, that is, non-A_{CR}, (e.g., B_{CR}). To predict and explain A_{CR}, we therefore need at the predictor side of the lens measures for both A_{PR} and non-A_{PR} (i.e., B_{PR}). If we are using the correct symmetric predictors at the same level of the constructs generality, testing our theory should lead to

$$r(A_{PR}, A_{CR}) = 1, \; r(B_{PR}, A_{CR}) = 0, \; r(A_{PR}, B_{CR}) = 0$$

and

$$r(B_{PR}, B_{CR}) = 1$$

as a strong and successful test. This is what is meant by perfect Brunswik symmetry. Unless our theory is strong and we already have a lot of additional knowledge about the hierarchical structures in pairs, we do not know what level of generality we have with that perfect pattern of convergent and discriminant validity. Contrasting Case 4 with Case 1 in Figure 4.1 illuminates that problem and suggests solutions. In Case 4 asymmetry is on both sides of the lens. Say our theory focuses now on a construct called $a1$ (cr1). At the predictor side, we have construct $A(PR_A)$ with facets a1, a2, a3 (pr1–pr3). Regarding the criterion construct a1, our predictor A_{PR} is contaminated by facets a2 and a3 (pr2 and pr3). However, the criterion a1 (cr1) we are interested in is also tied to a construct $B(CR_B)$, so pr2 and pr3 are non-a1 (pr1) and cr2 and cr3 are non-cr1. Here, non-a_{PR} is independent of non-a_{CR} (i.e., the correlation between non-a_{PR} and non-a_{CR} is zero). Therefore both the predictor and the criterion contain unwanted but psychometrically reliable variance, which are independent and unrelated to one another. To test the predictive validity of a_{PR} (pr1) relative to a_{CR} (cr1), we should remove the different unwanted parts. Set correlation with the bipartial variant for bivariate and multivariate cases does this (J. Cohen, 1982; J. Cohen & Cohen, 1983, Appendix 4). If our theory is true and perfect, the bipartial (set) correlation should be close to one after correcting for attenuation and restriction of range. In such a case, the resulting higher symmetry is related to a lower level of generality than to the one we started with constructs A and B. The virtues of hierarchical models can be used to investigate the correctness of lower level symmetries. Cases 2 and 3 denote one-sided asymmetries. Again, hierarchical models can give hints about what type of unwanted variances have to be suppressed to obtain higher symmetries. Profiting from these conceptualizations, we now can make some predictions to be tested in our research program.

We assume that intelligence is a broad disposition to solve problems. According to Brunswik symmetry, broad dispositions are only fairly validated by broad criteria. Therefore, we postulate that the predictive validity of intelligence goes up if we use several repeated criterion measures as aggregated performance in different problem-solving scenarios. We use three different computer-based complex scenarios and hypothesize that the predictive validity of our intelligence measures are highest with a performance aggregated over all three scenarios. Our first hypothesis is related to Case 2 in Figure 4.1. Our second hypothesis is concerned with path models based on g-type measures of working memory, intelligence, and knowledge compared with group factor models of these predictors. We postulate that group factor path models better predict and explain performance criteria than g-type path models. This prediction is based on independent research in which we found group factor models to be better than g-type models (Wittmann & Süß, 1996, 1997). The reason for that prediction is also derived from multivariate reliability theory (Wittmann, 1988), which distinguishes between wanted and unwanted variance. All intelligence assessments normally use time limits that introduce speed of information processing. Aggregation to g therefore leads to overrepresentation of speed as common variance to all tests. The true variance of complex problem solving may not be much related to reliable simple mental speed variance. This source actually could be totally unimportant. So the reliable simple mental speed variance can be regarded as unwanted reliable variance if we assume that thinking longer in complex problems pays off against being fast in the sense of simple mental speed (i.e., going very fast to a wrong solution). A third hypothesis deals with path models in which we capitalize on results by Hunter (1986), who found that knowledge is always the best predictor of performance and that intelligence has strong indirect effects on performance via knowledge.

The Mannheim Research Project

Many daily problems can be characterized as "complex" in various aspects, and a part of these problems can be described as interactions between a person and a dynamic system of interconnected variables. Problems of this kind can be simulated by computers, and we assume that the cognitive demands of simulated problems are comparable to realistic problems. This offers the opportunity to observe human behavior in environments under controlled laboratory conditions.

Research with computer-simulated complex problems has become an expanding field during the past 20 years. For example, the tasks of a small-town mayor (Dörner,

Kreuzig, Reither, & Stäudel, 1983), a business manager (Wolfe & Roberts, 1986), the head of a firefighting crew (Brehmer, 1986), and an air traffic controller (Ackerman, 1992) were simulated. Research topics included the prediction and explanation of individual differences, knowledge acquisition and application, effects of knowledge instruction, expert–novice comparisons, and the effects of task characteristics on task difficulty (Frensch & Funke, 1995).

The focus of the Mannheim Research Project and prior studies (Süß, 1996) is on the determinants of individual differences in complex problem performance. We investigate the meaning of and the relationship between intelligence and knowledge as determinants of performance in realistic simulations. We assume that many of the disappointing results of previous studies on this topic (Funke, 1995; Kluwe, Misiak, & Haider, 1991) were attributable to a lack of differentiation on both intelligence and knowledge as well as a lack of reliability on the criteria measures. According to Brunswik theory, there is a lack of symmetry between predictors and criteria. In many of the studies, the predictor was a highly general construct, g, and the criterion was a single-act criterion (Fishbein & Ajzen, 1975), that is, performance on a single trial of a single task with unknown reliability. In Germany, there has been heated debate about the utility of psychometric intelligence tests (e.g., Kluwe et al., 1991).

The Master Plan in a Path-Analytic Framework

Cognitive and noncognitive determinants of complex problem-solving performance are our main focus. Here, we discuss mainly cognitive aspects of individual differences, although personality, biodata, and gender were also included in our research. Testing the ecological validity of computer-based problem-solving performance related to real life was not possible.

In a path-analytic framework we assume that knowledge is the best direct predictor of performance. Knowledge is influenced by intelligence, personality, interests, and motivation; intelligence is influenced by WMC. WMC is exogenous to all other constructs used. It is one of the general features of the cognitive architecture that could function as a limiting factor for a wide range of abilities, foremost reasoning ability. Several researchers have found strong but not perfect relationships between WMC and reasoning (Fry & Hale, 1996; Kyllonen & Christal, 1990; Salthouse, 1992). In our own research there was empirical evidence for this assumption (Süß, Oberauer, Wittmann, Wilhelm, & Schulze, 1996). Complex problem solving requires simultaneous storage and processing as well as coordination of diverse information. Therefore, we expect strong relationships to such performances. An interesting question is whether reasoning or WMC is the better predictor, or whether both contribute unique variance in predicting performances. Kyllonen (1994) conceptualized a research program at the Armstrong Laboratory and developed a theoretical framework for cognitive abilities measurement (CAM), in which WMC plays a prominent role and is expected to improve on classical ability testing. The first endogenous construct influenced by WMC is intelligence. In our view, controlling complex systems make strong demands on reasoning ability, which is required to detect systematic patterns among the changing states and to develop hypotheses about the causal structure of a system. Speed of information processing or verbal fluency is not expected to be of utmost importance. Therefore, we expect reasoning to be the most important and symmetrical predictor to success given sufficient reliability of criteria (Süß, 1996; Süß, Kersting, & Oberauer, 1991). To satisfy our conceptual framework, we need an intelligence model that can be organized as a hierarchy. The Berlin intelligence structure model (BIS), developed by Jäger (1982, 1984), is such a model. In the classification of the intelligence models of Sternberg and Powell (1982), the BIS would be a third-stage model like Guttman's (1954, 1965) radex model, as a two-facet model. The BIS synthesizes assumptions of hierarchy, multimodality, and multifactorial dependencies of intelligence test performances. It also integrates creativity as part of intelligence (Guilford, 1967). There is now ample evidence of construct and criterion validity in German-speaking Europe (Jäger et al., 1997). An open question is whether WMC tasks are just another variant of intelligence tasks, for better or worse, thus questioning causal priority, and we have no good answer. However, we made that decision by sampling WMC tasks used by cognitive researchers and adapted them for measuring individual differences.

The next endogenous construct is knowledge. Specific demands in realistic complex problem solving are preknowledge structures that can be used in a domain. Simulation and reality are never exactly identical; the application of preknowledge requires considerable amounts of transfer. Intelligence is the precondition for the acquisition and application of knowledge (Cattell, 1971); such knowledge may be closely related to crystallized intelligence. Thus, knowledge structures tailored to a specific domain should be the most direct predictor. For the ultimate criterion we use performances in three different computer-based scenarios broadly sampling complex problem-solving behavior. Thus, the master plan of our Mannheim Research Project closely resembles Ackerman's (1996) process, personality, interests, and knowledge (PPIK) framework and is as ambitious as Kyllonen's (1994) CAM taxonomy.

Method

In this section we briefly describe how we assessed the different constructs. Tasks that are well-known are not described in detail; only references are given. For more extensive descriptions (see Oberauer, Süß, Schulze, Wilhelm, & Wittmann, 1996; Süß et al. 1996).

Participants.   One hundred thirty-six students from the University of Mannheim participated in this study. Their mean age was 25.9 years (*SD* = 4.76), and 37.5% were women.

Assessment of Constructs.

Complex problem solving.   Three computer-simulated scenarios were used: Tailorshop, PowerPlant, and Learn. All systems were run on a PC.

PowerPlant is a simulation of a coal-fired power plant (Wallach, 1997). PowerPlant is a system with four variables, two of which can be manipulated by the operator (coal input and valve opening), and the other two variables (energy output and steam pressure) depend on them. The goal is to continuously control the energy output of the plant according to a demand curve that changes over time. At the same time, steam pressure, a second output variable, must not surpass constant upper and lower limits. Participants completed two trials, each consisting of 50 discrete steps.

Tailorshop is a slightly modified version of a simulation originally developed by Dörner and first used by Putz-Osterloh (1981). Tailorshop simulates a shirt factory and has 24 variables. Ten variables are exogenous (e.g., which can be manipulated directly), and 14 are endogenous (e.g., which are computed by the simulation). After having planned all decisions, the operator runs the simulation for one "virtual" month. The goal is to maximize the overall gain of the factory. A complete trial consisted of 12 simulation cycles corresponding to 1 year of management. Participants completed two trials with different starting values to obtain retest reliability. Performance was measured by the total assets after 12 simulated months.

Learn was developed at the Institute of Physical and Chemical Technology at the University of Mannheim (Maier & Strohhecker, 1996; Milling, 1996a). Learn is a management simulator for innovation management and was developed by management experts (Milling, 1996b). The system has several hundred variables, and information is presented over several hierarchically organized screen displays. Participants have to manage a high-technology company in competition with three other companies simulated by the computer. The simulation runs over 60 cycles, with each cycle representing a 3-month period. Problem-solving performance was measured by a composite of two indicators corresponding to the two goals: cumulative gains and technological quality of the player's own company. Both measures, set in proportion to the corresponding mean of all four companies on the market, were averaged to give the problem solving score for Learn.

WMC.   WMC was assessed with a battery of nine computerized tasks. The tasks were selected on the basis of prior research investigating the relationship between WMC and intelligence (Oberauer et al., 1996). The nine tasks represent tests of two functions categories. The first category is simultaneous storage and processing, coordination of information, and supervision of cognitive processes (Sup). The second category is content: one verbal (V), one numerical (N), and one spatial (F) working memory task.

The simultaneous storage and processing and coordination of information tasks were as follows:

1. *Reading span (V) and computation span (N).* (Daneman & Carpenter, 1980; Turner & Engle, 1989).

2. *Short-term memory (F).* This task was constructed as a spatial equivalent to the reading span. At the beginning of each item, an instruction for a 90° rotation to the left or right is presented on the screen. Next, a series of 3 × 3 matrix patterns is presented sequentially. Participants have to mentally rotate the patterns according to the instruction and to remember the resulting pattern. After two or three successive matrix presentations, participants are asked to draw what they remember (in correct order) into empty 3 × 3 matrices.

3. *Memory updating: Short-term memory version (N).* For this task, another 3 × 3 matrix appears on the screen. Some cells are declared as "active" cells and others are shaded gray. A number appears successively in each of the active cells, and participants are asked to remember the numbers.

4. *Spatial coordination (F).* (Oberauer, 1993). For this task, the screen is divided into cells by a 10 × 10 matrix. Dots appear sequentially for 1 s in different cells.

Participants are asked to reproduce the dot pattern by placing crosses into the cells of an empty matrix on the answer sheet. Before placing crosses into the empty matrix, participants have to decide whether the pattern created by all dots is symmetrical along a vertical axis. Depending on their decision, they have to give their response in a matrix on the left or the right side of the answer sheet.

Supervision of cognitive processes was assessed as three versions of switching tasks, one numerical (Allport, Styles, & Hsieh, 1994), one figurative, and one verbal (Zimmermann & Fimm, 1993). Fast responses have to be given to successive displays on the computer screen. In the numerical version, each display contains a number of equal digits arranged at random. Participants have to alternate between reading the digits and counting the number of digits in the display. In the figural version, two geometrical figures appear in each display. One figure has sharp edges, and the other has a smooth outline. Participants have to respond "left" or "right" to indicate on which side the sharp-edged or the smooth figure appears. The figures are selected at random from a pool of nine sharp-edged and nine smooth figures, and their placements are randomly determined. In the analogous verbal version, two words belonging to two prespecified categories appear instead of the figures. The participants have to indicate the side of the screen to which the word of the first or the second category belongs. On all tasks, a one-word reminder indicating the next decision criterion was displayed on the top part of the screen.

Intelligence. A battery of tasks to map the BIS was used (Jäger et al., 1997). The two facets of the BIS model are called the *operative* mode and the *content mode*. For the operative mode, four functions are distinguished: reasoning (K), speed (B), short-term memory (M), and creativity (E). For the content mode, three categories —verbal (V), numerical (N), and figural (F)—are distinguished. Thus, a 4×3 taxonomy results in 12 cross-classified cells. Each task is assigned to a cell on the assumption that it has one operational and one content component. The tasks have been selected by extensive research sampling from the worldwide population of intelligence tasks used. The B and M cells contain three tasks, the E cells four tasks, and the K cells five tasks for each content category, resulting in a total of 45 tasks. Aggregating the tasks within cells leads to 12 cell components that are used as the lowest level in the BIS hierarchy. Taking an average of three tasks varying content categories leads to 15 parcels that, after factoring, lead to the four postulated operative factors K, B, M, and E. Averaging four tasks while varying the operative categories leads to parcels that after factoring lead to three content factors V, N, and F. Because of this parceling technique, unwanted variance associated with factors from the other facet is suppressed (Wittmann, 1988). These group factors build the next hierarchical level, but, because the same tasks are used in different ways, operative factors and content factors are not statistically independent. General intelligence is assessed by aggregating over all task scores and is at the top of the hierarchy. The postulated structure with the BIS tasks has been replicated many times by independent research.

Knowledge. General economics knowledge was assessed with a standardized questionnaire (Beck, 1993). The test consisted of 19 multiple-choice questions about economic laws and strategies such as "Which of the following strategies serves best to decrease inflation rate?"

For problem-specific knowledge, we developed tests for all three computer-simulated scenarios. The knowledge test for the Tailorshop was a modified version of a prior test by Süß et al. (1991). The specific knowledge tests for PowerPlant and for the Tailorshop have two parts, one for system-related and one for action-related knowledge. The test for Learn only has items to assess action-related knowledge.

Knowledge and experience with PCs could influence performance on the computer simulations. A questionnaire was developed to assess this experience. This questionnaire has items assessing how many years of computer experience one had and how much time one spent with working or playing on a computer during a week.

Procedure. Participants worked on Tailorshop and PowerPlant twice to increase reliability and on Learn only once because a single trial took more than 2 hr. Students answered the system-specific knowledge tests immediately after a general instruction and after a detailed introduction and guided exercise on how to use the system. In addition to the standard condition, participants had the opportunity to explore Learn for 15 min or 12 simulation cycles at maximum. Immediately after than, they attempted to control the systems.

The students took tests on 3 days, 5–6 hr each day. On the 1st day they worked on the BIS tests and the WMC battery alternating in three blocks. On the 2nd day they worked on Tailorshop, PowerPlant, and on the respective system-specific knowledge tests. On the 3rd day they worked on Learn.

Results

This conceptual framework allowed us to investigate several hypotheses related to the methodological principles derived from Brunswik symmetry in an exploratory study and in a confirmatory path-analytic study. The exploratory question was, "From what level of aggregation or generality is what level of generality to be best predicted?" Our intelligence model related to the BIS can be organized in a hierarchical framework described earlier. This hierarchical model is used as a predictor model. Looking at the criterion side we can use, at the lowest level, the performance on our three computer games, the knowledge specific to each game, general business knowledge, and computer experience and knowledge. Performance on the three games is aggregated to total computer games performance (PL3) and the specific game-related knowledge to total game knowledge (PL3know). Aggregating PL3know with general business knowledge and computer knowledge leads to total knowledge (Know-g). The highest level of generality at the criterion results after aggregation of all knowledge scores (Know-g) with all game performances (PL3) to a total performances score (Perf-g).

The reasoning for these variants of aggregation is derived from Cattell's (1971) investment theory and Ackerman's (1997) PPIK theory. The operative mode of the BIS is closer to fluid intelligence and the content mode closer to crystallized intelligence. The operative mode is also a good operationalization of what Ackerman meant by "intelligence as a process." Regressing the different levels of the criterion model onto different levels of the predictor model is a test of Cattell's investment theory and at least a partial test of the knowledge part of PPIK theory. Such a testing is completely exploratory if we are not explicit about what levels of generality are most highly related to one another. However, we can be a little more precise using the Brunswik lens-model equation and psychometric theory. The latter tells us that aggregation of at least partially parallel scales leads to higher psychometric reliability, so if we capitalize on the positive manifold hypothesis, the higher the level of generality at our predictor model, the higher the reliability of the respective score and the higher the predictive validity. The same reasoning applies to the criterion model if we make a similar assumption due to parallelism of performances. On the other hand, aggregation leads to composites of broader nomothetic span. Whether broader nomothetic span also leads to higher construct reliability is unclear because we are not sure which of the variance components are wanted or unwanted reliable variance.

Explorations will reveal what levels of generality are best related to one another. From prior exploratory research, we know that the most general level of our predictor model, namely g, is not the best predictor for school grades, knowledge, and performance (Süß, 1996; Wittmann & Matt, 1986; Wittmann & Süß, 1996, 1997). The reasoning group factor K often turned out to be a better predictor than g. Table 4.1 shows compact and condensed tests of our hypotheses.

The columns denote the different levels of generality of the predictor model, with the lower ones at the left and the higher ones at the right. The three right-most columns give the results of a commonality analysis (Cooley & Lohnes, 1976). The rows of Table 4.1 from up to down indicate lower-to-higher criteria levels.

The first three rows contain the three different performance scores on the computer-based scenarios. Rows 4–6 show the respective game-specific knowledge scores, Row 7 the general business knowledge, Row 8 the computer knowledge, Row 9 the performance aggregate over the three scenarios (PL3), Row 10 the knowledge aggregated over scenario-specific knowledge (PL3-Know), and Row 11 the total knowledge, aggregating over Rows 7, 8, and 10 as Know-g. The last row depicts the assumed result of total investments as general performance through aggregating over Rows 9 and 11. Each row contains two lines of squared multiple correlation coefficients, the first line the unadjusted and the second line the adjusted coefficients (i.e., adjusted for different numbers of predictors). The highest validity coefficients squared within each row are in boldface to facilitate interpretation. Thus, we find the majority of boldface numbers in the cell column. For the majority of our criteria used, the best prediction was related to the 12 cell scores, even making adjustments. We also found that criteria at higher levels of aggregation were better predicted from intelligence than lower level criteria. Perf-g was best predicted from all variants of intelligence, thus bolstering Cattell's (1971) investment theory as well as the knowledge part of Ackerman's (1997) PPIK theory. The adjusted 37.7% of variance explained with the 12 cell scores, compared with the 23.3% from the g level, is a late tribute to Guilford's (1967) structure-of-intellect model. Guilford brought nomothetic span to intelligence research, and psychologists should never forget to give him credit for that. Although his early claims of 120 different intelligence factors were somewhat overdrawn and resulted in strong criticism from his peers, it obviously pays off to differentiate the intelligence construct as subfacets, or at least group factors in a Thurstonian sense. If we compare the g-level column with all other levels of generality, we can state that it is never the best level to maximize prediction of knowledge and performance. This bolsters one of our central hypotheses derived from our earlier research published in German publications. The last three

TABLE 4.1 Brunswik-Symmetry Between Knowledge, Performance, and Intelligence

Variable	$R^2_{12cells}$	R^2_F	R^2_{OP}	R^2_{CON}	r^2_g	$CO_{OP,CON}$	U_{OP}	U_{CON}
1. PowerPlant	.286	.267	.203	.186	.150	.122	.081	.064
	.216	.227	.179	.167	.143	.199	.060	>.048
2. Tailorshop	.184	.186	.153	.126	.106	.093	.060	.033
	.104	.141	.127	.106	.100	.092	.035	>.014
3. Learn	.277	.169	.155	.121	.100	.107	.048	.014
	.207	.124	.129	.101	.093	.106	.023	>.005
4. PowerPlant knowledge	.265	.263	.210	.159	.144	.106	.104	.053
	.194	.223	.186	.140	.138	.103	.083	>.037
5. Tailorshop knowledge	.386	.272	.231	.185	.168	.144	.087	.041
	.326	.232	.208	.167	.162	.143	.065	>.024
6. Learn knowledge	.157	.093	.087	.024	.015	.018	.069	.006
	.075	.043	.060	.002	.008	.019	.041	>-.017
7. Business knowledge	.306	.280	.224	.159	.097	.103	.121	.056
	.239	.241	.201	.140	.090	.100	.101	>0.40
8. Computer knowledge	.215	.136	.053	.082	.025	-.001	.054	.083
	.138	.089	.024	.061	.018	-.004	.028	<-.065
9. PL3 knowledge	.392	.294	.269	.181	.172	.156	.113	.025
Σ of 4–6	.333	.255	.247	.162	.165	.154	.093	>-.008
10. PL3	.384	.337	.311	.244	.222	.218	.093	.026
Σ of 1–3	.324	.301	.290	.227	.216	.216	.074	>.011
11. Know-g	.373	.305	.285	.184	.165	.164	.121	.020
Σ of 7–9	.312	.267	.263	.165	.159	.161	.102	>-.004
12. Performance	.432	.376	.348	.263	.238	.235	.113	.028
g, Σ 10 and 11	.377	.342	.328	.246	.233	.232	.096	>.014

Note. Numbers in boldfaced type are the highest validity coefficients squared. $n = 136$.

columns in Table 4.1 show the results of a commonality analysis. The four operative factors are orthogonal in pairs, as are the three content factors. However, the operative and the content factors are correlated in pairs because of the special construction principles behind the BIS. Therefore, we can ask what the unique contribution of content factors is, given the operative factors and vice versa. U(op) and U(con) denote that incremental unique variance and CO(op, con) the commonality of both facets. All three add up to total variance explained by all seven group factors.

Comparing the commonality column with the g-level column, we find both highly similar in terms of variance explained. For all criteria substantial unique variance is added, profiting from the group factor level of generality. For the majority of criteria, the operative factors add the greater amount of unique variance; an exception is computer knowledge. Adding up both unique variance parts gives an increase in predictive validity using the seven group factors over g. If we accept the content validity of our criteria for real-life performance relevant to personnel selection research and apply Hunter and Schmidt's (1982) framework of cost–benefit analysis, we find that we will fool ourselves in using only g-type intelligence predictors in terms of opportunity costs. Admittedly, our results are in stark contrast to results from the Anglo American literature, especially concerning the ubiquity of g in personnel selection meta-analysis, but we discuss possible differences and explanations later.

In the next section we demonstrate benefits from hierarchical models using orthogonalized group factors not only to improve prediction but also understanding and explanation. For this purpose, we use the relationship between WMC and intelligence. Kyllonen and Christal (1990) pointed to the close similarity of both sets of constructs. Working memory resources are thought to be essential in explaining individual differences in higher cognitive functions traditionally mapped with psychometric intelligence. Baddeley's (1986) model distinguishing a central executive and two slave systems know as a "phonological loop," storing and processing verbal and numerical content and a visuospatial sketchpad doing the same with figural content, is one of the most prominent models in experimental research. Cognitive researchers have devised variants of working memory tasks to operationalize these different functions. The nine tasks we used for working memory described earlier were factored into three orthogonal components: One factor, labeled WMC-SPAT, loaded tasks with spatial content; the second factor, WMC-NV, encompassed tasks with verbal and numerical content; and the third factor, WMC-SUP, aggregated mainly the switching tasks that mapped processing speed. The general working memory factor WMC-g was an aggregate over all nine tasks. Higher scores indicated better working memory.

Table 4.2's columns are organized similarly to those in Table 4.1. No assumptions about causal priority are made here. The rows start with the general working memory factor followed by the three orthogonal factors. The last three rows test a special hypothesis related to Brunswik symmetry in Figure 4.1, Case 2. Focusing, for example, on WMC-SPAT as a criterion to be predicted from psychometric intelligence, we know that WMC-NV and WMC-SUP are not WMC-SPAT because they are orthogonalized components. Therefore, in explaining WMC-SPAT via intelligence, we should remove all variance in intelligence that may be related to these non-WMC-SPAT components. We call this principle "theory-derived suppression." Applying it, we assume that intelligence in its variants of different levels of generality

93

TABLE 4.2   Brunswik Symmetry Between Working Memory and Intelligence

Variable	$R^2_{12cells}$	R^2_F	R^2_{OP}	R^2_{CON}	r^2_g	$CO_{OP,CON}$	U_{OP}	U_{CON}
1. WMC-g	.680	.667	.613	.571	.538	.517	.096	.054
	.649	.649	.601	.561	.535	.513	.088	>.048
2. WMC-SPAT	.485	.390	.232	.294	.182	.136	.096	.158
	.435	.356	.209	.278	.176	.131	.078	<.147
3. WMC-NV	.408	.341	.311	.290	.229	.260	.051	.030
	.350	.305	.290	.274	.223	.259	.031	>.015
4. WMC-SUP	.294	.239	.236	.146	.135	.143	.093	.003
	.224	.197	.212	.126	.128	.141	.071	>-.015
5. WMC-SPAT with suppressors	.564	.506	.371	.378	.286	.243	.128	.135
	.513	.470	.342	.354	.270	.226	.116	>.128
6. WMC-NV with suppressors	.496	.470	.448	.372	.335	.350	.098	.022
	.437	.432	.422	.348	.320	.338	.084	>.010
7. WMC-SUP with suppressors	.357	.318	.305	.240	.229	.227	.078	.013
	.282	.269	.272	.210	.211	.213	.059	>-.003

Note.   Numbers in boldfaced type are the highest validity coefficients squared. $n = 135$. WMC-g = General factor of all working memory tasks; WMC-SPAT = Spatial working memory factor; WMC-NV = Verbal–Numerical working memory factor; WMC-SUP = Processing Speed working memory factor.

contains reliable systematic unwanted variance regarding the WMC-SPAT factor, namely WMC-NV- and WMC-SUP-related variance. If our assumption is true, both unwanted components, although not correlated with WMC-SPAT, should nevertheless get significant beta weights in combination with intelligence, indicating the suppression of irrelevant variance and thus leading to higher Brunswik symmetry and a substantial improvement in predictive validity. We can apply this reasoning only to the level below WMC-g simply because, at the highest level, we have no measures for non-WMC-g. Testing this suppression hypothesis, we compare rows 2–4 with rows 5–7 and find substantive improvements in predictive validity. Boldface numbers again indicate the highest validities within a row. For WMC-SPAT, the adjusted R^2 using the cell level improves from 43.5% to 51.3%, an increase of 7.8%. We also repeat the observation that, even with adjustments, the cell level leads to the best validities for most criteria. The commonality analysis in the last three columns again shows that commonality is highly similar in its results to the g-level column. Therefore, working memory is a little bit more and different from g, in effect somewhat contextualizing the conclusions of Kyllonen and Christal (1990). Nevertheless, the prediction of WMC-g from g is impressive given the 53.5% of variance explained. Except for WMC-SPAT, unique variance from the operative factors was higher than from content. Intelligence as a process in Ackerman's (1996) sense is more important with working memory. We also note that, after removing the non-WMC-SPAT variance from the group factors, the unique variances in predicting WMC-SPAT were equivalent; taken together, however, 20% more variance was explained with the group-factor level than with the g-factor level. In comprehending what components at what level of generality have the highest beta weights, we still strive for better explanations.

Using stepwise regression with WMC-SPAT on the seven BIS group factors, K received the highest weight (.463), followed by the figural content factor F (.263) and the operative creativity factor E (.160). The verbal content factor V had a negative weight (−.263), meaning that those who scored high on V scored lower on WMC-SPAT. Once we suppressed the non-WMC-SPAT variance from the seven BIS group factors, K (.434), F (.464), and N (.334) remained as the only significant ones; the suppressors WMC-NV (−.399) and WMC-SUP (−.253) had negative beta weights. Accepting WMC-SPAT as a good assessment of Baddeley's (1986) visuospatial sketchpad in an individual-differences framework, we would be pleased to see how closely related it is to reasoning with figures (K and F), but why the significant number factor N? Does this mean that some people visualize numbers, or can numbers also be processed without visualization in the visuospatial sketchpad? This is an interesting challenge for cognitive researchers. Why not ask participants what they do and prefer, or devise experiments manipulating this? Going to the cell level provides additional hints. We find the cell score KF (.663), BN (simple speed with numbers [.286]) with positive weights, and simple speed with verbal content BV (−.255) with a negative one. Applying suppressor principles sustains these explanations, denoting that reasoning with figures KF (.709) and numerical speed BN (.286) are still more important after removing unwanted variance and verbal speed BV (−.255) holds its significant negative weight. The suppressors WMC-NV (−.278) and WMC-SUP (−.186) also have a negative weight, meaning that at a given level of intelligence, those scoring high on both have lower spatial working memory resources. For the phonological loop and the working memory speed factor, we found conceptually similar results demonstrating that for WMC-NV reasoning with numbers and verbal content (i.e., KN and KV got the highest weights). For the supervision and switching factor WMC-SUP, the highest weights resulted for KN, BF, and BV.

Thus far, exploratory analysis with some emphasis on theory-derived confirmation has been the main focus of our analysis. Going further in the direction of confirmatory analysis, we tested the path-analytical framework suggested by our master plan. The first path model tested used the general factors in all constructs.

Figure 4.2A demonstrates that Know-g had the strongest effect on aggregated performance (PL3). WMC-g had a significant direct effect and substantial indirect effects on BIS-g and Know-g. General intelligence had only an indirect effect via knowledge but no direct effect. Such a result replicates findings by Hunter (1986). Going to the group-factor level (see Figure 4.2B), we did not get higher predictive validity but did see better explanations while disentangling the internal structure of the relationship within our predictors and criteria used. Know-g, WMC-SPAT, and K had direct effects on the performance aggregate PL3. Know-g received direct effects only from K and WMC-SPAT. Reasoning and spatial working memory improved knowledge, in which K had a strong effect, which also led to a strong indirect effect on performance. K, on the other hand, received significant paths from all three working memory factors, with WMC-NV and WMC-SPAT having the largest ones. The four operative BIS factors had been computed as orthogonal, but, for the non-K factors B, E, and M, the Lagrange multiplier module of structural equation modeling nevertheless (Bentler, 1995) suggested missing paths that again could be interpreted as suppressor effects. In the context of predicting and explaining knowledge and performance, variance related to non-K factors had to be removed from reasoning to get a better fit to the empirical data, thus confirming our exploratory results. Comparing prediction and explanation, at least general knowledge is better predicted from the group-factor level (32.76% vs. 20.79%; Figure 4.2A vs. Figure 4.2B).

General Discussion and Summary

The philosopher of science Ian Hacking (1983) distinguished two principal modes of inquiry: representing and intervening. The preferred mode of individual-differences research is representing. Hypothetical constructs are mapped, assessed, and related to one another, normally without experimental interventions. These two modes also distinguish Cronbach's (1957, 1975) two disciplines. Discussions about virtues and drawbacks of both go back to Brunswik (1952) and his conceptual framework. Brunswik favored the representative design over the systematic (intervening) of R. A. Fisher and either got heavy fire from experimental psychologists or was ignored by mainstream psychologists in his time. Hammond (1966) is an excellent guide to Brunswikian concepts and has expanded on them impressively (e.g., Hammond, 1996). The strengths of individual-differences research has always been in prediction; the weaknesses are assumed in explanations. The construct of intelligence, the outstanding monument of success in individual-differences research, has become a crucible for representing and intervening. Cognitive researchers have partitioned psychometric tasks into components and tried to explain the processes behind them. Differential researchers welcomed the promises of better explaining their construct via working memory resources.

Baddeley's (1986) working memory model has the potential to be a crucible. Differential psychologists prefer a causal priority of predictability. Only after successful prediction is explanation worthwhile. However, they do not want to get trapped by the old adage directed to psychometric intelligence research, namely being able to measure a construct but not knowing what it is. Looking around for the secrets of successes in prediction and explanation of our peers in science, we found that the principles of symmetry are the golden key. Applying them to hierarchical models of our predictors, we easily found their potential with explaining hierarchical criterion models using the framework of Brunswik's lens model and named that approach *Brunswik symmetry*. The gestalt principles of the Brunswikian framework forced us to acknowledge the paucity of criterion models we too often use for validating our constructs. Global supervisor ratings used to validate selection instruments may be such an example of paucity. What sample of behavior do supervisors draw? How do they aggregate their overall judgments? Does this lead to biases in favor of general intelligence in terms of predictive validity?

To circumvent that problem, we chose to concentrate on broader samples of complex problem-solving behavior. Successes and failures in managing a power plant, a tailorshop, and a high-technology company, even as computer-based games, assessing at the same time task-specific knowledge and general business knowledge as well as experience with computers, is, at least in our eyes, a strategy that can bring breadth and nomothetic span to a criterion model that is possibly more content valid than supervisor ratings. At least it is a better test bed to falsify what intelligence as a dispositional construct claims to be, namely a tendency to behave in a smarter direction. Neglecting British understatement for a moment, we are impressed by our empirical results!

Brunswik symmetry paid off in an unexpected harvest of predictions and explanations, but we know that our peers will ask what the BIS model is and whether these factors are similar to what is known from Carroll's (1993) impressive metaresearch. Is the Berlin *g* somewhat biased compared with traditional *g*, so that the group factors and the cell scores are at an advantage? So far, we can say only that all single tasks used in the BIS correlated positively but to different degrees, thus giving group factors a chance. The nomothetic span of the BIS is broad and is closely related to Guilford's (1967) structure-of-intellect model. To counterattack the *g* problem, Raven's Progressive Matrices often used as a proxy for *g* is classified and empirically proved to map only KF in the BIS, thus missing the other important components. Factoring the working memory tasks, we found components that suggested from their loading pattern a close resemblance to what Baddeley (1986) found in experimental research. Yet, readers may have noted our hesitation in drawing conclusions about strict identity. It is not known whether constructs derived from experimental research that mainly concentrates on mean differences will show up in the same way in correlational research that deliberately removes the means in relating constructs. We are aware of possible cross-level fallacies. Yet, finding a spatial working memory factor and not being able to separate a numerical from a verbal one, it is tempting to draw parallels between the two disciplines.

From the relationships of our spatial and phonological working memory factors to psychometric intelligence, however, we see that both cannot be understood as

98

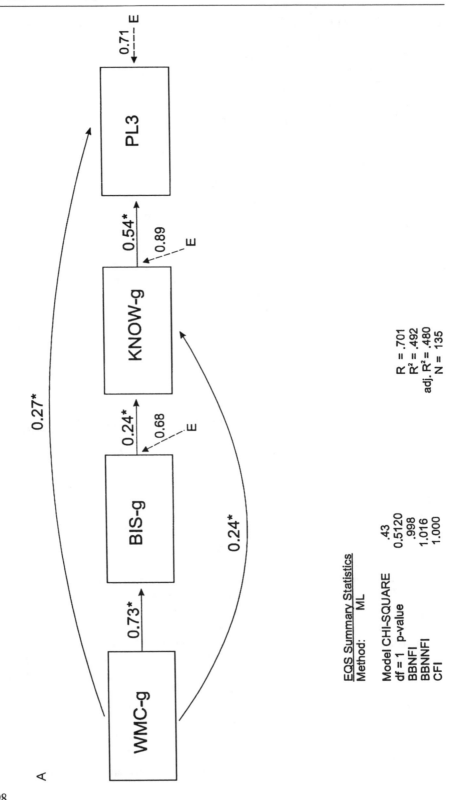

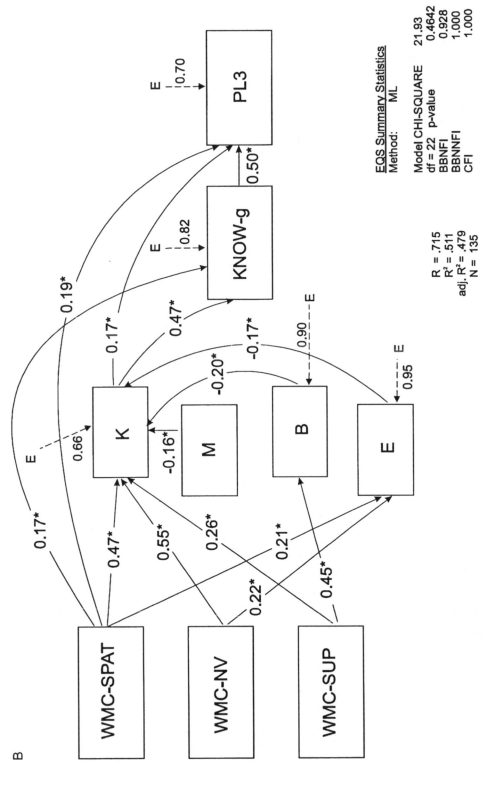

Figure 4.2. A: Prediction and explanation of performance from the *g* level. B: Prediction and explanation of performance from the group-factor level. WMC-*g* = General factor of all working memory tasks; BIS = Berlin intelligence structure; KNOW-*g* = total knowledge; PL3 = total computer games performance; WMC-SPAT = Spatial working memory factor; WMC-NV = Verbal-Numerical working memory factor; WMC-SUP = Processing Speed working memory factor; K = reasoning; M = short-term memory; B = speed; E = creativity.

slave systems that emphasize only passive storage of the respective content information. Both correlated highly with our reasoning factor K, which, in traditional differential parlance, is named as processing capacity of complex information derived from a content analysis of the intelligence tasks that are its markers. Therefore, it seems to us that what Baddeley (1986) conceptualized as a central executive is also incorporated into these factors. We would be eager to learn with functional magnetic resonance imaging studies what happens in the brain while solving our K markers and those of our working memory factors (see Posner & Raichle, 1997, for an overview of brain-imaging techniques and Gazzaniga, 1997, for overviews of application areas).

We could not fully present all our empirical results given the limits of a chapter. This applies especially to a more comprehensive test of Ackerman's (1996) PPIK theory framework. We can say, however, that we also found personality factors having independent paths related to our knowledge aggregate but not to the performance aggregate. The biodata also could be incorporated in a consistent way, and we found substantial gender differences in the performance, knowledge, and computer experience in favor of men but few in working memory and intelligence, which suggests different learning opportunities, interests, attitudes, motivations, self-concepts, and speculations about differential investment strategies of intelligence and time in the areas we chose as a criterion model.

Our overall results clearly underscore the importance of intelligence as a dispositional construct, which especially shows up after aggregation of criterion information. We believe that multiple-act criteria are more important to society than single-act ones and that the impact of intelligence is severely underestimated. This applies foremost to education. We hope that knowledge acquisition with due consideration of the limits set by intelligence, WMC, and all other trait complexes in PPIK will lead to better interventions and a bright future for learning and individual-differences research. We are also impressed by finding principles of symmetry to be an eternal golden braid (Hofstadter, 1979), even in psychology, and feel happy and comfortable back home in science.

REFERENCES

Ackerman, P. L. (1992). Predicting individual differences in complex skill acquisition: Dynamics of ability determinants. *Journal of Applied Psychology, 77*, 598–614.

Ackerman, P. L. (1996). A theory of adult intellectual development: Process, personality, interests, and knowledge. *Intelligence, 22*, 227–257.

Ackerman, P. L. (1997). Personality, self-concept, interests, and intelligence: Which construct doesn't fit? *Journal of Personality, 65*, 171–204.

Ackerman, P. L., & Heggestad, E. D. (1996). Intelligence, personality, and interest: Evidence for overlapping traits. *Psychological Bulletin, 121*, 219–245.

Ajzen, I., & Fishbein, M. (1980). *Understanding attitudes and predicting social behavior.* Englewood Cliffs, NJ: Prentice Hall.

Alderton, D. L., & Larson, G. E. (1994). Dimensions of ability: Diminishing returns? In M. G. Rumsey, C. B. Walker, & J. H. Harris (Eds.), *Personnel selection and classification* (pp. 137–144). Hillsdale, NJ: Erlbaum.

Alker, H. R. (1969). A typology of ecological fallacies. In M. Dogan & S. Rokkan (Eds.), *Quantitative ecological analysis in the social sciences.* Cambridge, MA: MIT Press.

Allport, A., Styles, E. A., & Hsieh, S. (1994). Shifting intentional set: Exploring the dynamic control task. In C. Umiltá & M. Moscovitch (Eds.), *Attention and performance XV* (pp. 421–452). Cambridge, MA: MIT Press.

Baddeley, A. D. (1986). *Working memory.* Oxford, England: Clarendon Press.

Beck, K. (1993). Dimensionen der ökonomischen Bildung: Meßinstrumente und Befunde. *DFG-Projekt: Wirtschaftskundlicher Bildungs-Test (WBT)* [Dimensions of economics education assessment: Instruments and results. Research report for the German research foundation]. Mainz, Germany: University of Mainz.

Bentler, P. M. (1995). *EQS structural equations program manual.* Encino, CA: Multivariate Software.

Brehmer, B. (1986). In one word: Not from experience. In H. R. Arkes & K. R. Hammond (Eds.), *Judgment and decision making* (pp. 705–720). Cambridge, England: Cambridge University Press.

Brunswik, E. (1952). The conceptual framework of psychology. In *International Encyclopedia of Unified Science* (Vol. 1, No. 10). Chicago: University of Chicago Press.

Brunswik, E. (1955). Representative design and probabilistic theory in functional psychology. *Psychological Review, 62,* 236–242.

Brunswik, E. (1956). *Perception and the representative design of psychological experiments.* Berkeley: University of California Press.

Campbell, D. T., & Fiske, D. W. (1959). Convergent and discriminant validation by the multitrait–multimethod matrix. *Psychological Bulletin, 56,* 81–105.

Carroll, J. B. (1993). *Human cognitive abilities: A survey of factor-analytic studies.* Cambridge, England: Cambridge University Press.

Cattell, R. B. (1971). *Abilities: Their structure, growth, and action.* Boston: Houghton Mifflin.

Cattell, R. B., & Tsujioka, B. (1964). The importance of factortrueness and validity, versus homogeneity and orthogonality in test scales. *Educational and Psychological Measurement, 24,* 3–30.

Cohen, J. (1982). Set correlation as a general multivariate data analytic method. *Multivariate Behavioral Research, 17,* 301–341.

Cohen, J., & Cohen, P. (1983). *Applied multiple regression/correlation analysis for the behavioral sciences* (2nd ed.). Hillsdale, NJ: Erlbaum.

Cohen, P. (1982). To be or not to be: Control and balancing of type I and type II errors. *Evaluation and Program Planning, 5,* 247–254.

Cooley, W. W., & Lohnes, P. R. (1976). *Evaluation research in education.* New York: Irvington.

Cronbach, L. J. (1957). The two disciplines of scientific psychology. *American Psychologist, 12,* 671–684.

Cronbach, L. J. (1975). Beyond the two disciplines of scientific psychology. *American Psychologist, 30,* 116–127.

Daneman, M., & Carpenter, P. A. (1980). Individual differences in working memory and reading. *Journal of Verbal Learning and Verbal Behavior, 19,* 450–466.

Dawes, R. M., & Corrigan, B. (1974). Linear models in decision making. *Psychological Bulletin, 81,* 95–106.

Dörner, D., Kreuzig, H. W., Reither, F., & Stäudel, T. (1983). *Lohhausen: Vom Umgang mit Unbestimmtheit und Komplexität* [Lohhausen: On dealing with uncertainty and complexity]. Bern, Switzerland: Huber.

Epstein, S. (1979). The stability of behavior: I. On predicting most of the people much of the time. *Journal of Personality and Social Psychology, 37,* 1097–1126.

Epstein, S. (1980). The stability of behavior: II. Implications for psychological research. *American Psychologist, 35,* 790–806.

Fishbein, M., & Ajzen, I. (1975). *Belief, attitude, intention, and behavior: An introduction to theory and research.* Reading, MA: Addison-Wesley.

Frensch, P., & Funke, J. (1995). *Complex problem solving: The European perspective.* Hillsdale, NJ: Erlbaum.

Fry, A. F., & Hale, S. (Eds.). (1996). Processing speed, working memory, and fluid intelligence. *Psychological Science, 7,* 237–241.

Funke, U. (1995). Using complex problem solving tasks in personal selection and training. In P. A. Frensch & J. Funke (Eds.), *Complex problem solving* (pp. 219–240). Hillsdale, NJ: Erlbaum.

Gazzaniga, M. S. (Ed.). (1997). *The cognitive neurosciences.* Cambridge, MA: MIT Press.

Gottfredson, L. S. (Ed.). (1997). Intelligence and social policy [Special issue]. *Intelligence, 24*(1).

Guilford, J. P. (1967). *The nature of human intelligence.* New York: McGraw-Hill.

Guttman, L. A. (1954). A new approach to factor analysis: The radex. In P. F. Lazarsfeld (Ed.), *Mathematical thinking in the social sciences* (pp. 258–348). Glencoe, IL: Free Press.

Guttman, L. A. (1965). A faceted definition of intelligence. In R. Eiferman (Ed.), *Studies in psychology: Scripta Hierosolymitana* (Vol. 14, pp. 166–181). Jerusalem, Israel: Magnes Press.

Hacking, I. (1983). *Representing and intervening: Introductory topics in the philosophy of natural science.* Cambridge, England: Cambridge University Press.

Hammond, K. R. (1966). *The psychology of Egon Brunswik.* New York: Holt, Rinehart & Winston.

Hammond, K. R. (1996). *Human judgment and social policy.* New York: Oxford University Press.

Harnqvist, K., Gustafsson, J.-E., Muthén, B., & Nelson, G. (1994). Hierarchical models of ability at class and individual levels. *Intelligence, 18,* 165–187.

Hays, W. L. (1994). *Statistics* (5th ed.). Orlando, FL: Harcourt Brace Jovanovich.

Herrnstein, R. J., & Murray, C. (1994). *The bell curve: Intelligence and class structure in American life.* New York: Free Press.

Hofstadter, D. R. (1979). *Gödel, Escher, Bach: An eternal golden braid.* New York: Basic Books.

Hunter, J. E. (1986). Cognitive ability, cognitive aptitudes, job knowledge, and job performance. *Journal of Vocational Behavior, 29,* 340–362.

Hunter, J. E., & Hunter, R. F. (1984). Validity and utility of alternate predictors of job performance. *Psychological Bulletin, 96,* 72–98.

Hunter, J. E., & Schmidt, F. L. (1982). Fitting people to jobs: Implications of personnel selection for national productivity. In E. A. Fleishman & M. D. Dunnete (Eds.), *Human performance and productivity: Vol. 1. Human capability assessment* (pp. 233–284). Hillsdale, NJ: Erlbaum.

Hunter, J. E., & Schmidt, F. L. (1990). *Methods of meta-analysis: Correcting error and bias in research findings.* Newbury Park, CA: Sage.

Jäger, A. O. (1982). Mehrmodale Klassifikation von Intelligenzleistungen: Experimentell kontrollierte Weiterentwicklung eines deskriptiven Intelligenzstrukturmodells [Multimodal classification of intelligence performance]. *Diagnostica, 28,* 195–226.

Jäger, A. O. (1984). Intelligenzstrukturforschung: Konkurrierende Modelle, neue Entwicklungen, Perspektiven [Research on the structure of intelligence: Competitive models, new developments, perspectives]. *Psychologische Rundschau, 35,* 21–35.

Jäger, A. O., Süß, H.-M., & Beauducel, A. (1997). *Berliner Intelligenzstruktur-Test: BIS-Test, Form 4.* [Test for the Berlin model of intelligence structure]. Göttingen, Germany: Hogrefe.

Kluwe, R. H., Misiak, C., & Haider, H. (1991). The control of complex systems and performance in intelligence tests. In H. Rowe (Ed.), *Intelligence: Reconceptualization and measurement* (pp. 227–244). Hillsdale, NJ: Erlbaum.

Kyllonen, P. C. (1994). CAM: A theoretical framework for cognitive abilities measurement. In D. K. Detterman (Ed.), *Current topics in human intelligence* (Vol. 4, pp. 307–359). Norwood, NJ: Ablex.

Kyllonen, P. C., & Christal, R. E. (1990). Reasoning ability is (little more than) working-memory capacity?! *Intelligence, 14,* 389–433.

Maier, F., & Strohhecker, J. (1996). Do management flight simulators really enhance decision effectiveness? In G. P. Richardson & J. D. Sterman (Eds.), *System dynamics '96: Proceedings of the 1996 International System Dynamics Conference* (Vol. 2, pp. 341–344). Cambridge, MA: MIT Press.

Milling, P. (1996a). Modeling innovation processes for decision support and management simulation. *System Dynamics Review, 12,* 211–234.

Milling, P. (1996b). A management simulator to support group decision making in a corporate gaming environment. In G. P. Richardson & J. D. Sterman (Eds.), *System dynamics '96: Proceedings of the 1996 International System Dynamics Conference* (Vol. 2, pp. 369–372). Cambridge, MA: MIT Press.

Mischel, W. (1968). *Personality and assessment.* New York: Wiley.

Nesselroade, J. R., & McArdle, J. J. (1997). On the mismatching of levels of abstraction in mathematical-statistical model fitting. In H. W. Reese & M. D. Franzen (Eds.), *Life-span developmental psychology: Biological and neuropsychological mechanisms* (pp. 23–49). Hillsdale, NJ: Erlbaum.

Oberauer, K. (1993). Die Koordination kognitiver Operationen: Eine Studie zum Zusammenhang von "working memory" und Intelligenz [The coordination of cognitive operations: A study on the relationship between working memory and intelligence]. *Zeitschrift für Psychologie, 201,* 57–84.

Oberauer, K., Süß, H.-M., Schulze, R., Wilhelm, O., & Wittmann, W. W. (1996). *Working memory capacity: Facets of a cognitive ability construct* (Research Rep. No. 7). University of Mannheim, Mannheim, Germany.

Posner, M. I., & Raichle, M. E. (1997). *Images of mind.* New York: Scientific American Library.

Putz-Osterloh, W. (1981). Über die Beziehung zwischen Testintelligenz und Problemlöseerfolg [On the relationship between test intelligence and success in problem solving]. *Zeitschrift für Psychologie, 189,* 79–100.

Ree, M. J., & Earles, J. A. (1994). The ubiquitous predictiveness of g. In M. G. Rumsey, C. B. Walker, & J. H. Harris (Eds.), *Personnel selection and classification* (pp. 127–135). Hillsdale, NJ: Erlbaum.

Robinson, W. S. (1950). Ecological correlations and behavior of individuals. *American Sociological Review, 15,* 351–357.

Rumsey, M. G., Walker, C. B., & Harris, J. H. (Eds.). (1994). *Personnel selection and classification.* Hillsdale, NJ: Erlbaum.

Salthouse, T. A. (1992). Working-memory mediation of adult age differences in integrative reasoning. *Memory and Cognition, 20,* 413–423.

Schmidt, F. L. (1994). The future of personnel selection in the U.S. Army. In M. G. Rumsey, C. B. Walker, & J. H. Harris (Eds.), *Personnel selection and classification* (pp. 333–350). Hillsdale, NJ: Erlbaum.

Schmidt, F. L., Ones, D. S., & Hunter, J. E. (1992). Personnel selection. *Annual Review of Psychology, 43,* 627–670.

Sternberg, R. (1994). The PRSVL model of person-context interaction in the study of human potential. In M. G. Rumsey, C. B. Walker, & J. H. Harris (Eds.), *Personnel selection and classification* (pp. 317–332). Hillsdale, NJ: Erlbaum.

Sternberg, R. J., & Powell, J. S. (1982). Theories of intelligence. In R. J. Sternberg (Ed.), *Handbook of human intelligence* (pp. 975–1005). Cambridge, England: Cambridge University Press.

Süß, H.-M. (1996). *Intelligenz, Wissen und Problemlösen: Kognitive Voraussetzungen für erfolgreiches Handeln bei computersimulierten Problemen* [Intelligence, knowledge, and problem solving: Cognitive prerequisites for successful performance on computer simulated problems]. Göttingen, Germany: Hogrefe.

Süß, H.-M., Kersting, M., & Oberauer, K. (1991). Intelligenz und Wissen als Prädiktoren für Leistungen bei computersimulierten komplexen Problemen [Intelligence and knowledge as predictors of performance in solving complex computer-simulated problems]. *Diagnostica, 37,* 334–352.

Süß, H.-M., Oberauer, K., Wittmann, W. W., Wilhelm, O., & Schulze, R. (1996). Working memory capacity and intelligence: An integrative approach based on Brunswik symmetry (Research Rep. No. 8). University of Mannheim, Mannheim, Germany.

Thorndike, E. L. (1939). On the fallacy of imputing the correlations found for groups to the individuals composing them. *American Journal of Psychology, 52,* 122–124.

Thorndike, E. L. (1940). *Human nature and the social science order.* New York: MacMillan.

Tucker, L. A. (1964). A suggested alternative formulation in the developments by Hursch, Hammond and Hursch, and by Hammond, Hursch and Todd. *Psychological Review, 71,* 528–530.

Turner, M. L., & Engle, R. W. (1989). Is working memory capacity task dependent? *Journal of Memory and Language, 28,* 127–154.

Wallach, D. (1997). Learning to control a coal-fired power plant: Empirical results and a model. In D. Harris (Ed.), *Engineering psychology and cognitive ergonomics* (Vol. 2, pp. 19–23). Hampshire, England: Ashgate.

Wiggins, J. S. (1973). *Personality and prediction: Principles of personality assessment.* Menlo Park, CA: Addison-Wesley.

Wittmann, W. W. (1987). Grundlagen erfolgreicher Forschung in der Psychologie [Foundations of successful research in psychology: Multimodal assessment, multiplism, multivariate reliability and validity theory]. *Diagnostica, 33,* 209–226.

Wittmann, W. W. (1988). Multivariate reliability theory: Principles of symmetry and successful validation strategies. In J. R. Nesselroade & R. B. Cattell (Eds.), *Handbook of multivariate experimental psychology* (2nd ed., pp. 505–560). New York: Plenum.

Wittmann, W. W., & Matt, G. E. (1986). Aggregation und Symmetrie: Grundlagen einer multivariaten Reliabilitäts- und Validitätstheorie, dargestellt am Beispiel der differentiellen Validität des Berliner Intelligenzstrukturmodells [Aggregation and symmetry: Foundations of a multivariate theory of reliability and validity, exemplified with the concept of differential validity of the Berlin structure of intelligence model]. *Diagnostica, 32,* 309–329.

Wittmann, W. W., & Süß, H.-M. (1996). Vorhersage und Erklärung von Schulnoten durch das Berliner Intelligenzstrukturmodell [Prediction and explanation of school grades through the Berlin structure of intelligence model]. In B. J. Ertelt & M. Hofer (Eds.), *Beiträge zur Arbeitsmarkt- und Berufsforschung: Theorie und Praxis der Beratung — Beratung in Schule, Familie, Beruf und Betrieb* (Bd.

AB203, S. 161–184). Nürnberg, Germany: Institut für Arbeitsmark- und Berufsforschung der Bundesanstalt für Arbeit.

Wittmann, W. W., & Süß, H.-M. (1997, July). *Challenging g-mania in intelligence research: Answers not given, due to questions not asked.* Paper presented at Eighth Biennial Meeting of the International Society for the Study of Individual Differences, Aarhus, Denmark.

Wolfe, J., & Roberts, C. R. (1986). The external validity of a business management game: A five-year longitudinal study. *Simulation and Games, 17*, 45–59.

Zee, A. (1989). *Fearful symmetry: The search for beauty in modern physics.* New York: Collier.

Zimmermann, P., & Fimm, B. (1993). *Testbatterie zur Aufmerksamkeitsprüfung (TAP), Version 1.02* [Attention test battery]. Würselen, Germany: Vera Fimm/Psychologische Testsysteme.

Discussion

Open discussion of Wittmann's paper centered around the importance of appropriate criteria for assessing individual differences in learning. Wittmann briefly described several additional investigations that showed how the development of new performance criteria can be especially useful in exploring the relations between abilities, personality, and learning. Additional discussion focused on gender differences in task performance on criterion tasks.

Dr. Baddeley: Just a rather general question. In terms of your different trajectories, I noted some work that Randy Engle did with working memory span tasks that seems to suggest that he got qualitatively different strategies adopted by different subjects. What's the effect on the sorts of analysis that you do if, in fact, people do something qualitatively different? Does it matter?

Dr. Wittmann: That's a very good question, but we have no good answer on that because we haven't looked at these qualitative differences. I have shown you some switching tasks, and we are working with a colleague of Freiburg University, Germany. The switching tasks are from him. He works in the neuropsych area. We are going to talk about these issues with him, but we don't have at the moment a good answer because all we did was quantitatively in terms of individual-differences research.

What we're going to do in the future is looking at training and things like that, hopefully we're going to get rid of these gender differences and things like that. Maybe this leads to showing up qualitative differences.

Dr. Kyllonen: I really like the work that you've done on the criterion tasks. I think that's really useful. And I have a question related to any kind of principles that you might derive out of the kinds of tasks you've developed and looked at or what principles you might have used in order to select domains in which to build these various tasks. I think that on the ability side we have lots of principles. On the criterion side we don't really have any.

Dr. Wittmann: Well, what we have at the criterion side, is a bunch of strategic principles, and I have to give credit to Martin Fishbein and Icek Ajzen. They have made an interesting distinction between single acts and multiple acts which I had picked up 10 years ago with in personality research. And if Gerald [Matthews] would do as I, I would predict that he'd get pretty much higher coefficients first only in terms of prediction, but then you can look what's going on to get better explanations. Fishbein and Ajzen also make an interesting distinction that you could use, namely, "principles of correspondence" is how they call it, which is a synonym for Brunswick symmetry. You could have a look at correspondence in terms of context, target, time and action. Time is one thing which I could refer to how to improve the criterion side (i.e., aggregating over time).

I'm embarrassed what we as psychologists do. We always use these short-term criteria, and you have seen on my transparencies question marks in referring to what kind of questions interest other disciplines. I've told you that I'm in a business-biased university at Germany. What do the business people do? Are they interested whether somebody is going to make a mistake or something good in a single situation? They are, but not predominately. They are interested at the wins and losses in the long run, the balances at the end of the fiscal year. So you have to aggregate over a longer time period. There are many different situations within 1 year related to the fortune of a company.

In the personality research area, we looked for such a comprehensive criterion. We had a look at the whole literature of Hans Eysenck, especially what he believed and found as differential indicators for extraverted and introverted behavior. We picked up all these indicators and looked at a study done by my academic teacher and mentor Jochen Fahrenberg. In that study students participated over 8 weeks in his psychophysiological lab. Jochen is first author of the German-speaking Freiburg Personality Inventory, which also assesses Eysenck's E and N dimensions. At the beginning of the 8-week study, E and N were assessed. The students kept diaries and were rated. We found eight indicators for E and 7 indicators for N compatible with Eysenck. Aggregating these indicators over 8 weeks led to the impressive convergent and discriminant validity coefficients of .70 for E and .82 for N while the E indicators correlated practically zero with N and the N indicators zero with E. I have shown you that with a transparency which is not in our paper. These results are published in Wittmann (1987). Well sometimes theories, good theories, like Hans Eysenck's theory, are going to pay off.

In the areas where we don't have good theories, we have to use trial and error or other things. But there are very good examples for the importance of context, for example, in advertising research which Icek Azjen and Martin Fishbein (1980) did. (The beer example is in chapter 12.) They found general attitude towards beer as the worst predictor asking in the context of what kind of beer do you buy for your friends or if you have an invitation. I guess you don't buy Bud. Maybe it depends on who you're going to invite. Probably better are international beers or premium ones. When they asked what's your attitude towards Beck's beer, German beer, for example, then this attitude was more closely related to buying beer for invitation and things like that. We used three different scenarios in our study. We deliberately varied the context and the content of these games, the task-specific knowledge, computer knowledge, and business knowledge.

We also could profit from taxonomies. In education we have Bloom's taxonomy. Are you interested in simple knowledge? I am not. I have a lot of examinations with the business students or sometimes with medical students, and they have the tradition to learn the phone book by heart. That's not a criterion we think to be important as an academic performance criterion. We want to have performances related to applications, analysis, synthesis, and evaluation. You see it depends on what kind of criteria, and there are many possibilities to construct the type of criteria you are asking for.

Dr. Alexander: I've got to bring up the gender issue. How many females were involved in helping you plan these tailor shop simulations? I keep thinking it would be hard for me to stay very much interested in keeping some factory going. I don't know.

Dr. Wittmann: The female part of gender in my hometown, Nürnberg, where I also used the tailor shop in a similar study outperformed the males in all two other towns (Berlin and Mannheim). But the differences between them were there in all three studies, females always on average performed worse than males within each of the three studies. We didn't specifically look after gender differences, we're simply not interested in the beginning for genders. Just by chance we stumbled over these differences. But if you look at the content of a shirt factory, shouldn't that be something interesting for a woman?

Dr. Alexander: Oh, no. We buy them. But we may not care about the industrial concerns related to their manufacture.

Dr. Ackerman: Werner, that does suggest a paradigm though. And Ruth Kanfer and I thought about this with our air traffic control task. And that is that if the underlying computer algorithm that runs these tasks is identical but the cover story is different — you know, a dress shop versus a tailor — you might end up with very different results if the cover story does appear to be gender specific.

Dr. Wittmann: Well probably you are right, but let me explain what the main causal variable or explanatory predictive variables was that we found after our appetite for explanation was whetted. It was computer literacy. The women just had lower scores on that computer experience scale. You have to handle that computer and make sense out of it. Maybe it's a lack of training they have. We want to do training studies and look what's going on. I have some promising results. If the instructor for that computer stuff is a woman, then the women profited much more than the men.

Dr. Wagner: How much training do people get on that?

Dr. Wittmann: You have to make a decision every month, 12 times.

Dr. Wagner: How many hours or minutes are people actually spending doing this game over the course of the study?

Dr. Süß: One game we used 90 minutes for 12 simulation months. Before we started, we have an introduction of about 20 minutes. They learned to handle the system. But I think it's perhaps not enough.

Dr. Wagner: For a total we're talking about maybe a couple of hours of experience with this task?

Dr. Süß: Yes. But we used this simulation game not only one time, we used it three times. And 1 year later we played the game again with the same pupils two times. So the performance aggregate in the studies Werner referred to with the gender differences consisted of five games aggregated over 1 year.

Dr. Stanovich: I want to go back to this content issue on the gender difference. And again, maybe someone who knows this literature better than I do, Rick Wagner or Phil Ackerman, can help me here. But didn't Steve Ceci a few years ago do just what you suggested in a comparison with learning disabled children in a multidimensional computer task and change the content? The underlying algorithm was just the same. It was just Phil's suggestion. And he found a really large difference, which would suggest that a similar thing might happen in the gender situation.

Dr. Wittmann: Okay. Goods hints. We will try. As often in the life of research projects, some very important facts show up, and you want to have the answers. But we didn't concentrate on these issues. This just happened. One last remark because I have to make an advertisement. We have one guy right here, Jan-Eric (Gustafsson). He contributed to a brilliant paper in *Intelligence* (Harnqvist, Gustafsson, Muthén, & Nelson, 1994), and his results are very much related to what I'm talking about. If you look at that paper you get a better understanding that how you aggregate is very important. First they aggregated over classes, then used only the class mean scores and doing a factor analysis and many schools from Sweden as a unit of analysis they found a crystallized intelligence factor first. When they analyzed the scores at the individual level as in classical individual-differences research, the first one was the fluid factor. You see how we aggregate our data has consequences for what variance parts show up or don't show up. That crystallized factor must be surely related to treatment differences between the classes, qualities of teachers, and so on. We really should pay attention to aggregate to a level we want. I guess these are the tasks we have to solve in the near future.

II

PROCESSES

5

Intelligence and Visual and Auditory Information Processing

IAN J. DEARY

Recently, Neisser (1997), in assessing the broad field of psychometric intelligence, stated that "as of now, the study of intelligence looks promising" (p. 80). This was (almost) his final word in answering the responses to the broad overview of IQ research produced by an American Psychological Association working party under his chairmanship (Neisser et al., 1996). Within that article, however, there were at least three different types of research on human intelligence. First, there was research based on studies of psychometric ability tests that attempted to find the number, nature, and organization of human mental abilities. Such research has a broad consensus in that about three levels of ability may be distinguished: (a) specific or narrow cognitive abilities such as were emphasized in the theories of Guilford or Thurstone; (b) group factors of ability—such as verbal, spatial, memory, or speediness—akin to those emphasized by Vernon, Burt, and Cattell; and (c) general intelligence (or *g*) proposed by Galton and discovered by Spearman (Carroll, 1993; Gustafsson, 1984). This type of intelligence research is what Sternberg (1990) called the *"geographical"* approach to intelligence; it tells us about the lie of the land (i.e., it describes the phenomena), but it fails to provide validity for the concepts of mental ability it describes.

There are at least two broad types of validity research on intelligence. The first is predictive validity, the type of research that takes mental ability scores and uses them as predictors of life outcomes. These outcomes often have to do with performance in educational or occupational settings (Neisser et al., 1996). These data render mental tests useful, but the tests remain scientifically unsatisfying. Predictive validity satisfied Binet (whose concern was the construction of a practical test), but not Spearman (whose concern was to discover the nature of human intelligence and the reasons for individual differences in mental abilities). Satisfying Spearman is the topic of this chapter, which brings me to the third type of research on human intelligence and the second type of validity research. Spearman wanted to know what it meant, in process terms, to be smarter than someone else. For Spearman, the specific content of the tests used to measure ability differences was of little importance, thus his doctrine of the "indifference of the indicator." Similarly, Kline (1997) recently stated that

> The leading psychometrists, such as Cattell and Eysenck, figures whom Cattell is keen to separate from mere itemetric moles, regard factors only as starting points for their investigations. . . . In the field of intelligence great efforts are being made to investigate the underlying nature of the g factors. Intelligence tests are not the end but the means of investigation. (pp. 385–386)

According to Spearman and Kline, mental tests were used merely to measure individual differences in mental ability; they formalized researchers' impressions that some people are smarter than others on some or most cognitive tasks. The most interesting question, according to those authors, is what constitutes the origins of mental ability differences. Spearman contributed a lot to how researchers might think about beginning the search for such origins. In his earliest empirical writings, Spearman (1904) proposed that the origins of intelligence differences might lie in the simplest psychological process, which, to him, was the discrimination of one sensation from another (Deary, 1994a). In this, he was in agreement with Galton (1883). However, if this was Spearman's psychological guess at the basic processes underlying intelligence, he also had a biological guess. That is, he also likened differences in g to the different amounts of energy that people had available for their engines (i.e., specific abilities). Thus, Spearman's writings indicate that there might be tractable physiological as well as psychological bases for intelligence differences.

There is no reason why researchers should not look for the understanding of intelligence differences in both psychological/cognitive parameters and in physiological indexes, and the choice reminds one about the issue of the correct level of description to be used for a reductionistic account of human intelligence. Put simply, to validate mental test differences by linking them to brain parameters, researchers must necessarily make a choice about which parameters are available. Therefore, the type of research examined here presupposes a model of brain operation with parameters that have individual differences related to mental test performance. Spearman (1923) thought that such a model was the sine qua non of proper research on intelligence differences. Thus, his first book on intelligence was not about the psychometrics of intelligence; rather, it was about the structure of intelligence and dealt with the processes that underlie intelligence and that contain the parameters of basic individual differences. Spearman's (1923) *Nature of "Intelligence" and the Principles of Cognition* has been called the first cognitive psychology textbook (Gustafsson, 1992). It was in this book that Spearman arrived at his principles of cognition: the apprehension of experience, the education of correlates, and the education of relations. These, it appears, were derived largely from his time in the armchair rather than in the laboratory, but it was his willingness to address the problem of the nature of intelligence rather than his specific answer that is informative.

Spearman (1923) thought that mental tests could not reveal anything interesting about the nature of intelligence: "Any search for 'the nature of intelligence' has shown itself to have a prospect of success when, and only when, it becomes merged into the greater quest after the scientific 'principles of cognition' " (p. 32). Indeed, Spearman (1923) described mental tests as "miners excavating forward into wonderfully rich new ground, but repeatedly missing the correct direction on account of labouring in darkness. The light they need is just that which irradiates from principles — from these alone" (pp. 35–36).

Finding such principles was the main job of psychology, and Spearman's (1923) view of the research required appears to be a cognitive rather than a differential psychology agenda. The way he articulated the problem makes it clear that, to satisfy his interest in discovering the nature of intelligence (the reasons why some people are smarter than others), researchers must first find out the structure of thinking:

> Whenever the make-up of any cognitive operation has to be analyzed, this is best done by resolving it into the unit-processes as its basal constituents. . . . Psychology, to obtain the much fuller measure of success awaiting it, must evolve towards a mental cytology. (Spearman, 1923, p. 59)

Given the rise of cognitive psychology and neuroscience, researchers should not have to make up their own model of cognitive functioning. They can expect to borrow measurement tools to index individual differences in validated cognitive and psychophysiological parameters from other areas of psychology.

Reductionistic Routes to the Nature of Intelligence

In seeking the nature of intelligence, one must make choices about the nature of the variables that are to bear the brunt of the explanatory burden. The choices that have been made may be organized into a rough-and-ready hierarchy from those that contain variables close to psychometric test items to those that contain basic biological variables. There is nothing wrong with being interested in variables at more than one level, although researchers do appear to have favorite strata. What is interesting is the information that different levels might give us with respect to intelligence. The modern-day "nature of intelligence" type of research is committed to some or all of the following four objectives: (a) establishing the extent of the association between psychometric intelligence test scores and variables from the chosen reductionistic measure; (b) establishing the direction of causation between psychometric intelligence and lower level variables; (c) finding a mechanistic explanation for the association between psychometric intelligence and information-processing variables; and (d) providing a tractable theory for the information-processing variable and the task in which it is embedded.

In the next main section of this chapter, I use visual and auditory processing tasks as case studies of the information-processing approach to intelligence. However, before that, it is instructive to enumerate some of the other choices that people have made in attempting an information-processing understanding of human intelligence differences. Those four questions may be asked of all of these approaches. Furthermore, one may use these to assess whether there has been any success in achieving understanding of the nature of intelligence or what Spearman (1923) called the "mental cytology."

A Psychometric Cytology

Some researchers hardly appear to obey the reductionistic call in looking for tools that might illuminate the nature of intelligence. Instead, they appeal in ingenious ways to psychometric tests themselves to get at what it means to be clever. Even within this approach, there are various routes taken. Sternberg (1977) used a partial item presentation–reaction time method to isolate — and quantify the temporal aspects of — the components of analogical reasoning items. He later extended this research to inductive reasoning and series completion (Sternberg & Gardner, 1983). Elsewhere, I have described and evaluated this approach (Deary, 1997a). The main concern with this approach is the validity of the components, that is, whether anything basic and general about brain–cognitive processing has been isolated using this method.

Some improvements to Sternberg's (1977) approach, in the light of the analyses of Raven's Progressive Matrices items by Carpenter, Just, and Shell (1990), were made by Embretson (1995). She rigorously tested a model of an abstract reasoning task that had working memory and general control processes (like Sternberg's, 1977, metacomponents) as the covert components of the task performance. Indeed, these two components accounted for 92% of the variance in task ability, and the components were able to fully mediate the effects of the abstract reasoning task on the four factors derived from the Armed Services Vocational Assessment Battery. However, once more, the question of the validity of the so-called components should be posed. A component model must be stipulated before the analyses — they are in no way a "discovery" of this type of research. The working memory component is essentially a task difficulty parameter, and it is a moot question whether there are cognitive primitives that are isomorphic with manipulable aspects of task difficulty. Therefore, although one can have some success in modeling task item success (especially IQ-type tasks), the fundamental question of whether such components exist inside the head as well as on the test paper remain unanswered. The same might be asked of the work of Kyllonen and Christal (1990), who appeared to find that intelligence was largely explained by differences in working memory. Again, recall that the tests of working memory are at the same level of analysis as IQ-type test items and that one must appeal to the respective tests' reductionistic nomological networks to make a judgment about whether working memory and intelligence are causal one to the other, mutually causal, reflections of a deeper set of causes, or just two names for much the same construct.

A Cognitive Cytology

Given Spearman's (1923) original attempt to identify the mental components underlying task performance, it is perhaps most natural that those interested in the nature of intelligence should look to cognitive and experimental psychology for a classification of mental processes and tasks that might index these. The growing enthusiasm in the late 1970s and early 1980s for this combining of differential and experimental and cognitive psychology was discussed at length by Deary (1997a). Examples of cognitive tasks applied to individual differences research are the Hick reaction time task, the Sternberg memory scan task, and the Posner letter matching task. Indexes from all of these tasks and many more correlate significantly with scores on psychometric intelligence tests (Jensen, 1987; Vernon, 1987). It is a different matter to ask whether researchers have identified the aspects of these tasks that lead to the correlations with intelligence. That is, one may demonstrate the association, but the direction of causation, the mechanism of association, and the essence of the performance parameters tend to be missing. For example, it was suggested originally that the increase in reaction time with increased stimulus uncertainty in the Hick task might be a measure of individual differences in a participant's "rate of gain of information." Similarly, it was said that the increment consequent on each additional stimulus element in the Sternberg memory scan task was an indication of the time needed to scan one element in working memory. The Posner task was supposed to be able to index the time it took to consult long-term stores. Such isolating of processes from experimental tests is exactly what might be wanted from cognitive psychology. However, such task decompositions have rarely stood up to further investigation. Results from the Hick task, for instance, suggest that correlations with psychometric ability tests can be obtained with most of its indexes, regardless of whether they are theoretically interesting (Deary, 1997a). However, given the vibrancy of the cognitive psychology community, it should be just a matter of time before validated models of aspects of cognition are available in the form of tests whose parameters might be related more revealingly to IQ-type test scores.

A Psychophysical Cytology

I say more about this level of the search for the nature of intelligence shortly. Note that this was the stratum within which Galton (1883) and Spearman (1923), with their interests in sensory discrimination, first assumed that researchers should search for those simple processes that might be the building blocks of intelligent performance (Deary, 1994a). Also at the level of sensory processing, there have been desultory and unsuccessful attempts to correlate critical flicker frequency and fusion with IQ-type test scores (Jensen, 1983). Others have borrowed established tasks from the field of auditory processing (Raz, Willerman, & Yama, 1987). By far the most studied task within this realm has been inspection time (IT), and it is discussed in the next main section.

A Physiological Cytology

With the difficulties of mechanistic interpretation and construct explication inherent in cognitive and even psychophysical measures, it is tempting to bypass them and go straight to physiological parameters. Here, it appears, that one can obtain tractable information about parameters of nervous system function and their individual differences. Potentially, however, there are many nervous system parameters that researchers might select, and, because they do not fully comprehend the functional complexity of the brain's neural networks, there are others they cannot even guess. Of those that have been chosen, one of the simplest is the conduction velocity of nerves (NCV). Although it is not yet settled, there is some evidence that this parameter has a slight correlation with psychometric intelligence (Rijsdijk & Boomsma, 1997). If this finding is reviewed in terms of the four criteria mentioned earlier, it might meet the correlation criterion and would seem to offer an unequivocal answer in terms of direction of causation, for it is hardly likely that high cognitive ability

115

would cause faster NCV. The interpretation of what NCV represents does not pose the same problems as cognitive or psychophysical tests, being much simpler. However, the question of the mechanism of the association between NCV and mental ability test scores remains. One hypothesis is that faster NCV might mediate the correlation between reaction time and psychometric intelligence. However, partialing out the NCV–IQ association from the reaction time–IQ association does not noticeably reduce the latter, thus rejecting the simple mechanistic interpretation (see Deary & Caryl, 1997).

The largest area of interest within the psychophysiology of intelligence is electro-encephalography, especially the study of brain-evoked electrical potentials. This has been extensively reviewed recently (Deary & Caryl, 1993, 1997), and it seems certain that indexes in this area meet the correlation criterion. It also seems that there are identifiable subareas of evoked potentials that are reliably associated with intelligence test scores, such as the latency of certain electrical peaks and the shape and complexity of the waveforms. Within this field, again, there has to be a question about the direction of causation because it is not clear whether the brain indexes that are associated with intelligence are causal to or elicited by the tasks that evoke them. Furthermore, there is no unequivocal mechanistic understanding of the association, reflecting the imperfect knowledge concerning the concepts that underlie evoked potential indexes and their individual differences.

The NCV is largely a peripheral nervous system measure that does not get at more integrated aspects of brain function. (Although that is a weakness in terms of the likely important aspects of brain function for intelligence, it is a strength in terms of clarity of interpretation.) A physiological approach that has begun to produce results and that will gather momentum is the measurement of functional aspects of brain function via various scanning techniques. Results of some small studies using positron–emission tomography (PET) (Haier, 1993; Haier et al., 1988) suggest that people who score better on psychometric intelligence tests have lower rates of cerebral metabolism while performing the tasks. This has led to the "efficient brain" hypothesis. The problem here, however, having established the correlation between, say PET and IQ-type measures, is that all other criteria are unclear. The direction of causation is not clear — performing a task might easily induce a brain state that is not in a deep sense causal to the score (the brighter person may be less anxious as a result of the test; see Deary et al., 1994) — and the mechanism of the association and the concepts inherent in the PET indexes are far from being understood.

An Anatomical Cytology

Whereas one might have to guess at the brain functions being indexed by cognitive and neurophysiological tasks, the direct measurement of structural aspects of the brain provide an unequivocal indicator of brain differences. Thus, the finding that brain volume — as indexed by structural magnetic resonance imaging — correlates at about .4 or more with differences in psychometric IQ-type tests gives a solid correlation and an unequivocal result with respect to the direction of the correlation (Rushton & Ankey, 1996). It will be much more difficult to discover why brain volume is associated with mental ability. There are several potential explanatory parameters to choose from, and the following have been suggested by the authors of the primary empirical reports: dendritic expansion, more synapses, myelin thickness, metabolic efficiency, efficient neurotransmitter production, release and uptake, and brain reserve capacity (summarized by Deary & Caryl, 1997).

A Genetic Cytology

Two things herald the promise of mechanisms of intelligence from genetic research. The first of these is the fact that mental abilities are moderately heritable. The second is the advances in molecular genetic technology and quantitative trait loci, which means that behavior phenotypes can be linked to multiple genes, each of which accounts for some of the variance in the individual differences. When polymorphisms of specific gene loci have been associated with individual differences in mental abilities, this will suggest some possible biochemical mechanisms contributing to different ability levels.

Visual and Auditory IT

IT belongs to the psychophysical levels and is used here as a case study in an attempt to get at a part of the nature of intelligence (Deary, 1996). IT is a name given to four things: a task, a parameter, an individual-differences measure, and a construct. As a construct it arose from ideas about visual perception that conceived of vision operating in a quantal fashion, such that elementary visual discriminations required a minimum amount of time (Vickers, Nettelbeck, & Willson, 1972). These ideas have had a resurgence in popularity with researchers such as Poppel (1994), who suggested that quanta of perceptual function are required to achieve multimodal sensory integration. In any case, the construct IT was intended to express this basic limitation in perceptual function. As a task, IT was designed to be free from all difficulties of discrimination other than temporal limitations. Given this remit, Vickers designed the commonly used task that involves discriminating which of two parallel, vertical lines of markedly different lengths is longer. To impose temporal limitations, the stimulus is presented for various durations, ideally extending below that duration at which the participant achieves chance (50%) responding and above that duration at which participants' responses are perfect. To prevent further processing of the stimulus after the nominal stimulus duration, the stimulus is backward masked. Therefore, unlike mental ability tasks, IT tasks are always solved correctly when there is no limitation to the stimulus IT. There is no requirement to respond quickly in IT tasks; only the correctness of the participant's response at the various stimulus durations are recorded. Thus, in IT tasks a graph may be produced in which the participant's probability of a correct response is plotted against the stimulus duration. Such a graph describes a cumulative normal ogive (Deary, Caryl, & Gibson, 1993; Vickers et al., 1972). A participant's IT — an individual-differences measure — is the duration at which the participant achieves a given (arbitrarily chosen) level of correctness (often 85%). The individual-differences measure correlates between .4 and .5 with psychometric ability tasks — especially performance-type task scores — in the general adult population. This is no longer the subject of much debate, having been established by qualitative reviews (Deary & Stough, 1996; Nettelbeck, 1987), meta-analyses (e.g., Kranzler & Jensen, 1989), and large single stud-

117

ies (e.g., Deary, 1993a). These studies tend to show that the correlation between IT and verbal intelligence is lower, at or above .2. More research is required on the association between IT and psychometric intelligence: IT has still not been tested in addition to a wide battery of tests to gauge IT's associations with broad and narrow abilities in the three-stratum model of psychometric intelligence (Carroll, 1993).

I just described IT as a task, a construct, and an individual differences measure. Also note that it is a parameter; indeed, the model of task performance assumes that IT is the only parameter needed to describe a participant's performance at different levels of task difficulty (i.e., levels of stimulus duration; Vickers et al., 1972). Recall that Embretson's (1995) novel approach to the modeling of psychometric tasks was aimed at isolating covert parameters according to prior theory. In IT, one has the unusual situation of a task (IT) that supposedly delivers individual differences (in IT) in a parameter (IT) that is an indicator of a basic psychophysical limitation and construct (IT)!

Because there is nothing that states that the original stimulus used in the IT task is essential, others have sought to record individual differences in the same parameter and thereby index the same construct using other techniques. In the visual modality, a tachistoscopic word identification task appears to have the same structure of associations with mental ability as did the original version of the IT task (compare McGeorge, Crawford, & Kelly, 1997, and Deary, 1993a).

Furthermore, reasoning that if IT as a construct is a basic sensory limitation then it should be measurable in auditory and visual forms, Deary (e.g., 1994b) devised a so-called auditory IT task. This task asks the participant to indicate the temporal order of two successive tones that differ markedly in pitch, typically by more than 100 Hz. The stimulus tones are played, one after the other, without any gap, and they are backward masked. Individual differences in this auditory task correlate with psychometric ability test scores at about the same level as do visual tests of IT (Deary, 1994b, 1995; Deary, Caryl, Egan, & Wight, 1989). Others have used slightly different auditory processing tasks, although they still used a temporal order and pitch-based discrimination involving two tones, and found similar levels of association (e.g., Raz & Willerman, 1985). However, the finding of a significant psychometric intelligence–auditory IT has not always been found, especially when the participants are of high mean ability and have an attenuated range (Langsford, Mackenzie, & Maher, 1994). It would strengthen the hypothesis of a general, cross-modal IT limitation if individual differences in auditory and visual IT were highly correlated. To date, this important question has attracted few studies, and those have typically showed only modest visual–auditory associations, from about .2 to .5 (Deary, Caryl, et al., 1989; Nettelbeck, Edwards, & Vreugdenhil, 1986). One group of researchers attempted to extend IT to the tactile mode but had little success (Nettelbeck et al., 1986).

Explanatory Problems

Having constructed simple, psychophysical tasks to measure IT parameters in visual and auditory contexts and results showing that both of these correlate significantly with cognitive ability test scores, what, if anything, can one say has been discovered about the nature of intelligence? As discussed by Deary (1996), some (call them "reductionists") have taken the correlations to mean that some form of mental speed is causal to individual differences and therefore that there is clear evidence about the nature of a modest amount of the variance in intelligence. Others (call them "nonreductionists") have interpreted the evidence in a contrary fashion and have taken the associations to mean nothing more than the fact that people with high intelligence can find cognitive strategies to "penetrate" IT tasks and perform relatively well on them. Many of these arguments have been conducted from the armchair rather than the laboratory bench, and, whereas those favoring a reductionist account of IT will brandish a handy epithet such as "mental speed" to capture the construct measured by IT differences, nonreductionists will appeal to the motivation, concentration, attention, personality, and strategies of the high-ability people that perhaps help them to achieve a better IT score.

After establishing a correlation between psychometric ability test scores and an apparently low-level cognitive–psychophysical index, the proper course of action is to address the other three objectives that must be performed to gain any credible understanding of the nature of intelligence (i.e., the causal direction of the association, the mechanism of the association, and the brain process indexed by the low-level measure must be explored). These tasks often overlap in practice, and experiments that address one of these also often bear on the other two. Such explanatory problems are being addressed actively in the case of IT and were summarized recently (Deary, 1996; Deary & Stough, 1996). Figure 5.1 shows the types of research that are being or have already been conducted to try to explain the IT–mental ability association; these fields are discussed by Deary (1996) and Deary and Stough (1996). This is a partial representation of the nomological net in which the phe-

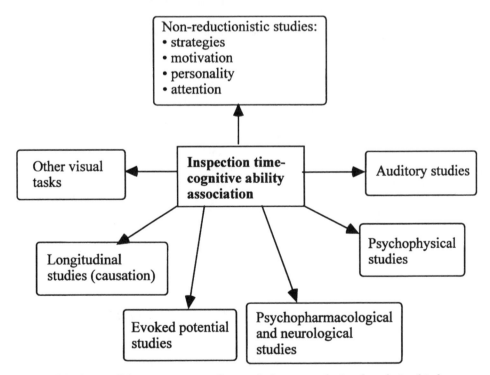

Figure 5.1. Some of the current areas of research that are exploring the relationship between inspection time and psychometric intelligence.

nomenon of IT exists. It is also an explicit statement of how much research remains to be completed; glaring holes in the data, such as the correlation between auditory and visual tasks and the detailed psychophysics of IT (Deary et al., 1993; Levy, 1992), require filling.

Ways Forward

Several trials and tribulations of IT research still exist, and some have been discussed elsewhere (Deary, 1996; Deary & Stough, 1996; Sternberg, 1997, with a reply by Deary & Stough). The aspect of current and future research that will be highlighted in this chapter harks back to Spearman's (1923) notion of the "indifference of the indication." That is, there is nothing important about the task that is used to index a construct; indeed, it is so much the better if the same parameter can be obtained from superficially different-seeming tasks (this leniency is what makes g such a powerful and counterintuitive phenomenon). It is better still if the tasks that are being used for this development come with a full research backing from their own area of interest. Therefore, whereas research on intelligence and information-processing limitations must still include IT measures using the best available tasks, a proper understanding of the contribution made by IT will involve the use of non-IT tasks that are thought to capture the same limitations of perceptual processing.

The general philosophy that drives this approach is that endless perusal of IT will not necessarily tell researchers why it correlates with psychometric intelligence. Presumably, IT is merely one example of a set of tasks that captures some processing variance that relates to differences in higher cognitive ability differences. Craik (1943) warned against too narrow a study of single instances when trying to discover lawfulness in nature:

> You can never prove the existence of any external thing, or its obedience to a particular law, by trying to wring the truth out of a particular example; you must vary the conditions, repeat the experiments, make a hypothesis and a remote inference from that hypothesis and test it out. In any particular experiment some unforeseen factor may be at work; you cannot safely pick up a single stone, pass it to a friend and say: "There, in your hand, you hold a perfect example of the law of gravitation; analyse its behaviour and you will know all." On the contrary, the earthward pull of that particular stone may be partly due to magnetic iron ore in it. . . . It is only by taking numerous examples and tracking down the problem from all sides that we can extract the truth; we can never wring it out of the particular example. (pp. 3–4)

Progress in Visual Processing

The Expanded Judgment Test and the Frequency Accrual Speed Test

From the arguments that have surrounded the interpretation of the IT–psychometric intelligence correlation, it is clear that one cannot assume identity between the IT task and the theoretical construct (an error made frequently in psychology). The originator of the IT theory and task — Douglas Vickers — has sought to develop other tasks that will capture the IT as a construct and allow the extraction of IT as a parameter. Among the more important problems that led to his taking this route were the problems with stimulus–mask interactions in IT tasks. The first task he wrote of was the expanded judgment task in which observers viewed a series of horizontal lines presented consecutively on one or other side of a midline on a computer monitor (Vickers, Foreman, Nicholls, Innes, & Gott, 1989). The lines were of different lengths and, after viewing a train of lines, the observers had to decide whether, on average, those on the left or right were longer. Two advantages might be seen as inherent to such a task over the original IT task. First, there was no need for a backward mask because the series of lines arrived at such a fast rate that each successive line effectively masked the previous one. Second, instead of relying on a single brief stimulus presentation, the observer was asked to make a cumulative judgment based on a stimulus train, the rate of which could be varied. One of the ideas behind the expanded judgment task was that the limiting factor in performance was the rate at which information could be accumulated.

Vickers (1995) subsequently developed a conceptually similar task on which he has done more theoretical, experimental, and correlational work: the frequency accrual speed task. In this task, the observer views a panel with two lights, one on each side of the midline of a special presentation device. Again, the observer sees a train of stimuli, with flashes coming successively from one or the other of the lights. The observer's task is to state which of the lights had more flashes. Various parameters may be manipulated: the ratio of flashes between the more and less numerous sides, the duration of each flash and the interflash interval, and the total number of flashes seen. Individual differences in the frequency accrual speed task have about the same correlations with cognitive ability test scores as does IT (Vickers, 1995; Vickers & McDowell, 1996). Moreover, individual differences in the task correlate moderately with IT differences. Experiments by Vickers have led him to conclude that the key parameter in the task is not speed of processing and that this might also be said of IT (Vickers, Pietsch, & Hemingway, 1995). Instead, Vickers now hypothesizes that limitations of working memory are the key to performance on the frequency accrual speed test.

However, Deary and Caryl (1997) have criticized Vickers's original conceptualization of the frequency accrual speed test and the parallels he has drawn with IT. The frequency accrual speed test involves making a judgment — which of two series of light flashes had more? — about two adjacent supraspan series of light flashes, obviously involving active memory processes in a way that IT does not. Second, Vickers has never taken the flash duration (including the long, unmasked interflash interval) to a duration that is low enough to impose speed-of-processing limitations. Therefore, his conclusion — the most damaging one to a speed-of-processing interpretation of IT that speed of processing is not the key parameter in frequency accrual speed test performance was judged by Deary and Caryl (1997) not to have been tested let alone refuted. They have posed some specific hypotheses for future frequency accrual speed test research: for example, that reducing the flash–interflash interval duration will successively make speed of processing the key parameter in the task, especially when the flash series is not so lengthy as to impose a large memory load. They have also suggested that the frequency accrual speed test correlates with IT because it is a high-level task, more akin to a psychometric ability task than a psychophysical task, and not because both IT and the frequency accrual speed test are low-level tasks indexing the same single parameter. These criticisms do not decry the attempts to construct new tasks that assess processing speed limitations; it is merely that each task must be analyzed according to the criteria set out earlier; in particular, researchers must carefully analyze whether parameters extracted from a task truly get at the construct being targeted. Deary and Caryl (1997) have concluded that the frequency accrual speed task, as it stands at present, is not appropriate for assessing the construct of IT.

Visual Change Detection and Latent Processing Traits

As stated earlier, Vickers's attempt to move from IT to the parallel development and study of new tasks aiming at the same information-processing construct is worthwhile and likely to be informative. Certain aspects of the IT task are problematic, especially the attainment of an effective mask to ensure that poststimulus processing does not occur (Deary, 1996). It seems certain, more so with some forms of the IT task than others, that some people use stimulus–mask artifacts to inform them about the position of the long line (Egan, 1994). However, strategies have not been found to cause the IT–cognitive ability correlation; if anything, they tend to reduce it. Another issue with the original IT task it that the chance of correct answer is 50%; lowering the rate of chance might provide more information in each trial. This was done using words as stimuli in the experiment by McGeorge et al. (1997). However, another route was taken by Deary, McCrimmon, and Bradshaw (1997). They adapted a psychophysical task developed by Phillips and Singer (1974): the visual change detection task. On this task, the observer attends to a computer monitor screen. On it they are warned by a cue, and there follows an array of 49 small rectangles set randomly in a virtual 10×10 matrix. After a variable duration, one more rectangle is added to the array. The observer's task is to indicate which of the (now) 50 rectangles was the one that was added later than the others. The full array of 50 remains on the screen until after the observer has made a response. There is no masking of the stimuli and, as with IT, the observer is under no pressure to respond quickly; only the correctness of the response and the duration between the appearance of the first 49 and the additional (target) stimulus is recorded. Like IT, the relationship between the probability of a correct response and the target stimulus onset delay (stimulus onset asynchrony) in the visual change detection task is described by a cumulative normal ogive. Furthermore, differences in the task correlate moderately highly — above .4 — with psychometric ability test scores. Deary et al. (1997) also used a third task, a visual movement detection task, that involved one of the small rectangles (the target) moving to the left or right instead of appearing later than the rest. The duration between the appearance of the array and the movement was the manipulated variable.

However, Deary et al. (1997) went further in their study of the visual change detection and movement detection tasks. They reasoned that key aspects of the visual change and movement detection tasks were significantly different from IT: The target was one stimulus among a large array, requiring broad, parallel attention rather than the narrower attention required by IT, and there was no backward mask, so no poststimulus information was available from that source. Nevertheless, there was one prominent shared aspect of IT and the visual change and movement detection tasks:

that stimulus onset asynchrony was manipulated and appeared to be a sufficient parameter to predict the correctness of responses on the tasks. Therefore, Deary et al. (1997) reasoned that if time limitations on processing were the key parameters that accounted for the correlations with psychometric intelligence tasks, then only the latent variable from the three visual processing tasks — IT visual change detection, and visual movement detection — should correlate with psychometric ability tasks. Whereas these associations would act as convergent validity data for a processing speed–time limitation hypothesis, Deary et al. also added a discriminant validity task. They reasoned that is was necessary to have a visual discrimination task that was similar in many respects to the duration-based tasks but that lacked the requirement for speeded processing. The task chosen was the contrast sensitivity test. This is a two-alternative, forced-choice discrimination task in which respondents are asked to nominate which of two adjacent stimulus arrays contains a grating. The stimulus arrays are inspected at leisure and responses are unspeeded. If the contrast level of the grating is plotted against the probability of a correct response, then the function approximates to a normal ogive, as for the other visual processing tests. The four visual tasks and three psychometric ability tests were given to 65 normal adults who had also been given the Alice Heim 4 Test of General Mental Ability and the National Adult Reading Test (a verbal ability test). The model shown in Figure 5.2 had a highly acceptable fit to the data. It may be seen that a latent trait— common to and highly associated with all three visual tasks — correlates at .46 with the latent trait common to the three mental ability tasks. It may be calculated from the paths in the model that the correlation with the nonverbal section of the Alice Heim 4 Test is .66. Furthermore, it may be seen from Figure 5.2 that there are no significant correlations among the residuals of the visual tests; that is, all of the visual test covariance that is shared is related to psychometric ability test scores. The contrast sensitivity test did not have any significant association with the other visual or psychometric ability tests. Deary et al. argued that one interpretation of these data is that temporal limitations in basic information processing represent one modest fraction of the nature of intelligence differences. As with any latent trait, other

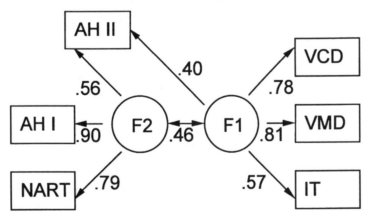

Figure 5.2. A structural model of the associations between three psychometric ability tests and three visual processing tasks. NART = National Adult Reading Test; AHI and AHII = Alice Heim 4 Verbal and Nonverbal scores, respectively; IT = inspection time; VCD = visual change detection; VMD = visual movement detection; F1 = Factor 1; F2 = Factor 2.

interpretations are possible. Nevertheless, this type of research can quickly answer the charge that the correlation between IT and psychometric intelligence is caused by some quirky aspect of the IT setup.

Deary (1997b) extended this latent trait approach by developing further tests that embody temporal processing limitations but whose phenotypic characteristics are different from those of IT. Vickers's notions of avoiding the mask-related problems of the original IT task and providing a task on which temporal limitations on processing could be examined in a setting that could allow repeated presentation of the stimuli were incorporated. Such a task appeared to have been developed in the auditory domain, where Warren (1993) had for years been examining participants' abilities to report correctly the order of elements in auditory loops that contained repeats of stimulus trains such as high and low tones and buzzes. He considered that the ability to detect temporal order was basic to higher order perception. Using this setup, Deary (1997b) developed a new visual temporal processing task called the "IT loop test." On this task the participant watches a computer monitor while a series of letters is repeated in the same order in the same screen location, time after time. For example, four loops of the stimulus train A, C, E, and I would appear as *ACEI*ACEI*ACEI*ACEI*, where left-to-right position equals time and the asterisk character is used as a loop separator. Each element of the loop is presented for identical and variable durations, including the separator. The participant's task is to state the order of the elements in the loop. The relation between the duration of the stimulus elements and the probability of reporting the correct order of the elements is described well by a cumulative normal ogive, and individual differences in the loop task are correlated with psychometric ability test scores (National Adult Reading Test and Wechsler Adult Intelligence Scale–Revised Performance test scores) at or above .5. To my knowledge, no one has examined the IT and the IT loop task in the same participant group at the same time. The intention is to add this task to others that assess visual information processing and to determine whether variance from this task also enters into a visual processing latent trait that relates to psychometric intelligence.

In summary, a general approach to advancing IT research is encouraged that is comparable to that used by Embretson (1995) in getting at covert cognitive compounds. Low-level processing tasks that purport to index the same or similar constructs and allow the extraction of parameters relevant to these constructs should be tested on the same group of participants, who should also be given a battery of psychometric mental tests. Thereafter, one should model the latent traits that express task covariance as correlates of latent psychometric traits. The idea driving this approach is that tasks — even well characterized psychophysical tasks — are generally impure, containing temporal processing variance as well as idiosyncratic variance related to the specific instantiation of the task. By combining tasks that are as dissimilar as possible and that share a parameter of interest the attempt is to distill the temporal processing construct and remove the task-specific variance. The latter might or might not be correlated with cognitive or other psychological individual differences. The question remains of truly identifying the nature of any such latent visual processing variable. It cannot blithely be assumed that some "speed of processing" has truly been extracted even from a series of phenotypically different tasks. Other possibilities must be kept in mind, such as some kind of general task difficulty or strategic variance.

124

Keeping batteries of information-processing tasks as heterogeneous as possible should minimize this problem. Furthermore, more experimental and physiological research validating the individual tasks should also answer such a concern. Indeed, apart from the latent trait approach to isolating performance parameters, the choosing of different tasks to arrive at similar processes offers at least one further benefit: Each task brings with it its own nomological network. In the case of visual change detection task of Phillips and Singer (1974), there is physiological as well as psychophysical research to support the interpretation of the task. It has been found that there is parallel activity in the lateral geniculate nucleus while cats performed the discriminations involved in the task, suggesting the possibility that the temporal limitations in detecting differences have a tractable neural basis (Singer & Phillips, 1974).

Progress in Auditory Information Processing

A similar process of varying the discrimination task to find different routes into the same processing limitations has gone on in the field of auditory IT research. Raz (discussed at length by Deary, 1994b) was the first to introduce variations on the auditory task. He and his colleagues used a more standard psychoacoustic procedure derived from the research of Massaro. This involved brief, unmasked (often 20 ms) tones of markedly different pitches played one after the other. The observer's task was to state the order (high–low or low–high) of the tones. This was made more easy or difficult by varying the quiet interstimulus interval. A longer period of silence between the two tones made the discrimination easier, whereas a short period produced chance-level responding. People scoring higher on IQ-type tests tended to be able to make accurate discriminations of temporal order at shorter interstimulus intervals. Such studies were interpreted at first as indicating that speed of processing was related to psychometric intelligence. However, Raz et al. (1987) used a variation on their procedure and, instead of varying the interstimulus interval, varied the pitch difference between the stimulus tones (I refer to this as the "Raz test"). In their study, they found moderately sized (around .5) correlations between psychometric intelligence tests and pitch discrimination threshold. This led them to suggest that it was the ability to achieve accurate stimulus representation, not speed of processing, that is responsible for the correlation with IQ-type tests.

This possibility was tested by Deary (1994b), who administered three different auditory tests to a group of more than one hundred 13-year-old schoolchildren. The Raz test and the previously used auditory IT test (Deary, Caryl, et al. 1989) were used, as was the Seashore Pitch Discrimination Test. Raven's Progressive Matrices and the Mill Hill Vocabulary Scale were also given. Deary (1994b) argued that the auditory IT emphasized the speed of information processing (i.e., having a large pitch difference between its stimulus tones and manipulating the stimulus duration), whereas the Seashore task emphasized unspeeded sensory discrimination. It was argued that the Raz task tested both the speed of processing and the pitch discrimination because it had various degrees of pitch difference in the stimulus tones and it played the tones for only 20 ms. Thus, a so-called speed factor was extracted from the Raz and auditory IT tasks and a pitch factor from the Raz and Seashore tasks. It was found that both related to psychometric intelligence but that the speed factor was the stronger associate. However, it was noted in the article's discussion that the association between a general factor extracted from the three auditory tests and that from Raven's Progressive Matrices and the Mill Hill Vocabulary Scale was .52 ($p < .001$).

Although Deary (1994b) was testing a specific hypothesis, there was a reason for not forcing the three auditory tasks into separate factors — they showed universally high intercorrelations — but instead attempting to fit a similar model to that used for the visual tests. This was attempted for the first time here. The data that were used in the previous article were used in this new model. However, a third mental test, the Culture-Fair Intelligence Test, was included. This was not used in previous analyses because it had not been used in the first wave of testing with the sample (Deary, Head, & Egan, 1989). The 107 participants who had complete data in Deary (1994b) were used in this reanalysis. The descriptions of participants, tests, and procedures, except for the Culture-Fair Intelligence Test, are given in the previous article. In the present analyses mental test raw scores, not IQ data, were used in the models. The correlation matrix and descriptive statistics used to model the data in this chapter are shown in Table 5.1. The model stipulated simply that a latent factor from the auditory processing tests correlated with a latent factor from the psychometric ability tests (see Figure 5.3).

The model was tested using the EQS structural equations modeling program via the maximum-likelihood method. The average of the off-diagonal absolute standardized residuals was .029, $\chi^2(8, N = 107) = 5.94$, $p = .65$, indicating a good fit. The fit indexes were as follows: Bentler–Bonett normed fix index = 0.98, Bentler–Bonett nonnormed fit index = 1.01, and comparative fit index = 1.00, all also indicating a good fit. All of the parameters in the model were significant, and the Wald and the Lagrange multiplier tests did not indicate that any parameters should be removed from or added to the model, respectively. A more economical model was tested, one that stated that all of the six tests — the three psychometric

TABLE 5.1 Correlations Among Three Psychometric Ability Tests and Three Auditory Processing Tests

Measure	Psychometric ability tests			Auditory processing tests		
	Mill Hill Vocabulary	Raven's Progressive Matrices	Cuture-Fair Test	Seashore Pitch	Auditory inspection time	(log) Raz auditory test
Mill Hill Vocabulary	—					
Raven's Progressive Matrices	.439	—				
Culture-Fair Test	.398	.536	—			
Seashore Pitch	.315	.333	.342	—		
Auditory inspection time	.425	.383	.295	.596	—	
(log) Raz Auditory Test[a]	.422	.445	.394	.688	.755	—
M	44.7	50.6	34.1	38.7	75.1	1.1
SD	5.641	5.007	4.375	6.980	15.851	0.477

Note. N = 107; participants as in Deary (1994b).

[a]Correlations with this test have been reversed in sign from Deary (1994b).

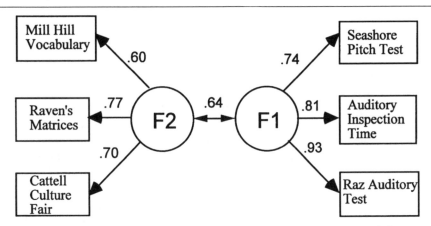

Figure 5.3. A structural model of the associations among three psychometric ability tests and three auditory processing tasks. F1 = Factor 1; F2 = Factor 2.

tests and the three auditory processing tests — were the result of a single factor. This reflected the fact that, in a principal-components analysis, the first unrotated principal component accounted for 54.8% of the total variance. However, a single-factor model fits the covariance matrix poorly: The residuals, as above, averaged .069, $\chi^2(9, N = 107) = 36.4$, $p < .001$, and the fit indexes were all below 0.9.

Note that unlike the visual experiment that used this latent trait approach, there is no task that fails to load on the auditory processing factor. Therefore, it is more difficult to articulate the latent parameter that these tests share and that is responsible for the association with psychometric ability test scores. Certainly, all of the tests involve pitch discrimination and the comparisons of tones, played consecutively, in working memory. Also, because the participants were 13-year-olds, one cannot discount some factor associated with sustained concentration, especially with respect to the psychophysical tasks. These possibilities — the possible strong association between some kind of general discrimination or general concentration factor with general mental ability or that some factor such as concentration or attention was at work in the whole correlation matrix — is almost a replay of the argument between Spearman (1904) and Thorndike, Lay, and Dean (1909), who addressed similar possibilities from similar data sets. It is just these types of dilemmas that necessitate more reductionistic research into the psychophysical tasks used in individual-differences research. Just as I said earlier, that psychometric tests cannot be used to get at the nature of intelligence, so it seems that at the psychophysical level one cannot dissect the latent constructs in the psychophysical tasks without appealing to yet lower levels of reduction.

In fact, such further reduction has already begun. Caryl (1994; Caryl & Harper, 1996) has studied the brain's electrical evoked responses to IT tasks. His studies have shown that individual differences in the steepness of the rise from the N140 trough to the P200 peak are associated with performance on the visual and auditory IT tasks with mental ability tasks. Furthermore, there was no association between pitch discrimination and this aspect of the evoked response. This type of "triangulation" (i.e., linking performance on psychometric and different psychophysical tasks through psychophysiological parameters) is a promising route for advancing information-processing understandings of the nature of intelligence.

Conclusion

In this chapter I have adopted a reductionistic structure. I have described three broad types of research on human intelligence: psychometric, predictive, and reductionistic, with the latter type concerned with the nature of intelligence differences. With respect to reductionist research on human intelligence, there is a range of responses, ordered here into a broad hierarchy: psychometric, cognitive, psychophysical, physiological, anatomical, and genetic. I might have put biochemical approaches between the physiological and anatomical to accommodate the occasional report, such as that which relates IQ to the pH of the brain (Rae et al., 1996). With respect to the psychophysical level of the hierarchy, I chose to discuss the study of IT. There are several current areas of research on the association between IT and psychometric intelligence. Of these, the research that has attempted to construct related but distinct psychophysical tasks to identify the construct within IT that relates to psychometric intelligence differences was discussed and some new analyses were presented. Because of the difficulties in devising tasks whose parameters are easily equated with cognitive constructs, I recommend that a latent trait approach to information-processing constructs offers a useful way forward.

REFERENCES

Carpenter, P. A., Just, M. A., & Shell, P. (1990). What one intelligence test measures: A theoretical account of processing in the Raven's Progressive Matrices test. *Psychological Review, 97*, 404–431.

Carroll, J. B. (1993). *Human cognitive abilities: A survey of factor-analytic studies.* Cambridge, England: Cambridge University Press.

Caryl, P. G. (1994). Early event-related potentials correlate with inspection time and intelligence. *Intelligence, 18*, 15–46.

Caryl, P. G., & Harper, A. (1996). Event related potentials (ERPs) in elementary cognitive tasks reflect task difficulty and task threshold. *Intelligence, 22*, 1–22.

Craik, K. (1943). *The nature of explanation.* Cambridge, England: Cambridge University Press.

Deary, I. J. (1993a). Inspection time and WAIS–R IQ subtypes: A confirmatory factor analysis study. *Intelligence, 17*, 223–236.

Deary, I. J. (1993b, April). *Speed of information processing and verbal ability.* Paper presented at the Rodin Remediation Conference, London.

Deary, I. J. (1994a). Sensory discrimination and intelligence: Postmortem or resurrection? *American Journal of Psychology, 107*, 95–115.

Deary, I. J. (1994b). Intelligence and auditory discrimination: Separating processing speed and fidelity of stimulus representation. *Intelligence, 18*, 189–213.

Deary, I. J. (1995). Auditory inspection time and intelligence: What is the direction of causation? *Developmental Psychology, 31*, 237–250.

Deary, I. J. (1996). Reductionism and intelligence: The case of inspection time. *Journal of Biosocial Science, 28*, 405–423.

Deary, I. J. (1997a). Intelligence and information processing. In H. Nyborg (Ed.), *The scientific study of human nature: Tribute to Hans Eysenck at eighty* (pp. 282–310). Elmsford, NY: Pergamon Press.

Deary, I. J. (1997b, July). *Intelligence and the discrimination of temporal order.* Paper presented at the Fifth European Congress of Psychology, Dublin, Ireland.

Deary, I. J., & Caryl, P. G. (1993). Intelligence, EEG and evoked potentials. In P. A. Vernon (Ed.), *Biological approaches to human intelligence* (pp. 259–315). Norwood, NJ: Ablex.

Deary, I. J., & Caryl, P. G. (1997). Not so F.A.S.T., Dr. Vickers! *Intelligence, 24*, 397–404.

Deary, I. J., Caryl, P. G., Egan, V., & Wight, D. (1989). Visual and auditory inspection time: Their interrelationship and correlations with IQ in high ability subjects. *Personality and Individual Differences, 10*, 525–533.

Deary, I. J., Caryl, P. G., & Gibson, G. J. (1993). Nonstationarity and the measurement of psychophysical response in a visual inspection time task. *Perception, 22,* 1245–1256.

Deary, I. J., Ebmeier, K. P., MacLeod, K. M., Dougall, N., Hepburn, D. A., Frier, B. M., & Goodwin, G. M. (1994). PASAT performance and the pattern of uptake of 99mTC-exametazine in brain estimated with single photon emission tomography. *Biological Psychology, 38,* 1–18.

Deary, I. J., Head, B., & Egan, V. (1989). Auditory inspection time, intelligence and pitch discrimination. *Intelligence, 13,* 135–148.

Deary, I. J., McCrimmon, R. J., & Bradshaw, J. (1997). Visual information processing and intelligence. *Intelligence, 24,* 461–479.

Deary, I. J., Parker, D. M., Campbell, L. J., & Nicolson, C. (1997, April). *Intelligence and visual and auditory inspection times: Two independent studies.* Paper presented at the Eighth Biennial Conference of the International Society for the Study of Individual Differences, Aarhus, Denmark.

Deary, I. J., & Stough, C. (1996). Intelligence and inspection time: Achievements, prospects, and problems. *American Psychologist, 51,* 599–608.

Di Lollo, V., Hanson, D., & McIntyre, J. S. (1983). Initial stages of information processing in dyslexia. *Journal of Experimental Psychology: Human Perception and Performance, 9,* 923–935.

Egan, V. (1994). Intelligence, inspection time and cognitive strategies. *British Journal of Psychology, 85,* 305–316.

Embretson, S. E. (1995). The role of working memory capacity and general control processes in intelligence. *Intelligence, 20,* 169–189.

Galton, F. (1883). *Inquiries into human faculty and its development.* London: Dent.

Gustafsson, J.-E. (1984). A unifying model for the structure of intellectual abilities. *Intelligence, 8,* 179–203.

Gustafsson, J.-E. (1992). The relevance of factor analysis for the study of group differences. *Multivariate Behavior Research, 27,* 239–247.

Haier, R. J. (1993). Cerebral glucose metabolism and intelligence. In P. A. Vernon (Ed.), *Biological approaches to human intelligence* (pp. 101–175). Norwood, NJ: Ablex.

Haier, R. J., Siegel, B., Neuchterlein, K. H., Hazlet, E., Wu, J., Pack, J., Browning, H., & Buchsbaum, M. S. (1988). Cortical glucose metabolic rate correlates of abstract reasoning and attention studied with positron emission tomography. *Intelligence, 12,* 199–217.

Jensen, A. R. (1983). Critical flicker frequency and intelligence. *Intelligence, 7,* 217–225.

Jensen, A. R. (1987). Individual differences in the Hick paradigm. In P. A. Vernon (Ed.), *Speed of information processing and intelligence* (pp. 101–175). Norwood, NJ: Ablex.

Kline, P. (1997). Commentary on "Quantitative science and the definition of measurement in psychology." *British Journal of Psychology, 88,* 385–387.

Kranzler, J. H., & Jensen, A. R. (1989). Inspection time and intelligence: A meta-analysis. *Intelligence, 13,* 329–347.

Kyllonen, P. C., & Christal, R. E. (1990). Reasoning ability is (little more than) working memory capacity?! *Intelligence, 14,* 389–434.

Langsford, P. B., Mackenzie, B. D., & Maher, D. P. (1994). Auditory inspection time, sustained attention, and the fundamentality of mental speed. *Personality and Individual Differences, 16,* 487–497.

Levy, P. (1992). Inspection time and its relation to intelligence: Issues of measurement and meaning. *Personality and Individual Differences, 13,* 989–1002.

McGeorge, P., Crawford, J. R., & Kelly, S. W. (1997). The relationship between WAIS-R abilities and speed of processing in a word identification task. *Intelligence, 23,* 175–190.

Neisser, U. (1997). Never a dull moment. *American Psychologist, 52,* 79–81.

Neisser, U., Boodoo, G., Bouchard, T. J., Boykin, A. W., Brody, N., Ceci, S. J., Halpern, D. F., Loehlin, J. C., Perloff, R., Sternberg, R. J., & Urbina, S. (1996). Intelligence: Knowns and unknowns. *American Psychologist, 51,* 77–101.

Nettelbeck, T. (1987). Intelligence and inspection time. In P. A. Vernon (Ed.), *Speed of information processing and intelligence* (pp. 295–346). Norwood, NJ: Ablex.

Nettelbeck, T., Edwards, C., & Vreugdenhil, A. (1986). Inspection time and IQ: Evidence for a mental speed–ability association. *Personality and Individual Differences, 7,* 633–641.

Phillips, W. A., & Singer, W. (1974). Function and interaction of on and off transients in vision: I. Psychophysics. *Experimental Brain Research, 19,* 493–506.

Poppel, E. (1994). Temporal mechanisms in perception. *International Review of Neurobiology, 37,* 185–202.

Rae, C., Scott, R. B., Thompson, C. H., Kemp, G. J., Dumughn, I., Styles, P., Tracey, I., & Radda,

G. K. (1996). Is pH a biochemical marker of IQ? *Proceedings of the Royal Society of London, Series B-Biological, 263,* 1061–1064.

Raz, N., & Willerman, L. (1985). Aptitude-related differences in auditory information processing: Effects of selective attention and tone duration. *Personality and Individual Differences, 6,* 299–304.

Raz, N., Willerman, L., & Yama, M. (1987). On sense and senses: Intelligence and auditory information processing. *Personality and Individual Differences, 8,* 201–210.

Rijsdijk, F. V., & Boomsma, D. I. (1997). Genetic mediation of the correlation between peripheral nerve conduction velocity and IQ. *Behaviour Genetics, 27,* 87–98.

Rushton, J. P., & Ankey, C. D. (1996). Brain size and cognitive ability: Correlations with age, sex, social class, and race. *Psychonomic Bulletin and Review, 3,* 21–36.

Singer, W., & Phillips, W. A. (1974). Function and interaction of on and off transients in vision: II. Neurophysiology. *Experimental Brain Research, 19,* 507–521.

Spearman, C. (1904). "General intelligence," objectively determined and measured. *American Journal of Psychology, 15,* 201–293.

Spearman, C. (1923). *The nature of "intelligence" and the principles of cognition.* London: Macmillan.

Sternberg, R. J. (1977). Component processing in analogical reasoning. *Psychological Review, 84,* 353–378.

Sternberg, R. J. (1990). *Metaphors of mind.* Cambridge, England: Cambridge University Press.

Sternberg, R. J. (1997). Inspection time for inspection time: Reply to Deary and Stough. *American Psychologist, 52,* 1144–1150.

Sternberg, R. J., & Gardner, M. K. (1983). Unities in inductive reasoning. *Journal of Experimental Psychology: General, 112,* 80–116.

Thorndike, E. L., Lay, W., & Dean, P. R. (1909). The relation of accuracy in sensory discrimination to general intelligence. *American Journal of Psychology, 20,* 364–369.

Vernon, P. A. (Ed.). (1987). *Speed of information processing and intelligence.* Norwood, NJ: Ablex.

Vickers, D. (1995). The frequency accrual speed test (FAST): A new measure of "mental speed?" *Personality and Individual Differences, 19,* 863–879.

Vickers, D., Foreman, E. A., Nicholls, M. E. R., Innes, N. J., & Gott, R. E. (1989). Some experimental tests of the application of an interval of uncertainty model to a time-limited expanded judgment task. In D. Vickers & P. L. Smith (Eds.), *Human information processing: Measures, mechanisms and models* (pp. 253–265). Amsterdam: North-Holland.

Vickers, D., & McDowell, A. (1996). Accuracy in the frequency accrual speed test (FAST), inspection time and psychometric intelligence in a sample of primary school children. *Personality and Individual Differences, 20,* 463–469.

Vickers, D., Nettelbeck, T., & Willson, R. J. (1972). Perceptual indices of performance: The measurement of "inspection time" and "noise" in the visual system. *Perception, 1,* 263–295.

Vickers, D., Pietsch, A., & Hemingway, T. (1995). Intelligence and visual and auditory discrimination: Evidence that the relationship is not due to the rate at which sensory information is sampled. *Intelligence, 21,* 197–224.

Warren, R. M. (1993). Perception of acoustic sequences: Global integration versus temporal resolution. In S. McAdams & E. Bigand (Eds.), *Thinking in sound: The cognitive psychology of human audition* (pp. 37–68). Oxford, England: Oxford University Press.

Discussion

Deary, perhaps the consummate debater, fielded a barrage of questions at the end of his presentation, which mostly focused on the controversial aspects of the implications of results from the inspection time paradigm. Brief discussion about the meaning of intelligence for dyslexia followed.

Dr. Stankov: You have done a lot of very good interesting work in inspection time. You have been a prime mover in emphasizing the importance of it. And then I think you have addressed some of the concerns that I had in the past about it today. But then I still am not enthused about it all. And the reasons for that are as follows:

I have problems with the psychometric work that people like yourself are doing. In that the batteries of test that you use are very limited. You have usually one test of fluid intelligence, another test of crystallized intelligence. Sometimes you will then include the spatial test, but nothing more than that. And that is limited from my point of view. And in particular, because with your visual inspection time, a Spatial Ability factor might be particularly relevant. And also, there is the perceptual speed component that is measured in typical tests of intelligence. So in terms of Carroll's model or Gf–Gc theory model, you are perhaps limited in your definition of psychometric domain.

In auditory domain . . . you might be doing it, but I have no recollection at this stage. Checking the sensitivity, the acuity, auditory acuity of your subjects, and that might be critical. I also have concerns about psychophysics.

Now, I know that in auditory domain it had to do with your decision to toss out the subjects because of tone deafness which is a very poorly defined construct. And tone-deaf people cannot sing, but they can hear tones. They can speak to us and understand — hear us talk. So they distinguish tones, and that sounds a little bit questionable to me as a procedure of tossing them out. And I'm worried about the fact that one of the originators of that theory has moved on to another model instead of inspection time. And he is using the interpretation in terms of working memory rather than in terms of the speed.

Dr. Deary: There are different questions there, and thanks for giving me the opportunity to talk in reference to some of these other issues. The first is a proper comment, that one can make about almost any area, which is the complaint of incompleteness. That is, there isn't a study to date with, say, a full French and Ekstrom Kit of Factor-Referenced abilities and inspection time. However, there are now dozens of studies of inspection time with different psychometric ability tasks and batteries including studies with the WAIS [Wechsler Adult Intelligence Scale] and studies with the WISC [Wechsler Intelligence Scale for Children]. While there's no doubt about this association between inspection time and psychometric ability, you can always make the comment that you haven't used absolutely every mental ability task in association with IT [inspection time]. One could certainly encourage more extensive batteries with better factor-referenced kits. I don't accept that as a criticism except that it's always better to do more extensive work in an area. But if one compares it with every other information-processing measure, IT has got more extensive correlations with different types of mental ability tasks at the psychometric level than others.

The second comment was about checking for acuity. In the inspection time task which involved visual stimuli, we worked with the othalamic people in Edinburgh, and we don't just take visual acuity into account. We take near point and contrast sensitivity at times into account also (e.g., Deary, McCrimmon, & Bradshaw, J., 1997). In visual acuity people can proceed with corrected vision, usually "six–six" or better. Therefore, nobody's ever left out unless they can't see. Because almost all people can do these studies, there's absolutely no problem with leaving people out there.

The auditory thing. As you know, I have said at great length in my papers that there is this problem that given very, very long durations there's still a substantial minority of people who cannot tell two tones 110 Hertz apart. We've adopted various strategies to try and take account of this. One, as you say, is to use measures of pitch discrimination; and leaving out people with poor pitch discrimination (Deary, Head, & Egan, 1989). We've tried putting pitch discrimination in as a covariate and we've tried putting both in and trying to extract latent traits (Deary, 1994b). There is a new task that uses phase shifted sine waves to produce a directional movement in tones. Subjects have to detect whether a tone appears on the left or the right before a mask appears in the middle (Deary, Parker, Campbell, & Nicolson, 1997).

You mentioned the frequency accrual speed test of Doug Vickers where, in fact, Doug Vickers has gone over to a working memory description. Let me just say two things about that. Doug, as you know, Lazar, and I are in contact a lot. And I said to Doug, "Well, Doug, why did you move from inspection time on to some of these new tasks?" And he said, "Well, this is the reason." He said, "Psychologists are a bit like water buffaloes. They find a new parameter or a new task and that's a bit like water buffaloes coming across a beautiful, clean, clear pool in a desert. They all realize it's the only one around, so they all rush around it. And as soon as they've got to it, this becomes muddy and disturbed. I thought my IT was like this pool. It just got all muddied up and disturbed." So he said, "I'm going off to a new water hole and find my own new clear pool." So he's developed these new tasks.

And I'll just describe very briefly the frequency accrual speed task. It's a little panel in the visual modality with two light emitting dials. And what you see — if you just look at my fingers and pretend they are the light emitting dials — you get flashes alternating like flash–flash, flash–flash, flash, flash–flash–flash–flash, flash. And over a while you've got to decide which side had more flashes.

Now, in a critique we've got coming out in *Intelligence* (Deary & Caryl, 1997), we said at least two things about his task which, in fact, he's now accepted. One is the train of flashes is so long it's very, very supraspan: it's a memory task. And it shows characteristics of memory tasks. It's got a recency effect. The second is that the duration for which each flash is presented is 50 milliseconds with a 50-millisecond gap: well beyond what we would expect for any processing limitation on an unmasked stimulus. So what we're essentially saying is: The task doesn't tap processing limitations because the stimuli are never brief enough for any to be missed and for individual differences to be measured in that. And the second thing is that it's such a long span before you actually make the response it probably does tap memory. So for those two reasons — yes, it probably is a different task, and it's probably irrelevant rather than contradictory to inspection time research.

Dr. Stanovich: Ian, on your list of other temporal and masking tasks, you had the Lovegrove spatial frequency work. And I was wondering what your interpretation of that work is, showing differences in a population and with the reading disabled population where there's a dissociation between that disability and intelligence.

Dr. Deary: I'm reminded of a talk I gave to the Royal Society in London (Deary, 1993) at a dyslexia conference. There were those who saw dyslexia as basically a problem of phonological encoding. And people like John Stein from Oxford and Lovegrove from Australia said, "Well, basically it's a problem of visual information processing." And, of course, somebody at some point asked a very good question. How can it be the case that people with reading disabilities have got very poor backward masking but are said to have normal mental abilities? And I think that's a difficult question to answer. Not one that I could answer here.

Dr. Stanovich: That's the essence of the paradox I'm getting at. I mean you have an indicator of a kind of a global *g*; and then you have an indicator of a disability that's been analyzed in modular terms. How do you have both?

Dr. Deary: Yes. Well, that's precisely what I'm trying to articulate as well. Di Lollo, Hanson, and McIntyre's (1983) work as well might indicate that kind of thing in dyslexia. There is a possible contradiction. But, of course, if we can explain 98% of the population, that will do for a wee while.

6

Individual Differences in Priming: The Roles of Implicit Facilitation From Prior Processing

DAN J. WOLTZ

The term *memory priming* refers to measurable facilitation in task performance that is attributable to a prior processing event. Whereas all learning could be described as facilitation from prior experience, priming is unique in two respects. First, the term *priming* generally refers to facilitation from a single and well-defined prior event (e.g., exposure to a word or a picture or a specific problem to be solved) rather than multiple events or a multifaceted event (e.g., completing an academic course, listening to a lecture, reading a book). Second, priming is presumed to be independent of conscious recollection of the learning episode. In most other forms of cognitive learning, the effect of prior experience is measured with deliberate recall of events or information presented in events. Priming measures assess facilitation in performance without reference to the event thought to be responsible for the facilitation, and evidence of priming is often accompanied by a demonstration of its independence from event recall (e.g., Tulving, Schacter, & Stark, 1982). For these reasons, priming is described as an implicit rather than explicit memory measure.

Priming as defined here might be considered an elementary learning event in memory. It is elementary in that it represents learning from a single exposure to a stimulus or event and because it represents measurable memory phenomena for which the learner has little or no conscious control. The underlying question addressed in this chapter is whether priming is also an elementary component of more complex forms of learning. This question is difficult to answer, and it eventually will require a variety of research approaches to address adequately. The question is approached here by investigating individual differences in priming relative to several forms of learning. I first describe distinctions among several forms of priming along with theoretically driven predictions concerning the roles of different priming processes in more complex forms of learning. I then review empirical evidence related to these predictions, along with a discussion of how these ideas fit into broader conceptualizations of learning aptitude.

Priming Distinctions

Direct or Repetition Priming Versus Indirect or Semantic Priming

One distinguishing feature among priming tasks is whether the priming events directly or indirectly correspond to the target events on which facilitation is measured. The term *direct priming* or *repetition priming* refers to performance facilitation (i.e., shorter processing time or fewer errors) observed on a target processing event that is identical, or nearly identical, to a previous processing event. For example, if individuals are asked to read a word list, their subsequent tachistoscopic identification of those words in the same typography is facilitated relative to new words (e.g., Jacoby, 1983). Similarly, prior exposure to words in a list facilitates word fragment completion, such as recognizing the solution to _O_Q__TO as the word MOSQUITO (e.g., Tulving et al., 1982). Repetition priming effects such as these have been shown to be relatively long-lasting (weeks and months in some studies), dependent on the repetition of stimulus-specific perceptual features (i.e., encoding modality, typography, and so forth) and independent of participants' recognition that the stimuli had been seen before (see Schacter, 1987, 1992, for reviews).

In contrast to this, the term *indirect priming* or *semantic priming* refers to performance facilitation on a target processing event that is only conceptually or semantically related to a previous priming event. For example, reading the word *bread* typically facilitates the subsequent reading time of semantically related words such as *butter*. Although there have been alternative views postulated, this facilitation is generally thought to reflect the automatic spread of activation among semantically associated elements in a memory network (Anderson, 1983a; Collins & Loftus, 1975; McNamara, 1994; Neely, 1977, 1991).

Although repetition priming can persist for week or months, indirect or semantic priming is relatively short-lived. One set of studies demonstrated this persistence difference within the same processing task (Woltz, 1990; Woltz & Shute, 1995). The task involved repetitions of word meaning comparisons (*big = gigantic?*). In Woltz's (1990) study, repetitions were manipulated to be either identical repetitions (*big gigantic* repeated as *big gigantic*) or semantically related repetitions (*big gigantic* repeated as *large huge*). Priming was defined as latency reductions on repeated compared with nonrepeated trials. Whereas semantic priming effects were only marginally evident after five intervening trials, identity repetition priming effects were large and stable over the maximum lag investigated (15 trials). In another study, identity repetition priming effects were found to be remarkably strong after 1 month (Woltz & Shute, 1995).

Perceptual Versus Conceptual Repetition Priming

Within the category of direct or repetition priming measures, the distinction between perceptual (data-driven) priming and conceptual priming has become increasingly important in recent years. Repetition priming can be primarily perceptual in nature in that facilitation from repeated processing events depends on the perceptual similarity of the prime and target events (e.g., Blaxton, 1989; Jacoby, 1983; Roediger & Challis, 1992; Toth, Reingold, & Jacoby, 1994; Weldon & Roediger, 1987). Conversely, repetition priming can be largely conceptual in nature, or it can be a mix of perceptual and conceptual facilitation (e.g., Blaxton, 1989; Hamann, 1990; Rappold & Hashtroudi, 1991; Srinivas & Roediger, 1990; Weldon, 1993; Woltz, 1996). In other words, repetition priming can depend as much or more on the repetition of nonperceptual processes (e.g., meaning retrieval, semantic comparisons, etc.) as on the repetition of perceptual processes. Indirect or semantic priming effects are necessarily conceptually driven in nature because prime and target trials share few if any perceptual features.

The vast majority of implicit memory research has relied on perceptually driven repetition priming measures to define implicit memory functions (Roediger, 1990; Srinivas & Roediger, 1990). Correspondingly, theories of separate memory systems for implicit and explicit memory phenomena primarily reflect the distinction between perceptual repetition priming and episodic memory for the perceptual priming events (Schacter, 1990; Tulving & Schacter, 1990). Despite this past focus on perceptual priming, I believe that the eventual impact of implicit memory theory and research for understanding real-world complex behavior will ultimately depend on the understanding of conceptual priming (both direct and indirect). Although perceptual priming may play an important role in complex perceptual performances, it seems less likely that it plays a major role in cognitively complex tasks such as language comprehension, problem solving, and complex cognitive skill acquisition. On the other hand, it seems plausible that conceptual priming could play a considerable role, but one that has not yet been fully understood. Consistent with this view, in this chapter I focus on evidence regarding individual differences in both conceptually driven repetition priming and semantic priming and their relationships to differences in more complex forms of learning.

Most priming evidence reviewed in this chapter comes from the repeated meaning comparison task described earlier. Although identity repetitions in this task conceivably could reflect perceptual priming, earlier work has demonstrated that only about 10%–15% of the repetition priming effects in this task are attributable to perceptual overlap (Woltz, 1990, 1996). Instead, a majority of the priming effect is due to the repetition of meaning comparisons (Woltz, 1996).[1] Thus, individual differences in repetition priming in this task are presumed to primarily reflect conceptual priming differences. Individual differences that are specific to perceptual priming are not addressed here, and I know of little work that has been done in this area (see Perruchet & Baveux, 1989).

---

[1] Other evidence suggests that priming in the meaning comparison task does not depend on explicit recognition of prior trials (Woltz & Madsen, 1998).

Repetition Priming and Learning From Repetitive Practice

Theoretical Links Between Repetition Priming and Skill Acquisition

As described, typical measures of repetition priming assess performance facilitation attributable to an identical recurrence of one prior processing event. Similarly, a broad class of skill acquisition paradigms represents the accumulated facilitation from repeated processing events that are identical or differ only slightly from one another. Identity repetitions within the practice of a skill constitute a high degree of consistent mapping of task demands, a characteristic that is fundamental to performance improvements (Ackerman, 1988; Schneider & Shiffrin, 1977; Shiffrin & Schneider, 1977).

At least two current learning theories of skill acquisition emphasize the role of memory changes that are due to identical or nearly identical processing repetitions. Most notably, Logan's (1988) theory of skill acquisition is entirely instance based. According to this theory, the development of skilled performance depends on the shift from algorithm-based performance (i.e., application of verbal performance rules) to the direct retrieval of specific instances that have been encountered during practice. Logan (1990) linked the phenomenon of repetition priming from a single event to the gradual accumulation of instance representations. Similarly, Anderson's (1983b, 1993) adaptive character of thought theories of learning include knowledge compilation and tuning mechanisms that allow for general-purpose knowledge to become highly specialized with respect to instance-specific task demands that are repeated during skill acquisition. Consistent with repetition priming phenomena, Anderson (1983b, 1993) has suggested that this proceduralization can occur with a single repetition.

Not everyone, however, has agreed that skill acquisition and repetition priming represent the same underlying memory processes. Schwartz and Hashtroudi (1991) reviewed clinical neuropsychological evidence and concluded that different forms of neurological impairment selectively affect priming and skill acquisition. They also produced evidence using the fragment completion task that was inconsistent with evidence on this issue produced by Logan (1988, 1990) using different tasks.

Kirsner and Speelman (1996) also reported evidence that is inconsistent with the notion that repetition priming and skill acquisition reflect common processes. Using a lexical-decision task, they found that power functions fitted both preexperimental practice data (i.e., performance differences for words with different word frequency estimates) and experimental data (i.e., repetition priming performance). However, the slope estimates were inconsistent across these two forms of data. They also failed to find the gradual increase in priming with practice reported by Logan (1988, 1990). Thus, there is some debate about the relationship between repetition priming and skill acquisition.

One form of evidence not considered by either Logan (1988), Kirsner and Speelman (1996), or Schwartz and Hashtroudi (1991) is the relationship between individual differences in repetition priming and skill acquisition. Although this form of evidence alone cannot resolve the issue, it can provide an alternative test of the various positions. If priming and skill performance are correlated at stages of skill acquisition where instance-based learning is presumed to occur, this would be consistent with the common process stance. A potentially more informative result would

138

be if no correlation were found or if the pattern of correlation over time did not correspond to predictions of instance representation. Such findings would be difficult to reconcile with a common process explanation of repetition priming and skill acquisition.

The correlation between repetition priming and skill acquisition was initially investigated by Woltz (1988). This research showed a relationship between conceptual repetition priming measures (both meaning comparisons and category membership decisions) and a hierarchical if–then rule application task that involved repetitive practice. Repetition priming contributed to explaining skill acquisition performance beyond that of working memory, verbal knowledge, and task-specific processing speed measures. Furthermore, the pattern of correlations between repetition priming and skill performance over practice was distinct from that of knowledge and working memory. Although the knowledge and working memory measures explained more learning variance early in practice, priming and processing speed explained more variance late in skill practice. Chaiken (1993) qualified this finding by demonstrating that the temporal proximity of measures affected the magnitude of the relationships, but he also replicated the general finding.

Relations Among Priming, Recognition, and Skill Acquisition

Following Woltz's (1988) and Chaiken's (1993) work, a more comprehensive test of the relationship between repetition priming and later stages of skill acquisition was conducted by Woltz (1993). The study included measures of repetition priming, episodic recognition, and skill acquisition in three content domains: numeric, spatial, and verbal. This design provided the opportunity to address questions about the generality of priming differences across notably different tasks, the relationship of individual differences in priming and recognition, and the relationship of priming and episodic memory, both domain-specific and general, to skill acquisition.

Overview of the method. In that study, 305 Air Force recruits performed three conceptual repetition priming tasks, one each with verbal, numeric, and spatial item content. The verbal task used repeated meaning comparison trials, as described earlier. The numeric task involved repeated addition and subtraction problems (e.g., $42 - 11$; $17 + 32$). The spatial task used repeated mental rotation problems. Both the numeric and spatial tasks resembled the verbal priming task in that responses were L (for *like*) or D (for *different*), corresponding to conceptual comparisons. In each priming task the repeated trials occurred at lags of 1, 6, 36, and 144 trials. Positive mean priming effects were evident in each measure, and they declined systematically with lag.

For analysis of individual differences in priming, speed scores from second occurrence trials were regressed on speed scores from first occurrence trials within lag.[2] The residuals were used as the index of priming magnitude. Positive residuals

[2] Speed scores were computed as follows: For each trial type, a performance index was computed as the number of correct trials per unit time (i.e., response speed adjusted for errors). This index for contrasting first- and second-occurrence trials had the advantage of combining priming variance that was otherwise distributed across two variables (latency and errors). Also, as a speed rather than time metric, the sample distributions more closely approximated normal distributions.

reflected greater speed on the second occurrence trials than was expected given first occurrence speed, and negative residuals reflected lower speed on second occurrence trials than expected. As was the case in previous research using similar measures (Woltz, 1988, 1990; Woltz & Shute, 1993), residuals were more reliable indexes of priming than simple differences or the percentage of change scores.

After each priming task, participants performed old–new recognition probes that were in the same format as the priming trials. Rather than responding to the similarity of the stimuli, participants responded as to whether they had seen the trial during the previous task (half of all trials were new). Recognition performance as indexed by d' was reliably above chance in each task. The recognition data provided a test of the interpretation that priming effects and their relationship to learning may represent a general memory ability for prior processing events rather one that is specific to implicit memory measurement.

Finally, participants in this study performed three cognitive skill acquisition tasks modeled after the if–then task used earlier (Chaiken, 1993; Woltz, 1988). A verbal skill task represented a simplified version of that used in the earlier studies. Spatial and numeric skill tasks were developed to have the same hierarchical rule structure as the verbal task but requiring evaluations of figural and numeric stimuli, respectively. According to Chaiken's (1993) evidence, fixing the skill acquisition tasks after the priming and recognition tasks meant that task proximity effects would work against the hypothesized increase in correlation with later skill blocks. Data from all three skill acquisition tasks were well fitted by two-parameter power functions (Newell & Rosenbloom, 1981), even at the individual level. They therefore appeared to be reasonable skill learning tasks on which to test the hypothesized relationships.

The relationship between priming and recognition.   The first question of interest in this study was whether individual differences in priming magnitude were correlated with recognition. As described earlier, independence of priming from recognition is a hallmark of implicit memory phenomena. However, most of this evidence comes from data-driven rather than conceptually driven priming measures, and independence is typically assessed in ways other than sample correlations between measures. The most widely cited form of evidence is that patients with amnesia who had severely impaired memory for recent events performed within normal limits on certain implicit memory tasks (e.g., Graf, Squire, & Mandler, 1984; Warrington & Weiskrantz, 1970). Conditional or stochastic independence of implicit and explicit memory task performance has also been demonstrated in studies using participants with normal memory for recent events (e.g., Jacoby & Dallas, 1981; Tulving et al., 1982). In those studies, the likelihood of performance facilitation on a given item was shown to be independent of correct recognition of that item. Finally, some studies with normal individuals have provided evidence that implicit and explicit measures are functionally independent with respect to task manipulations (e.g., Jacoby, 1983; Roediger & Challis, 1992; Weldon & Roediger, 1987).

These various findings of independence, however, do not necessarily support a prediction that implicit and explicit measures will be uncorrelated in the normal adult population. The rank orderings of individuals on priming magnitude and recognition accuracy could be similar, despite the fact that the measures are functionally and stochastically independent. Furthermore, the lack of correlation between implicit and explicit measures when patients with amnesia and normal participants are compared (i.e., a mean difference in explicit measures but no difference in implicit measures) indicates little about the correlation of the two measures within these groups before the onset of the memory disorder (or what the relationship is within the normal group). Unfortunately, prior estimates of the correlation between implicit and explicit memory measures within normal populations are scarce and inconsistent (Perruchet & Baveux, 1989). The importance of estimating the relationship between priming and recognition in normal populations is not simply to test the same independence assumption that has been tested with other methods. It tests a conceptually different form of independence.

The relationship between episodic recognition and priming in this study was estimated with confirmatory factor analysis (Bentler, 1995). Figure 6.1 shows a factor model that includes general priming and recognition factors as well as domain- and task-specific factors for both priming and recognition. There were four recognition variables in each domain (d' for positive match and negative match trials at two levels of exposure). There were also four priming variables in each domain (residual scores for repetitions at the four lags). The model shown in Figure 6.1 was contrasted with alternative models in a manner consistent with more conventional multitrait–multimethod investigations (Widaman, 1985). The model in Figure 6.1 had a significantly better fit than alternative models that contained (a) no general factors, (b) no task-specific factors, (c) perfectly correlated general recognition and general priming factors, and (d) perfectly correlated task-specific factors for recognition and priming (i.e., perfectly correlated within but not across task domains).

The model and parameter estimates shown in Figure 6.1 suggest several conclusions. First, performance facilitation from prior events and recognition of those events constitute separate but correlated factors. Furthermore, there is a general priming ability and a general episodic recognition ability that exist after accounting for task- or domain-specific priming and recognition. For the 12 priming measures, the general and domain-specific priming factors contributed about equally. For the 12 recognition measures, the domain-specific factors contributed somewhat more than the general factor.

As can be seen in Figure 6.1, general recognition and priming factors had a notable correlation. The task-specific recognition and priming factors were also positively correlated. A zero correlation between recognition and priming would be most easily interpreted vis-à-vis other evidence for independence between implicit and explicit memory measures. Conversely, the presence of a positive correlation has several possible interpretations. First, a significant correlation could reflect a causal relationship between recognition and priming processes, and the direction of causation could be in either direction. Performance facilitation in priming could be due to explicit item and response recognition. Alternatively, perceived performance fluency associated with priming could influence recognition judgments, especially when explicit recollection is poor (see Johnston, Hawley, & Elliott, 1991). Evidence from another study suggested that the later of these interpretations is possibly true, but it is more likely that neither is true.

In a recent study by Woltz and Madsen (1998), participants made recognition judgments immediately after performing word meaning comparison items used to measure priming. Repetition lags in this study ranged from a few minutes to 1 month. Results showed that participants responded more quickly on priming trials that they said were old, but this was the case regardless of whether the item actually

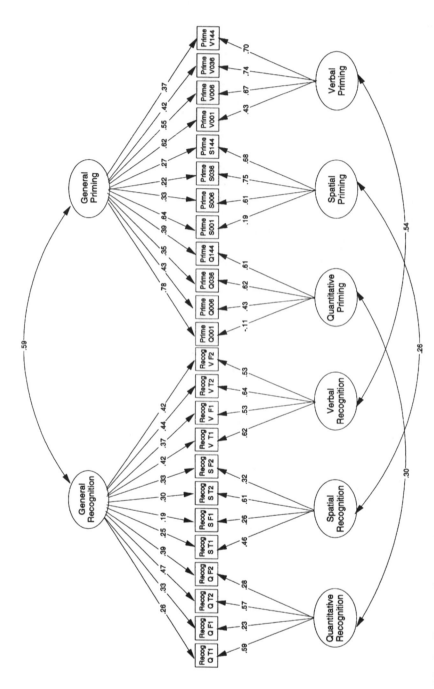

Figure 6.1. Confirmatory factor analysis model for priming and recognition (Recog) measures. A standardized solution is shown. For simplicity, error in the model is not shown. Errors for negative match recognition variables were allowed to correlate within content domain. Model fit statistics: $\chi^2 = 301.80$ (221, $N = 305$); comparative fit index (CFI) = .964. Q = quantitative; S = spatial; V = verbal; T = time.

was old (primed) or new (unprimed). This outcome is least compatible with the interpretation that recognition drives the performance facilitation seen in repeated trials (i.e., priming). It is potentially compatible with the interpretation that recognition judgments are helped by perceived facilitation from priming. However, if participants used perceived fluency in making recognition judgments, it could produce a positive correlation between the two measures only if this strategy improved recognition performance. Counter to this, recognition judgments were no more accurate when they followed performance of the trial than when they were made without performance. Even if using perceived fluency was a common strategy for making recognition judgments, it probably was not helpful because the variation in item complexity was large relative to the typical magnitude of priming.

In contrast to a causal interpretation, the correlation between priming and recognition could simply reflect a common processing factor influencing both measures. Given the findings of Woltz and Madsen (1998), this seems to be the most plausible interpretation. Interpreting the estimated correlation as a shared influence on priming and recognition is not necessarily incompatible with the other evidence for independence of these memory phenomena. The prior evidence has led some to postulate separate memory systems for implicit and explicit memory processes (Schacter, 1990; Tulving & Schacter, 1990).[3] However, even neurologically distinguishable memory systems reside within the same nervous system and are likely to be subject to general physiological or psychological characteristics that may affect all processes. Given the long history of finding positive correlations among a wide variety of ability measures, it seems unreasonable to expect two memory measures to yield distributions that are completely uncorrelated, even if the measures are dissociated in other ways.

Relationships of priming to skill acquisition and other abilities. The Armed Services Vocational Aptitude Battery (ASVAB) scores were available on all but 8 of the participants in this study (Department of Defense, 1984). Of the 10 subtests, seven (all but the technical knowledge tests) were used to estimate two factors that were based on prior analyses of ASVAB subtests (Kyllonen & Christal, 1990). A perceptual speed factor had two simple speeded tasks as indicators: Code Speed and Numerical Operations. A general ability factor had reasoning, knowledge, and language indicators: Arithmetic Reasoning, Math Knowledge, Word Knowledge, General Science, and Paragraph Comprehension.

Neither the general recognition nor general priming factors had strong relationships to the ASVAB factors. The only statistically significant correlation ($p < .05$) was .19, between general priming and perceptual speed. Therefore, consistent with previous evidence, recognition and priming abilities appear to have little in common with conventional ability constructs (see Underwood, Boruch, & Malmi, 1978; Woltz, 1990).

A question of primary interest in this study concerned the relationship of priming and recognition to skill acquisition after varied amounts of practice. The contrast of priming and recognition as predictors was important because prior evidence of the relationship of priming to skill acquisition could reflect instance recognition (recall that priming and episodic recognition were correlated).

---

[3] Note that the proposals for separate memory systems pertain exclusively to perceptual priming.

Figure 6.2 shows correlation estimates for the priming and two ASVAB factors with skill performance by block for each of the three skill tasks.[4] Correlations for the general recognition and task-specific factors are not shown because they rarely approached statistical significance. Several findings were noteworthy in these estimates. First, the general priming factor was correlated with all three skill acquisition tasks (and as mentioned, the domain-specific factors were not). This suggests that prior evidence of priming predicting skill learning did not reflect merely task-specific variance or method overlap. It appears that general ability to benefit from repeated events is what predicts performance differences associated with repetitive practice in cognitive skill acquisition. Second, although the recognition and priming factors were themselves correlated, only priming had consistent, statistically significant relationships with skill performance. Thus, performance facilitation from repeated events appears to be distinct from recognition of repeated events in its relationship to this class of learning task. Third, the pattern of relationships over the observed time course of learning replicated prior findings for relatively simple skills (Ackerman, 1988; Chaiken, 1993; Woltz, 1988). In all three learning tasks, general ability had its strongest relationships in the early or middle stages of observed practice, whereas perceptual speed had a steadily increasing relationship with performance except in the spatial skill task, where it had no appreciable relationship. Of primary importance, the general priming factor had an increasing relationship over the observed practice blocks.

Together, these patterns of correlation suggest that different learning and aptitude processes are instrumental at various phases of the cognitive skill acquisition studied here. General knowledge and reasoning skill, perhaps including working memory, appear to be instrumental in early learning blocks when rules must be remembered and applied.[5] As the declarative rules become proceduralized and their application demands less verbal recall and working memory, general ability relationships drop. Coinciding with this, performance most likely becomes increasingly dependent on procedural memory and, in these tasks, probably instance-specific memory.[6] This presumably drives the increasing relationship between repetition priming and skill performance in the later blocks observed in these tasks. Perceptual speed also increases in its relationship to performance in two of the three tasks. This presumably reflects the fact that performance efficiency relies more on speed of encoding and responding after the general ability and working memory demands subside (see Ackerman, 1988).

Summary of findings and interpretations. Repetition priming and episodic recognition measures yielded separate but correlated factors that were general across

---

[4]For analysis of individual differences in the skill tasks, latency and error by block were combined into adjusted speed indexes as described for the priming measures.

[5]This study did not include a separate measure of working memory. However, prior evidence has shown the same pattern of results for working memory as was found for the general ability factor here (Woltz, 1988), and Kyllonen and Christal (1990) found a strong relationship between factors defined by the Armed Services Vocational Aptitude Battery subtests and working memory factors.

[6]Unpublished evidence for the numeric skill learning task used in this study suggests that instance memory is important to learning. A subset of instances was withheld from practice and then introduced at different times for different participants. Old–new instance differences were evident as early as Block 4, and they systematically increased as practice increased.

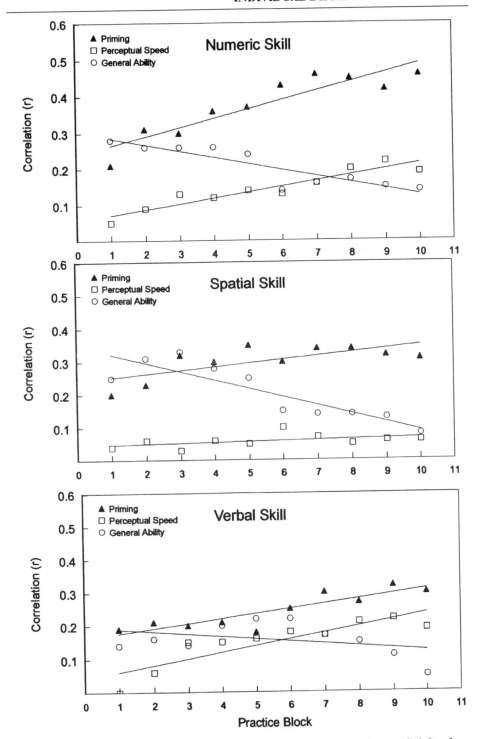

Figure 6.2. Estimated correlations of priming, perceptual speed, and general ability factors with skill acquisition tasks by practice block.

145

verbal, spatial, and numeric content domains. The correlation between these two general factors probably represents common underlying influences on priming and recognition performance rather than a causal influence from one to the other. However, additional evidence is needed to test this interpretation. Neither the priming nor the recognition factor was related to conventional ability factors of general ability and perceptual speed. Finally, as predicted, the priming factor alone correlated with skill performance, and the relationship increased through later stages of skill practice, when learners are presumed to make transitions to instance-based representations of the skills.

Priming and Other Forms of Repetitive Learning

The evidence just described is consistent with the notion that individual differences in facilitation from single events in part determines who benefits most from multiple exposures during extended practice. This interpretation is consistent with instance-based skill learning theories (e.g., Anderson, 1983b, 1993; Logan, 1988), but it is not the only interpretation possible. An alternative explanation is that priming represents a type of processing speed measure and that processing speed measures increase in their relationship to learning over moderate amounts of practice on consistently mapped tasks (Ackerman, 1988, 1990, 1992). However, evidence reported by Woltz and Shute (1993) is inconsistent with this alternative interpretation. They demonstrated that individual differences in priming are related to other forms of learning that involve repetitive practice and that the relationship does not always parallel that of processing speed.

In one study by Woltz and Shute (1993), 274 Air Force recruits performed a computerized associative learning task modeled after the digit symbol task common to individual intelligence tests. At the top of the computer display, there was a row of six consonant–vowel–consonant (CVC) trigrams. Each CVC was presented above a one-syllable word with which it was to be associated (e.g., GUK might be associated with *coat*). At the bottom of the display, single probes were presented (*GUK = coat?*). Participants had to press L (for *like*) or D (for *different*) depending on whether the probe matched an association at the top of the display. Task instructions emphasized response speed without errors.

Initially, participants had to look to the top of the display to verify each probe. However, as in the digit symbol task, practice provided an opportunity to learn the associations, eventually eliminating the need for a visual search on each trial. To emphasize the learning character of this task, the location of the six CVC–word pairs was shuffled on each trial, thus making the visual search more difficult and the learning of associations more advantageous (see Ackerman & Woltz, 1994, for a more complete characterization of the demands of this learning paradigm). However, time to respond to each trial was limited so that overt memorization strategies would be difficult to use.

In contrast to the late relationship of repetition priming to simple procedural skill performance, here the relationship was greater in early trials and declined with practice. This pattern was different from both processing speed and working memory, both of which increased in their relationship to performance over the trials investigated. This demonstrated that repetition priming is not related universally to repetitive learning at later stages of practice when other processing speed variables tend to predict performance. Instead, it suggests that repetition priming predicts performance at any stage in which instance memory is important to learning.

Repetition priming rather than working memory was probably important in the early stages of learning in this paradigm because there was little or no declarative knowledge to apply. Instead, performance efficiency depended on how quickly one could acquire instance-specific associative information to replace simple visual search.[7] Working memory apparently became important to performance when most associations had been learned later in practice (i.e., working memory is not important to visual search, but it is important to the retrieval and verification of many newly learned associations).

In total, the correlational evidence from both skill acquisition and associative learning studies are consistent with the idea that individual differences in repetition priming reflect memory processes that are important to forms of learning that depend on repetitive practice. Furthermore, these memory processes do not appear to be tapped well by conventional ability measures. However, this conclusion must be tempered somewhat by the lack of evidence on priming and complex forms of skill acquisition that are acquired over longer learning periods.

Semantic Priming and Language Comprehension

Theoretical Links

As noted in the introduction, semantic priming is a temporary form of facilitation compared with repetition priming, and it is generally thought to reflect spreading activation in long-term memory. When a processing event (e.g., *moist = damp?*) is preceded by a recent prior event that is semantically related (e.g., *soggy = wet?*), the facilitation is presumed to reflect activation that has spread across associative links between the related terms' memory representations. This facilitation declines rapidly over a few intervening trials, which presumably reflects activation decay (see Woltz, 1990). Because of the temporary nature of this form of priming, it is not likely that individual differences would be related to the long-term buildup of skill over multiple repetitions. However, there are other forms of complex learning that theoretically depend as much or more on temporary activation processes as on the long-term strengthening of instance-based memory representations.

Reading comprehension, or language comprehension in general, has been postulated as a learning and performance domain that depends in part on spreading activation (e.g., Just & Carpenter, 1992; Just, Carpenter, & Keller, 1996). Connecting information from one unit of meaning to the next within and across sentences is thought to depend on specific comprehension processes acting on newly encoded information that is available in working memory. Some relevant information may be the focus of conscious attention or explicit rehearsal, but in reading all but the simplest passages, there is too much information for such attention-driven mainte-

---

[7] In further investigations, Ackerman and Woltz (1994) found that the reliance on retrieval versus visual search depended on both ability and volitional–motivational factors. More individuals could be induced into using retrieval with periodic memory tests and with a combination of goal-setting and self-focus instructions.

nance to suffice. Activation of elements stored in long-term memory is postulated to account for the remaining storage demands in complex domains such as language comprehension (Anderson, 1983b; Cantor & Engle, 1993; Just & Carpenter, 1992).

The central feature of Just and Carpenter's (1992; Just et al., 1996) theory is that comprehension is constrained by working memory. Working memory is defined somewhat differently in this theory than by Baddeley (1986). Rather than a central executive and storage systems that are largely attention driven, Just and Carpenter (1992) defined working memory as storage and processing elements that are all fueled by activation, which is a limited resource. Working memory capacity is equated with the amount of available activation.

Individual-Differences Evidence Linking Semantic Priming and Comprehension

Although Just and Carpenter (1992) postulated a capacity model of reading that described activation as the limiting factor in working memory, there have been few direct tests of this aspect of their theory. There are numerous demonstrations of how individual differences in specific measures of working memory capacity predict reading differences (e.g., Cantor & Engle, 1993; Daneman & Carpenter, 1980, 1983; King & Just, 1991), but there are viable alternatives to the activation interpretation of the working memory differences.

Daneman and Carpenter's (1980, 1983) reading span task has been the defining measure of working memory capacity in most research investigating working memory and reading. In this task, participants are presented with unrelated sentences to read and comprehend one at a time. The participant must also remember the final word of each sentence. Thus, like most measures of working memory, this task demands concurrent storage (the final words) and processing (the sentence comprehension). A person's reading span is indexed by how many words can be retained under these task demands. The correlation between reading span and reading comprehension measures has generally been taken to support the capacity theory of comprehension that relies on activation to define capacity (Cantor & Engle, 1993; Just & Carpenter, 1992). However, this may be an overinterpretation of the evidence because it has never been demonstrated that the reading span task measures activation more than it measures attention-driven storage and processing abilities (also see Waters & Caplan, 1996).

Engle and his colleagues provided the most direct test of the activation capacity notion in reading. In one set of experiments, Cantor and Engle (1993) investigated the interrelationships of a span measure modeled after Daneman and Carpenter's (1980, 1983) work, a fan measure of activation following earlier work by Anderson (1974), and a general reading measure. The activation definition of working memory capacity was tested by assessing whether variance in the activation measure would account for the relationship between the span measure and the reading measure. The evidence suggested that the fan measure of activation did indeed account for most of the predictive power of the working memory measure.

Support of this evidence for the activation theory of capacity rests on the assumption that the fan task primarily measured individual-differences in activation processes. Anderson (1974) first investigated the fan effect and demonstrated that the time needed to verify a fact about a subject is a positive function of how many facts are

148

known about that subject.[8] This phenomenon has been interpreted as reduced activation for each fact in accord with the number of associative links through which a finite amount of activation must spread (Anderson, 1983b). The slope representing response time as a function of fan size (the number of facts known) has been taken as an index of activation capacity. The shallower the slope, the greater the activation capacity (i.e., the less the learner's retrieval time is affected by additional associative links).

However, if this measure assesses attention-driven storage and retrieval mechanisms more than automatic activation processes, then the finding of Cantor and Engle (1993) says little about the activation capacity theory. Instead, the evidence would merely indicate that two different measures of attention-based working memory capacity (span and fan) overlap considerably in their relationship to verbal comprehension abilities. Conway and Engle (1994) in fact demonstrated in a series of experiments that an attention resource explanation of fan slope differences was more appropriate than an activation explanation. They showed that high and low working memory groups as defined by a span measure differed in fan slopes only when the subjects of the fan sentences had partially overlapping predicates (i.e., "The artist was in the boat" and "The doctor was in the boat"). Such a memory set produces interference effects that apparently require attentional resources to overcome. Consequently, empirical support was weakened for the notion that activation processes define a capacity limit in language comprehension.

In another attempt to address this issue, Larkin (1996; Larkin, Woltz, Reynolds, & Clark, 1996) conducted research investigating the relationship of activation to reading by using semantic priming rather than the fan task as an index of activation. There is no compelling reason to suspect that facilitation from semantically related word comparisons is attributable to conscious strategies or attention-driven memory processes, as appears to be the case in the fan measure. Semantically related repetitions are varied within and across trial blocks such that they are unpredictable. Furthermore, task instructions make no reference to repeated trials. During postexperimental interviews, most participants report no awareness of the semantic relatedness of trials, and those who do notice it report no performance strategies related to this awareness. It is presumed that those who show greater facilitation from semantically related repetitions do so because they have experienced a greater degree of spreading activation from prime to target trial representations in memory.

The first study (Larkin et al., 1996) investigated both repetition and semantic priming differences in 60 sixth-grade children and correlated these measures with reading ability. Both forms of priming were measured with a version of the meaning comparison task used in earlier research (Woltz, 1990). However, item content was simplified. Repetition priming lags included both within-sessions lags of a few minutes as well as 2- and 3-day lags, whereas semantic priming was assessed with lags of only one, two, and three trials. Finally, recognition of previously presented trials was also assessed both within sessions and over lags of 2 and 3 days.

Several findings in this study were important. First, semantic priming had a sig-

---

[8]A fan effect of this type appears to be present only with unrelated facts about a subject (e.g., "The lawyer is in the park"; "The lawyer is in the boat"; and "The lawyer is in the church"). When facts are related and can be organized into a schema, response times do not always increase with the number of facts known (Reder & Anderson, 1980).

nificant correlation with two reading indexes obtained: the Stanford Achievement Test (SAT) reading composite ($r = .51$) and teacher ratings of reading ability ($r = .49$). This finding suggested that, as predicted by recent reading theories, individual differences in activation are associated with differences in reading ability.

The second finding of interest was that the correlations of repetition priming with the same two indexes of reading were not statistically significant ($rs < .17$). This was true for repetition priming measured at both short and long lags. The lower relationships of repetition priming compared with semantic priming could not be explained by reliability differences. This finding suggested that repetition and semantic priming may represent distinct memory mechanisms, even when measured within the same semantic processing task.[9] Although repetition priming appears to be an important predictor of learning under repetitive practice conditions, it does not appear to be related to reading skill in children.

Finally, this study addressed the relationship of recognition memory to both reading and priming. Similar to the semantic priming measure, the recognition measure had substantial relationships with the reading measures ($rs = .45$ and $.51$, respectively, for SAT and teacher ratings). However, the semantic priming and recognition measures correlated only modestly ($r = .33$). More important, they each made statistically significant ($p < .05$) contributions to explaining reading variance in multiple regression. Thus, individual differences in semantic priming and episodic recognition of the priming events appeared to represent different aptitudes that both contributed to explaining reading differences. Priming presumably represents the activation processes described as being central to language comprehension by Just and Carpenter (1992) and others. By contrast, recognition performance may represent the more effortful recall of prior processing events that is important to reading processes such as comprehension monitoring.

This research was pursued further by Larkin (1996) to contrast the role of semantic priming in reading comprehension with that of working memory. Another goal was to investigate whether individual differences in semantic priming were distinct from differences in verbal knowledge and general processing speed. In that study, 94 sixth-grade children were administered a battery of computerized reading measures that included passages demanding disambiguation (e.g., Daneman & Carpenter, 1983) and comprehension of anaphoric references (e.g., Gernsbacher, 1989). The children also performed the semantic priming measure used by Larkin et al. (1996), a simplified version of the alphabet recoding working memory task (Woltz, 1988), the SAT Vocabulary test, and a letter-matching processing speed task (Posner, Boies, Eichelman, & Taylor, 1969).

Daneman and Carpenter's (1980, 1983) working memory measure was not used because of its heavy demand on reading. It was decided that reading differences among sixth-grade children might dominate the measure of general working memory capacity in that task. Furthermore, Engle and colleagues have demonstrated comparable relationships in adults between reading and working memory using nonreading working memory measures (see Cantor & Engle, 1993; Turner & Engle, 1989). The alphabet recoding working memory task assumed only prior knowledge of the alphabet. Each trial of this task presented the child with two noncontiguous

---

[9]This is supported by the modest correlation between semantic and repetition priming measures, which ranged from .23 at short identity repetition lags to .31 at long lags.

letters (e.g., *T K*) and a recoding distance (e.g., Forward 3). In this example, participants would have to advance *T* and *K* by three letters and select the answer (*W N*) from eight alternatives. The answer had to be computed before seeing the alternatives, so response elimination strategies were not possible. Recoding distances ranged from one to three letters. Adult versions of this task have been shown to correlate well with other working memory measures (Kyllonen & Christal, 1990).

Larkin (1996) replicated the earlier finding that semantic priming differences are important predictors of reading comprehension in children. Semantic priming correlated .60 with a composite of the computerized comprehension measures. Working memory, processing speed, and verbal knowledge measures were also correlated with comprehension (rs = .44, .33, and .62, respectively).[10] Of primary importance, semantic priming made a statistically significant ($p < .05$) contribution when all predictors were entered into a multiple regression analysis. Vocabulary and working memory also had significant regression weights, but processing speed did not.

Thus, in children aged 11–12 years, semantic priming differences appear to be an important predictor of reading comprehension. Furthermore, much of the variance in reading performance that is explained by semantic priming cannot be attributed to more general aptitude constructs such as working memory, processing speed, and verbal knowledge.

These findings are inconsistent with the notion that working memory capacity differences are equivalent to differences in activation (Cantor & Engle, 1993; Just & Carpenter, 1992). Priming and working memory measures had a modest correlation with one another, and both made unique contributions to explaining reading variance. Instead, this evidence is consistent with conclusions by Conway and Engle (1994) that working memory differences as assessed by conventional working memory measures represent a different set of capacity limits than activation (also see Waters & Caplan, 1996). Working memory limits probably reflect attention processes as described by Baddeley (1986, 1993) more than automatic activation limits.

Finally, semantic priming appears to represent activation differences that are not captured in repetition priming. The correlation between semantic and repetition priming measures was modest. Furthermore, although semantic priming predicted reading, repetition priming did not.

Summary and Conclusion

There is relatively little published evidence on individual differences in priming, either repetition or semantic. The vast majority of evidence about priming comes from experimental and clinical studies, not correlational studies. There have even been suggestions that individual differences are unimportant for processes that are outside of attentional control (e.g., Hasher & Zacks, 1979, 1984). Yet, given the major impact that experimental and clinical priming research has had on theories of the organization of human memory (e.g., Schacter, 1992; Tulving & Shacter, 1990), it seems imperative to explore the possibility that important individual differences exist for these processes within nonclinical populations.

---

[10] Semantic priming correlated with working memory only .25 but had higher correlations with vocabulary (r = .45) and processing speed (r = .48).

The evidence reviewed here suggests that there are measurable individual differences in priming, at least in conceptual priming. It remains to be seen whether this conclusion will hold for perceptual priming.

Two forms of conceptual priming were considered. Direct or repetition priming represents the degree of performance facilitation from an identical repetition of a single processing event. Individual differences presumably reflect the ability to store or strengthen event-specific memory traces that function in an implicit fashion. Indirect or semantic priming represents the degree of performance facilitation from a semantically related prior processing event. Individual differences here presumably reflect an ability or capacity for the temporary spread of activation to make long-term memory contents more available. The current evidence suggests that there are reliable individual differences in both forms of priming within both adults and children.

The evidence described here suggests that individual differences in both forms of conceptual priming may be consequential to understanding differences in certain types of learning. Repetition priming differences were shown to predict learning differences in two classes of repetitive learning tasks. In one class of skill acquisition tasks, learning proceeds from a working memory intensive application of declarative knowledge to a proceduralized application of well-practiced instances or routines. Here, repetition priming differences predicted skill performance at the point where working memory and general ability measures declined in their predictive ability. It is postulated that measuring differences in the benefit from a single repeated event taps the same ability construct that is displayed in learning, which depends on the cumulative benefit of consistent procedural repetitions. By contrast, semantic priming differences were shown to predict reading comprehension differences, a relationship not found for repetition priming. Of importance, the semantic priming relationship to reading appeared to be largely independent of the relationships between reading and working memory, episodic memory, verbal knowledge, and processing speed. This is consistent with current theories of language comprehension that postulate a central role of temporary memory activation in comprehension. However, the evidence was inconsistent with claims that working memory capacity differences are simply activation differences.

In the study of learner differences, investigations on the role of simple cognitive processes (i.e., specific and narrowly defined processes) have generally been disappointing in their ultimate impact compared with research on more general or broad ability constructs that encompass many processes. This may be due in part to measurement problems inherent in attempts to capture individual differences in highly specific processes, wherein differences may be relatively small, context specific, and represented by difference scores or unreliable model parameters (Lohman, 1994). More important, by definition, highly specific and isolated cognitive processes do not affect the variety of learning and performance domains that general aptitude constructs do. Some theorists have suggested that the most meaningful variability among learners cannot be captured by isolating individual processes but that it requires looking more interactively at the selective use and coordination of cognitive, affective, and conative processes in response to situational demands (e.g., Ackerman, 1996; Kanfer & Ackerman, 1989; Snow, 1992; Sternberg, 1994). Given these broad and compelling views of theory and research on learner differences, it seems important to consider the utility of future investigations on priming as a learning ability.

The study of individual differences in priming has two potential benefits to psychological theory. First, the advancement of detailed cognitive theories of learning depends on understanding well-defined processes. Strengthening memory elements, in both temporary and persistent ways, plays a crucial role in several prominent learning theories. Tests of the existence and importance of these postulated memory processes is often seen as the domain of experimental research. However, investigating individual differences in cognitive processes can be an important adjunct to experimental tests of theories (see Cronbach, 1957; Snow & Lohman, 1989; Underwood, 1975). Thus, investigating the role of priming in learning through the study of individual differences may benefit the development and refinement of cognitive learning theories. Note in this context that contributions of correlational evidence to general learning theories depends as much or more on the pattern of correlations across theoretically meaningful task facets as on the overall magnitude of correlations between the process and learning measures.

Second, current evidence suggests that priming measures may prove to be important predictors in their own right of differences in specific forms of learning (i.e., they may explain as much or more variance as conventional ability measures) and in this way they may contribute to cognitive ability theory. Although one might not expect priming to account for large amounts of variance in many forms of learning, its conceptual overlap with some specific learning processes make it a noteworthy candidate for selected learning paradigms. Furthermore, evidence suggests that priming differences have only modest relationships with traditional aptitude constructs. Thus, priming differences may potentially explain learning variance that is unaccounted for by more commonly investigated cognitive ability constructs.

REFERENCES

Ackerman, P. L. (1988). Determinants of individual differences during skill acquisition: Cognitive abilities and information processing. *Journal of Experimental Psychology: General, 117,* 288–318.

Ackerman, P. L. (1990). A correlational analysis of skill specificity: Learning, abilities, and individual differences. *Journal of Experimental Psychology: Learning, Memory, and Cognition, 16,* 883–901.

Ackerman, P. L. (1992). Predicting individual differences in complex skill acquisition: Dynamics of ability determinants. *Journal of Applied Psychology, 77,* 598–614.

Ackerman, P. L. (1996). A theory of adult intellectual development: Process, personality, interests, and knowledge. *Intelligence, 22,* 227–257.

Ackerman, P. L., & Woltz, D. J. (1994). Determinants of learning and performance in an associative memory/substitution task: Task constraints, individual differences, volition, and motivation. *Journal of Educational Psychology, 86,* 487–515.

Anderson, J. R. (1974). Retrieval of propositional information from long-term memory. *Cognitive Psychology, 6,* 451–474.

Anderson, J. R. (1983a). A spreading activation theory of memory. *Journal of Verbal Learning and Verbal Behavior, 22,* 261–295.

Anderson, J. R. (1983b). *The architecture of cognition.* Cambridge, MA: Harvard University Press.

Anderson, J. R. (1993). *Rules of the mind.* Hillsdale, NJ: Erlbaum.

Baddeley, A. D. (1986). *Working memory.* Oxford, England: Clarendon Press.

Baddeley, A. D. (1993). Working memory or working attention? In A. Baddeley & L. Weiskrantz (Eds.), *Attention: Selection, awareness, and control* (pp. 152–170). Oxford, England: Clarendon Press.

Bentler, P. M. (1995). *EQS: Structural Equations Program manual.* Encino, CA: Multivariate Software.

Blaxton, T. A. (1989). Investigating dissociations among memory measures: Support for a transfer appropriate processing framework. *Journal of Experimental Psychology: Learning, Memory, and Cognition, 15,* 657–668.

Cantor, J., & Engle, R. W. (1993). Working-memory capacity as long-term memory activation: An individual-differences approach. *Journal of Experimental Psychology: Learning, Memory, and Cognition, 19,* 1101–1114.

Chaiken, S. R. (1993). Test-proximity effects in a single-session individual differences study of learning ability: The case of activation savings. *Intelligence, 17,* 173–190.

Collins, A. M., & Loftus, E. F. (1975). A spreading activation theory of semantic processing. *Psychological Review, 82,* 407–428.

Conway, A. R. A., & Engle, R. W. (1994). Working memory and retrieval: A resource-dependent inhibition model. *Journal of Experimental Psychology: General, 123,* 354–373.

Cronbach, L. J. (1957). The two disciplines of scientific psychology. *American Psychologist, 12,* 671–684.

Daneman, M., & Carpenter, P. A. (1980). Individual differences in working memory and reading. *Journal of Verbal Learning and Verbal Behavior, 19,* 450–466.

Daneman, M., & Carpenter, P. A. (1983). Individual differences in integrating information between and within sentences. *Journal of Experimental Psychology: Learning, Memory, and Cognition, 9,* 561–584.

Department of Defense. (1984). *Test manual for the Armed Services Vocational Aptitude Battery* (DoD 1304.12AA). North Chicago, IL: U.S. Military Entrance Processing Command.

Ericsson, K. A., & Kintsch, W. (1995). Long-term working memory. *Psychological Review, 102,* 211–245.

Gernsbacher, M. A. (1989). Mechanisms that improve referential access. *Cognition, 32,* 99–156.

Graf, P., Squire, L. R., & Mandler, G. (1984). The information that amnesic patients do not forget. *Journal of Experimental Psychology: Learning, Memory, and Cognition, 10,* 164–178.

Hamann, S. P. (1990). Level-of-processing effects in conceptually driven implicit tasks. *Journal of Experimental Psychology: Learning, Memory, and Cognition, 16,* 970–977.

Hasher, L., & Zacks, R. T. (1979). Automatic and effortful processes in memory. *Journal of Experimental Psychology: General, 108,* 356–388.

Hasher, L., & Zacks, R. T. (1984). Automatic processing of fundamental information. *American Psychologist, 39,* 1372–1388.

Jacoby, L. L. (1983). Perceptual enhancement: Persistent effects of an experience. *Journal of Experimental Psychology: Learning, Memory, and Cognition, 9,* 21–38.

Jacoby, L. L., & Dallas, M. (1981). On the relationship between autobiographical memory and perceptual learning. *Journal of Experimental Psychology: General, 110,* 306–340.

Johnston, W. A., Hawley, K. J., & Elliott, J. M. (1991). Contribution of perceptual fluency to recognition judgments. *Journal of Experimental Psychology: Learning, Memory, and Cognition, 17,* 210–223.

Just, M. A., & Carpenter, P. A. (1992). A capacity theory of comprehension: Individual differences in working memory. *Psychological Review, 99,* 122–149.

Just, M. A., Carpenter, P. A., & Keller, T. A. (1996). The capacity theory of comprehension: New frontiers of evidence and arguments. *Psychological Review, 103,* 773–780.

Kanfer, R., & Ackerman, P. L. (1989). Motivation and cognitive abilities: An integrative/aptitude-treatment interaction approach to skill acquisition. *Journal of Applied Psychology, 74,* 657–690.

King, J., & Just, M. A. (1991). Individual differences in syntactic processing: The role of working memory. *Journal of Memory and Language, 30,* 580–602.

Kirsner, K., & Speelman, C. (1996). Skill acquisition and repetition priming: One principle, many processes? *Journal of Experimental Psychology: Learning, Memory, and Cognition, 22,* 563–575.

Kyllonen, P. C., & Christal, R. E. (1990). Reasoning ability is (little more than) working-memory capacity?! *Intelligence, 14,* 389–433.

Larkin, A. A. (1996). *Semantic priming and working memory capacity: A test of distinctive roles in reading comprehension.* Unpublished doctoral dissertation, University of Utah, Salt Lake City.

Larkin, A. A., Woltz, D. J., Reynolds, R. E., & Clark, E. (1996). Conceptual priming differences and reading ability. *Contemporary Educational Psychology, 21,* 279–303.

Logan, G. D. (1988). Toward an instance theory of automatization. *Psychological Review, 95,* 492–527.

Logan, G. D. (1990). Repetition priming and automaticity: Common underlying mechanisms? *Cognitive Psychology, 22,* 1–35.

Lohman, D. L. (1994). Component scores as residual variance (or why the intercept correlates best). *Intelligence, 19,* 1–11.

McNamara, T. (1994). Theories of priming: II. Types of primes. *Journal of Experimental Psychology: Learning, Memory, and Cognition, 20,* 507–520.

Neely, J. H. (1977). Semantic priming and retrieval from lexical memory: Roles of inhibitionless spreading activation and limited-capacity attention. *Journal of Experimental Psychology: General,* *106,* 226–254.

Neely, J. H. (1991). Semantic priming effects in visual word recognition: A selective review of current findings and theories. In D. Besner & G. Humphreys (Eds.), *Basic processes in reading: Visual word recognition* (pp. 264–336). Hillsdale, NJ: Erlbaum.

Newell, A., & Rosenbloom, P. S. (1981). Mechanisms of skill acquisition and the law of practice. In J. R. Anderson (Ed.), *Cognitive skills and their acquisition* (pp. 1–55). Hillsdale, NJ: Erlbaum.

Perruchet, P., & Baveux, P. (1989). Correlational analysis of explicit and implicit memory performance. *Memory and Cognition, 17,* 77–86.

Posner, M. I., Boies, S. J., Eichelman, W. H., & Taylor, R. L. (1969). Retention of physical and name codes of single letters. *Journal of Experimental Psychology Monograph, 79,* 1–16.

Rappold, V. A., & Hashtroudi, S. (1991). Does organization improve priming? *Journal of Experimental Psychology: Learning, Memory, and Cognition, 17,* 103–114.

Reder, L. M., & Anderson, J. R. (1980). A partial resolution of the paradox of interference: The role of integrating knowledge. *Cognitive Psychology, 12,* 447–472.

Roediger, H. L., III (1990). Implicit memory: Retention without remembering. *American Psychologist, 45,* 1043–1056.

Roediger, H. L., III, & Challis, B. H. (1992). Effects of exact repetition and conceptual repetition on free recall and primed word-fragment completion. *Journal of Experimental Psychology: Learning, Memory, and Cognition, 18,* 3–14.

Schacter, D. L. (1987). Implicit memory: History and current status. *Journal of Experimental Psychology: Learning, Memory, and Cognition, 13,* 501–518.

Schacter, D. L. (1990). Perceptual representation systems and implicit memory: Toward a resolution of the multiple memory systems debate. *Annals of the New York Academy of Sciences, 608,* 543–572.

Schacter, D. L. (1992). Understanding implicit memory: A cognitive neuroscience approach. *American Psychologist, 47,* 559–569.

Schneider, W., & Shiffrin, R. M. (1977). Controlled and automatic human information processing: I. Detection, search, and attention. *Psychological Review, 84,* 1–66.

Schwartz, B. L., & Hashtroudi, S. (1991). Priming is independent of skill learning. *Journal of Experimental Psychology: Learning, Memory, and Cognition, 17,* 1177–1187.

Shiffrin, R. M., & Schneider, W. (1977). Controlled and automatic human information processing: II. Perceptual learning, automatic attending, and a general theory. *Psychological Review, 84,* 127–190.

Snow, R. E. (1992). Aptitude theory: Yesterday, today, and tomorrow. *Educational Psychologist, 27,* 5–32.

Snow, R. E., & Lohman, D. L. (1989). Implications of cognitive psychology for educational measurement. In R. L. Linn (Ed.), *Educational measurement* (pp. 263–331). Phoenix, AZ: Oryx Press.

Srinivas, K., & Roediger, H. L., III. (1990). Classifying implicit memory tests: Category association and anagram solution. *Journal of Memory and Language, 29,* 389–412.

Sternberg, R. J. (1994). PRSVL: An integrative framework for understanding mind in context. In R. J. Sternberg & R. K. Wagner (Eds.), *Mind in context: Interactionist perspectives on human intelligence* (pp. 218–232). Cambridge, England: Cambridge University Press.

Toth, J. P., Reingold, E. M., & Jacoby, L. L. (1994). Toward a redefinition of implicit memory: Process dissociations following elaborative processing and self-generation. *Journal of Experimental Psychology: Learning, Memory, and Cognition, 20,* 290–303.

Tulving, E., & Schacter, D. L. (1990). Priming and human memory systems. *Science, 247,* 301–306.

Tulving, E., Schacter, D. L., & Stark, H. A. (1982). Priming effects in word-fragment completion are independent of recognition memory. *Journal of Experimental Psychology: Learning, Memory, and Cognition, 8,* 336–342.

Turner, M. L., & Engle, R. W. (1989). Is working memory capacity task dependent? *Journal of Memory and Language, 28,* 127–154.

Underwood, B. J. (1975). Individual differences as a crucible in theory construction. *American Psychologist, 30,* 128–134.

Underwood, B. J., Boruch, R. F., & Malmi, R. A. (1978). Composition of episodic memory. *Journal of Experimental Psychology: General, 107,* 393–419.

Warrington, E. K., & Weiskrantz, L. (1970). Amnesia: Consolidation or retrieval? *Nature, 228,* 628–630.

Waters, G. S., & Caplan, D. (1996). The capacity theory of sentence comprehension: Critique of Just and Carpenter (1992). *Psychological Review, 103,* 761–772.

Weldon, M. S. (1993). The time course of perceptual and conceptual contributions to word fragment completion priming. *Journal of Experimental Psychology: Learning, Memory, and Cognition, 19*, 1010–1023.

Weldon, M. S., & Roediger, H. L., III. (1987). Altering retrieval demands reverses the picture superiority effect. *Memory and Cognition, 15*, 269–280.

Widaman, K. F. (1985). Hierarchically tested covariance structure models for multitrait–multimethod data. *Applied Psychological Measurement, 9*, 1–26.

Woltz, D. J. (1988). An investigation of the role of working memory in procedural skill acquisition. *Journal of Experimental Psychology: General, 117*, 319–331.

Woltz, D. J. (1990). Repetition of semantic comparisons: Temporary and persistent priming effects. *Journal of Experimental Psychology: Learning, Memory, and Cognition, 16*, 392–403.

Woltz, D. J. (1993). *The relationship between repetition priming and skill acquisition* (Tech. Rep. No. 1). Salt Lake City: University of Utah, Department of Educational Psychology Project on Skill Learning.

Woltz, D. J. (1996). Perceptual and conceptual priming in a semantic reprocessing task. *Memory and Cognition, 24*, 429–440.

Woltz, D. J., & Madsen, J. G. (1998). *Independence in implicit and explicit memory measures for semantic processing events.* Manuscript submitted for publication.

Woltz, D. J., & Shute, V. J. (1993). Individual difference in repetition priming and its relationship to declarative knowledge acquisition. *Intelligence, 17*, 333–359.

Woltz, D. J., & Shute, V. J. (1995). The time course of forgetting exhibited in repetition priming of semantic comparisons. *American Journal of Psychology, 108*, 499–525.

Discussion

The focus of the discussion of Woltz's paper was about the specific aspects of his assessment of working memory, differences in assessment of priming in children and adults, and implications for individual differences in reading skills.

Dr. Wittmann: Could you please be a little more precise how you measured working memory — is it possible to prime to the phonologic level? Is it possible to prime to the spatial one? And it struck me that you get an additional significant beta weight in that study.

Dr. Woltz: It was just a single measure of working memory. We're trying to do a follow-up study where we have a number of measures of working memory; but that particular measure was called *alphabet recoding*, and it's something that has shown up in a lot of the Armstrong Laboratory studies of working memory in the past. People are given one, two, or three letters of the alphabet and then a recoding number like +2 or −1, and they have to go forward or backward in the alphabet. If it's +2, each letter must be incremented forward in the alphabet by two. With children we didn't want to have a working memory measure that depended on knowledge. We thought the alphabet was a safe bet. So this requires a phonological loop for rehearsing the initial letters — you get shown the stimuli, and then they're taken away, so you have to remember those letters, and then you have to do the recoding forward or backward in the alphabet, and then you have to give your answer all at once. That task has been given with a battery of other working memory measures, and it has a reasonably high loading on a General Working Memory factor.

Dr. Baddeley: I really like your results, and I wondered if you'd thought of them as analogous to the long-term working memory concept that Ericsson and Kintsch

157

[in their 1995 *Psychological Review* article] have presented, which is I think somewhat related to our interpretation of recency effects. Namely, that they represent a passive activation of existing structures.

Dr. Woltz: Yes. I think the semantic priming thing is very much like that, and I think it's interesting that in the correlations it's somewhat distinct from the more short-term working memory.

Dr. Baddeley: And related to that, we've been doing some experiments where we've been having random generation in conjunction with comprehension and finding that we get very little relationship between the difficulty of the comprehension of passages ranging from fairy stories to philosophy and the concurrent random generation task.

Dr. Lohman: First, I appreciate the carefulness with which you've done this work. It's really excellent. I did have a couple of concerns though. As you moved from the older subjects to these grade school children, did you find that your tasks behaved the same? For example, in the semantic priming task, was there any variability in probability of answering correctly to the semantic prime in the first place?

Dr. Woltz: We adjusted the content of the items for reading level—the words were within the capability of the sample.

Dr. Lohman: But there was no variability in determining whether the terms were related?

Dr. Woltz: Well, there were priming effects in both latency and errors.

Dr. Lohman: One of the things I was concerned about was if, in fact, some of the variance you're seeing in priming reflects whether subjects vary in their understanding of the connection between the words in the first place. If a subject did not understand that the words were synonyms, then how could priming take place? That was one concern.

And the second issue had to do with the correlations with math and with reading. With one exception, they looked about the same. And so I was wondering to what extent you felt that these results were peculiar to reading or math, and to what extent they reflect more Gc types of skills or even something beyond that.

Dr. Woltz: Well, to answer your first question . . . the error rates were relatively low. We didn't have anybody who had error rates beyond about 10%. And so I really don't know how much the priming measure could be reflecting that. But in general, people did not make many errors.

Your second question was math? I think you're absolutely right that that—that standardized achievement measure is pretty general. I think the repetition-priming measure did not correlate with any of those achievement measures, which is consistent with what was found in the adult study where it was just repetition priming measured and it didn't have a correlation with the general ASVAB [Armed Services Vocational Aptitude Battery] measure. I think you're absolutely right that the standardized achievement measures were pretty general. The repetition using the Reading subscale of the SAT [Stanford Achievement Test] really captured reading comprehension, and that was part of the motivation for the second study where we tried to measure comprehension in a real focused way. So I agree that the interpretation probably ought to be broadened for the first study.

Dr. Stankov: When you look at the loadings—in particular, the general priming level—going from the tasks that define, let's say, numeric priming, they go down from .78, .43, .35, and so on. And the same happens with most of the others. I find that fascinating. That is the kind of data that I look at when I talk about complexity. And it probably has some implications for the skill learning in the literature. I think it is worthwhile paying attention to the logic. Not just the general structure of the model, but also the patterns within the loadings, and they try to fix them. . . .

Dr. Woltz: I think that's a really interesting point. I didn't explain the priming variables, but they represent the repetition lag, and the loadings are higher with the shorter repetition lags.

Dr. Widaman: I have one comment and one question. The comment is you mentioned difference scores, and it seems like we keep beating ourselves up with comments about difference scores. But there's a fair amount of recent research or publications on difference scores that argue the different scores can be quite reliable. And so the classic findings on different scores are being overturned by recent research showing that different scores can be more reliable than people ever thought they would be so — and I think what you're showing with your priming effects is that they are reliable. They are much more reliable and potentially more reliable still if you increase trials and do all the things that psychometricians would recommend that we do.

The question pertains to the fact that you've drawn similarities between the relationships between repetition priming and skill acquisition and between semantic priming and reading comprehension. And when I heard your talk about reading comprehension, it struck me that you're stressing the similarities between the two kinds of models. With repetition priming, it seems like if there are individual differences in that, that might indeed be a precursor of skill acquisition. That in order to acquire skills, one needs some level of repetition priming. But with semantic priming I wonder which is the chicken and which is the egg, and whether you only get semantic priming with reading comprehension and whether reading comprehension drives semantic priming.

Dr. Woltz: I think there is a real difference between repetition priming and semantic priming in that sense. Another way that this shows up is in the fact that semantic priming has correlations with all the other things that were measured. It has a pretty high correlation with knowledge. It has a modest correlation with speed and some correlation with working memory. And so untangling where it fits in all that is quite complicated. I think the fact that it made a unique contribution to explaining reading differences suggests that it isn't simply due to the knowledge, the acquisition of knowledge that accompanies reading. I mean vocabulary development goes along with reading. You develop vocabulary and reading skill concurrently. But the fact that semantic priming made a unique contribution to reading beyond vocabulary I think suggests that there might be something distinct but it's obviously intertwined in some way.

7

Learning, Automaticity, and Attention: An Individual-Differences Approach

EDWARD NĘCKA

The goal of the research reported in this chapter was to examine the relationships among general intelligence, the automatization of cognitive processes, and the attentional mechanisms of cognitive control. This research was part of a broader research project aimed at investigating individual differences in cognition, with particular emphasis on the fundamental cognitive prerequisites of general intelligence. Initial research established that intelligence could be accounted for partly by the specificity of working memory functioning (Nęcka, 1992). Three basic aspects of working memory were identified: speed, storage capacity, and retention capability. The findings indicated that neither speed nor storage capacity alone (see Kyllonen & Christal, 1990) could account for general mental ability. Rather, they indicated that some combination of, or interaction among, the three aspects of working memory showed a stronger relationship to measures of general mental ability. This idea was further developed by Polczyk and Nęcka (1994, 1997). Later studies investigating the attentional bases of intelligence (Nęcka, 1996) supported the limited-resource theory of attention proposed by Kahneman (1973) and further elaborated by others (e.g., Hunt & Lansman, 1982, 1986; Norman & Bobrow, 1975). It appears that measures of attentional resources best account for individual differences in general mental ability. Guided by these findings, I have recently developed a cognitive model of intelligence in which general mental ability is defined as a process of oscillation within the acceptable limits of ever-changing states of arousal and within the traitlike, structural limits posed by the mechanisms of working memory and attention (Nęcka, 1997).

The general assumption on which this project was based is that there are many elements of intelligence (in contrast to Sternberg, 1990). In other words, it is understood that general mental ability is a statistical and psychometric phenomenon

161

rather than a genuine psychological entity. However, there are undoubtedly individual differences in the ability to understand concepts, plan one's actions, solve problems, and perform other important cognitive functions. Understanding these individual differences requires the identification of all the important cognitive correlates of intelligence and the analysis of their role in the organization of intelligent behavior. Attentional mechanisms of cognitive control, generally investigated with interference tasks (e.g., the Stroop task), are likely one of the sought-after cognitive prerequisites of intelligence. Although systematic study of such relationships is scarce, the importance of the efficiency of cognitive control to the theoretical understanding of human intelligence seems worth examining. One study investigating such relationships in gifted children (Nęcka, Gruszka, & Orzechowski, 1996) has produced encouraging results. The two experiments reported in this chapter are primarily a continuation of the Nęcka et al. study. In these later experiments, however, I used the Navon task, which appears to be more important for the investigation of intellectual giftedness than the classical Stroop task.

The rationale behind my research is rooted in five basic theoretical assumptions. First, I assumed that attention is a system of cognitive control in which the vast amount of information processed by the cognitive system is reduced to a tolerable extent. The term *cognitive control* refers to the regulation of both the initial stage of stimulus elaboration and the final stage of response production. By definition, cognitive control is the ability to inhibit distracting response alternatives to permit some target response. According to the resource theory of attention (Kahneman, 1973; Norman & Bobrow, 1975), cognitive control is regulated by specific allocation of attentional resources. Because the efficiency of cognitive control requires attentional resources, it is assumed that such processing is best assessed using tasks that tax such resources (i.e., those involving incongruity between response tendencies, such as the Navon task).

Second, I assumed that the more automatic a particular action is, the fewer attentional resources are required for its performance. The division of cognitive processing into controlled, conscious, and effortful on the one hand and automatic, unconscious, and effortless on the other (Hasher & Zacks, 1979; Schneider & Shiffrin, 1977; Shiffrin & Schneider, 1977) is not a concise one. However, the concept of a continuum between totally controlled and entirely automatic processes seems to preserve its theoretical soundness. It is therefore acceptable to assume that while becoming increasingly automatic, a process requires a decreasing amount of attentional resources, which may thus be allocated to other ongoing processes. In other words, automatization allows the reallocation of attentional resources from a previously effortful process to others (Hunt & Lansman, 1982; Norman & Bobrow, 1975). As a consequence, automatization allows the performance of several actions simultaneously.

Third, I assumed that automatization occurs as a function of learning. Consecutive learning trials result in two concurrent effects: (a) the transition of cognitive processing from being controlled at the highest conscious level of cognitive organization to a more local level of organization and (b) increased efficiency of response production and performance, understood in terms of speed, accuracy, or both. Consequently, learning permits an investment of attentional resources in other processes that are not yet automatized. As automatization proceeds, these newly automatic processes in turn require less conscious effort, and so on (Ackerman, 1986, 1987, 1988; Ackerman & Schneider, 1985).

Fourth, I assumed that the speed of automatization is connected to psychometric intelligence. The process of automatization is understood here as a rudimentary one, referring to the elementary cognitive processes that — in the case of highly intelligent people — become less dependent on the central distribution of attentional resources relatively quickly as skill acquisition proceeds. In the case of less intelligent people, the liberation of attentional resources due to automatization is assumed to occur more slowly. It follows that less intelligent people require more attentional resources to process and control initial action and that they therefore cannot invest them in another action or to additional demands of the ongoing task. The connection between intelligence and speed of automatization of cognitive processes has been proposed on the theoretical level (Sternberg, 1985), but some empirical findings are also available (e.g., Neubauer, 1990).

Fifth, I assumed that psychometric intelligence is related to the increased efficiency of cognitive control. In general, cognitive control permits the suppression of unnecessary responses as well as the execution of consecutive actions in their appropriate order. Increased strength of cognitive control likely results in enhanced proficiency of various cognitive tasks, and the performance of individuals labeled *bright* or *intelligent* is characterized by such proficiency. In this way, cognitive control might be treated as a rudimentary mechanism underlying the trait of intelligence rather than just an accidental correlate of high IQ.

These assumptions have already been verified by many separate studies, including the ones mentioned earlier, but not by way of a unified experimental approach. A unified approach to understanding the relationships among intelligence, automaticity, and attention requires an experimental design that would jointly take into account the variables pertaining to attentional mechanisms of cognitive control, learning and automatization, and individual differences in general cognitive ability. Moreover, the previous researchers did not investigate the process of automatization in tasks that reflect the basic functions of attention, particularly cognitive control and resource allocation. Hence, it might be interesting to examine how learning, with its consequences related to automatization of cognitive processes, affects the performance of a task that measures the efficiency of cognitive control. In my research, I sought to address these previously neglected problems and asked the following questions:

1. Is the importance of cognitive control attenuated by the process of learning and by the consequent automatization of mental processes? How and to what extent can learning influence the performance of a task that measures the efficiency of cognitive control?
2. Is psychometrically assessed intelligence related to the speed of automatization of task performance if the task itself reflects the efficiency of cognitive control?
3. Is intelligence related to the efficiency with which cognitive control is exerted over task performance?
4. Can learning and automaticity weaken the strength of the relationship, if there is one, between intelligence and efficiency of cognitive control?

163

Experiment 1

Method

Participants.   The sample consisted of 101 participants, 57 of whom were men, who were students of various departments except psychology. Their mean age was 23.9 years. Participation was voluntary. Participants were informed that they would take part in the psychological study of "how the human mind operates."

Computerized Task.   A modified version of the task originally proposed by Navon (1977) was used in this study. In this task, a global figure composed of an aggregate of local elements was presented on the computer screen. The global stimulus (4.75 × 2 cm) was either a rectangle or a letter presented at a distance of approximately 40 cm. The local elements composing the global figure were either asterisks or letters, shown in Figure 7.1. There were four experimental conditions arranged in a 2 × 2 experimental design: the local congruent condition (a rectangle composed of letters); the global congruent condition (a letter composed of asterisks); the local incongruent condition (a letter composed of letters); and the global incongruent (same stimulus as the local incongruent condition). There were two independent variables: congruency (congruent vs. incongruent) and orientation (local vs. global). The task consisted of 96 trials, 24 for each condition, presented in random order.

Participants were asked to respond to one aspect of the stimulus and to ignore the second. In the local condition they were required to respond to the local ele-

```
RRRRRRRRRRR          * * * * * * * * * * * *
RRRRRRRRRRR          * * * * * * * * * * * *
RRRRRRRRRRR                  * * *
RRRRRRRRRRR                  * * *
RRRRRRRRRRR                  * * *
RRRRRRRRRRR                  * * *
RRRRRRRRRRR                  * * *
RRRRRRRRRRR                  * * *
RRRRRRRRRRR                  * * *


KKK      KKK          ZZZ          ZZZ
KKK      KKK          ZZZZ         ZZZ
KKK      KKK          ZZZZZ        ZZZ
KKK      KKK          ZZZ ZZ       ZZZ
KKKKKKKKKKK           ZZZ    ZZ    ZZZ
KKK      KKK          ZZZ      ZZ ZZZ
KKK      KKK          ZZZ        ZZZZZ
KKK      KKK          ZZZ         ZZZZ
KKK      KKK          ZZZ          ZZZ
```

Figure 7.1. Example stimuli used in the modified Navon task.

ments of the global letter, whereas in the global condition they were to respond to the global letter itself. The required type of response was enforced by including only the target aspect of the given stimulus in the response key. For example, when the letter A, composed of uppercase Bs, was presented on the screen, the lowercase letters c, m, u, and b were shown in the response key, which appeared at the bottom of the screen. In this way, participants were forced to respond to the local aspect of the stimulus because a response to the global aspect of the stimulus was unavailable. Consequently, participants had to ignore the global aspect of the stimulus because their attention was "forcefully" drawn to the local aspect of the stimulus. If the letter a instead of b was included in the response key, participants had to process the global aspect of the stimulus because there was no way to respond to the local aspect. In this case, their attention would be drawn to the global aspects of the stimulus. This example involved an element of conflict, in that the two different aspects of the stimulus invoked contradictory response tendencies. Correct responding requires suppression of one tendency (e.g., response to the global aspect) to execute the other (e.g., response to the local aspect). This means that participants had to select some aspects of the stimulus at the expense of others in a situation that might have changed completely in the next experimental trial.

Paper-and-Pencil Tests. Two measures of general intelligence were administered: Raven's Advanced Progressive Matrices (RAPM; 5 min plus 40 min [for the two parts]) and the Verbal Analogy Test (VAT; 25 min). As contrast measures, which were used to determine whether intelligence would account totally for the expected differential effects, I used Urban and Jellen's (1986) Test for Creative Thinking— Verbal Production (TCT — VP) and its new nonverbal version, the Test for Creative Thinking–Drawing Production (TCT — DP; K. Urban, personal communication, June 10, 1994). The Polish adaptation (Brzozowski & Drwal, 1995) of the Eysenck Personality Questionnaire–Revised (EPQ — R; see Eysenck & Eysenck, 1975) was used to assess three basic dimensions of personality: extraversion, neuroticism, and psychoticism. To my knowledge, the effect of personality on the automatization of cognitive processes has not been studied systematically, although the differential relationships among learning, automaticity, and cognitive control may not be solely a function of intelligence.

Procedure. Four consecutive series of the Navon task were interpolated with the paper-and-pencil tests in a fixed sequence. The sequence of events during the experimental session was as follows: TCT — DP, Navon Series 1, RAPM, Navon Series 2, the VAT, Navon Series 3, TCT — VP, Navon Series 4, and EPQ — R. Each series of the Navon task required 5–7 min to complete. The whole experimental session took about 2½ hr depending on the participant's pace.

Results and Discussion

I analyzed the results with a repeated measures multivariate analysis of variance, (MANOVA). Response latencies on the Navon task dramatically decreased with series $F(3, 291) = 136.53$, $p < .001$. They were also much greater in the incongruent condition than in the congruent one, $F(1, 97) = 1,440.96$, $p < .001$, and greater for global orientations than for local ones, $F(1, 97) = 11.87$, $p < .001$. Congruency appeared to be the most important task characteristic influencing response latencies, explaining the majority of total variance, followed by the much weaker influence of task series. The general pattern of relationships between reaction time (RT) and all independent variables is shown in Figure 7.2, which represents the significant three-way interaction, $F(3, 291) = 7.56$, $p < .001$. Post hoc comparisons using the Tukey method revealed that, in both the congruent and incongruent conditions, the first series significantly differed from all others. In other words, the decrease of RT observed in Series 2, 3, and 4 was statistically insignificant regardless of condition. It also appeared that the differences between the global and local conditions were significant only in Series 2, 3, and 4 of the incongruent condition.

The MANOVA also revealed a Series × Condition interaction, $F(3, 291) = 8.76$, $p < .001$. It appeared that RT, although decreasing over the four consecutive series, differed significantly between the congruent and incongruent conditions in every series (see Figure 7.3). However, the post-hoc comparisons using the Tukey method showed that the difference between Series 3 and 4 lost its significance in the congruent condition. The interaction may also be interpreted in terms of the differences between the congruent and incongruent conditions. These differences, although highly significant in every series, appeared to become less salient in the last series. For instance, the difference between conditions was 840 ms in Series 1 and only 710 ms in Series 4.

To examine whether the effect of incongruity declined with practice, I decided to estimate the relative strength of this effect independently in Series 1 and 4 (i.e., at the beginning and the end of the learning session). It appeared that this effect was significant in both Series 1, $F(1, 100) = 629.48$, $p < .001$, and Series 4, $F(1,$

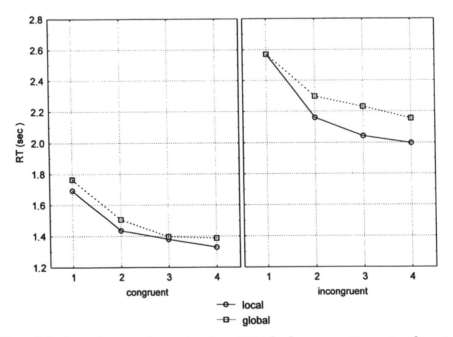

Figure 7.2. General patterns in reaction times (RTs) for four consecutive series of practice on the Navon task in all conditions in Experiment 1: Series × Condition × Orientation, $F(3, 291) = 7.56$, $p < .0001$.

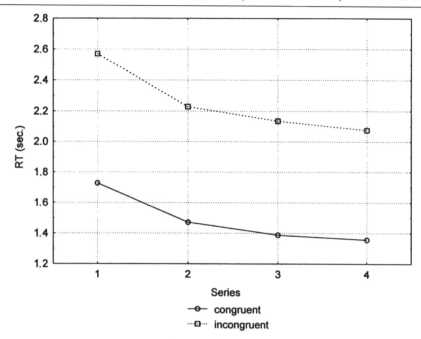

Figure 7.3. The decline of reaction times (RTs) throughout practice in both the congruent and incongruent conditions of the Navon task in Experiment 1: Series × Condition, $F(3, 291) = 8.76$, $p < .0001$.

98) = 1134.87, $p < .001$, but not at the same level. This means that this task characteristic explained more variance in RT in Series 4 than in Series 1. Thus, in spite of the fact that RT significantly decreased with series and plateaued quickly, and despite the diminutive effect of series on the influence of congruency on RT, the relative importance of the main experimental condition of incongruity rose with series. Evidently, the strength of cognitive control, operationalized as the relatively small increase in RT occurring with incongruity, appears to be resistant to skill acquisition. It also appeared that the effect of orientation, which was insignificant in the first series, reached the highest level of significance in the fourth series, $F(1, 98) = 14.98$, $p < .001$. The average difference between response latencies in the global and local conditions was about 100 ms in the fourth series.

Intraindividual standard deviations were also influenced by the main experimental task characteristics. Variance decreased with series, $F(3, 291) = 34.78$, $p < .001$, and was much smaller in the congruent condition than in the incongruent one, $F(1, 97) = 344.40$, $p < .001$. The orientation variable was not significant. However, it is worth examining the three-way interaction among series, condition, and orientation shown in Figure 7.4. In this analysis, individual standard deviations behaved similarly to responses latencies (compare with Figure 7.2). The most prominent change took place between Series 1 and 2, after which no effect of learning was found (post hoc comparisons using the Tukey method). Contrary to response latencies, standard deviations were greater for local orientation, but only in the incongruent condition, Series 1. Otherwise, they were greater for global orientation. Therefore, the effects

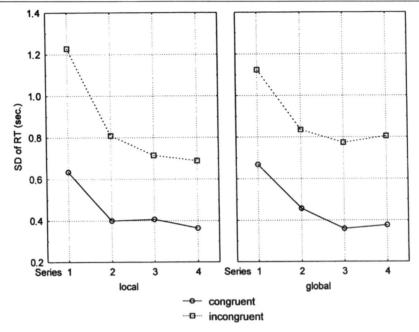

Figure 7.4. Intraindividual standard deviation of reaction times (RTs) in the four consecutive series of practice on the Navon task in all conditions in Experiment 1: Series × Condition × Orientation, $F(3, 291) = 3.01$, $p < .03$.

of series and condition were similar for RT and its standard deviations, whereas the effect of orientation was different for every dependent variable.

The main effects of condition and orientation were assessed independently for Series 1 and 4 to ascertain whether skill acquisition, shown in Figure 7.4, eliminated the influence of these main effects. In Series 1, only the effect of condition appeared to be significant, $F(1, 100) = 71.19$, $p < .001$; the effect of orientation, as well as its two-way interaction with condition, did not reach the .05 level of significance. In Series 4, on the other hand, both task characteristics appeared to be significant, as was their interaction, showing that Series 4 global orientation was more demanding, as evidenced by an increased variation in RT. Interestingly, the relative importance of congruity increased significantly compared with the first series, $F(1, 98) = 287.39$, $p < .001$. It accounted for much more of the total variance in intraindividual RT standard deviations in Series 4 than it accounted for in Series 1. As I found in the case of response latencies, skill acquisition did not eliminate the influence of main effects; to the contrary, the importance of these effects was even greater as learning proceeded.

Accuracy was not the best dependent variable to analyze because of an apparent ceiling effect and skewed distribution (mean number of errors = 0.299, $SD = 0.56$). This finding is important in itself because it justifies the conclusion about almost errorless performance of the Navon task. However, I found that the number of errors was significantly higher in the first series than in the next three series, $F(3, 291) = 6.98$, $p < .001$. The effects of condition and orientation were not significant.

Analysis of the relationship between the experimental variables and individual differences revealed that participants scoring high on RAPM responded faster:

The average difference of 225 ms was highly significant, particularly in the first series, $F(1, 96) = 15.06$, $p < .001$. These relationships were also investigated with a correlational approach (see Table 7.1). As can be seen, both intelligence tests correlated negatively with response latencies regardless of condition and series. However, the correlation coefficients were highest in Series 1, suggesting that learning may have attenuated the strength of the RT–IQ relationship. The correlation between the RAPM and the VAT was high ($r = .60$, $p < .001$), thus accounting for the similarity between the patterns of relationships concerning the two ability measures.

The analysis of the interaction, shown in Figure 7.5, may suggest that the high scores on the RAPM were not accompanied with the increased speed of automatization. Rather, low-scoring participants showed more salient effects of practice between Series 1 and 2, perhaps because their initial performance was relatively lower. In other words, low-scoring participants had "more to improve" and therefore took the opportunity to learn more effectively. Therefore, if gain scores serve as indexes of automaticity, one can conclude that intelligent individuals automatized with less speed relative to less intelligent individuals. Furthermore, the two-way interaction between ability test scores and condition revealed that high-scoring participants were generally faster and outperformed their low-scoring peers particularly in the incongruent condition, $F(1, 96) = 13.24$, $p < .001$. The same effects were found when the VAT served as the criterion of intelligence, although the statistical significance of these effects was slightly lower in this case. These findings clearly suggest that intelligence is related to more efficient cognitive control because intelligent participants showed less disruption as a result of incongruity.

To investigate the relationships between intelligence and experimental effects without the loss of information connected with the median-split procedure, I used a correlational approach. Six variables were calculated as the differences in RT between later versus earlier series (e.g., RT in Series 2 minus RT in Series 1; see

TABLE 7.1 Correlation Coefficients Between Ability Measures and Experimental Variables in Experiment 1

Condition and measure	Series			
	1	2	3	4
Congruent local				
Raven's	−.38***	−.29**	−.28**	−.25*
Analogy	−.33**	−.31**	−.30**	−.20*
Congruent global				
Raven's	−.47***	−.25*	−.37***	−.34**
Analogy	−.45***	−.32**	−.34**	−.33**
Incongruent local				
Raven's	−.39***	−.25*	−.24*	−.26**
Analogy	−.44***	−.29**	−.25*	−.19
Incongruent global				
Raven's	−.51***	−.42***	−.37***	−.35***
Analogy	−.39***	−.38***	−.34**	−.30**

*$p < .05$.   **$p < .01$.   ***$p < .001$.

169

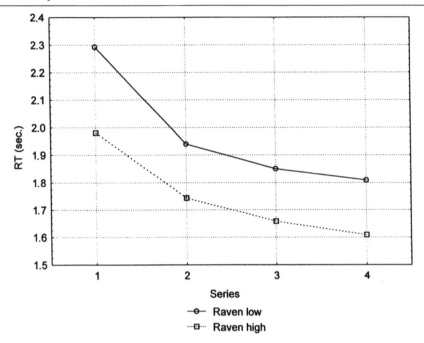

Figure 7.5. Reaction times (RTs) over practice obtained by participants differing in Raven's Advanced Progressive Matrices scores in Experiment 1: Intelligence × Series, $F(3, 288) = 3.11, p < .03$.

Table 7.2). These difference scores served as indexes of the relative decrease in RT between Series 1 and 2, 2 and 3, and so forth. I computed the difference scores only for the incongruent global condition (i.e., the most demanding one) to evaluate more revealing gain scores. Table 7.2 shows the positive correlations of three of these measures with RAPM scores. These relationships suggest that less intelligent participants showed greater effects of practice and automatization, as indicated by the differences in RTs between Series 1 and all subsequent series. This was also evident in that the difference scores for these participants were mostly negative, and their absolute values were assumed to represent the magnitude of learning effects. Therefore, when automatization is operationalized as the relative reduction of RT as a function of practice, the strength of its relationship with low- rather than high-ability test scores becomes evident. Note, however, that the VAT results did not indicate such a relationship.

I also sought to examine whether the Intelligence × Congruity interaction, representing the efficiency of cognitive control found in the case of intelligent participants, would disappear with practice. Therefore, I conducted separate analyses of variance (ANOVA) for the Series 1 and 4. This interaction was significant in both cases regardless of the intelligence test applied, and its relative strength even increased with practice, $F(1, 99) = 5.54, p < .02$; RAPM, first series, $F(1, 97) = 11.97, p < .001$, RAPM, fourth series; VAT, first series, $F(1, 99) = 4.04, p < .05$, and fourth series, $F(1, 97) = 6.03, p < .02$. Therefore, the importance of psychometric intelligence for the efficiency of cognitive control did not disappear with skill acquisition.

This finding was confirmed with regression and correlation analyses, which I

TABLE 7.2 Correlation Coefficients of Six Measures of
Automatization, Obtained Through Subtraction of Mean RTs From
Four Series of Learning, With Ability Test Scores in Experiment 1

Variable	Raven's	VAT
2-1	.31**	.17
3-2	.04	.03
4-3	.10	.12
3-1	.31**	.17
4-2	.10	.11
4-1	.34***	.23*

Note. Variables 2-1 through 4-1 were calculated as the differences between reaction times (RTs) observed in respective series (e.g., Series 2 minus Series 1) in the most difficult incongruent global condition. These indexes are mostly negative because greater RTs were generally subtracted from shorter RTs. Thus, the more negative such an index is, the greater the apparent effect of automaticity. Therefore, positive correlations indicate that the lower ability measures (e.g., Raven's Advanced Progressive Matrices scores) are related to a greater decrease of RT (and greater automaticity effects). VAT = Verbal Analogy Test.
$*p < .05.$ $**p < .01.$ $***p < .001.$

performed to avoid the loss of information connected with splitting the sample at the median point. I operationalized the efficiency of cognitive control as the difference between RTs observed in the congruent condition and RTs observed in the congruent condition. Such difference scores were calculated only for the global condition (in which RTs were generally greater) and independently for the four series. It appeared (see Table 7.3) that RAPM scores correlated negatively and significantly with the indexes of the efficiency of cognitive control in every series. In the case of the VAT, the correlations were significant only in Series 2 and 3.

The data were also subjected to a regression analysis. In a stepwise hierarchical model, the indexes of the efficiency of cognitive control served as dependent variables, whereas two ability measures and their interaction were used as predictor variables. After examining the model in which both tests served as two separate independent variables, I entered the RAPM × VAT interaction variable into the

TABLE 7.3 Correlation Coefficients Between Psychometric
Intelligence and Indexes of the Strength of Cognitive Control in
Experiment 1

Variable	Raven's	VAT
I-C Series 1	−.28**	−.13
I-C Series 2	−.33***	−.22*
I-C Series 3	−.25*	−.24*
I-C Series 4	−.21*	−.16

Note. I-C is a difference score. This variable was calculated as the difference between reaction times (RTs) observed in the incongruent and RTs observed in the congruent condition. Greater differences indicate lower efficiency of cognitive control. VAT = Verbal Analogy Test.
$*p < .05.$ $**p < .01.$ $***p < .001.$

equation. In this way, it was possible to determine whether the interaction variable was able to increase the regression parameters, mainly the beta indexes and the adjusted R^2 statistics. The results show that only the RAPM scores were able to predict the cognitive control measures, such that high scores were related to small congruency differences. This relationship, however, was weak. The adjusted R^2s were only .07, .10, .07, and .03, respectively, in the consecutive series. The beta indexes (only for the RAPM) were in their 20s, except those in the second series, in which beta was -0.33. The hierarchical blocked analysis did not show any significant influence of the interaction variable, which was introduced after the single predictors were analyzed. I am thus justified in concluding that psychometric intelligence is related to the increased efficiency of cognitive control and that this relationship — although weak in nature — does not disappear with practice.

The pattern of results was similar for the standard deviations of the RTs but not identical to with the one observed for RTs. RAPM scores accounted for a significant amount of variance, $F(1, 96) = 14.56$, $p < .001$. However, they did not enter into any interaction with series, condition, or orientation. It also appeared that these scores improved their relative importance between Series 1 and 4, $F(1, 97) = 4.64$, $p < .04$, Series 1; $F(1, 99) = 20.21$, $p < .001$, Series 4. The three-way interaction of RAPM scores, condition, and orientation reached the required level of significance only in the fourth series, $F(1, 97) = 5.51$, $p < .02$. According to this interaction, low-scoring participants responded with decreased regularity, particularly in the incongruent condition and when the global orientation was required.

The data also indicated the general importance of verbal ability as assessed by the VAT, $F(1, 96) = 13.13$, $p < .001$, and lack of significant interactions with the VAT. However, I observed the increasing overall importance of verbal ability in consecutive sessions, $F(1, 99) = 6.67$, $p < .01$, Series 1; $F(1, 99) = 11.16$, $p < .01$, Series 4. Moreover, the interaction between verbal ability and condition, $F(1, 97) = 7.24$, $p < .01$, and orientation, $F(1, 97) = 3.96$, $p < .04$, was significant only in Series 4. The nature of these interactions suggested that the advantage of greater intelligence was more salient in the incongruent condition and with global orientation (i.e., when the task was relatively more demanding). I therefore concluded that individual differences in both RT and its intraindividual standard deviation became more strongly related to intelligence as participants proceeded from Series 1 to Series 4.

The differential effects on RT and variance hitherto described seemed to be solely a function of intelligence. As measured by the TCT — DP, more creative participants responded generally faster than less creative ones, $F(1, 96) = 4.07$, $p < .05$. A similar advantage was found when RT standard deviations served as a dependent variable, $F(1, 96) = 4.81$, $p < .03$. However, the TCT — VP did not indicate any significant differences. The tendency for creative individuals to respond faster and more regularly in a task that requires selective attention is interesting in and of itself, but the effect of creativity does not compare to the influence of mental ability test scores. No interaction between creativity and series and between condition and orientation was found, nor were there any two-way or three-way interactions. Regarding personality dimensions, only psychoticism entered into a three-way interaction with series and condition, $F(3, 285) = 3.62$, $p < .02$. The analysis of this interaction revealed that participants scoring high on psychoticism responded faster, but only in the incongruent condition, Series 1. Otherwise, there were no significant differences between high- and low-scoring groups. No effects of extraversion and neuroticism were found, simple or interactive.

Experiment 2

Method

Participants. Seventy 7th and 8th graders, equally divided into girls and boys, served as participants. Their mean age was 14.6 years. Although they were recruited through the psychological counseling unit supervised by their school, there was no pressure to participate.

Computerized Task. I used the same modified Navon task that was used in Experiment 1 in this experiment.

Paper-and-Pencil Tests. General intelligence was assessed with the RAPM, standard version, Series A, B, C, D, and E. The time limit for the RAPM was 20 min. As a second measure of intelligence, I used the Vocabulary Test developed by Choynowski (1967). It consists of 40 multiple-choice items that require the selection of one proper synonymous relation with some target word out of four possibilities. The time limit for the Vocabulary Test was 5 min. The personality structure of each participant was assessed with the Polish version of the EPQ — R (Brzozowski & Drwal, 1995). Creativity was not assessed in this experiment.

Procedure. Four series of the Navon task were interpolated with the administration of the paper-and-pencil tests, as in Experiment 1. The experimental sessions took about 2 hr.

Results and Discussion

Mean RT in the Navon task was 1.96 s, and the mean intraindividual standard deviation was 0.67 s, compared with the respective values in Experiment 1: 1.87 and 0.68 s. It is clear that Experiment 2's participants did not perform worse than those in Experiment 1 in spite of the age difference and the presumed inequality in general mental ability.

Response latencies were significantly greater in Series 1 than in the Series 2, 3, and 4, $F(3, 207) = 64.78$, $p < .001$. They were also greater in the incongruent condition than in the congruent one, $F(1, 69) = 1019.96$, $p < .001$, and greater for global orientation than for local, $F(1, 69) = 79.95$, $p < .001$. The three-way interaction, $F(3, 207) = 3.75$, $p < .02$, revealed that the differences between local and global orientations disappeared in Series 3 and 4, but only in the congruent condition. In the more demanding incongruent condition, they were significant regardless of series (see Figure 7.6). The other dependent variables (i.e., the standard deviation of RT and accuracy) indicated similar but weaker effects.

The strength of all experimental effects was examined independently in Series 1 and 4 of the Navon task to assess the influence of practice on the efficiency of

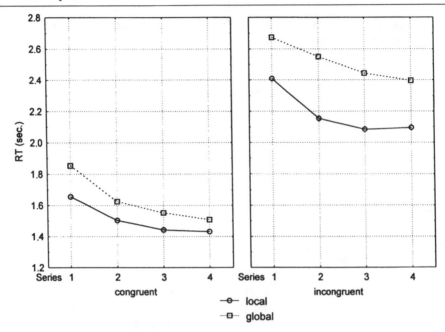

Figure 7.6. Reaction times (RTs) over practice relative to the task's conditions in Experiment 2: Series $\times$ Condition $\times$ Orientation, $F(3, 207) = 3.75$, $P < .02$.

cognitive control. Table 7.4 indicates no significant differences between Series 1 and 4. The effect of congruency was the most influential one regardless of the dependent variable. Contrary to in Experiment 1, the strength of this effect did not increase substantially during practice but maintained its significance in accounting for individual differences in RT. The Condition $\times$ Orientation interaction with regard to RT was significant only in Series 4. This interaction resulted from the lack of differences between local and global orientations in the congruent condition and the existence of such differences in the incongruent condition. In the case of the stan-

TABLE 7.4 Comparison of the Strength of Experimental Effects Observed in Series 1 and 4 of the Navon Task in Experiment 2

Condition	Series 1		Series 4	
	F	p	F	p
RT	981.63	.001	839.85	.001
Orientation	34.53	.001	36.88	.001
Condition $\times$ Orientation	ns		14.68	.001
SD	149.39	.001	234.87	.001
Orientation	8.40	.01	ns	
Condition $\times$ Orientation	ns		ns	
ER	13.67	.001	10.81	.01
Orientation	ns		ns	
Condition $\times$ Orientation	ns		ns	

Note. RT = reaction time; ER = error rate.

174

dard deviations of RTs, the importance of condition increased in Series 4. The weaker effect of orientation, however, lost its significance with series. In the case of response accuracy, only the effect of condition was significant, both in Series 1 and 4. However, the error rate was low in this experiment, indicating a substantial ceiling effect and a skewed distribution.

High-scoring participants obtained shorter response latencies regardless of whether the RAPM, $F(1, 68) = 5.37$, $p < .03$, or the Vocabulary Test, $F(1, 68) = 7.38$, $p < .01$, served as the mental ability assessment tool. The correlation between the RAPM and the Vocabulary Test was .40. Similar effects, both in terms of the strength and the nature of the relationship, were observed when examining the standard deviations of the RTs. In the case of accuracy, no effects of intelligence were found, probably because of the ceiling effect. Intelligence measured with RAPM also entered into an interaction with series, $F(3, 204) = 2.94$, $p < .04$, shown in Figure 7.7. The post hoc comparisons (Tukey method) revealed that the difference between the two ability groups lost its significance in Series 4, although it was significant in Series 1, 2, and 3. It also appeared that, in the case of high-scoring participants, it was the first series that differed significantly from all others. In the case of low-scoring participants, however, the mean RT was greater in Series 1 than in Series 2 and greater in Series 2 than in Series 3. Only the difference between the Series 3 and 4 was not significant. Therefore, it seems that less intelligent participants had steeper learning curves, probably because their initial level of performance was low. However, in Series 4, both ability groups responded with comparable speed. Note, however, that no analogous interaction was found when the Vocabulary Test was

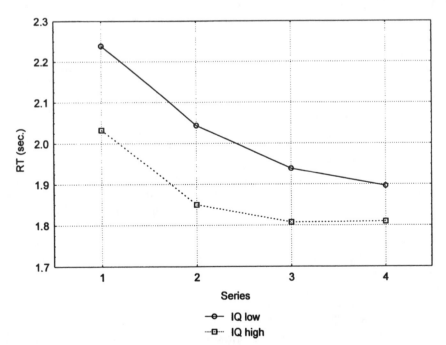

Figure 7.7. Reaction times (RTs) obtained by high- and low-scoring participants in the four consecutive series of the Navon task in Experiment 2: Intelligence × Series, $F(3, 204) = 2.94$, $p < .04$.

used. The three-way interaction showed that the advantage of intelligence in shortening RT was particularly salient in the global incongruent condition. No similar effects were found concerning the standard deviations of RTs and error rate, and the two-way interaction was also significant. The effects of personality were also insignificant, except that high scores on neuroticism were related to greater RTs.

The importance of ability measures throughout skill acquisition was investigated through the independent comparisons of critical statistics in Series 1 and 4. It appeared that the simple effect of mental ability (RAPM), although being a weak but significant source of variance in the first series, $F(1, 68) = 6.34$, $p < .02$, lost its significance in Series 4. In the case of the Vocabulary Test, the respective statistics were as follows: Series 1, $F(1, 68) = 5.61$, $p < .02$, and Series 4, $F(1, 68) = 4.99$, $p < .03$. This pattern of findings was the same for response latencies and their standard deviations. Intelligence measured by the RAPM accounted for a significant amount of variance in the first series, $F(1, 68) = 8.89$, $p < .01$, but was insignificant in the fourth series. On the other hand, intelligence assessed by the Vocabulary Test accounted for a significant amount of variance in the first series, $F(1, 68) = 5.33$, $p < .03$, and the fourth series, $F(1, 68) = 6.28$, $p = .02$. Interactive effects were not significant in either series regardless of dependent variable. The error rate was not significant for any effects regardless of series, assessment tool, or dependent variable. I therefore concluded that, as far as the results of Experiment 2 are concerned, learning eliminated the influence of psychometric intelligence on Navon task performance. This conclusion seems to apply only to the general intelligence assessed by the RAPM, but not to the verbal intelligence assessed by the Vocabulary Test. A comparison of the strength of the Intelligence × Incongruity interaction between Series 1 and 4 was not possible because these effects were too weak to reach significance regardless of the assessment tool.

As in Experiment 1, I used regression and correlation analyses to investigate more subtle relationships between intelligence and performance. Scores on the Vocabulary Test did not correlate significantly with RTs in Series 3 and 4; in the first two series, the correlation coefficients ranged from $-.10$ ns to $-.29$ ($p < .05$). The RAPM scores, on the other hand, significantly correlated with RTs in all series and conditions, particularly in the global incongruent condition, Series 2 ($r = -.51$) and 3 ($r = -.46$). Other coefficients ranged from $-.18$ to $-.37$. Thus, the relationship between fluid intelligence (assessed by the RAPM) and RT was strongest in the most difficult condition of the Navon task and in the intermediate stages of practice. The intraindividual standard deviations of RT correlated with RAPM scores (but not with the Vocabulary test scores) mostly in the incongruent conditions and across series. Thus, the variability of RTs was inversely related to ability test scores mainly in the experimental conditions, which were characterized by the incongruity of stimuli.

The indexes of automaticity, calculated the same way as in Experiment 1, revealed a relationship with the RAPM scores and no relationship with Vocabulary Test scores. There was a negative ($-.32$) relationship between RTs in Series 1 and 2. There was a positive relationship, however, between RTs in Series 2 and 3 (.26) and between Series 2 and 4 (.34). Note that the indexes of automaticity were difference scores having, in most cases, negative values because the RTs observed in an earlier series (e.g., Series 1) were generally higher than the RTs observed in the later series (e.g., Series 2) from which it was subtracted. The negative correlation of this index with RAPM scores showed that high-scoring individuals had better indexes of automaticity between Series 1 and 2. However, high-scoring individuals had worse indexes of automaticity, as indicated by positive correlations between RT differences in Series 2 and 3 as well as Series 2 and 4. In other words, the data suggest that intelligent people automatized their responses more efficiently than low-scoring individuals at the initial stage of learning but not at the later stages of skill acquisition. This interpretation therefore suggests that intelligent participants made substantial, stable progress during the first series, whereas participants with low ability showed improvements throughout practice.

The indexes of the efficiency of cognitive control were operationalized separately in the four series as the RT differences between incongruent and congruent conditions (global orientation only). The RAPM scores showed a relationship with these indexes in Series 2 ($r = -.47$, $p < .001$), 3 ($r = -.39$, $p < .001$), and 4 ($r = -.30$, $p < .01$), but not in Series 1. The Vocabulary Test did not show any relationship to the efficiency of cognitive control regardless of series. Hierarchical, blocked approach, regression analyses did not reveal a different pattern of relationships. The joint influence of the two ability measures did not influence the regression parameters. Except for neuroticism in Series 2, the personality variables did not enter the equations. In this case, the beta indexes were -0.53 (RAPM) and 0.26 (Neuroticism scale), whereas the equation parameters were as follows: $R = .54$, $R^2 = .29$, adjusted $R^2 = .26$. Thus, Series 2 appeared to be critical for assessing the efficiency of cognitive control. The data suggest that general intelligence, but not verbal ability, is related to increased resistance to incongruity. This relationship does not seem to disappear with learning, although its strength depends on the stage of skill acquisition.

General Discussion and Conclusion

At the beginning of this chapter, I asked whether learning could attenuate the importance of cognitive control in determining individual differences. The data obtained in Experiments 1 and 2 convincingly indicate that the answer is no: The efficiency of cognitive control remained important in determining individual differences because of the acquisition of Navon task skill and the subsequent automatization of cognitive processes determined that task's performance. Such a decisive answer is based on the thorough examination of the relationships shown in Figures 7.2–7.4 and 7.6. Undoubtedly, practice affected performance because the indexes of performance improved with the consecutive series of skill acquisition. However, learning did not erase the *relative difficulty* of the incongruent condition compared with the congruent one. In some cases, this relative difficulty was even greater in Series 4 (i.e., in the final stages of skill acquisition). Therefore, participants showed the benefit of practice through shortened RTs, decreased intraindividual variance, and, to some extent, reduced error rate. However, participants showed persistent disruptions in all three dependent variables in conditions that created incongruous response tendencies.

It is not the absolute level of performance that matters in the Navon task, then. The most informative and interesting indicator of the attentional mechanisms of cognitive control is the relative difficulty of the incongruent condition. If skill acquisition eliminated this relative difficulty, one could infer that learning increased the level of cognitive control. On the contrary, if learning increased this relative difficulty, one could argue that automatization attenuated the level of cognitive control. This appears to be the case because the increased efficiency of cognitive control is best measured by reduced disruption caused by incongruent response tendencies, when one response alternative must be actively suppressed to allow selection of another response alternative. Participants in both experiments showed almost errorless performance, even in the incongruent condition. However, they showed disruptions in RT, as measured relative to the congruent condition in which no response suppression (and thus only weak cognitive control) was necessary.

Regarding the second question formulated earlier on the relationship between intelligence and speed of automatization, the answer also appears to be no. The methodology of assessment of the relative speed of automatization is a critical issue here. When the slope of the learning curve is to be taken into account, one may not conclude that intelligent participants showed a faster rate of automatization. Examination of Figures 7.5 and 7.7 shows that low-scoring participants obtained steeper learning curves, presumably because their initial level of performance was lower. In other words, less intelligent individuals had more to learn and therefore took the opportunity to improve with the four series of repeated practice provided to them. More intelligent participants also took this opportunity, but apparently to a lesser degree, probably because their initial level of performance was already somewhat advanced. However, the results of the regression analysis indicate a slightly different pattern of results. In Experiment 1, as indicated by smaller gain scores between consecutive trials, less intelligent participants showed quicker automatization regardless of series (see Table 7.2). In Experiment 2, more intelligent participants showed more rapid automatization at the beginning of the learning process. As practice proceeded, however, less intelligent participants showed more rapid automatization. In other words, higher levels of fluid intelligence may be connected with faster rates of automatization only at the initial stages of skill acquisition provided that the sample consists of high school students (Experiment 2). In the case of the generally more intelligent participants showing restricted variance in mental ability (college students, Experiment 1), higher levels of intelligence seem to be associated with slower rates of automatization regardless of the stage of learning.

These findings challenge Sternberg's (1985) theory of the relationship between intelligence and speed of automatization, although they do not justify rejection of the theory either. If the Navon task permitted identical level of performance of both ability groups at the beginning of skill acquisition, more intelligent participants might show steeper learning curves within a few initial trials. Perhaps Sternberg's thesis would hold if one takes into account different levels of automatization. This may be acceptable only when the task is completely new; if it is at least moderately automatized, intelligence does not appear to be related to the speed of further automatization. However, such a conclusion is not consistent with the data obtained by Tetewsky and Sternberg (1986), who found that moderately novel tasks best reflected individual differences in general mental ability.

Another interpretation pertains to the theory of three phases of skill acquisition proposed by Ackerman (1988) and further elaborated by Kanfer and Ackerman (1989). Perhaps the first (cognitive) phase of learning, for which intelligence may be critically important, included only a few initial trials, immediately after which the second (associative) phase followed. I was not able to split a few initial trials

178

from the rest of the block of 24 trials constituting the experimental conditions of the Navon task. If I were, this hypothesis would have been investigated already.

The tentative answer to the third question, concerning the relationship between intelligence and cognitive efficiency, is yes: intelligent individuals likely exert more cognitive control over responding than less intelligent individuals. Although all participants showed disruptions in RT in the incongruent condition, intelligent participants were considerably less affected. This conclusion is evidenced by the Intelligence × Condition (congruent vs. incongruent) interaction, which was significant regardless of the intelligence assessment tool. Moreover, this interaction did not diminish because of learning, and in some instances it increased its significance in the final series, as opposed to the initial series. However, these effects were not found in Experiment 2, in which general intelligence in the incongruent condition accounted for individual differences only in the case of global orientation, as if the two task characteristics determining the task's difficulty (incongruity and global orientation) operated jointly to disrupt performance. These results do not exclude the positive answer to the question of whether intelligence is related to the increased efficiency of cognitive control. The regression analyses performed on the data obtained in Experiment 2 indicated further encouraging results. The zero-order correlations of RAPM scores with the incongruent minus congruent difference scores were negative and strong. Again, the stage of skill acquisition appears to matter. More intelligent individuals obtained higher indexes of cognitive control in all series except Series 1, the initial phase of learning. Although the strength of this relationship slightly decreased with practice, the correlations and the beta indexes were statistically significant at least at the .01 level.

I am justified in formulating a negative answer to the fourth question posed earlier: The processes of learning and automatization do not eliminate the relationship between intelligence and the strength of cognitive control. In other words, intelligent individuals are probably characterized by their greater efficiency in cognitive control, notwithstanding the reduction in variability attributable to skill acquisition. Learning reduces the variability both between and within individuals, but the relative advantage of intelligent people in the incongruent condition maintained meaningful differences. It would be worth examining the effects of increased practice (i.e., more than four series) because my data do not provide a conclusive answer to the question of whether the relationship between intelligence and cognitive control depends on automatization.

Finally, I emphasize that the findings reported in this chapter are consistent with the literature. First, the data support the thesis that elementary cognitive tasks (ECT) correlate with fluid rather than crystallized intelligence (Roberts & Stankov, 1997; also see chapters 1 and 19 in this book). In my study, the Vocabulary Test (presumed to assess only crystallized intelligence) did not produce any consistent results concerning the relationships under investigation, whereas the VAT (presumed to assess a combination of fluid and crystallized intelligence) appeared to be a much weaker correlate of the ECT variables. Second, the RT literature dealing with the problem of stimulus–response compatibility (e.g., Kornblum, Hasbroucq, & Osman, 1990) also showed that the effect of incongruity did not disappear with practice (see Fitts & Seeger, 1953). Roberts (1997) showed that incongruent responses correlated more significantly with intelligence than congruent ones. In this way, my findings supplement some existing theoretical positions.

179

In general, the results of my research allow me to draw several conclusions concerning the relationships among cognitive control, automatization, and individual differences. It appears that the strength of cognitive control is well assessed with the modified Navon task. The processes of learning and automatization showed the expected effects on the basic indexes of Navon task performance (i.e., the absolute values of RT, the standard deviation of RT, and error rate). They did not, however, influence the efficiency of cognitive control, which was operationalized as the relative difficulty of the incongruent condition versus the congruent one. It was impossible to discern a clear relationship between intelligence and speed of automatization; maybe this relationship does not exist, or maybe its character depends on the learning phase. However, intelligence appeared to be a significant correlate of the efficiency of cognitive control, which is a result worth further examination regarding the cognitive bases of the general mental ability. It also appears that the relationship between intelligence and the efficiency of cognitive control is probably not attenuated by automatization. Hence, this relationship appears to be a basic one, not interpretable in terms of the increased ability of intelligent people to familiarize a novel computerized task. On the other hand, the alleged relationship between intelligence and speed of automatization probably *is* interpretable in this way, as my data seem to suggest.

REFERENCES

Ackerman, P. L. (1986). Individual differences in information processing: An investigation of intellectual abilities and task performance during practice. *Intelligence, 10*, 101–139.

Ackerman, P. L. (1987). Individual differences in skill learning: An integration of psychometric and information processing perspectives. *Psychological Bulletin, 102*, 3–27.

Ackerman, P. L. (1988). Determinants of individual differences during skill acquisition: Cognitive abilities and information processing. *Journal of Experimental Psychology: General, 117*, 288–318.

Ackerman, P. L., & Schneider, W. (1985). Individual differences in automatic and controlled information processing. In R. F. Dillon (Ed.), *Individual differences in cognition* (Vol. 2). Orlando, FL: Academic Press.

Brzozowski, P., & Drwal, R. (1995). *Kwestionariusz osobowości Eysencka: Polska adaptacja EPQ-R.* Warsaw, Poland: Pracownia Testów Psychologicznych Polskiego Towarzystwa Psychologicznego.

Choynowski, M. (1967). *Test znajomości słów.* Warsaw, Poland: Pracownia Psychometryczna PAN.

Eysenck, H. J., & Eysenck, S. B. G. (1975). *Manual for the Eysenck Personality Questionnaire.* San Diego, CA: Educational and Industrial Testing Service.

Fitts, P. M., & Seeger, C. M. (1953). S-R compatibility: Spatial characteristics of stimulus and response codes. *Journal of Experimental Psychology, 46*, 199–210.

Hasher, L., & Zacks, R. T. (1979). Automatic and effortful processes in memory. *Journal of Experimental Psychology: General, 108*, 356–388.

Hunt, E., & Lansman, M. (1982). Individual differences in attention. *Advances in the Psychology of Human Intelligence, 1*, 207–254.

Hunt, E., & Lansman, M. (1986). Unified model of attention and problem solving. *Psychological Review, 93*, 446–461.

Kahneman, D. (1973). *Attention and effort.* Englewood Cliffs, NJ: Prentice Hall.

Kanfer, R., & Ackerman, P. L. (1989). Dynamics of skill acquisition: Building a bridge between intelligence and motivation. *Advances in the Psychology of Human Intelligence, 5*, 83–134.

Kornblum, S., Hasbroucq, T., & Osman, A. (1990). Dimensional overlap: Cognitive basis for stimulus–response compatibility — A model and taxonomy. *Psychological Review, 97*, 253–270.

Kyllonen, P. C., & Christal, R. E. (1990). Reasoning ability is (little more than) working memory capacity?! *Intelligence, 14*, 389–433.

Navon, D. (1977). Forest before trees: The precedence of global features in visual perception. *Cognitive Psychology, 9*, 353–383.

Nęcka, E. (1992). Cognitive analysis of intelligence: The significance of working memory processes. *Personality and Individual Differences, 13*, 1031–1046.

Nęcka, E. (1996). The attentive mind: Intelligence in relation to selective attention, sustained attention, and dual task performance. *Polish Psychological Bulletin, 27*, 3–24.

Nęcka, E. (1997). Attention, working memory, and arousal: Concepts apt to account for the "process of intelligence." In G. Matthews (Ed.), *Cognitive science perspectives on personality and emotion* (pp. 503–554). Amsterdam: Elsevier Science.

Nęcka, E., Gruszka, A., & Orzechowski, J. (1996). Selective attention in gifted children. *Polish Psychological Bulletin, 27*, 39–51.

Neubauer, A. C. (1990). Coping with novelty and automatization of information processing: An empirical test of Sternberg's two-facet subtheory of intelligence. *Personality and Individual Differences, 11*, 1045–1052.

Norman, D. A., & Bobrow, D. J. (1975). On data-limited and resource-limited processes. *Cognitive Psychology, 7*, 44–64.

Polczyk, R., & Nęcka, E. (1994). Not the speed, so what? Capacity and retention capability of working memory as cognitive roots of intelligence. *Polish Psychological Bulletin, 25*, 97–110.

Polczyk, R., & Nęcka, E. (1997). Capacity and retention capability of working memory modify the strength of the RT/IQ correlation: A short note. *Personality and Individual Differences, 23*, 1089–1091.

Roberts, R. D. (1997, July). *Processing speed, stimulus-response compatibility, and intelligence.* Paper presented at the Eighth Biennial Meeting of the International Society for the Study of Individual Differences, Aarhus, Denmark.

Roberts, R. D., & Stankov, L. (1997). *Individual differences in speed of mental processing and human abilities.* Manuscript submitted for publication.

Schneider, W., & Shiffrin, R. M. (1977). Controlled and automatic human information processing: I. Detection, search, and attention. *Psychological Review, 84*, 1–66.

Shiffrin, R. M., & Schneider, W. (1977). Controlled and automatic human information processing: II. Perceptual learning, automatic attending, and a general theory. *Psychological Review, 84*, 127–190.

Sternberg, R. J. (1985). *Beyond IQ: A triarchic theory of human intelligence.* Cambridge, England: Cambridge University Press.

Sternberg, R. J. (1990). *Metaphors of mind: Conceptions of the nature of intelligence.* Cambridge, England: Cambridge University Press.

Tetewsky, S. J., & Sternberg, R. J. (1986). Conceptual and lexical determinants of nonentrenched thinking. *Journal of Memory and Language, 25*, 202–225.

Urban, K. K., & Jellen, H. G. (1986). Assessing creative potential via drawing production: The Test for Creative Thinking–Drawing Production (TCT — DP). In A. J. Cropley, K. K. Urban, H. Wagner, & W. Wieczerkowski (Eds.), *Giftedness: A continuing worldwide challenge* (pp. 163–169). New York: Trillium Press.

Discussion

Discussion following Nęcka's presentation sought clarification about the details of his studies, specifically with respect to the presence or absence of automaticity and on the advantages and disadvantages to particular data-analysis tactics.

Dr. Hunt: In your procedure, the subject could not anticipate whether the trial was going to be a local trial?

Dr. Nęcka: They couldn't. It changed every trial.

Dr. Hunt: The point I want to make about that is that it's not a consistent mapping task. And in the sense of automatization, I think it's misleading. You're using a term here for a task which is always going to be a controlled processing task and always going to require the inhibitions of erroneous responses. I really have a feeling of what you may be seeing is learning a familiarity with the apparatus rather than the task because of the nature of the task. In fact, it's very close to the Wonderlic test of intelligence where in a 10-minute test you keep a shifting set in each trial.

Dr. Nęcka: Well, in fact, the participant learned how to operate the apparatus earlier. There were training sessions before. So the participants would respond about 10 times in advance and obtained feedback. Only after we ensured that they understood everything and they didn't commit errors, we allowed them to proceed to the experiment proper. So they had the opportunity to learn the basics in advance.

Dr. Hunt: But I'm talking about automatization. I'm talking about really getting those motor tasks down to where you're touch typing.

Dr. Nęcka: In a previous study, in the private study, we checked the blocked design — the trials were blocked into global/local — global/congruent, and so forth. And it was very difficult to obtain any stable consistent relationship with anything.

My position is that blocking allows automatization and speedy response, but it confuses the differential effects and correlations with other measures.

Dr. Stankov: Well, just a thing on Buz's [Hunt] question. You're saying that from any trial they get only certain options indicating what it is. So they would have to look on the keyboard and find out what is the alternative that they can answer, and then address that alternative.

Dr. Nęcka: Well, in fact, they were not required to look at the keyboard because the response alternatives were indicated on the screen, too, just below the stimulus proper. They had the four response alternatives. And they only were supposed to choose the direction which is up, down, left, right on the keyboard. So they learned how to operate this up, down, left, right keys. They just pressed the left button. That's all.

Dr. Widaman: I have a couple of comments. One of them is, I've done some work with reaction time tasks where in certain conditions reaction times have larger variability than in others, and it appeared that one way of portraying learning on this task was the decrease in standard deviation as a function of practice on the task. And I think that speaks to a point that came up earlier about the strength of relationship between intelligence and performance in different conditions. And what you've shown us that means appear to converge to a certain extent, but means can converge (if response variability is decreasing), it could even lead to higher correlations of intelligence at later stages of practice than at earlier stages of practice. So one issue is instead of dividing and doing a median split and looking at high and low groups, I think a key aspect of your hypotheses would be to look at the correlation of intelligence with performance at each of the four stages of practice. And again, it's entirely consistent mathematically that a slight convergence of means can be consistent with an increase in the correlation. So that's one point.

And a second point is that with a task like this when it's fairly well behaved — I'm not sure what it looks like with individuals. But it might be also interesting to try characterizing whether it's with structural equation modeling and looking at growth curve models or trying to estimate some parameters of nonlinear growth curve models for individuals and then look to see how the parameters or the growth functions change. If it were growth curve modeling, you could set up one index which would represent sort of an initial level, and then the curve for the individuals would be some kind of downward negatively accelerated curve. And it's possible that if you isolated that as a latent variable, you'd be able to look at the relationships of intelligence to parameters that describe the change over time. And I just encourage you to get away from doing median splits and so on and leaving the intelligence scores in the metric in which they come and look at how they relate to performance with conditions and then to parameters of curves like that.

Dr. Nęcka: I should do that probably, but the reason I didn't is that the Navon task is built according to the 2 × 2 design. So it's ideal for the MANOVA analysis. With correlations it would be it will be difficult. I cannot imagine how could I do it.

Dr. Ackerman: I want to amplify what Keith [Widaman] was saying. That part of the problem is (and this is something that Cronbach and Snow point out in their classic work) is that when you do a median split you're making an underlying assumption that there is a joint for the phenomenon that happens to be the median of whatever sample that you've obtained. Given the two different samples that you have, the median for ability has different meaning for our college sample than it does for your school-age sample. And so you may actually have very different meaning to high and low intelligence for those two groups, even though you've adopted the same methodology.

Dr. Nęcka: Definitely, yes.

Dr. Juan-Espinosa: I wonder if you compared the rating score on the comprehension score in the series. What did you find?

Dr. Nęcka: Well, the effects were mostly the same, very similar. I mean the Raven and the verbal analogy test behaved in a very similar manner. The vocabulary tests brought about somewhat different results in the second experiment. For instance, some effects were not visible entirely in reference to the Raven scores. However, they were found in reference to vocabulary tests. But it appeared that the vocabulary test, which is not a power test, which is based on the crystallized knowledge, appeared sometimes more in the revealing in terms of the individual differences and learning connections. But the verbal analogy and the Raven behave in the same manner.

Dr. Süß: I think this experiment will be a good foundation to test the skill acquisition series. That's the only one missing link for speed tests. You review the speed tests and in the first session you have high correlation with the Raven. But at the end of the second experiment, there are only high correlations with speed tests. And I think it is necessary to use correlational analysis because otherwise you lose information.

III

METHODOLOGICAL STRATEGIES

8

The Structure of Ability Profile Patterns: A Multidimensional Scaling Perspective on the Structure of Intellect

MARK L. DAVISON, HAIJIANG KUANG, and SE-KANG KIM

Cluster analysis, factor analysis (FA), and multidimensional scaling (MDS) have been used to study the structure of human abilities. As reflected in Gustafsson and Undheim's (1996) review and elsewhere, FA has been the most common. In his comparison of FA and MDS, MacCallum (1974) suggested one reason why FA has been so dominant. MacCallum noted that FA is based on an explicit model linking the observed test scores to model parameters. This model-based link between observed data and parameters makes FA a far richer method for the study of Person × Test (or item) data matrices. In the absence of an explicit model, MDS parameter estimates are far less rich in meaning.

The purpose of this chapter is to describe and illustrate an explicit model for test scores, one that leads to an MDS analysis (Davison, 1994; Davison, Gasser, & Ding, 1996; Davison & Skay, 1991). The model also leads to an interpretation of MDS dimensions in terms of profile patterns. Conceptually, the MDS representation is based on a decomposition of an individual's profile into two aspects.

The first aspect is profile level here defined as an unweighted average of the scores in the profile. If M_{pt} is the measurement of person p ($p = 1, \ldots, P$) on test t ($t = 1, \ldots, T$) and the profile of person p is the T-length vector $\mathbf{M}_p = (M_{pt})$, then the profile level is $M_{p.} = (\Sigma_t M_{pt})/T$. The second aspect is the profile pattern defined as deviations about the profile level, that is, a T-length vector $\mathbf{m}_p = (m_{pt} = M_{pt} - M_{p.})$. The MDS model uses a single parameter to represent individual differences

---

This research was supported by Grant R999B40010 from the National Center for Education Statistics in the U.S. Office of Education. We thank Kevin S. McGrew and Richard W. Woodcock for the data used in the example.

in observed profile levels and one or more dimensions to represent individual differences in ability patterns. In effect, the MDS dimensions are a structural representation of the ability profile patterns (as distinct from profile level).

The profile pattern interpretation has been foreshadowed in the literature. For instance, in criticizing Spearman's (1904) two-factor theory, Thurstone (1936) recommended using "a profile of mental abilities to describe each individual instead of a single index of intelligence" (p. 133). In his multiple-factor theory, however, Thurstone emphasized separate ability factors over which profiles could be defined, but not profiles or profile patterns per se. In effect, Thurstone's separate ability factors appeared in the foreground of his theory with profile patterns remaining in the background. The MDS model discussed shortly reverses this by moving profile patterns to the foreground and relegating separate ability constructs to the background.

Wechsler (1974) foreshadowed this perspective to an even greater extent than did Thurstone (1936). As summarized by McDermott, Fantuzzo, and Glutting (1990) and by Zachary (1990), Wechsler did not believe that specific ability scales existed primarily to assess specific abilities per se. Rather, according to Wechsler, one purpose of subtests was to assess the global capacity of the individual. The second purpose was to identify the highs and lows of single subtest variations within an individual. Whereas Thurstone (1936) kept ability patterns in the background and specific abilities in the foreground, Wechsler relegated the specific abilities to the background and moved global ability level and ability pattern into the spotlight.

We begin our chapter by describing the MDS model and interpretation of the model parameters. An application of the model is briefly illustrated. Results of MDS analyses based on the model can be used to study hypotheses about the relationship between profile patterns and external variables, and such an application of MDS results is briefly illustrated. Selected prior MDS analyses are then briefly reexamined in light of the profile pattern interpretation. Finally, the concept of a profile pattern as embodied in MDS is compared with related concepts from the literature.

An Explicit Model for Test Scores

We take the factor model and Figure 8.1 as our point of departure. Figure 8.1 shows a Person × Test data matrix, in which each column represents an observed variable and each row represents a person. Each data point is an element, M_{pt}, the measurement of person p using test t. The basic assumption of the factor model is that we can posit a small set of latent variables, represented by the columns of dots in Figure 8.1, so that the observed variables can be accounted for as linear combinations of the latent ones. We can do the same thing, however, by persons (or by rows) instead of by variables (or by columns).

Each row of the data matrix constitutes a person's profile. We can posit a small set of latent profiles, represented by the rows of dots in Figure 8.1, such that the observed profiles can be accounted for as linear combinations of the latent ones. This leads to a model that is linear and hence looks much like the factor model:

$$M_{pt} = c_p + \Sigma_k w_{pk} x_{tk} + e_{pt}. \tag{8.1}$$

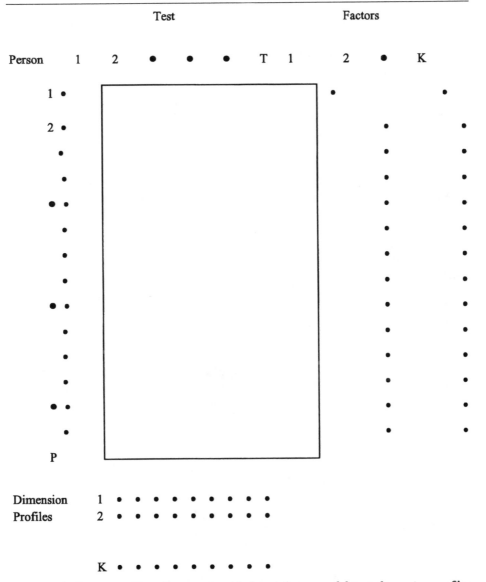

Figure 8.1. Persons × Test data matrix with latent factors and latent dimension profiles. From "Identifying Major Profile Patterns in a Population: An Exploratory Study of WAIS and GATB Patterns," by M. L. Davison, M. Gasser, and S. Ding, 1996, *Psychological Assessment*, 8, p. 27. Copyright 1996 by the American Psychological Association. Adapted with permission of the authors.

Here M_{pt} designates an observed data point, the score of person p on test t. The parameter c_p equals the mean score in row p, that is, $c_p = M_{p.} = (\Sigma_t M_{pt})/T$, indexes the overall height of person p's profile, and it is hereafter called the *level parameter*.

Each term in the sum on the right side of Equation 8.1 refers to a latent profile pattern k. Because latent profiles will later correspond to MDS dimensions, one can think of k as designating either a latent profile pattern or the corresponding MDS dimension. Each term in the sum is the product of a person parameter, w_{pk}, and a test parameter, x_{tk}. The test parameter, x_{tk}, equals the score of test t in latent profile k. The person parameter, w_{pk}, is a weight for person p on latent profile k. Roughly speaking, w_{pk} indexes the degree of correspondence between the actual profile of person p and the latent profile k. Finally, e_{pt} is an error term representing measurement error and systematic deviations from the model.

Implicit in this model is the idea that individual differences in profile levels, represented by c_p in Equation 8.1, determine the grand mean of the test intercorrelation matrix. Individual differences in profile patterns, represented by $\Sigma_k w_{pk} x_{tk}$ in Equation 8.1, determine the patterning of test intercorrelations about their grand mean. This patterning of correlations about their grand mean is what Snow, Kyllonen, and Marshalek (1984) called the "topography of ability and learning correlations."

Although the profile interpretation of Equation 8.1 has seldom been recognized, it is not a new model. It has been around long enough to acquire several other names that are useful in locating the relevant literature. Bechtel, Tucker, and Chang (1971), Carroll and Chang (1968), Davison (1994), Davison and Skay (1991), and Tucker (1960) called it the "vector" model. The French psychometrician Benzecri (1969), Weller and Romney (1990), and Greenacre (1984) called it the "correspondence analysis" model. It is one of Nishisato's (1980) "dual scaling" models because it leads to the scaling of both tests and people. Cattell's (1967) Q-factor model is a special case of Equation 8.1 in which the observed data are standardized by row and c_p drops from the model because it equals zero for every person p. Furthermore, it is the model underlying Skinner's (1979) modal profile analysis.

Assumptions and Restrictions

Having described the model, we now need some way to estimate the parameters. There is a variety of methods (Benzecri, 1969; Weller & Romney, 1990). The estimation method chosen leads to a new interpretation of the literature in which MDS has been applied to the intercorrelations of tests.

To develop the estimation method, however, we first need to add some assumptions and restrictions to uniquely identify the parameters:

$$\Sigma_t x_{tk} = 0.0 \text{ for all } k \tag{8.2}$$

$$(1/P)\Sigma_p w_{pk}^2 = 1.0 \text{ for all } k \tag{8.3}$$

$$\Sigma_p w_{pk} w_{pk'} = 0 \text{ for all } (k, k') \tag{8.4}$$

$$(1/P)\Sigma_p e_{pt} = 0 \text{ for all } t \tag{8.5}$$

$$(1/P)\Sigma_p e_{pt}^2 = \sigma^2 \text{ for all } t \tag{8.6}$$

and

$$\Sigma_p w_{pk} e_{pt} = 0 \text{ for all } (k, t). \tag{8.7}$$

Here, P refers to the number of people in the data matrix and σ^2 equals the variance of the deviations, e_{pt}, in Equation 8.1. For the most part, Equations 8.2–8.7 are variations on standard assumptions and side conditions. Note that in Equation 8.2, each latent profile, k, is ipsative, that is, the mean of the scores in each latent profile equals zero. Consequently, latent profiles will reproduce observed profile patterns (scatter plus shape), but not the level of observed profiles that is reproduced by the level parameters c_p. Equation 8.6 implies that the error variances are equal for all tests. This is an unduly strong assumption, but one that seems necessary to justify the kinds of scaling analyses most commonly available in existing statistical packages.

Estimation of Parameters

Equations 8.1–8.7 lead to the following result concerning the squared Euclidean distance proximity measure defined over all possible pairs of tests (Davison, 1996; Davison & Skay, 1991), a result on which parameter estimation can be based:

$$\delta_{tt'}^2 = (1/P)\Sigma_p(M_{pt} - M_{pt'})^2 \tag{8.8}$$

$$= \Sigma_k(x_{tk} - x_{k'})^2 + 2\sigma^2 \tag{8.9}$$

$$= d_{tt'}^2 + 2\sigma^2.$$

As shown in Equation 8.9, under the assumptions of Equations 8.1–8.7 (Davison, 1996) and except for an additive constant ($2\sigma^2$) $\delta_{tt'}^2$ will equal the squared Euclidean distance between pairs of tests (t, t') expressed in terms of the test parameters x_{tk} in the model of Equation 8.1. This implies that the squared Euclidean distance proximity measure satisfies the fundamental assumption of common MDS analyses. Hence, we can estimate the test parameters in the model by computing the squared euclidean distance matrix for all possible pairs of tests and submitting that matrix to an MDS analysis. The MDS analysis should yield one dimension for each latent profile. Along a given dimension k, the scale value for test t along dimension k is our estimate of the score for test t in latent profile k, x_{tk}.

This leads to an analysis that closely parallels FA as shown in Table 8.1. The first step in FA and MDS is to compute a proximity matrix. Whereas in FA, the proximity

TABLE 8.1   Schematic Comparison of Factor Analysis and Multidimensional Scaling of Test Data

Step	Factor analysis	MDS
Estimate proximity matrix	Covariance matrix or correlation matrix	Squared Eculidean distances or correlation matrix
Estimate test parameters	Factor algorithm: Factor loading matrix	Nonmetric MDS: MDS scale value matrix (x_{tk})
Estimate person parameters	Regress data on loading matrix: Factor loadings	Regress data on scale values: Corrected weights (w_{pk})

Note.   MDS = multidimensional scaling.

matrix is a covariance or correlation matrix, in MDS it would be a squared Euclidean distance matrix or a correlation matrix. When the observed variables are in standardized form (standardized by variable), the squared Euclidean distances will be monotonically related to the correlation coefficients. Therefore, in a nonmetric MDS, we would get the same solution using either squared Euclidean distances or correlation coefficients, and that solution provides estimates of the test parameters in our model.

As with FA, the second step is to submit the proximity matrix to an analysis that will yield estimates of the test parameters in our model. In the case of FA, any of several well-known algorithms has been used to estimate the test parameters, the factor loadings. For the MDS analysis, the squared Euclidean distances (or correlations) would be submitted to an MDS analysis. If the assumptions of the model are satisfied, the analysis should yield one dimension for each latent profile. Along dimension k, the scale value x_{tk} will be our estimate of the score for test t in latent profile k.

The third step involves estimating the person parameters, factor scores in factor analysis and person correspondence indexes w_{pk} in MDS. Because Equation 8.1 is linear, once the test parameters, x_{tk}, have been estimated, the person parameters (c_p, w_{pk}) can be obtained by regressing person p's observed score profile onto the test parameters (e.g., the MDS scale values). Roughly speaking, each correspondence coefficient w_{pk} will index the correspondence between the actual profile of participant p and the latent profile k. The paper by Davenport, Davison, Bielinski, and Ding (1995) contains SPSS and SAS algorithms for performing the analysis in Table 8.1.

Example: MDS Analysis of Cognitive Ability Scales

Participants

The data for the illustration come from 176 25- to 39-year-old adults in the norming sample of the Woodcock–Johnson Psychoeducational Battery—Revised (WJ–R; Mcgrew, Werder, & Woodcock, 1991; Woodcock & Johnson, 1989).

Instruments

The cognitive ability portion of the WJ-R contains 14 subtests arranged into ability clusters of 2 subtests each. The ability clusters and the 2 subtests in each (in parentheses) are as follows: Long-Term Memory (Visual–Auditory Learning and Memory for Names), Short-Term Memory (Memory for Sentences and Memory for Words), Speed of Processing (Visual Matching and Cross Out), Auditory Processing (Incomplete Words and Sound Blending), Visual Processing (Visual Closure and Picture Recognition), Comprehension–Knowledge (Picture Vocabulary and Oral Vocabulary), and Fluid Reasoning (Analysis–Synthesis and Concept Formation).

Profile Interpretation of Test Parameter Estimates

Table 8.2 shows a 3-D MDS solution obtained using ALSCAL (Young & Lewyckyj, 1979). To aid interpretability, the original ALSCAL solution was rotated to optimize

TABLE 8.2   Three-Dimensional MDS Solution Based on WJ–R COG Extended Battery Data Intercorrelations (X_{tk})

Test	Processing speed vs. long-term memory (Dimension 1)	Auditory vs. visual processing (Dimension 2)	Comprehension–knowledge vs. visual processing (Dimension 3)
MEMNAM	−1.27	−0.26	−0.49
V-A-LRNG	−1.05	−0.60	0.04
MEMSEN	0.05	0.99	0.25
MEMWRD	1.48	**1.85**	−1.08
VISMATCH	**2.54**	−0.42	−0.02
CROSOUT	**1.29**	−0.19	−0.13
INCOMWRD	−0.26	**1.56**	−0.87
SOUNBLEN	−0.03	0.46	−0.02
VISCLOS	−0.56	**−2.14**	−0.90
PICRECOG	−0.58	**−1.09**	−1.49
PICVOC	−0.51	−0.30	**2.11**
ORALVOC	−0.50	0.53	**1.65**
ANALSYNT	0.32	−0.16	0.44
CONCFORM	−0.90	−0.24	0.51

Note.   Boldface numbers identify the major scales used to interpret dimension profiles. WJ–R COG = Woodcock–Johnson Psychoeducational Battery — Revised cognitive ability; MEMNAM = Memory for Name; V-A-LRNG = Visual–Auditory Learning; MEMSEN = Memory for Sentence; MEMWRD = Memory for Words; VISMATCH = Visual Matching; CROSOUT = Cross Out; INCOMWRD = Incomplete Words; SOUNBLEN = Sound Blending; VISCLOS = Visual Closure; PICRECOG = Picture Recognition; PICVOC = Picture Vocabulary; ORALVOC = Oral Vocabulary; ANALSYNTH = Analysis–Synthesis; CONFORM = Concept Formation.

the varimax criterion (Kaiser, 1974). Figure 8.2A shows the scale values for the first dimension plotted as a profile pattern. The 14 subtests are shown along the horizontal axis. Above each subtest we have plotted its coordinate along Dimension 1 in Table 8.2. Somewhat arbitrarily, we have paid particular attention to scale values above 1.00, the root-mean-square coordinate.

In the profile pattern of Figure 8.2A, there are marked peaks for the two Speed of Processing subtests: Visual Matching and Cross Out. In addition, the scale value for one of the Short-Term Memory tests, Memory for Words, also exceeded 1.00. These tests seem to assess skills for which speed is critical, either because they involve processing speed per se or temporary short-term memory storage. The lowest points in the profile, the only two values below −1.00, occur for the two Long-Term Memory tests, Memory for Names and Verbal–Auditory Learning. People with this profile performed better on the Speed of Processing subtests and on the Memory for Words test than on the Long-Term Memory tests. Given the high points for Visual Matching and Cross Out, coupled with the low points for Memory for Names and Verbal–Auditory Learning, we have called this the "processing speed versus long-term memory profile." We are not, however, wedded to the interpretation contained in this label.

In MDS, the dimensions can be reflected without loss of fit. That is, it is completely arbitrary which end of a dimension is positive and which is negative. Therefore, for each dimension profile, there is a mirror image profile obtained by reversing all the signs. In the case of Dimension 1 in Table 8.2, reflecting the

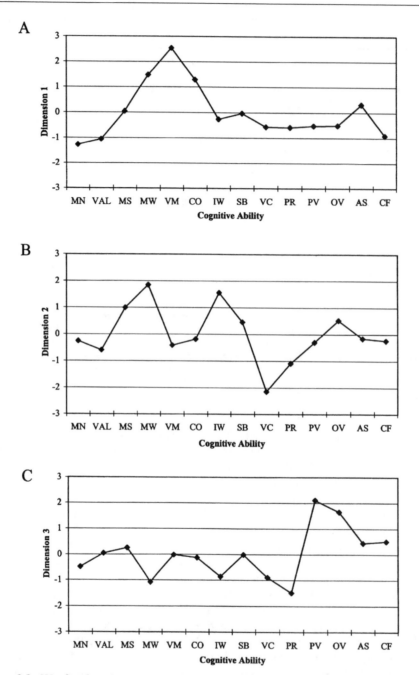

Figure 8.2. Woodcock–Johnson Psychoeducational Battery — Revised dimension profile patterns. A: Dimension 1, processing speed versus long-term memory. B: Dimension 2, auditory versus visual processing. C: Dimension 3, visual processing versus comprehension–knowledge. MN = Memory for Names; VAL = Visual–Auditory Learning; MS = Memory for Sentences; MW = Memory for Words; VM = Visual Matching; CO = Cross Out; IW = Incomplete Words; SB = Sound Blending; VC = Visual Closure; PR = Picture Recognition; PV = Picture Vocabulary; OV = Oral Vocabulary; AS = Analysis–Synthesis; CF = Concept Formation.

signs of all tests, yields a profile with peaks for Long-Term Memory tests and low points for the two Processing Speed tests and Memory for Words. People with this mirror-image profile would have higher scores on Memory for Names and Visual–Auditory Learning than on Memory for Words, Visual Matching, and Cross Out.

Figure 8.2B shows the second dimension of Table 8.2 plotted as a profile pattern. Again, each subtest is plotted along the horizontal axis. Above each subtest, its scale value appears along Dimension 2 in Table 8.2. Figure 8.2B's profile has a peak above the two Short-Term Memory tests, Memory for Sentences and Memory for Words, and a second peak above Incomplete Words, one of the Auditory Processing tests. The interpretation of this grouping is unclear. Two of the tests are short-term memory tests; all three are presented orally and all three involve verbal material. "Troughs" occur above the Visual Processing subtests, Visual Closure and Picture Recognition. Despite the fact that the point for one of the auditory subtests is not terribly high (Sound Blends), we have labeled this an "auditory versus visual processing dimension" because it seems to involve the auditory processing of meaningful verbal material. In any case, people who resemble this profile would perform better on three tests containing verbal material presented orally (Memory for Sentences, Memory for Words, and Incomplete Words) than on two Visual Processing tests (Visual Closure and Picture Recognition). People with the mirror-image profile would perform better on the Visual Processing subtests than on the three tests presented orally.

Figure 8.2C shows Dimension 3 plotted as a profile pattern. There is a clear peak over the two Comprehension–Knowledge tests, Picture Vocabulary and Oral Vocabulary. Likewise, there is a clear trough below the Visual Processing subtests (Visual Closure and Picture Recognition), although the first of these with a scale value of $-.90$ fails to meet our cutoff of -1.00. There is a second trough below Memory for Words that involves remembering a string of unrelated words. An individual with this profile would perform better in Comprehension–Knowledge test than in Visual Processing and Memory for Words test. Conversely, someone with the mirror-image profile would have displayed a stronger performance in the area of Visual Processing and Memory for Words test than in Comprehension–Knowledge test.

Profile Interpretation of Person Parameters

Table 8.3 shows the estimates of the person parameters for 14 participants. Column 1 shows their correspondence indexes for the processing speed versus long-term memory profile pattern shown in Figure 8.2A. Those with positive correspondence indexes, such as Participant 85, have observed profile patterns that displayed a trend similar to the processing speed versus long-term memory pattern shown in Figure 8.2A. Those with negative correspondence indexes, such as Participant 16, had observed profile patterns that displayed the mirror-image trend, higher on Long-Term Memory tests than on the Processing Speed tests (and Memory for Words). Columns 2 and 3 show the correspondence indexes for Dimensions 2 and 3, respectively: auditory versus visual processing and comprehension–knowledge versus visual processing.

For some participants, there was only one dimension with a correspondence index

TABLE 8.3   Person Parameters for 14 People: WJ–R COG Profiles

Participant No.	Processing speed vs. long-term memory Dimension 1 w_{p1}	Auditory vs. visual processing Dimension 2 w_{p2}	Comprehension–knowledge vs. visual processing Dimension 3 w_{p3}	Level c_p	R^2
15	.01	.03	.10	0.17	.06
27	.00	.01	.15	−0.61	.06
26	.63	.04	.62	0.32	.72
80	.12	.00	.00	0.69	.09
54	.23	.22	.37	1.22	.41
19	−.43	−.38	−.59	−0.49	.81
16	−.74	.39	.34	0.28	.81
168	.69	−.45	−.52	−0.84	.72
42	−.56	−.14	0.3	0.37	.57
85	.87	−.12	−.08	0.10	.71
119	−.08	−.80	.03	−0.36	.62
164	.09	.84	.29	0.29	.76
130	−.05	.06	−.70	−2.09	.46
149	.07	−.05	.79	0.73	.89
VAF	1.24	1.29	1.84	5.47	

Note.   VAF = variance accounted for by the 14 Woodcock–Johnson Psychoeducational Battery—Revised (WJ–R) cognitive ability (COG) subtests. w_{p1}, w_{p2}, w_{p3}, and c_p are statistical symbols defined in the text.

that was large in absolute value (e.g., Participant 119 or 130). Their observed patterns resembled only one of the three dimensions. Others had weights that were substantial in absolute value on more than one dimension (e.g., Participant 26 or Participant 19). Their observed profiles were a blend (linear combination) of the patterns reflected by two or more dimensions.

Column 4 shows the level parameter for each participant. Because the raw test scores in this analysis were standardized to have a mean of zero and a variance of one, level parameter estimates above zero, such as that for Participant 54, indicate an above-average profile level. Negative-level parameter estimates, such as that for Participant 130, indicate a below-average profile level.

Column 5 shows the proportion of variance in each participant's profile accounted for by the three dimensions. The profiles of some participants were recovered well, such as those of participants 19 and 16, for whom more than 80% of the profile variance could be accounted for. For other participants, notably 15 and 27, virtually none of the variance in their profiles was accounted for by the three dimensions. The average R^2 for this sample was .38. On average, less than half of the profile pattern variance could be accounted for by the three dimensions.

In comprehending the meaning of the correspondence indexes, examination of individual profiles can be instructive. Consider Participant 85, whose profile was accounted for reasonably well (R^2 = .71). The correspondence index for Dimension 1 was large in absolute value, whereas the other two correspondence indexes were small. This suggests that the observed profile of Participant 85 should resemble the Dimension 1 profile pattern shown in Figure 8.2A. The triangles in Figure 8.3 show

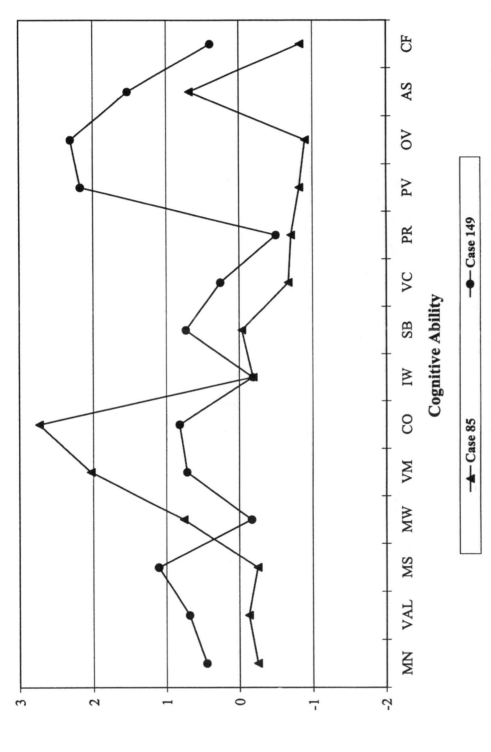

Figure 8.3. Observed Woodcock–Johnson Psychoeducational Battery – Revised cognitive profile of Participant 85 (triangles) and Participant 149 (Circles). MN = Memory for Names; VAL = Visual–Auditory Learning; MS = Memory for Sentences; MW = Memory for Words; VM = Visual Matching; CO = Cross Out; IW = Incomplete Words; SB = Sound Blending; VC = Visual Closure; PR = Picture Recognition; PV = Picture Vocabulary; OV = Oral Vocabulary; AS = Analysis–Synthesis; CF = Concept Formation.

the observed profile of Participant 85. It is only slightly elevated, as reflected by the level parameter estimate of .10. Furthermore, it shows the expected peaks for the Speed of Processing tests and the expected valley for the Long-Term Memory tests. This particular participant scored somewhat above average overall and showed greater strength on the Speed of Processing than on the Long-Term Memory subtests.

As another example, consider Participant 149, whose data were well accounted for ($R^2 = .89$). This individual also had a somewhat elevated profile, as reflected in the level parameter estimate (.73). Participant 149's correspondence index was high for Dimension 3 and negligible for Dimensions 1 and 2, suggesting that this participant's observed profile would resemble the comprehension–knowledge versus visual processing pattern shown in Figure 8.2C. The circles in Figure 8.3 show this person's observed profile. It is clear from a comparison of Figures 8.2C and 8.3 that Participant 149's observed profile does indeed bear a marked resemblance to the comprehension–knowledge versus visual processing pattern.

As can be seen in Table 8.4, the correspondence indexes were largely uncorrelated with each other. Correspondence indexes for Dimensions 1 and 2 were virtually uncorrelated with the level parameter ($rs = -.05$ and .06, respectively), but there was a modest correlation between correspondence indexes for Dimension 3 and the level parameter ($r = .42$). Those with higher profiles showed a tendency toward a particular pattern, a pattern marked by higher scores on the Comprehension–Knowledge than on the Visual Processing subtest. Conversely, those with lower profiles showed a tendency toward patterns with higher scores on the Visual Processing than on the Comprehension–Knowledge subtest. Note that individual differences in overall profile levels could be correlated with individual differences in profile patterns.

Table 8.5 shows the correlations of model parameters with scores on the achievement subtests of the WJ–R: Letter Word Identification, Passage Comprehension, Calculation, Applied Problem Solving, Dictation, Writing Sample, Science, Social Studies, Humanities, Word Attack, Reading Vocabulary, Quantitative Concepts, Proofing, and Written Fluency. Correspondence indexes for the first two dimensions had nonsignificant ($p > .05$) correlations with all of the achievement tests. None of the correlations for these first two dimensions exceeded .14 in absolute value. Particular ability in processing speed compared with long-term memory (Dimension 1) or auditory compared with visual processing (Dimension 2) carried no advantage for measured achievement in school subjects.

Correspondence indexes for Dimension 3, comprehension–knowledge versus

TABLE 8.4 Intercorrelations of Person Parameter Estimates

Dimension	Processing speed vs. long-term memory Dimension 1	Auditory vs. visual processing Dimension 2	Comprehension– knowledge vs. visual processing Dimension 3	Level
1	—	−.18	.05	−.05
2	−.18	—	−.01	.06
3	.05	−.01	—	.42
Level	−.05	.06	.42	—

TABLE 8.5   Correlations of Achievement Tests With Person Parameters

Test	Processing speed vs. long-term memory Dimension 1	Auditory vs. visual processing Dimension 2	Comprehension– knowledge vs. visual processing Dimension 3	Level
Letter/Word Identification	.04	.13	.48	.72
Passage Comprehension	.00	.07	.50	.71
Calculation	.09	−.01	.48	.57
Applied Problem	−.03	.05	.57	.67
Dictation	.17	.05	.47	.68
Writing Sample	.01	.06	.48	.68
Science	−.12	.07	.57	.56
Social Studies	−.08	.09	.62	.65
Humanities	−.11	.01	.56	.67
Word Attack	.12	.13	.38	.69
Reading Vocabulary	.01	.10	.61	.70
Quantitative	.02	.04	.57	.65
Proofing	.11	.04	.44	.72
Writing Fluency	.14	−.08	.47	.66

visual processing, however, were consistently correlated with all of the measures of achievement ($p < .01$). These correlations ranged from a high of .62 for the Social Studies test to a low of .38 for the Word Attack test. Ability profile level was also consistently correlated with achievement ($p < .01$). Correlations with the level parameter ranged from a low of .56 on the Science test to a high of .72 on the Proofing test. Overall, these correlations suggested that those who did well on the achievement tests tended to have ability profiles that were higher overall (profile level) and were somewhat higher in the Comprehension–Knowledge test than in other areas.

As this example illustrates, within the context of the model in Equation 8.1, scale values are test parameter estimates and can be interpreted in terms of prototypical profile patterns (and mirror-image patterns) corresponding to dimensions. Observed profile patterns are represented as linear combinations of the prototypes. Person parameters are interpreted with respect to these same prototypical profile patterns. Profile-level parameters quantify individual differences in overall profile height. Correspondence indexes quantify the degree of match between observed profiles and dimension prototypes. As illustrated earlier, correspondence indexes can be used to study associations between match to prototypes and external variables, achievement tests in our example.

Prior MDS Analyses

Various authors (e.g., Ackerman, Kanfer, & Goff, 1995; Guttman, 1954, 1965; Guttman & Levy, 1991; Silverstein, 1987; Snow et al., 1984) have applied MDS to associations among ability measures. We now turn to a brief reexamination of these results in light of the profile interpretation for MDS.

Guttman (1954) predicted that content and complexity differences among the tests would lead to a circumplex structure with more complex tests at the periphery

199

of the space and less complex ones at the center. Instead, Guttman (1965) found that the more complex tests from Thurstone's (1936) studies appeared at the center and that less complex test appeared at the periphery. Snow et al. (1984) analyzed a larger number of ability tests. They, too, concluded that the more complex tests fell to the center of the solution and cognitively less complex tests to the periphery. Snow et al. also noted content distinctions: verbal, numerical, and figural, distinctions that were further supported by Ackerman's (1988) reanalysis of Allison's (1960) data. Ackerman (1988) also suggested a fourth content area, mechanical, and a performance level versus speed contrast (Marshalek, Lohman, & Snow, 1983).

When MDS dimensions are viewed as profile patterns, it is the tests at the periphery that define the patterns. At least with respect to the tests analyzed by Guttman (1965) and Snow et al. (1984), it would seem to be the cognitively less complex tests that were at the periphery of the solution and hence that were the best markers of profile patterns. It remains to be seen whether this is a general phenomenon. If so, it would seem to have major implications for those constructing ability test batteries who want the battery to distinguish various profile patterns clearly. Complex tests may be good markers for global ability (or overall profile level) but less useful in defining patterns of ability.

Guttman and Levy (1991) and Silverstein (1987) have applied multidimensional scaling to the structure of Wechsler tests. Silverstein's first dimension clearly distinguished between Verbal and Performance subtests. Thus, it represented a profile pattern marked by a discrepancy between Verbal and Performance subscales, a much discussed, controversial discrepancy in the assessment literature (Bannatyne, 1974; Kaufman, 1979). Silverstein labeled his second dimension "freedom from distractibility." It was marked by highest scores on the Digit Span, Arithmetic Reasoning, and Digit Symbol subtests. Valleys in the profile occur for the Picture Completion and Picture Arrangement subtests. It may in fact represent a difference between numerical and figural material, a distinction also noted by Snow et al. (1984). These two dimensions are virtually identical to those identified by Moses and Pritchard (1995) in their modal profile analysis (Skinner, 1979) of Wechsler Adult Intelligence Scale–Revised data (Wechsler, 1981). They also seem similar to the first two dimensions of Guttman and Levy, although Guttman and Levy gave a much different interpretation to their solution.

Interpreted as profile patterns, MDS dimensions represent performance contrasts (e.g., verbal vs. performance or auditory vs. visual). After reviewing the MDS literature, the results seem to suggest a contrast between level and speed of processing (Ackerman, 1988; Marshalek et al., 1983). It also suggests contrasts along a content facet with four levels: verbal, figural, mechanical, and numerical (e.g., Ackerman, 1988; Guttman & Levy, 1991; Snow, Corno, & Jackson, 1996). WJ-R Dimension 2 and Guttman and Levy's Dimension 3 hint at contrasts between two levels of a sensory–modality facet: visual versus auditory. There may be other facets, such as process, with at least three facets: long-term memory, short-term memory, and fluid reasoning. Combining the profile pattern interpretation with results from prior studies would lead to a structure represented by global ability (profile level) and profile patterns, patterns marked by performance contrasts within and between Guttman-like facets.

Discussion

Profile Patterns and Other Constructs

Although MDS dimensions can represent bipolar traits, the dimensions discussed earlier are *not* bipolar in the sense of having mutually exclusive end points. For instance, consider the verbal versus performance dimension from Silverstein's (1987) analysis of the Wechsler Adult Intelligence Scale. Verbal and performance ability are positively correlated and hence anything but mutually exclusive. One can be high in both or low in both. However, verbal and performance ability are imperfectly correlated, and therefore one can readily be higher in one than the other. Rather than reflecting bipolarity, Silverstein's verbal versus performance dimension reflects tendencies to be higher in one than the other, consistent with an imperfect correlation between verbal and performance abilities.

If one defines the term *construct* as broadly as have some authors (e.g., Snow et al., 1996), then profile patterns are indeed constructs. A profile pattern is not, however, a homogeneous construct of the factor-analytic type. Researchers use multiple items or multiple indicators to assess homogeneous constructs, but they expect the multiple indicators to be reasonably internally consistent. If a person scores high on one indicator, researchers expect that person to score high on all of the indicators within the limits of measurement error. When researchers quantify a homogeneous construct, what they quantify is the person's standing along that construct.

A profile pattern is *not* homogeneous. Inherently, one cannot specify a pattern in terms of a single element because a pattern is by definition an arrangement of two or more elements. A psychological pattern, therefore, can be specified only in terms of two or more homogeneous constructs. Although one must use multiple indicators to specify a profile pattern, those indicators will not be internally consistent because they will reflect two or more distinct constructs. The pattern itself is a specified arrangement of scores among the several indicators. When one quantifies a profile pattern, what one quantifies is the degree of match between the specified pattern and a person's actual profile.

In that they cut across two or more constructs, ability profile patterns resemble the aptitude complexes of Snow et al. (1996) and the trait complexes of Ackerman and Heggestad (1997). However, unlike aptitude or trait complexes, profile patterns contrast performance in two or more areas (e.g., the verbal vs. performance dimension of the Wechsler subscales). In this respect, the profile patterns resemble Messick's (1994) "within-person contrasts," a phrase he used to describe intraindividual differences. Profile patterns can contrast performance on two or more abilities or traits or on two or more ability or trait complexes.

In short, a profile pattern is a psychological construct in the broadest sense, but not a homogeneous construct of the factor-analytic type. Psychologically, it is "contrastive," not bipolar, and it bears more resemblance to an aptitude complex or a within-persons contrast than to an ability factor or trait.

Hierarchical Structures of Ability

Elements in the MDS model correspond loosely to elements in hierarchical factor models of ability. Although there are various forms of hierarchical models

(Gustafsson & Undheim, 1996), we ignore the distinctions between them here for the sake of brevity. Most hierarchical models include a general ability factor. This general ability factor corresponds roughly to the component of variance represented in the MDS model as individual differences in profile level. The MDS profile level parameter is an equally weighted average of scores in the person's ability profile, whereas the general factor score is usually an unequally weighted sum (Davison, 1985).

At lower levels, hierarchical models refer to more specialized ability factors. The MDS representation of structure replaces specialized ability factors with patterns of ability (see also Marshalek et al., 1983). Whereas hierarchical factor models place specialized abilities per se in the foreground of the theory, the MDS model places patterns defined over those specialized abilities in the foreground, relegating specific abilities per se to the background.

Factor and MDS Models

The complementary role of MDS and FA in the study of human abilities can be understood partly through this distinction between specialized abilities per se and profile patterns defined over those specialized abilities. As a tool of psychological theory, FA aims to yield a representation of general and specialized ability constructs. MDS yields a representation of the major profile patterns defined over those specialized abilities.

When based on the model of Equation 8.1, MDS becomes particularly useful when the research questions concern profile patterns. For instance, what are the major ability profile patterns in a population? How are those patterns related to performance on outcome variables? Are there subgroup differences on those profile patterns? What are the developmental antecedents of those patterns?

Because it is framed in terms of patterns, the MDS model may provide an important link between psychometric research on one hand and the psychological assessment literature, including the neuropsychology literature, on the other (e.g., Moses & Pritchard, 1995). The applied psychological literature on assessment has long been concerned with profile patterns. The major psychometric models have not been framed in terms of profile patterns; therefore, they have been ill-suited to the study of some questions arising in applied assessment. Because the MDS model of Equation 8.1 is so framed, it can provide a vehicle for studying assessment hypotheses concerning profile patterns. Models framed in terms of profile patterns may be particularly important in trying to provide a research base for profile interpretations of applied assessments.

Compared with the factor model and FA, the MDS model and analysis are more uniquely appropriate for the study of profile patterns. The MDS model may well provide a link between psychometric methods on one hand and the applied assessment literature on the other.

Conclusion

At the beginning of this century, Spearman (1904) proposed his two-factor theory with one general factor and one specific factor for each test in the battery. He formulated that theory in terms of homogeneous constructs. In so doing, he established a precedent that psychometric research has followed faithfully through the present day in multiple-factor models, item response theories, and structural equations models. His precedent has influenced more than just psychometric research. It has had an impact on test and test battery construction, the dependent variables used in experimental studies, the covariates used in Aptitude × Treatment interaction research, and the predictor and criterion variables used in correlational studies.

Spearman's (1904) model helped launch an extremely productive century of individual-differences research. Despite that productivity, however, his precedent is one that researchers should not and need not follow blindly. From a statistical perspective, psychometric models can be formulated in terms of either homogeneous constructs of the factor type or profile patterns as needed. If researchers are to fully realize the potential of assessment batteries and psychometric methods for the study of individual differences, they must recognize how and when to reformulate those models in terms of profile patterns.

For most of this century, researchers have been perfecting their methods for the study of homogeneous constructs of the factor type. As researchers move into the next century, they should bring their methods for studying profile patterns to the same level of sophistication as their methods for the study of homogeneous constructs.

REFERENCES

Ackerman, P. L. (1988). Determinants of individual differences during skill acquisition: Cognitive abilities and information processing. *Journal of Experimental Psychology: General, 117,* 288–318.

Ackerman, P. L., & Heggestad, E. D. (1997). Intelligence, personality, and interests: Evidence for overlapping traits. *Psychological Bulletin, 121,* 219–245.

Ackerman, P. L., Kanfer, R., & Goff, M. (1995). Cognitive and noncognitive determinants and consequences of complex skill acquisition. *Journal of Experimental Psychology: Applied, 1,* 270–304.

Allison, R. B. (1960). *Learning parameters and human abilities* (Office of Naval Research Tech. Rep.). Princeton, NJ: Educational Testing Service.

Bannatyne, A. (1974). Diagnosis: A note on recategorization of the WISC scaled scores. *Journal of Learning Disabilities, 7,* 272–274.

Bechtel, G. G., Tucker, L. R., & Chang, W. C. (1971). A scalar product model for the multidimensional scaling of choice. *Psychometrika, 36,* 369–388.

Benzecri, J. P. (1969). Statistical analysis as a tool to make patterns emerge from data. In S. Watanabe (Ed.), *Methodologies of pattern recognition* (pp. 35–74). New York: Academic Press.

Carroll, J. D., & Chang, J. J. (1968). *How to use MDPREF, a computer program for multidimensional analysis of preference data.* Unpublished manuscript, Bell Telephone Laboratories, Murray Hill, NJ.

Cattell, R. B. (1967). The three basic factor analysis research designs: Their interrelations and derivatives. In D. N. Jackson & S. Messick (Eds.), *Problems in human assessment* (pp. 300–304). New York: McGraw-Hill.

Davenport, E. C., Jr., Davison, M. L., Bielinski, J., & Ding, S. (1995). *SPSS and SAS templates for profile analysis via multidimensional scaling.* Minneapolis: University of Minnesota, Department of Educational Psychology.

Davison, M. L. (1985). Multidimensional scaling versus components analysis of test intercorrelations. *Psychological Bulletin, 97,* 94–105.

Davison, M. L. (1994). Multidimensional scaling models of personality responding. In S. Strack & M. Lorr (Eds.), *Differentiating normal and abnormal personality* (pp. 196–215). New York: Springer.

Davison, M. L. (1996). *Addendum to "Multidimensional scaling and factor models of test and item responses."* Unpublished manuscript, University of Minnesota, Department of Educational Psychology.

Davison, M. L., Gasser, M., & Ding, S. (1996). Identifying major profile patterns in a population: An exploratory study of WAIS and GATB patterns. *Psychological Assessment, 8,* 26–31.

Davison, M. L., & Skay, C. L. (1991). Multidimensional scaling and factor models of test and item responses. *Psychological Bulletin, 110,* 551–556.

Greenacre, M. J. (1984). *Theory and application of correspondence analysis.* New York: Academic Press.

Gustafsson, J.-E., & Undheim, J. O. (1996). Individual differences in cognitive functions. In D. C. Berliner & R. C. Calfee (Eds.), *Handbook of educational psychology* (pp. 186–242). New York: Macmillan Library Reference.

Guttman, L. (1954). A new approach to factor analysis: The radex. In P. F. Lazarsfeld (Ed.), *Mathematical thinking in the social sciences* (pp. 216–257). Glencoe, IL: Free Press.

Guttman, L. (1965). A faceted definition of intelligence. *Scripta Hierosolymitana, 14,* 166–181.

Guttman, L., & Levy, L. (1991). Two structural laws for intelligence tests. *Intelligence, 15,* 79–104.

Kaiser, H. F. (1974). An index of factorial simplicity. *Psychometrika, 39,* 31–36.

Kaufman, A. S. (1979). *Intelligent testing with the WISC-R.* New York: Wiley.

MacCallum, R. C. (1974). Relations between factor analysis and multidimensional scaling. *Psychological Bulletin, 81,* 505–516.

Marshalek, B., Lohman, D. F., & Snow, R. E. (1983). The complexity continuum in the radex and hierarchical models of intelligence. *Intelligence, 7,* 107–127.

McDermott, P. A., Fantuzzo, J. W., & Glutting, J. J. (1990). Just say no to subtest analysis: A critique on Wechsler theory and practice. *Journal of Psychoeducational Assessment, 8,* 290–302.

Mcgrew, K. S., Werder, J. K., & Woodcock, R. W. (1991). *WJ-R technical manual.* Allen, TX: DLM.

Messick, S. (1994). The matter of style: Manifestations of personality in cognition, learning, and teaching. *Educational Psychologist, 29,* 121–136.

Moses, J. A., Jr., & Pritchard, D. A. (1995). Modal profiles for the Wechsler Adult Intelligence Scale–Revised. *Archives of Clinical Neuropsychology, 11,* 61–68.

Nishisato, S. (1980). *Analysis of categorical data: Dual scaling and its applications.* Toronto, Ontario, Canada: University of Toronto Press.

Silverstein, A. B. (1987). Multidimensional scaling vs. factor analysis of Wechsler's intelligence scales. *Journal of Clinical Psychology, 43,* 381–386.

Skinner, H. (1979). Dimensions and clusters: A hybrid approach to classification. *Applied Psychological Measurement, 3,* 327–341.

Snow, R. E., Corno, L., & Jackson, D., III (1996). Individual differences in affective and conative functions. In D. C. Berliner & R. C. Calfee (Eds.), *Handbook of educational psychology* (pp. 243–310). New York: Macmillan Library Reference.

Snow, R. E., Kyllonen, P. C., & Marshalak, B. (1984). The topography of abilty and learning correlations. In R. J. Sternberg (Ed.), *Advances in the psychology of human intelligence* (Vol. 2, pp. 47–104). Hillsdale, NJ: Erlbaum.

Spearman, C. (1904). "General intelligence" objectively determined and measured. *American Journal of Psychology, 15,* 201–293.

Thurstone, L. L. (1936). A new conception of intelligence and a new method of measuring primary abilities. *Educational Record, 17*(Suppl. 10), 124–138.

Tucker, L. R. (1960). Intra-individual and inter-individual multidimensionality. In H. Gulliksen & S. Messick (Eds.), *Psychological scaling: Theory and applications* (pp. 107–121). New York: Wiley.

Wechsler, D. (1974). *Wechsler Intelligence Scale for Children–Revised.* New York: Psychological Corporation.

Wechsler, D. (1981). *WAIS-R manual: Wechsler Adult Intelligence Scale–Revised.* New York: Psychological Corporation.

Weller, S. C., & Romney, A. K. (1990). *Metric scaling: Correspondence analysis.* Newbury Park, CA: Sage.

Woodcock, R. W., & Johnson, M. B. (1989). *Woodcock–Johnson Psychoeducational Battery — Revised.* Allen, TX: DLM.

Young, F. W., & Lewyckyj, R. (1979). *ALSCAL-4 user's guide.* Carrboro, NC: Data Analysis and Theory Associates.

Zachary, R. A. (1990). Wechsler's intelligence scales: Theoretical and practical considerations. *Journal of Psychoeducational Assessment, 8,* 276–289.

Discussion

Several participants questioned Davison about the relative advantages and the difficulties of interpreting the scaling solutions he demonstrated. Discussion ranged widely, with examples from previous attempts to resolve profiles and multivariate representations of abilities.

Dr. Alexander: First of all, I'm very pleased with the analysis. I think it's very promising. But I want to go to something a little bit more conceptual. You said that in looking across your profiles, particularly when you were looking at [Table 8.4] there were individuals who did well on achievement that had a certain profile, and I think you were talking about individuals particularly like participant Number 149. And I want to jump back to the discussions about whether the notion of intelligence has to change over the course of one's lifetime. Do you think that what you have is a particular configuration that's generalizable to other ages, or are you looking at a profile pattern particularly powerful for older adults?

Dr. Davison: The norming data with which we're working go all the way down to preschool. This analysis was just our first cut at the data, and so I don't know whether these same patterns are going to emerge at the early ages. We have done some analyses where we tried to fit a common set of profiles, four profiles or three, and we found that the fit was noticeably less good with our youngest age group, which would have been a preschool group, and with our oldest adults who would have been over 55 or 60. So while we haven't gone very far with this kind of analysis, it is beginning to look like the structure of those ability profile patterns may be somewhat different at those two extremes.

Dr. Ackerman: If your profile analysis yields this sort of analog to a bifactor analysis where we're contrasting different sets of abilities in a sense, what does that mean if you add another ability to your battery? Does that really throw off the whole inter-pretation of the dimensions?

Dr. Davison: Inherently when you're dealing with profile patterns, everything is very context bound. The pattern itself is very specific to the particular configuration of tests that you have in that particular battery. And that's an aspect of profiles that just gets carried over into any analysis like the one we have. So yes, the interpre-tations of things do tend to be rather contextually bound to a particular configuration of tests.

Dr. Gustafsson: I have a question along similar lines. The structure of this kind of scaling approach is hierarchical. You pull out the general factor first and then you look at profiles, and I really enjoyed that. What I find somewhat problematic is that you tend to bring in an entirely new set of constructs. I would be much more pleased to see the profile differences formulated in terms of our established ability constructs. Would it be possible to rotate the solution so that we would see the structures that we normally get out?

Dr. Davison: Any alternative analysis like this does risk interjecting confusion. It looks like we're talking about something totally unrelated to traditional factors — as if profiles are from Mars and factors are from Venus. But in fact our model is a linear model, so factors and patterns are all within the same space. And while I haven't done it here, it is quite possible to express profile patterns in terms of factors, because they share this common framework of a linear model, and there's a mapping from one to the other. So it is possible to draw exactly the kinds of connections that you were talking about. I did not draw them here. I share your concern. I don't want to talk about profiles in a way that's going to spread confusion.

Dr. Wright: I was just wondering if you could sort of characterize the factor analysis model with a hierarchical model and then use factor scores and disturbances to recreate these profiles. I don't know whether you've tried that.

Dr. Davison: I haven't tried it. Obviously, there's not exactly a one-to-one mapping but a connection between general ability and the profile level that you see here. I think it is possible to relate the specific factors to profiles and express the patterns in terms of some underlying factors that are your frame-of-reference so to speak.

That was the idea that I was trying to convey in those first remarks where I talked about Thurstone with his specific abilities in the foreground. Patterns remained in the background of his thinking. But you can do the opposite. You can bring the patterns into the foreground, which is what I did today, and put the specifics in the background. But the important point is that they are two aspects of the same picture. It's just a question of what's in the foreground and what's in the background.

Dr. Deary: I'd just like to comment that, far from factors and profiles coming from two separate planets, the profile analysis looked very much like an unrotated principal components or factor analysis with the general factor first and then a bipolar factor. I just thought it'd be interesting to see whether in fact the factors further down came out similarly too because they looked very similar.

Dr. Davison: I have an article in *Psychological Bulletin* in 1985 which pointed out a mapping similar to the one you describe between unrotated factors and the dimensions that come out of a multidimensional scaling.

Dr. Gustafsson: I have one more question which is about the homoscedasticity assumption. Did I understand it correctly that there is a restriction in your model such that the amount of profile variance is constant, or could you study that as an empirical question? It would, for example, be very interesting from a differentiation hypothesis point of view if you would have a correlation between the amount of profile variance and the level parameter.

Dr. Davison: I think it's a little bit different than the way you just expressed it. It would be more like the assumption that the unique variances are equal across tests. It's a necessary assumption only to justify certain kinds of analyses, those being the most common multidimensional scaling analyses in statistical packages. The assumption is not inherent to the model in any sense. It's just a restriction you have to place on it to get to a proximity measure which satisfies the usual assumptions.

Dr. Wittmann: What you are doing is basically using Raymond Cattell's covariation chart and partitioning it. And it really refers to one of my favorite things, aggregation and what happens using aggregation. Is the way we aggregate our scores really that what we want? Look at Lee Cronbach's distinction between level, scatter, and shape. You had been concentrating on scatter. And what are the questions for scatter?

Dr. Davison: As you say, Cronbach divided profiles into level, shape, and scatter. This model partitions level, but it keeps shape and scatter combined. Is there a model which separates level, shape, and scatter distinctly? And it turns out that there is. The model in my talk contains parameters which are expressed with respect to a Cartesian coordinates system. For every model expressed in a Cartesian coordinates system, there is a corresponding model expressed in terms of polar coordinates. If you take this model, and reexpress it in terms of polar coordinates, what you get is one parameter which represents level. You get one parameter which represents individual differences in scatter. And then you get one or more parameters which represent individual differences in profile shape. The resulting model expressed in polar coordinates gives the complete breakdown of the kind that Cronbach was talking about.

Dr. Wittmann: Can I add a bit more substantive interpretation? You used the kind of memory tasks which are related to cognitive psychology and the classical ability stuff. And then you used the scatter. What you found out, the majority of the scatter in all these interesting cognitive tasks which means differences in encoding, memory, and other stuff has nothing to do with the traditional ability tasks. Only the third dimension, the scatter between the figural factor and the verbal factor. Would you agree with such an interpretation?

Dr. Davison: What you're pointing to is the fact that the first two patterns were uncorrelated with the academic achievement variables. Yes. I think that is the implication of it. Except as those tasks are related to global ability, they were unrelated to school achievement — I think that's what you're getting at, and I think that's a fair interpretation.

9

Investigating Theoretical Propositions Regarding Mental Abilities: Their Structure, Growth, and Influence

KEITH F. WIDAMAN

The domain of human mental abilities is central to the understanding of the lives of individuals. Individual differences in mental abilities contribute to many of the successes that people enjoy and the failures they endure. Mental abilities are frequently invoked to explain near-term outcomes, such as school grades and achievement test scores, as well as longer-term outcomes, including occupational success and income (e.g., Tomlinson-Keasey & Little, 1990). The reach of mental abilities is broad, and research and theory should not constrict the conception of abilities and their importance for the development of the individual.

Research and theory about mental abilities often focus on the years of formal schooling, from kindergarten through college. These years encompass a time in every person's life during which a wide array of intellectual skills are fostered, nurtured, inculcated, or stymied in systematic and unsystematic ways by parents, educators, and the educational system (Horn, 1988). Young children enter kindergarten with a substantial number of highly developed skills already in place, however, and a considerable array of contextualized and specialized skills are acquired after formal schooling, with the entry into the world of work and throughout the vital years of adulthood. As a result, any adequate theory of the life span growth, maintenance, and decline of mental abilities must be multifaceted, and musing about the next steps that research on abilities should pursue is a decidedly difficult and complex undertaking (Horn, 1988; Horn & Hofer, 1992; Schaie, 1996).

Thinking about the future of research on mental abilities encourages one to ponder broad issues. The investigator's task here is to understand where research on abilities has been, where it currently stands, and, most crucially, where the field is headed during the years to come. In 1997, researchers stand on a temporal threshold, opening onto a new millennium, the twenty-first century. Researchers stand on another threshold — a methodological one — opening onto a new and exciting era in the study of human abilities. The measurement operations used in the study of mental abilities are increasing in both breadth and depth. Increasingly, researchers supplement paper-and-pencil tests with reaction time (RT) paradigms, electroencephalographic techniques, positron emission tomography, both structural and functional magnetic resonance imaging, and other state-of-the-art techniques to shed light on mental skills and their biological substrates. Additionally, advances in statistical models and methods, most notably in the area of structural equation modeling, enable more adequate statistical representations of theoretical conjectures. As a result, future research on mental abilities is almost sure to be even more exciting and varied than has been the case during the 20th century.

In this chapter, I emphasize the need for a close interplay between theoretical propositions regarding mental abilities, the measures of abilities that researchers obtain, and the mathematical and statistical models researchers use to represent their data. I first state and discuss several theoretical propositions regarding human abilities. Next, I describe several recent studies and analyses that I have conducted, noting the implications of each study for the theoretical propositions stated initially. I close with some general observations on the future of research on mental abilities.

Theoretical Propositions Regarding Mental Abilities

In this section, I offer five theoretical propositions that apply to the domain of mental abilities. The propositions offered are implicit or explicit bases for much research and theory regarding mental abilities; as such, dispute on these issues would be unlikely. However, I believe the full implications of these propositions are often overlooked. Only by carefully considering the theoretical and methodological implications of these propositions will a comprehensive understanding of the domain of mental abilities be possible.

Proposition 1: Mental abilities are the phenotypic expression of interacting, interpenetrating genetic and environmental influences. Genetic influences on human abilities are difficult to dispute. Accumulating evidence from behavioral genetic studies provide converging evidence of the genetic determination of variance in many mental abilities (Plomin, 1990; Plomin, DeFries, & McClearn, 1990). A host of issues arise when considering the results of behavior genetic studies, issues including (a) the consistency or replicability of estimates of genetic and environmental influences, (b) the proper interpretation of heritability estimates, and (c) the implications of large or small estimates of heritability of a trait for remediation efforts or for educational and curriculum design. Despite their importance, virtually all of these issues are beyond the scope of this chapter.

One issue deserving attention here is the place of genetic and environmental sources of variance in mental abilities. The present Zeitgeist encourages researchers to presume that genetic sources of variation on many abilities "drive" the development of these traits to a far greater extent than do environmental sources of variation (e.g., Scarr, 1992; Scarr & McCartney, 1983). However, researchers must not lose sight of the fact that disentangling the influences of genetic and environmental sources of variance is a most difficult matter, almost certainly more complex than typically assumed. Estimates of high heritability for a trait frequently lead to presumptions that the trait is resistant to environmental influence, despite warnings about the tenuous nature of such a conclusion. A trait with a high heritability in one generation may have a modest heritability in the next, however, if a potent change in the environment occurs. The future is likely to foster a view in which neither genetic nor environmental sources of variance are considered to have clear causal priority over the other with regard to the development of human abilities.

Proposition 2: Mental abilities rely on and are supported by biological and brain processes and by environmental and educational processes that structure one another. The mind–brain problem is one of the oldest in the philosophical literature and one that is still current. Human mental abilities operate in the realm of mind, yet the structures, functions, and circuitry of the brain provide the physiological substrate for the cognitive operations that make up abilities. Given the dependence of mental abilities on electrical and other physiological processes in the brain, such as blood flow, many researchers presume that the future holds the possibility of a theoretical reduction of mental abilities into constituent brain processes (cf. Stankov & Roberts, 1997). In a fashion analogous to that regarding whether genetic or environmental sources "drive" the development of mental abilities, the ontogenesis of brain processes is presumed to drive the development and expression of mental abilities, with events in the realm of mind and the environment being of little importance.

However, a considerable body of research on nonhuman primates and other mammals has shown that environmental manipulations have profound effects on brain structure and function (e.g., Greenough & Black, 1992; Greenough, Black, & Wallace, 1987). Enriched environments lead to higher levels of certain critical neurotransmitters in the brain as well as positive changes in neuronal structures, and impoverished environments have the opposite effects, when compared with levels found in organisms in their typical environments. Even simple learning leads to changes in receptive fields in the brain (Weinberger, Ashe, & Edeline, 1994). When environmental and learning effects of these sorts are taken into account, the prudent view is that the state of brain structures and processes at any point in the life span may be at least as much a function of the environmental and educational conditions the organism has enjoyed or endured as the result of preprogrammed development of biological structures during development.

Proposition 3: Mental abilities develop along an ontogenetic temporal continuum that spans the prenatal, perinatal, and postnatal periods, a continuum that continues throughout the individual's life span. This proposition is a virtual truism, yet two principal reasons exist for presenting it. The first is to draw attention to the fact that researchers must remain aware that the appearance of any particular aspect of mental ability may have precursors whose causal effects were initiated at earlier ages, perhaps much earlier ages. The second is this: The ontogenetic continuum provides a dimension along which changes in ability may be charted. When charting changes in ability during development, however, the researcher should remain alert to opportunities to investigate hypotheses about the basis for and mechanisms of developmental change (Siegler & Crowley, 1991). For example, is chronological age the proper metric for charting developmental change? Or would some other metric —

such as physiological indexes (e.g., skeletal maturity, neural myelinization) or environmental experiences (Schroots & Birren, 1990) — provide a more valid index for representing the basis for developmental change?

Proposition 4: Mental abilities can be represented at several levels, including the latent trait, cognitive process, and metacognitive levels; any adequate theory of mental abilities must represent the interplay of these levels and how this interplay changes during development. One reason for restating this obvious point is the lack of centrality of these issues in current research on mental abilities. After the first rush of research in the mid-1970s on individual differences in cognitive processes and mental abilities (e.g., Sternberg, 1977), interest appears to have flagged. Interest may have diminished for any of several reasons, including the presence of several notable failures to find predicted relations and the difficulties accompanying the design of such studies and analyses of resulting data (e.g., Keating, List, & Merriman, 1985). Regardless of the reasons for the reduced interest, research on the cognitive bases of mental abilities must regain prominence to fulfill the promise of a full understanding of the processes underlying abilities and changes in these mental skills.

Proposition 5: Mental abilities are dynamic traits that grow, stabilize, and then decline across the life span; mental abilities are affected by specifiable factors and in turn influence many aspects of human behavior and development. Mental abilities might be relatively fixed or unchanging, malleable, or somewhere in between. The position that individual differences in mental abilities are relatively fixed and unchanging has waxed and waned over the course of this century. The "fixed" position has often predominated, buttressed by consistent findings of high levels of stability of individual differences in mental abilities across time. Indeed, Eysenck (1987) argued that individual differences in unchanging genotypes lead directly to individual differences in ability test scores. In a methodological vein, Collins and Cliff (1990) claimed that latent-variable models, commonly used to represent human abilities, use constructs that are nondynamic (i.e., not changing) in nature, due to invoking the notion of a *true score* for each latent variable.

However, the proposition that mental abilities are malleable and changeable is also consistent with accumulated empirical data (Horn, 1988). Here, the position of an individual on a given dimension of mental ability is interpreted as that person's "accumulated level of skill developed to date." If one accepts the contention that ability at a given point in time may predict both ability at a later point in time as well as change in ability between times of measurement, then high levels of stability of scores across time are consistent with clear malleability of abilities. Individual differences in intelligence are highly stable between 5 and 18 years of age (Bloom, 1964), suggesting that intelligence is at best slowly changing. However, the stability of individual differences across time can be observed at the same time as massive changes, hence malleability, of the mean level of ability across time. Mental abilities at age 5 years bear little resemblance to the myriad skills exhibited by the senior graduating from high school, even in the face of substantial stability of individual differences in ability across this wide age span. When theorizing about these matters, one must attend to changes in mean level as well as changes in relative standing within the group at any given point in time.

Empirical Studies of Mental Abilities: Their Structure, Growth, and Influence

In the preceding section, I presented five propositions that provide a basic backdrop for the study of mental abilities. In this section, I describe a series of studies I have conducted or analyses I have pursued that provide evidence relating to the five propositions just stated. Research results are often interpreted within fairly narrow bounds. However, just as frequently, empirical results have implications for broad issues underlying research in a domain, implications that remain implicit and unstated. In this section, I attempt to draw out these broader implications.

Children of Mothers With Phenylketonuria

The presence and potentially devastating effects of phenylketonuria (PKU) have been well-known for many years. Before the discovery of the biological basis for the condition, however, children with PKU presented an interesting, perplexing problem. Normal in all respects at birth, children with PKU showed a pronounced decline in mental ability during the first 2–6 years of life, a decline that proved permanent. PKU is an inborn error of metabolism, consisting of a deficiency of liver phenylalanine hydroxylase, an enzyme necessary for metabolizing phenylalanine (PHE) into tyrosine. If not properly metabolized, PHE builds up in the blood, and the resulting high levels of PHE cause damage to the central nervous system. Even though the precise damage to the brain has not yet been established, the practical outcomes are not at question: If untreated, children with PKU often decline to the level of severe mental retardation.

In the mid-1950s, a treatment for PKU was developed consisting of dietary restrictions to reduce the level of PHE in the blood. Then, in 1963, a newborn screening test was developed to identify infants with PKU, and newborn screening is currently practiced worldwide. Although the genetic defect underlying PKU was not discovered until 1983, the disastrous effects of PKU had already been eradicable for 20 years. Indeed, within one generation, the heritability of phenotypic traits associated with the PKU genotype was reduced from a high level to approximately zero, with the elimination of the negative behavioral sequelae of PKU.

The foregoing sounds like a wonderful success story. However, researchers and practitioners did not foresee the potentially devastating effects of prenatal exposure to high levels of PHE. Beginning in the late 1950s, many female infants with PKU were identified with the disorder, were treated with the proper diet, and developed normal levels of intelligence. These infants proceeded through childhood and adolescence, entered young adulthood, and began to have offspring of their own. Many of the infants born to these mothers with PKU exhibited symptoms of PKU, such as microcephaly and low intelligence regardless of whether the infants themselves had PKU. The high level of PHE in the mother's blood passed the placental barrier into the fetus, whose liver was too immature to metabolize the PHE. The resulting buildup of PHE in the blood of the fetus damaged the brain and other developing fetal systems before birth, leading to irreversible disabilities including low intelligence.

To study the parameters of this problem, the Maternal PKU Collaborative (MPKUC) Study was initiated in 1984, with Richard Koch as the principal investigator. The MPKUC Study is a comprehensive study of the progress of each of more than 400 pregnancies of mothers with PKU as well as a wide range of outcomes by the offspring.

In recent research (Widaman, 1998), I examined the relations among maternal background characteristics, variables related to the course of the pregnancy, and the Mental Development Index (MDI) and the Psychomotor Development Index (PDI) scores on the Bayley Scales of Infant Development obtained by infants at 12 months of age. The three maternal background characteristics were mother's intelligence, mother's socioeconomic status (SES), and mother's age. If one considers only the three maternal background variables and the two child outcome variables of the MDI and PDI at 12 months of age, a structural model with paths shown in Figure 9.1 is adequate to explain the relations among these variables. Mother's IQ related strongly to MDI scores (β = .30) and to PDI scores (β = .25), mother's SES related only to MDI scores (β = .21), and mother's age had no direct effects on MDI and PDI scores. Taken at face value, the results presented in Figure 9.1 might be interpreted as being consistent with a simple genetic transmission model, with mother's IQ as a prominent cause of both mental and psychomotor development of the infant at 1 year of age.

However, I also had access to potential mediator variables that might explain how or why the maternal background variables of IQ and SES related to the MDI and PDI scores. These mediator variables included (a) indicators of the PHE level in the mother's blood during pregnancy; (b) mother's weight gain during pregnancy; (c) the number of weeks of gestation from conception to birth; and (d) a set of birth

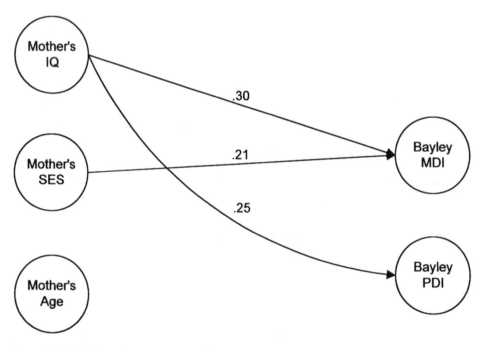

Figure 9.1. Relations between maternal background characteristics and child outcomes from the Maternal PKU Collaborative Study. MDI = Mental Development Index; PDI = Psychomotor Development Index; SES = socioeconomic status.

measurements, including length, weight, and head circumference. A final model representing relations among these variables is shown in Figure 9.2 Although the model in Figure 9.2 appears complex, the major pathways of influence are easy to discern. Proceeding from left to right in Figure 9.2, the higher the mother's IQ and SES, the lower the level of PHE in her blood, presumably because of better dietary control. Also, the higher the mother's IQ and SES, the higher the weight gain by the mother during pregnancy, probably resulting from selection of better dietary foodstuffs. Finally, mother's SES also had an effect on weeks gestation, perhaps because of better prenatal care.

In the middle of the figure, one can see that the Birth Measures latent variable was affected directly by five latent variables. Three of these influences were proximal: (a) a negative effect of PHE level ($\beta = -.21$), with higher levels of maternal PHE leading to infants with smaller birth measurements; (b) a positive effect of weight gain ($\beta = .22$), with higher weight gain leading to larger birth measurements; and (c) a strong positive effect of gestational age ($\beta = .51$), with longer gestation leading to larger infant birth measurements. The two remaining positive effects on birth measurements — .18 from SES and .12 from maternal age — were based on more distal measures.

Finally, to the right of the figure, one can see the MDI and PDI scores at 12 months of infant age. The MDI was influenced by five latent variables. Only one of these paths was of substantial magnitude, the effect of maternal PHE level during pregnancy ($\beta = -.39$). Thus, the higher the level of maternal PHE, the lower the infant MDI score at 12 months of age. The remaining paths were of modest value, ranging from .09 to .13; each was of at best borderline statistical and practical significance. Notably, the direct effect of mother's IQ was reduced from .30 to .10, and the direct effect of mother's SES was reduced from .21 to .09. Maternal PHE level and weight gain mediated most of the effects of mother's IQ and SES on MDI scores. A similar pattern of results held for PDI scores, which were affected by three latent variables.

These results from the MPKUC Study provide substantiation for four of the five theoretical propositions stated earlier. With regard to Proposition 1, the effects of mother's IQ on infant MDI and PDI scores appeared at first to fit with notions of simple, basic genetic influence. However, these effects were mediated largely by variables that reflected prenatal environmental influences that were or might easily have been under environmental control or manipulation. Some might argue that the effects of mother's IQ and SES on PHE level and weight gain reflected the influence of genetic sources of variance, representing dietary selection that was influenced by genetics (e.g., Scarr & McCartney, 1983). However, diet may be varied or controlled independently of genetics, and dietary variables were clearly the primary influences on the MDI and PDI scores. In related fashion, per Proposition 2, the brain processes on which MDI and PDI scores depend did not develop solely according to a preprogrammed biological program but were strongly influenced by maternal physiological and dietary processes. Environmental influences, in the form of PHE level during the prenatal period, had strong effects on infant abilities at 12 months of age.

The results are also clearly consistent with Proposition 3, as the effects of maternal physiological variables during the prenatal period affected the prenatal environment of the fetus, which, in turn, had strong influences on infant outcomes at 1 year of

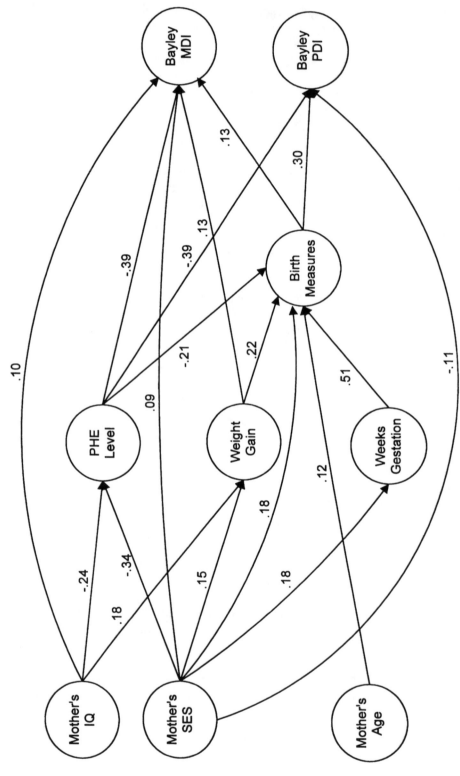

Figure 9.2. Relations among maternal background characteristics, prenatal mediators, and child outcomes from the Maternal PKU Collaborative Study. PHE = phenylalanine; SES = socioeconomic status; MDI = Mental Development Index; PDI = Psychomotor Development Index.

age. Finally, the results support Proposition 5, as the maternal physiological variables during pregnancy had clear and important effects on the level of mental and psychomotor functioning of the infant a full year after birth. These findings suggest that mental and psychomotor abilities are malleable during the prenatal period, and future research on intelligence scores at later ages will investigate the continuing influence of pregnancy-related and later variables on more mature levels of mental ability for the children in the MPKUC Study.

Studies of Cognitive Processes Underlying Mental Abilities

Shifting gears, I now provide a brief overview of several research studies that my students and I conducted on the cognitive processes underlying performance required by batteries of mental abilities. In these studies, we explored the cognitive components underlying certain forms of simple numerical processing. When we initiated our program of research, virtually all research had concentrated on modeling RTs for verifying simple addition problems, and analyses were based on average, group-level data obtained from college students. The primary focus of the prior research was to define what was known as the "search and compute" stage of processing. That is, when confronted with a simple addition problem, the solver was hypothesized either to search through a memory network of addition facts for the correct sum of the two digits or to compute anew the correct sum. Once the correct answer was obtained, the sum was compared with the stated answer, and an appropriate "correct" or "incorrect" response was made by a corresponding buttonpress.

Given the state of research, many extensions were possible. These included consideration of (a) complex addition; (b) cognitive components required for problem solution in addition to those making up the search and compute stage; (c) other forms of numerical problems (e.g., multiplication); (d) individual differences; (e) the developmental context; and (f) other ways of formatting problems (e.g., production tasks). My students and I provided some of these extensions; other researchers initiated other extensions. In all, much has been learned about numerical processing during the past 12 years.

In the first study, Widaman, Geary, Cormier, and Little (1989) developed a general processing model for simple and complex addition. They found that the best predictor representing the search and compute stage for simple addition problems was the product of the two single-digit addends (PROD). That is, for the problem 1 + 2, the product of addends is 2; for the problem 8 + 9, the product of addends is 72. Widaman et al. argued that the product of addends is consistent with a network retrieval process; the larger the value of the product, the longer the necessary search through the memory network. Interestingly, any problem involving the addition of zero (e.g., 6 + 0) has a zero product, implying an absence of memory network search, consistent with the heuristic that addition of zero leaves a number unchanged.

Widaman et al. (1989) found that RTs by the average participant to simple and complex addition problems were well captured by a straightforward equation with the following basic terms: about 7 ms for each unit increase in the PROD term, 53 ms to encode each digit and to reencode or verify digits in incorrect sums, 205 ms to carry a unit to the 10s column, 130 ms to verify the incorrectness of problems,

217

and 760 ms to execute all processes that did not differ across problem types (i.e., basic encoding, decision, and response time).

In a second study, Geary and Widaman (1987) extended their research in two ways: considering simple and complex multiplication problems and modeling individual differences in parameter estimates. The results from that study related to individual differences are summarized most succinctly in Figure 9.3. On the left, there are four latent variables defined by indicators from the arithmetic problems in the RT format: (a) Memory Search rate, with the PROD estimate; (b) Carry, or the speed of executing a carry to the 10s column; (c) Truth, or the RT difference between correct and incorrect problems; and (d) time to Encode, Decide, and Respond, times that are a component of responding to every problem. The Memory Search Rate and Carry latent variables were highly correlated, and Geary and Widaman specified a second-order Arithmetic Processes factor to subsume these first-order processes, unique to responding to simple numerical problems. Similarly, the Truth and Encode, Decide, and Respond latent variables were highly correlated, so they specified a second-order Speed factor for these two first-order factors, which reflected processes required when responding to many types of problems in the RT format. On the right of the figure are three latent variables that were based on a battery of nine paper-and-pencil tests.

Consistent with their a priori hypotheses, the Arithmetic Processes latent variable was highly negatively related to the Numerical Facility factor ($\beta = -.88$), and the Speed latent variable was highly negatively related to the Perceptual Speed factor ($\beta = -.71$). Thus, the faster one executes a search of memory for arithmetic facts and the faster one executes a carry (leading to lower scores on the Arithmetic Processes factor), the higher the score on the Numerical Facility latent variable. In a similar fashion, the more quickly one executes basic encoding and responding to problems and the faster one resolves the correctness of problems, the higher one's position on the Perceptual Speed factor.

In another study, Widaman, Little, Geary, and Cormier (1992) extended their prior research in yet another direction, to the developmental context. One of the most intriguing findings was the outcome of modeling the relationship between cognitive component parameter estimates and student characteristics marking development. For students in elementary school through college, chronological age and grade in school are highly correlated, virtually perfectly correlated. However, age and grade — placed in nonlinear statistical models — make differential predictions. Widaman et al. found that grade in school was a better predictor of the cross-sectional developmental trends than was chronological age. For example, PROD parameter estimates were best represented by the following equation: PROD = $200(\text{grade})^{-1.16}$. That is, PROD estimates were approximately 200 times the inverse of grade. Widaman et al. argued that grade in school is a proxy for time spent on learning addition facts and that this practice on addition tasks accounted for the superior predictive power of grade in school relative to chronological age.

These findings on studies of numerical facility support several of the propositions stated earlier. The most obvious connection is to Proposition 4, which holds that dimensions of ability may be represented at different levels, including the latent trait and cognitive component levels. Widaman et al. (1989) demonstrated the ability to isolate a number of cognitive components underlying responding to addition problems. Geary and Widaman (1987) then showed that individual differences on cog-

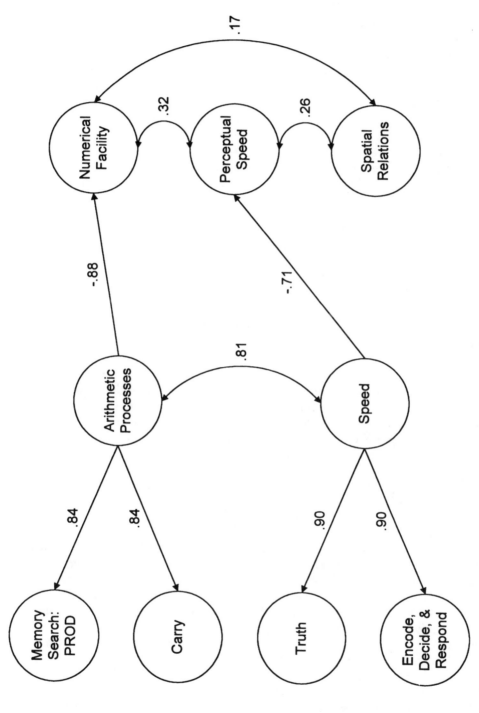

Figure 9.3. Relations among reaction time parameter estimates and traditional constructs based on paper-and-pencil tests. From "Individual Differences in Cognitive Arithmetic," by D. C. Geary and K. F. Widaman, 1987, *Journal of Experimental Psychology: General, 116*, p. 168. Copyright 1987 by the American Psychological Association. Adapted with permission of the authors. PROD = product of the two single-digit addends.

nitive components unique to addition responding are strongly related to, and therefore account for, individual differences in numerical facility, findings replicated in later studies (e.g., Little & Widaman, 1996; Widaman et al., 1992). Interestingly, these studies also showed that individual differences on certain cognitive components underlying addition responding were not directly related to numerical facility but had strong, predicted relations with other dimensions of ability.

The findings also relate to other propositions. Proposition 2 states that both environmental and biological sources of variance may contribute to mature levels of mental abilities. The systematic relationship between grade in school and cognitive component scores supports this notion with regard to environmental inputs, suggesting that the systematic inculcation of numerical skills during schooling leads to improvements in ability. The relationship between parameter estimates and grade in school also suggests, relative to Proposition 3, that chronological age may not always be the optimal indicator along which developmental change should be charted. Many environmental and biological indicators are highly correlated with chronological age yet offer intriguing and straightforward alternative explanations of developmental trends. Finally, the results relate to the aspects of Proposition 5 that pertain to factors that influence growth and development of abilities. Abilities are dynamic traits influenced by environmental experiences such as schooling; in turn, abilities potentially affect a wide array of other psychological phenomena, a topic to which I now turn.

Modeling Change in Skills as a Function of Practice and External Variables

One of the more enduring topics regarding mental abilities is representing change in mental abilities and skills as a function of time and studying the influence of external variables that influence or moderate this change. Theories and empirical results have accumulated on this topic for more than 50 years. Among many others, Anderson (1939) and Ferguson (1954, 1956) proposed theories for macroscopic development, or development across extended periods of time. Werner (1957) developed principles to account for macroscopic development and then extended these to more microscopic trends in development, a topic that has been reinvigorated by Fischer and colleagues (e.g., Fischer, 1980) and Siegler and Crowley (1991).

About 40 years ago, Fleishman (1960; Fleishman & Hempel, 1954, 1955) undertook a series of studies of learning of psychomotor tasks or skills. The general form of each of these studies included the collection of data on a psychomotor task across trials, to study the acquisition of skill on the task as a function of practice, as well as collection of data on a battery of ability tests, to study the influence of abilities on psychomotor learning at various stages of practice. The data from these classic studies provided the basis for theories of skill learning for many years. Concerns have been voiced about the analyses of data from these studies, however; the advances in statistical models and methods since the original publication of these data can provide more informative looks at the results.

In Fleishman and Hempel's (1954) study, a battery of 18 tests of ability was administered to 197 participants. This battery included tests of several different types, including 12 paper-and-pencil tests (involving numerical operations, mechanical principles, pattern comprehension, etc.) and 6 apparatus tests (involving RT and other motor tasks). The participants also completed 64 two-minute trials on the Complex Coordination Test (Form E), which required complex hand and foot movements in response to patterns of visual stimuli. The score for each 2-min trial was the number of correct hand–foot responses. Performance on the 64 trials was collapsed into scores representing skill at eight stages of practice. For example, Stage 1 subsumed Trials 1–5, Stage 2 comprised Trials 12–16, and so forth, through Stage 8, which reflected skill shown during Trials 60–64.

With 18 ability test scores and scores at eight stages of practice on the psychomotor task, Fleishman and Hempel (1954) reported a 26 × 26 matrix of correlations among all variables. This correlation matrix has an interbattery form, with three submatrices: (a) the symmetric 18 × 18 matrix of correlations among the 18 ability tests in Battery 1, a matrix that may be denoted R_{11}; (b) the symmetric 8 × 8 matrix of correlations among scores at the eight stages of practice in Battery 2, or R_{22}; and (c) the asymmetrical 8 × 18 matrix of correlations between the eight stages of practice and the 18 ability tests, or R_{21}. Thus, the full matrix $\mathbf{R}$ may be represented as

$$\mathbf{R} = \begin{bmatrix} R_{11} & R_{21} \\ R_{21} & R_{22} \end{bmatrix}.$$

Fleishman and Hempel (1954) performed a traditional common factor analysis of the entire 26 × 26 correlation matrix. This approach may be represented as

$$\mathbf{R} = \begin{bmatrix} P_1 \\ P_2 \end{bmatrix} [P_1' \quad P_2'] + \begin{bmatrix} U_1^2 & 0 \\ 0 & U_2^2 \end{bmatrix},$$

where P_1 and P_2 are the common factor pattern matrices for Batteries 1 and 2, respectively, and U_1^2 and U_2^2 are diagonal matrices and represent the unique factor variance matrices for the two batteries, respectively. This approach is justified only if one assumes that a single set of factors underlies measured variables in both matrices, that these factors are collinear across batteries, and that the standard factor-analytic model holds for variables in both batteries.

Given their analytic approach, Fleishman and Hempel (1954) analyzed the 26-variable matrix, extracting and rotating 10 factors to an orthogonal simple structure. The loadings on the first three factors came primarily from the eight psychomotor task variables, reflecting the attempt of common factor analysis to represent the simplex pattern of correlations among these variables. The loadings of the 18 ability tests on these first three factors were sparse and difficult to interpret. Of the remaining seven factors, six had interpretable loadings from ability tests, but few if any loadings from psychomotor task variables, and the last was an uninterpretable residual factor. As Ackerman (1987) argued, consistent with previous commentators (e.g., Humphreys, 1960), Fleishman and Hempel's solution was difficult to justify. The factors reported by Fleishman and Hempel represented combinations of ability tests and psychomotor tasks, and factors reflecting primarily one battery (e.g., ability factors) may have been misrepresented to some or great degree by the presence of variables from the other battery in the analysis. Clearly, batteries of measures should be analyzed separately.

Following an earlier suggestion by Humphreys (1960), Ackerman (1987) reanalyzed Fleishman and Hempel's (1954) data by first factor analyzing only the correlations among the 18 ability tests, or R_{11}. This factor-analytic solution may be represented as

$$R_{11} = P_1 P_1' + U_1^2,$$

where all symbols are as defined earlier. Then, Ackerman used the Dwyer extension to estimate the loadings of the eight psychomotor variables on the ability factors in P_1. Recall that the correlations between the eight psychomotor variables and the 18 ability tests are shown in the R_{21} matrix. Given the factor-analytic model for R_{11}, it can be shown that

$$R_{21} = P_2 \Phi P_1',$$

where Φ is the matrix of correlations among common factors and other symbols are as defined earlier. The matrix P_2 is a key matrix in this representation because it contains the factor pattern coefficients for the psychomotor task variables on the ability factors. Given the preceding equation, one may solve for P_2 as

$$P_2 = R_{21} P_1 (P_1' P_1)^{-1} \Phi^{-1},$$

where all symbols are as defined earlier. If factors are orthogonal, as was the case for Ackerman, then $\Phi = \Phi^{-1} = I$, an identity matrix, in which case that component drops out, leaving

$$P_2 = R_{21} P_1 (P_1' P_1)^{-1}.$$

In his analysis of the 18 ability tests in Battery 1, Ackerman (1987) extracted and rotated three factors to orthogonal simple structure; the three factors were named Perceptual Speed (Visual), Rate of Movement/Motor RT, and Practical/Mechanical Ability. The Dwyer extension results showed that the first and third factors tended to correlate highest with psychomotor task performance at early stages of practice and to correlate less and less as practice ensued. By contrast, the Rate of Movement/ Motor RT factor showed the opposite trend, correlating higher with psychomotor task performance at later stages of practice.

Ackerman's (1987) approach was a clear improvement on Fleishman and Hempel's (1954) procedures, producing a factor solution for the 18 ability tests that was uncontaminated by the psychomotor task variables. Shortcomings remain with this approach, however. Perhaps the most important problem is the failure to model explicitly the relations among the eight psychomotor task scores. If a latent-variable structure exists for the psychomotor tasks, the omission of this model would bias the pattern matrix P_2, which was the basis for conclusions regarding ability trait–psychomotor learning relations.

Still other approaches to analyzing Fleishman and Hempel's (1954) data may be pursued, one of which is presented here for the first time. In this approach, which is similar to that taken by Rogers, Fisk, and Hertzog (1994) with an original data set, I extend the prior analyses to follow the suggestion by Humphreys (1960) more completely: One should attempt to represent separately the correlations among the ability tests and the correlations among the stages of practice, proposing separate testable and theoretically justified models for these two sets of correlations. Only after well representing the within-battery relations for each battery should one proceed to model between-battery relations, and these should be consistent with the statistical representations of within-battery structures. Thus, this approach improves on the Ackerman (1987) procedures by respecting the within-battery structure of each of the two batteries of measures instead of respecting the within-battery structure of the first battery alone.

As Humphreys (1960) noted, common factor analysis is a rank reduction technique and tends to be an appropriate model for batteries of ability tests. However, the eight psychomotor task scores reflect performance on the same task across time. The correlations among these variables exhibit the simplex pattern, with high correlations just off the diagonal, and systematically lower correlations as one moves farther from the diagonal. Rank reduction techniques, such as factor analysis, do not fit simplex data well; indeed, simplex correlation matrices are often fit best by models that are full rank models, albeit with restricted forms. Jöreskog (1970) discussed several types of models that might be fit to simplex data, and more recent contributions (e.g., Browne & Du Toit, 1991; McArdle, 1989; Meredith & Tisak, 1990) have proposed other models.

To follow the logic of this new approach, I use the common factor model to represent relations among the 18 ability tests in R_{11}. Thus, one may write

$$R_{11} = P_1\Phi_1P_1' + U_1^2,$$

where Φ_1 is a matrix of correlations among the factors for Battery 1, and all other symbols are as defined earlier.

Following Jöreskog (1970), a standard model for simplex data may be written as

$$R_{22} = P_2(I - B_{22})^{-1}\Phi_2(I - B_{22}')^{-1}P_2' - U_2^2,$$

where P_2 is the matrix of loadings of Battery 2 measures on the factors for this battery, B_{22} is a matrix of directed relations among the factors in Battery 2, Φ_{22} is a diagonal matrix of residual variances of the latent variables, and other symbols are as defined earlier. With eight variables in a simplex-patterned matrix, B_{22} would have seven regression weights, with Stage 1 affecting Stage 2, Stage 2 affecting Stage 3, and so on, ending with Stage 7 affecting Stage 8. The remaining matrices — P_2, Φ_{22}, and U_2^2 — are diagonal matrices. Interested readers are referred to Jöreskog (1970) for specific requirements for patterns of fixed and free elements in all matrices to identify the models.

The separate models for Battery 1 and Battery 2 may then be placed within a more comprehensive model for the full interbattery matrix. This model has the form

$$\mathbf{R} = \begin{bmatrix} P_1 & 0 \\ 0 & P_2 \end{bmatrix} [I - B]^{-1} \begin{bmatrix} \Phi_{11} & 0 \\ 0 & \Phi_{22} \end{bmatrix} [I - B']^{-1} \begin{bmatrix} P_1' & 0 \\ 0 & P_2' \end{bmatrix} + \begin{bmatrix} U_1^2 & 0 \\ 0 & U_2^2 \end{bmatrix},$$

where

223

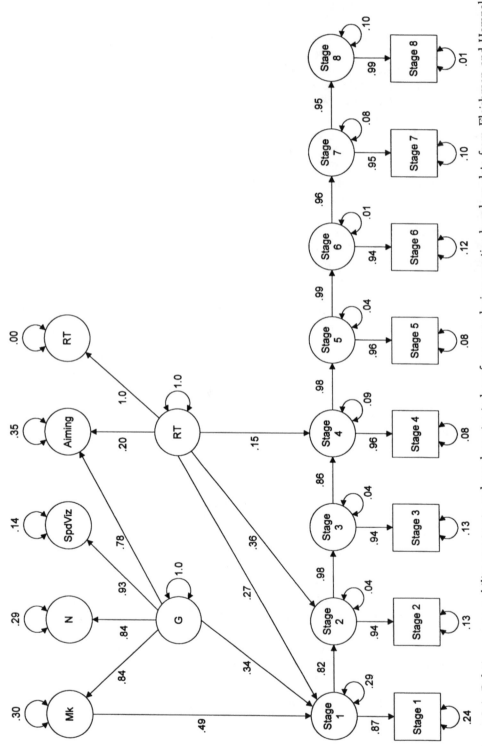

Figure 9.4. Relations among ability constructs and psychomotor task performance during practice based on data from Fleishman and Hempel (1954). Mk = Mechanical Experience; N = Numerical Facility; SpdViz = Speed/Visualization; RT = reaction time.

$$\mathbf{B} = \begin{bmatrix} 0 & 0 \\ B_{21} & B_{22} \end{bmatrix}.$$

B_{21} contains directed paths from factors in Battery 1 to factors in Battery 2, and all other symbols are as defined earlier.

When this model was fit to the data from Fleishman and Hempel's (1954) study, the first decision concerned the number of factors in Battery 1. Maximum-likelihood factor analysis suggested five factors; a priori specification of a five-factor structure, supplemented by a small number of post hoc modifications resulted in five interpretable factors. These five factors were labeled *Mechanical Experience, Numerical Facility, Perceptual Speed* (or *Speed/Visualization*), *Aiming,* and *Reaction Time.* Two second-order factors, labeled *G* and *RT*, were specified and adequately represented the correlations among the first-order factors. These higher order factors are shown at the top of Figure 9.4.

For Battery 2, one latent variable was specified for each of the eight stages of practice. As noted earlier, a first-order autoregressive pattern of directed relations was specified for these latent variables. That is, Stage 2 was predicted from Stage 1, Stage 3 from Stage 2, and so forth. This model fit the data for Battery 2 well.

Given the successful modeling of within-battery relations for both Battery 1 and Battery 2, attention switches to the relations between batteries. As shown in Figure 9.4, three factors from Battery 1 had significant effects on Stage 1, the earliest stage of performance on the psychomotor task, Mechanical Experience, G, and RT. The second-order RT factor also had a moderate additional influence on Stage 2 (β = .36) and a minor effect on Stage 4 (β = .15). No other paths from Battery 1 factors to performance at any of the eight stages of practice on the psychomotor tasks were statistically significant.

These results have implications primarily for Proposition 5, that mental abilities are influenced by specifiable factors and in turn influence other variables. In the present application, mental abilities influenced the course of psychomotor learning. In doing so, the primary effects of abilities were demonstrated at the earliest stage of practice on the psychomotor task. The only ability factor that affected psychomotor performance at later stages of practice was a factor reflecting basic speediness of motor responses, and the direct effect of this factor was felt around the middle of the stages of practice at the latest. This approach was able to provide a succinct picture of the nature of the relations between ability factors and performance on the psychomotor task at various stages, both with regard to the small number of required estimates as well as the location of the effects on psychomotor learning. Although the conclusions based on Figure 9.4 may differ little from those offered by Ackerman (1987), the current analytic approach is able to identify better precisely when influences on learning occur. The proposed analytic approach should be of broad utility, enabling researchers to study the effects of both abilities and background variables on the development of skills across time.

Conclusion

Studies of mental abilities, learning, and individual differences are usually designed to provide precise answers to specific questions. However, researchers should attempt to keep key, broader theoretical propositions regarding mental abilities and learning at the forefront of their research. Despite the tendency to concentrate on specific issues, researchers should remember that their research may have clear and direct implications for broader issues that fall outside the restricted theoretical framework within which the research is conducted. If they do not monitor the ties between their research results and these broader issues, others will. To ensure that proper conclusions on broader issues are drawn, researchers should draw them.

Moreover, researchers should ensure that their statistical models relating mental abilities and learning well represent their theoretical conjectures. At times, researchers use new, state-of-the-art statistical methods simply because the methods are "hot," not because they offer better insights into the phenomena under study. In general, researchers should use the simplest and most direct methods that provide the greatest consistency between their theoretical conjectures and their data. At times, this will lead them to develop new statistical models, or adapt existing statistical models, to provide the best match between models fit to data and the central hypotheses guiding their studies; at times, these methods may be complex. Still, their methods should illuminate the phenomena under study, not simply dazzle the eyes of readers. An aim to illuminate is the surest path to progress in research on mental abilities and learning.

REFERENCES

Ackerman, P. L. (1987). Individual differences in skill learning: An integration of psychometric and information processing perspectives. *Psychological Bulletin, 102*, 3–27.

Anderson, J. E. (1939). The limitations of infant and preschool tests in the measurement of intelligence. *Journal of Psychology, 8*, 351–379.

Bloom, B. S. (1964). *Stability and change in human characteristics.* New York: Wiley.

Browne, M. W., & Du Toit, S. H. C. (1991). Models for learning data. In L. M. Collins & J. L. Horn (Eds.), *Best methods for the analysis of change: Recent advances, unanswered questions, future directions* (pp. 47–68). Washington, DC: American Psychological Association.

Collins, L. M., & Cliff, N. (1990). Using the longitudinal Guttman simplex as a basis for measuring growth. *Psychological Bulletin, 108*, 128–134.

Eysenck, H. J. (1987). Speed of information processing, reaction time, and the theory of intelligence. In P. A. Vernon (Ed.), *Speed of information-processing and intelligence* (pp. 21–67). Norwood, NJ: Ablex.

Ferguson, G. A. (1954). On learning and human ability. *Canadian Journal of Psychology, 8*, 95–112.

Ferguson, G. A. (1956). On transfer and the abilities of man. *Canadian Journal of Psychology, 10*, 121–131.

Fischer, K. W. (1980). A theory of cognitive development: The control and construction of hierarchies of skills. *Psychological Review, 87*, 477–531.

Fleishman, E. A. (1960). Abilities at different stages of practice in rotary pursuit performance. *Journal of Experimental Psychology, 60*, 162–171.

Fleishman, E. A., & Hempel, W. E., Jr. (1954). Changes in factor structure of a complex psychomotor test as a function of practice. *Psychometrika, 19*, 239–252.

Fleishman, E. A., & Hempel, W. E., Jr. (1955). The relation between abilities and improvement with practice in a visual discrimination reaction task. *Journal of Experimental Psychology, 49*, 301–312.

Geary, D. C., & Widaman, K. F. (1987). Individual differences in cognitive arithmetic. *Journal of Experimental Psychology: General, 116*, 154–171.

Greenough, W. T., & Black, J. E. (1992). Induction of brain structure by experience: Substrates for cognitive development. In M. R. Gunnar & C. A. Nelson (Eds.), *Developmental behavioral neuroscience: The Minnesota symposium on child psychology XXIV* (pp. 155–200). Hillsdale, NJ: Erlbaum.

Greenough, W. T., Black, J. E., & Wallace, C. S. (1987). Experience and brain development. *Child Development, 58*, 539–559.

Horn, J. (1988). Thinking about human abilities. In J. R. Nesselroade & R. B. Cattell (Eds.), *Handbook of multivariate experimental psychology* (2nd ed., pp. 645–685). New York: Plenum.

Horn, J. L., & Hofer, S. M. (1992). Major abilities and development in the adult period. In R. J. Sternberg & C. A. Berg (Eds.), *Intellectual development* (pp. 44–99). New York: Cambridge University Press.

Humphreys, L. G. (1960). Investigations of the simplex. *Psychometrika, 25,* 313–323.

Jöreskog, K. G. (1970). Estimation and testing of simplex models. *British Journal of Mathematical and Statistical Psychology, 23,* 121–145.

Keating, D. P., List, J. A., & Merriman, W. E. (1985). Cognitive processing and cognitive ability: A multivariate validity investigation. *Intelligence, 9,* 149–170.

Little, T. D., & Widaman, K. F. (1996). A production task evaluation of individual differences in mental addition skill development: Internal and external validation of chronometric models. *Journal of Experimental Child Psychology, 60,* 361–392.

McArdle, J. J. (1989). A structural modeling experiment with multiple growth functions. In R. Kanfer, P. L. Ackerman, & R. Cudeck (Eds.), *Abilities, motivation, and methodology: The Minnesota Symposium on Learning and Individual Differences* (pp. 71–117). Hillsdale, NJ: Erlbaum.

Meredith, W., & Tisak, J. (1990). Latent curve analysis. *Psychometrika, 55,* 107–122.

Plomin, R. (1990). *Nature and nurture: An introduction to human behavioral genetics.* Pacific Grove, CA: Brooks/Cole.

Plomin, R., DeFries, J. C., & McClearn, G. E. (1990). *Behavioral genetics: A primer* (2nd ed.). New York: Freeman.

Rogers, W. A., Fisk, A. D., & Hertzog, C. (1994). Do ability–performance relationships differentiate age and practice effects in visual search? *Journal of Experimental Psychology: Learning, Memory, and Cognition, 20,* 710–738.

Scarr, S. (1992). Development theories for the 1990s: Development and individual differences. *Child Development, 63,* 1–19.

Scarr, S., & McCartney, K. (1983). How people make their own environments: A theory of genotype environment effects. *Child Development, 54,* 424–435.

Schaie, K. W. (1996). *Intellectual development in adulthood: The Seattle longitudinal study.* New York: Cambridge University Press.

Schroots, J. J. F., & Birren, J. E. (1990). Concepts of time and aging in science. In J. E. Birren & K. W. Schaie (Eds.), *Handbook of the psychology of aging* (3rd ed., pp. 45–64). San Diego, CA: Academic Press.

Siegler, R. S., & Crowley, K. (1991). The microgenetic method: A direct means for studying cognitive development. *American Psychologist, 46,* 606–620.

Stankov, L., & Roberts, R. D. (1997). Mental speed is not the "basic" process of intelligence. *Personality and Individual Differences, 22,* 69–84.

Sternberg, R. J. (1977). *Intelligence, information processing, and analogical reasoning: The componential analysis of human abilities.* Hillsdale, NJ: Erlbaum.

Tomlinson-Keasey, C., & Little, T. D. (1990). Predicting educational attainment, occupational achievement, intellectual skill, and personal adjustment among gifted men and women. *Journal of Educational Psychology, 82,* 442–455.

Weinberger, N. M., Ashe, J., & Edeline, J.-M. (1994). Learning-induced receptive field plasticity in the auditory cortex: Specificity of information storage. In J. Delacour (Ed.), *The memory system of the brain* (pp. 590–635). River Edge, NJ: World Scientific.

Werner, H. (1957). The concept of development from a comparative and organismic point of view. In D. B. Harris (Ed.), *The concept of development: An issue in the study of human behavior* (pp. 125–148). Minneapolis: University of Minnesota Press.

Widaman, K. F. (1998, March). *Effects of maternal demographic and biological variables on infant intelligence at one year of age: Outcomes from the Maternal PKU Collaborative Study.* Paper presented at the Gatlinburg Conference on Mental Retardation and Developmental Disabilities, Charleston, SC.

Widaman, K. F., Geary, D. C., Cormier, P., & Little, T. D. (1989). A componential model for mental addition. *Journal of Experimental Psychology: Learning, Memory, and Cognition, 15,* 898–919.

Widaman, K. F., Little, T. D., Geary, D. C., & Cormier, P. (1992). Individual differences in the development of skill in mental addition: Internal and external validation of chronometric models. *Learning and Individual Differences, 4,* 167–213.

Discussion

Discussion of Widaman's paper first centered around the interpretation of his modeling results and on the utility of examining higher order ability factors. Other interactions concerned the substantive meaning of the results, with respect to individual differences in the solving of math problems.

Dr. Lohman: Do you believe that you are obtaining high correlations between parameters in addition to the intercept, whereas others have not, because you're using methods that are superior to others or that you're doing things others were not doing?

Dr. Widaman: What we try to do is do a thorough task analysis of this processing task. When you present people with numeric problems, what indeed do they do? And I think something like inspection time, paradigms like that, and there are others. Hick's law or Hick's paradigm and so on. Procedures such as this, people have not done close task analyses of them, and what they've tried to do is get a theoretically driven parameter like how quickly individuals resolve bits of information. And then they relate that to general intelligence. There's no clear theoretical link between the two. It would be nice if it worked. But there's no task analysis of general intelligence such that you would say this is where inspection time comes in. Mental abilities all tend to be correlated.

Dr. Lohman: But you're answering a different question. Specifically, I refer to Bob Sternberg's work with analogies. None of the component scores in his models — with the notable exception of the intercept — showed correlations of this magnitude.

Dr. Widaman: In the whole raft of studies, the intercept and the encoding parameter correlated; but the components of reasoning, inference, mapping, and application did not. I think there were various problems. And finally, in 1983 he [Sternberg] published a paper where the reasoning components actually then did correlate with reasoning ability. I think that's a more complex domain, and they were dealing with complex sets of stimuli, and the cuing conditions they used were a miraculous way of trying to use additive factors or subtractive method to isolate different parameters. I think there was still enough variability in what was going that things were not terribly well conditioned in the experiment. And I think that this is a simpler process. I think numerical facility is psychologically a simpler process than reasoning is and. . .

Dr. Lohman: Might it have something to do with the fact that these are 0 or 1 variables [binary]? For example, carry is carry or not? Truth is truth or not?

Dr. Widaman: And what we did with carry, carry was coded as 0/1. And what we're using as score — that's the way the original variable scored. And what we get out is an estimate — an estimate for each individual and how long he or she took to carry. And the average carry parameter is between 200 and 250 milliseconds we found across several studies. But some people carry much faster than others. And so scores do vary. On the component estimates they vary over a wider range than that. And so we get a considerable amount of variance in both the carry parameter and in memory search rates that vary quite a lot.

One clarification. And that is, in essence each parameter estimate is a mean estimate for that individual, but it varies across individuals. So it's not a 1-trial estimate of how fast you take to carry. It's an average based on (in most of our studies) between 150 and 200 reaction time trials. So there is some aggregation going on. But we do estimate those parameters, and we've done psychometrics on those parameters. So we can divide our reaction time trials into even and odd trials and estimate the parameters separately. For each individual we estimate them on separate halves and then correlate them. And we find that certain parameters — in fact, the memory search rate parameter itself — come out looking not huge. It's around 7 to 10. That doesn't look large, but the product parameter estimate varies between 0 and 72. Eight plus 9 is the largest problem we use. And if you have a predictor variable that varies between 0 and 72 and you multiply that times 8 for the average person, his or her reaction times to 0 plus 1 would give you no search rate, no time to search. Because there's so much variability on that predictor variable, it represents a huge amount of processing time differences.

Dr. Gustafsson: I was going to comment a bit on the great idea of doing higher order models as you do and using them as a set of predictors. And here it really works out great, and I think it does that in your last model too. But I think that there is a slight problem in that particular model. The problem is that when you're using the first-order factor as a predictor as is the case for mechanical knowledge, the arrow should go from the residual variable towards the dependent variable because otherwise you get an indirect relationship between the G factor going over mechanical knowledge up to Stage 1, and that causes the direct estimate between G and Stage 1 to go down forcefully. So what you have here is an underestimation of the actual effect of G on Stage 1.

Dr. Widaman: And actually, I would like to do it correctly. And I was aware of that problem. What will happen then is that from the residual for mechanical knowledge there will be a direct effect there. The fit of the model would remain unchanged, but we would have a much better estimate of the relationship between G and Stage 1 and the relationship between the residual of mechanical and Stage 1, and that would be a much improved representation.

Dr. Deary: Keith, I was glad you raised the inspection time thing and the context of the modeling of arithmetic because I've been wrestling with what exactly the constructs are from these type of analyses and those of, say, Susan Embretson. A psychophysical measure would be assessed in terms of to what degree it's a valid parameter of a brain processing limitation. That's the theoretical interest, and the mechanism of the correlation is to be explained.

In your case I'm not sure to what extent these processes exist on the test paper or in the person's head. What do you think the sort of essential status of these parameters is that you're extracting? Are there modules of the brain that conduct these separate bits of a computation, or are they arbitrary splitting up of the psychometric tasks themselves?

Dr. Widaman: I think that the reaction time approach allows you to isolate some components that are required to perform, and those components required to perform are the same components whether they are paper and pencil or not. I think people did have to search through a memory network for the correct answer and mark that down. And if it's a multicolumn problem, they have to carry to the next column and do that. One or two components might not be involved, and that may account for the less than perfect relationship between the two. One is that there would be no truth parameter. If you were trying to do a task analysis of what it takes to perform on a paper-and-pencil test, the traditional paper-and-pencil test merely puts a box underneath a problem and you supply the answers of production task paradigm. And so there would be no true versus false kind of component on that task.

But otherwise, what we're trying to get at with the cognitive processing models, all we have from a paper-and-pencil test is an answer that specifies the number of problems correctly answered in a particular amount of time. What we're trying to do with the cognitive processing model is say what are the processes involved — and if someone is deficient in numerical facility, and you would know it from a low score on a paper-and-pencil test, but you wouldn't know why. There's the potential with cognitive processing models to say it's in search rate or it's in some other component. And this sort of model fit to an individual's reaction times to a differentiated set of problems would have at least the hope of being more definitive in saying what a deficiency in a numerical facility is.

10

Exploiting the Speed–Accuracy Trade-Off

DAVID E. WRIGHT and IAN DENNIS

The work presented in this chapter was motivated by two practical testing problems. One is the need to deal with the speed–accuracy trade-off problem. The other is the need for an item generative testing technology that is based on models that index item characteristics in terms of item facets.

This speed–accuracy trade-off problem arises when tests are affected by between-subjects variation in the speed–accuracy compromise adopted by different participants. One approach to dealing with this problem is to develop scoring procedures that combine speed and accuracy in a strategy-independent way. This approach was explored in some detail by Dennis and Evans (1996). However, as they pointed out, no scoring procedure will separate participants who work at the extremes of accuracy. The approach investigated in this chapter, proposed by Evans and Wright (1993), is to pace the participants as they work through the test by placing time allowances on items (not strictly time limits because participants are not permitted to respond earlier than the time allowed). Controlling time in this way has the added benefit of simplifying data structure and making item–response theory (IRT) methods and the associated testing technology applicable. Moreover, the times associated with items can be considered as item facets and used to adjust item difficulty. As a concrete example, in this article we consider a timed item version of a two-term transitive inference test.

The remainder of the chapter is organized as follows: In the next section, we describe the test data and the study population. Descriptive statistics for the test are also presented there. After that, we describe the IRT models and the results of fitting

We thank Hilary Sanders and Julian Stander for their comments and suggestions. We are also grateful to Phillip Ackerman, Pat Kyllonen, and Richard Roberts for their helpful comments.

these models using Markov chain Monte Carlo methods. We then discuss the problem of ability estimation and adaptive testing. We conclude with a discussion of the limitations of the study and briefly review some recent methodology.

Test Data and Study Population

The Two-Term Transitive Inference Test

Transitive inference is a form of deductive reasoning that is based on relationships between dimensions that have the property of transitivity (see Evans, 1982). Specifically, a relation $>$ is transitive if whenever $A > B$ and $B > C$, then $A > C$. The inverse $<$ of such a relationship is such that if $A < B$, then $B > A$.

There are many dimensions in the real world that are known to be transitive (e.g., goodness, height, weight, brightness, etc.). In natural language, the relationships $>$ and $<$ can be expressed by pairs of comparatives such as better–worse, taller–shorter, or heavier–lighter. The items used in the British Army Recruit Battery (BARB) transitive inference test derive from the problem forms, comparatives, and names shown in Table 10.1. The first four problem forms are *positive comparative* forms, whereas the last four are *negative equatives*.

TABLE 10.1   Problem Form and Content Used in the BARB
Transitive Inference Task

Problem forms

1. A is better than B	Who is better?
2. A is better than B	Who is worse?
3. A is worse than B	Who is better?
4. A is worse than B	Who is worse?
5. A is not as bad as B	Who is better?
6. A is not as bad as B	Who is worse?
7. A is not as good as B	Who is better?
8. A is not as good as B	Who is worse?

Comparatives

Taller–shorter
Better–worse
Stronger–weaker
Heavier–lighter
Happier–sadder
Older–younger
Brighter–dimmer
Faster–slower

Names

Fred, Bill, Tom, John, George, Paul, Mike, Steve, Bob, Phil, Ian, Dave, Sid, Pete, Joe, Chris

Note. BARB = British Army Recruit Battery.

In the standard BARB transitive inference, test items are generated in blocks of eight by forming a randomized blocks of the eight problem forms. Comparatives are selected randomly, and, for each item, names are selected at random without replacement. The timing is under the control of the participant who receives the instruction "Work as fast as you can but try to remain accurate."

In the experimental timed item version of the test, participants were presented with a fixed set of 44 items. Each item was presented for a controlled period of time, 2, 3, 4, or 5 s. During this period they had no opportunity to respond. After this period the response buttons on the touch screen were presented, and they were required to give their response by touching one of the buttons.

Participants

The experimental timed item version of the test was delivered to 1,273 British Army applicants between July and November of 1996. These applicants took the standard BARB recruitment tests followed by the experimental timed item transitive inference test, which was placed in the BARB experimental window.

Test Reliabilities

When a simple guessing adjusted score was used, the reliability, which was based on an even–odd split, of the timed item test was .79. This was identical to the test immediate–retest reliability of the current transitive inference test in BARB. However, the correlation between the scores on the two tests was .65, indicating that although the tests were equivalent in terms of their reliability, they were measuring different abilities.

IRT Modeling

IRT models are used to represent the relationship between the probability of a correct item response and an unknown ability θ (see Hambleton & Swaminithan, 1985). These models are generally of a sigmoidal form, rising from some guessing level to unity as ability increases. Figure 10.1 is an example of a normal ogive model. Apart from the guessing parameter, this model has parameters that index item difficulty and item discrimination. In most applications of IRT, separate parameters are used for each item. However, with structured populations of items, such as those in the task considered here, more parsimonious models that exploit the structure of the item population are of interest. By indexing item characteristics in terms of item facets, these models provide a basis for tailored and adaptive item generation. Because they can be used to represent psychological theories about the item populations, they are of some interest from a purely scientific perspective: They provide a formal framework for comparison of different psychological theories. In this context, the structured models are somewhat analogous to confirmatory factor analysis models.

One approach to fitting these models is to fit separate item characteristic curves to each item and then to model structure by regressing item parameter estimates

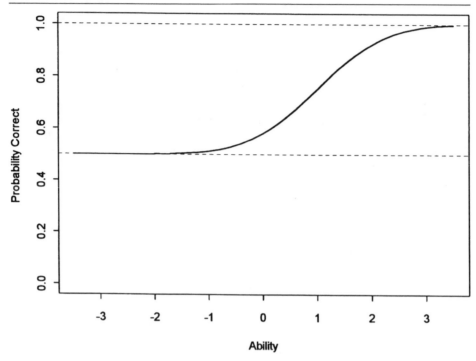

Figure 10.1. Normal ogive item characteristic curve ($\alpha = 0.5$, $\beta = 1$, and $\gamma = 1$).

on item facets (see, e.g., Mislevy, Sheehan, & Wingersky, 1993). However, it is more efficient to fit the model in one step with structured parameters. Moreover, this enables standard inferential procedures to be applied to the comparison of models.

We took a Bayesian approach using Markov chain Monte Carlo (MCMC) methods (see Gilks, Richardson, & Spiegelhalter, 1996) to sample from the posterior distribution of unknown parameters. The implementation of MCMC used was essentially the same as that presented by Albert (1992), with modifications to incorporate a guessing parameter and structured relationships across items. The MCMC algorithms were programmed using the package S-Plus (Statistical Sciences).

For applications of the EM (Dempster, Laird, & Rubin, 1977) algorithm, the logistic IRT models offer computational advantages over normal ogive IRT models. However, the converse is true within the framework of MCMC, and for this reason we use normal ogive models in this chapter. In the models the probability that an individual with ability θ gives a correct response to the i-th item $P_i(\theta)$ is given by

$$P_i(\theta) = \alpha_i + (1 - \alpha_i)\Phi(\beta_i\theta - \gamma_i), \tag{10.1}$$

where Φ denotes the standard normal distribution function. The item parameters α_i, β_i, and γ_i represent guessing, discrimination, and difficulty, respectively. In the analysis presented here, the guessing parameters α_i are fixed at .5, and the discrimination parameters β_i are assumed to be the same for all items. Rather than having a separate difficulty parameter for each item, we model item difficulty in terms of facet effects. Our model for item difficulty can be represented symbolically by the following formula:

$$\text{difficulty} = \text{problem form} + \text{time}, \tag{10.2}$$

where problem form is the eight-level facet shown in Table 10.1 and time is a four-level facet with levels corresponding to 2, 3, 4, and 5 s. Equation 10.2 simply states that item difficulty is modeled in terms of the main effects of the facets *problem form* and *time*. The difficulty structure of the items is thus modeled in terms of 11 parameters rather than the 44 parameters in the full model for item difficulty. If the problem form is denoted by j by j ($j = 1, 2, \ldots, 8$) and the level of the time facet by k ($k = 1, 2, 3, 4$, corresponding to item times of 2, 3, 4, and 5 s, respectively), the probability of a correct response given θ, which we denote by $P_{jk}(\theta)$, is given by

$$P_{jk}(\theta) = 0.5 + 0.5\Phi[\beta\theta - (\tau_j + \pi_k)], \tag{10.3}$$

where τ_j denotes the effect of problem type j and π_k denotes the effect of level k of time. To make the parameters identifiable, the constraint $\pi_4 = 0$ is imposed.

The prior distribution of ability was assumed to be standard normal. Noninformative independent uniform priors were assumed for all unknown model parameters. Convergence of the chain to the posterior distribution was assessed graphically after the first 500 iterations were discarded as burn-in (see Gilks et al., 1996, chap. 1). Posterior means and standard deviations for these parameters obtained from 1,000 MCMC iterations are given in Table 10.2.

The posterior means of the item characteristic curves with times of 2 and 5 s are shown in Figure 10.2. The full curves show the probability of a correct response for the eight problem types with a time of 2 s, whereas the broken curves show the probability of a correct response for the eight problem types with a time of 5 s. The structure in our model means that the latter were the same as the former translated to the left at a distance that represented the effect of changing from a time 2 s to 5 s. From Figure 10.2, one may note that except for Problem Types 5 and 8, the negative equative problem forms had virtually the same item characteristics as their positive comparative counterparts.

TABLE 10.2   Posterior Means and Standard Deviations

Parameter	Posterior M	Posterior SD
τ_1	−1.569	0.0743
τ_2	−1.341	0.0657
τ_3	−1.287	0.0735
τ_4	−1.752	0.0674
τ_5	−0.458	0.0722
τ_6	−1.040	0.0689
τ_7	−1.101	0.0642
τ_8	−0.963	0.0650
π_1	1.459	0.0299
π_2	0.509	0.0289
π_3	0.213	0.0322
π_4	0.0	0.0
β	0.740	0.0208

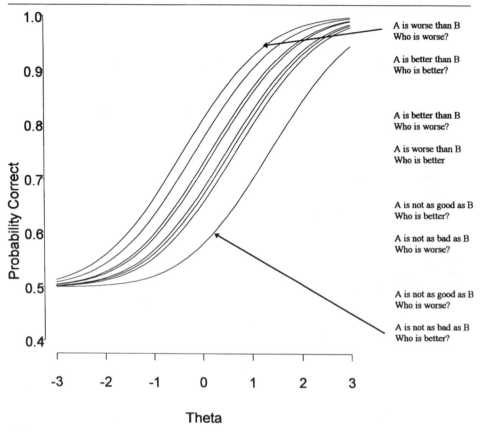

Figure 10.2. Item characteristic curves for the eight problem forms. The order of the curves top to bottom is the same as the order of the problem forms shown on the right.

Modeling Time Effects

The full curves shown in Figure 10.3 are the posterior mean item characteristic curves for different times with problems of Form 1. As might be expected, item difficulty decreased with increases in time. Moreover, the benefit of increasing the time limit diminished as the time limit increased.

Models incorporating time as a factor are of limited use in item generation because they cannot be used to predict item characteristics for items with times other than those used in the available data. For this reason and for parsimony, models in which difficulty is a smooth function of time are preferable to models with qualitative levels for time. In choosing an appropriate functional form for the effect of time t, it is reasonable to assume that difficulty declines as t is increased. However, it seems unrealistic to expect difficulty to decline without limit as t increases, and the effect of time would be expected to approach an asymptote representing the difficulty of the item when no time constraints are placed on it. A simple way that this effect is achieved is to incorporate a regression term for the variate $1/t$ in the model. This leads to a nine-parameter model for the difficulty structure symbolically represented in the following form:

236

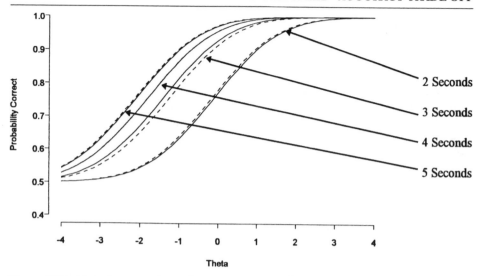

Figure 10.3. Posterior mean item characteristic curves for problems of Type 1. Models with time as a factor are shown as full curves. Models with time as a variate are shown as broken lines. Note that with $t = 4$ s, and that the two curves are coincident.

$$\text{difficulty} = \text{problem form} + 1/t. \tag{10.4}$$

If we introduce the regression coefficient λ, the probability of a correct response given ability θ, which we denote by $P_{jt}(\theta)$, is given by

$$P_{jt}(\theta) = 0.5 + 0.5\Phi[\beta\theta - (\tau_j + \lambda/t)]. \tag{10.5}$$

Posterior means and standard deviations for these parameters obtained from 1,000 MCMC iterations are given in Table 10.3.

The dashed curves shown in Figure 10.3 are the posterior mean item characteristic curves under Model 5. Figure 10.4 shows the posterior mean item characteristic curves for times 1.5, 2, 2.5, ..., 5.5 s. Note that curves for 1.5 and 5.5 s represent extrapolations beyond the range of data and are therefore of questionable reliability.

TABLE 10.3   Posterior Means and Standard Deviations

Parameter	Posterior M	Posterior SD
τ_1	−2.5910	0.1226
τ_2	−2.3520	0.0931
τ_3	−2.3390	0.0825
τ_4	−2.7632	0.0809
τ_5	−1.4886	0.0701
τ_6	−2.0208	0.0792
τ_7	−2.1653	0.0750
τ_8	−1.9993	0.0669
λ	4.8322	0.0967
β	0.7390	0.0213

Item Generation and Random Effects

In principle, the models described earlier could be used as a basis for tailored or adaptive item generation. However, in item generation, facets such as comparatives and names were allocated at random, and the effects of these facets were excluded from our IRT models. Although these effects were small compared with the effects of problem form and time, they were statistically significant. This is illustrated in Figure 10.5, which shows the posterior mean item characteristic curves for the following four items from the test that had the same time limit and the same problem form.

Item 5:	*Dave is not as short as Sid. Who is shorter?*	*Dave Sid*
Item 21:	*George is not as dim as Dave. Who is dimmer?*	*Dave George*
Item 25:	*Fred is not as young as Paul. Who is younger?*	*Paul Fred*
Item 37:	*Steve is not as sad as Bill. Who is sadder?*	*Steve Bill*

The bold curve shows the model in which these four items were assumed to have the same difficulty structure according to the model difficulty = problem form + $1/t$. The other item characteristic curves shown were obtained from the model in which each item had its own difficulty parameter.

One approach to dealing with the problem would be to extend the model to include additional facets. This would require a more extensive set of sample items, and ultimately it would require trial data on the full population of potential items. A more practical alternative is to follow a similar approach to that taken by Mislevy et al. (1993) and introduce a random effect ε on item difficulty. Symbolically, the model then takes the form

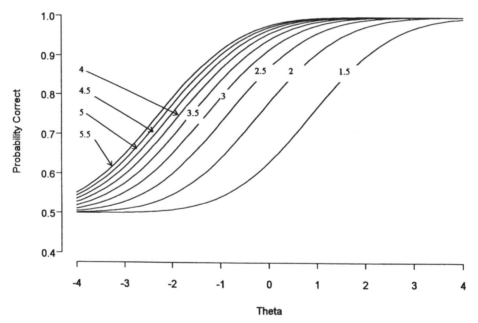

Figure 10.4. Posterior mean item characteristic curves for problems of Type 1 with times 1.5, 2, 2.5, . . . , 5.5 s.

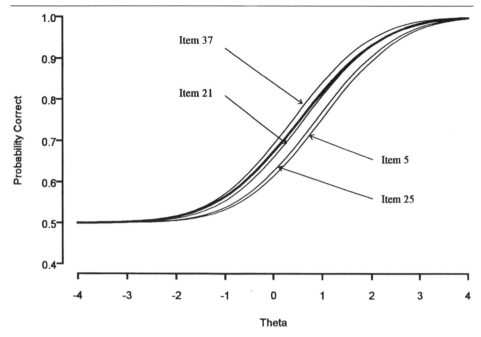

Figure 10.5. Posterior mean item characteristic curves for four items of the same problem form and a 2-s time allowance.

$$\text{difficulty} = \text{problem form} + 1/t + \varepsilon, \tag{10.6}$$

where ε represents a random effect drawn independently from a normal distribution with mean zero and variance σ^2. The estimation of the variance parameter σ^2 is easily incorporated into the MCMC algorithm. The magnitude of σ^2 is a measure of the adequacy of the model for item difficulty and affects inferences about ability.

Ability Estimation

Consider now a participant who has completed a specific sequence of items resulting in a vector of responses $y = (y_1, y_2, \ldots, y_n)^T$. If we denote the corresponding vectors of item guessing discrimination and difficulty parameters by α, β, and γ, respectively, for the moment assumed to be known, the posterior distribution of ability is obtained from Bayes theorem as

$$p(\theta|y, \alpha, \beta, \gamma, \sigma^2) \propto p(\theta) \prod_i \int_{-\infty}^{\infty} p(y_i|\theta, \alpha_i, \beta_i, \varepsilon_i) p(\varepsilon_i|\sigma^2), \tag{10.7}$$

where σ^2 denotes the error variance. Of course, in practice the parameters α, β, γ and σ^2 will be unknown. A fully Bayesian approach would be to compute values of $p(\theta|y, \alpha, \beta, \gamma, \sigma^2)$ for appropriate MCMC iterations and use the average of these as an MCMC-based estimate of the posterior distribution. Alternatively, some form

239

of approximation, with the simplest being the posterior mode of $p(\theta|y, \alpha, \beta, \gamma, \sigma^2)$, could be used.

Posterior distributions of ability were obtained for a sample of 5 participants chosen to reflect a large range of abilities by taking the average. These were obtained under the following three model specifications: (a) The full 45 (44 difficulty + 1

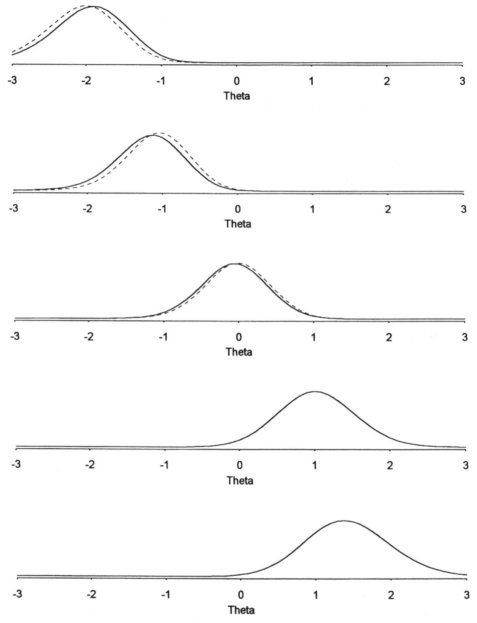

Figure 10.6. Posterior distribution of ability for selected participants. Full curve is for facet model with time as a variate. The broken curves are for Model 1. The full curves are for Models 2 and 3 (these are indistinguishable on the graph).

TABLE 10.4   Posterior Means and Standard Deviations of Ability

Participant No.	Posterior M			Posterior SD		
	Model 1	Model 2	Model 3	Model 1	Model 2	Model 3
1	−2.030	−1.939	−1.939	0.446	0.459	0.463
2	−1.079	−1.179	−1.184	0.424	0.444	0.450
3	−0.020	−0.068	−0.058	0.439	0.443	0.452
4	1.035	1.032	1.043	0.511	0.513	0.522
5	1.426	1.425	1.430	0.553	0.556	0.588

discrimination) parameter model with a common discriminating parameter and a separate difficulty parameter for each item (the error variance σ^2 was fixed at zero); (b) the 10 (9 for difficulty + 1 discrimination) parameter model with a common discriminating parameter and the model, difficulty = problem type + $1/t$ (the error variance was fixed at zero); and (c) the same model as the second one but with a random effect with variance σ^2 estimated from the data. The posterior distributions are shown graphically in Figure 10.6. Summaries of these are given in Table 10.4.

In this example, it is notable that incorporating a random effect on item difficulty to account for differences between items not captured in the model (5) has an imperceptible effect on inferences about ability. The error standard deviation is about 0.3 in this model. The error variation in this illustration is minimal and there is very little difference between the first and second models. The effect of artificially increasing the error variance is to increase the posterior standard deviation toward its previous value of unity and shrink the posterior mean ability toward zero.

Adaptive Testing

A major advantage of the IRT approach to modeling timed items tests is that it provides a basis for an adaptive procedure. This would not be feasible without timed items for two reasons: First, the complexity of the responses that make up latency as well as accuracy means that the IRT models and the established adaptive testing technology are inappropriate. Even if suitable models for dealing jointly with latency and accuracy data were available, the limited number of problem forms would mean that any adaptive algorithms would try to focus on a small subset of problem forms that participants would quickly begin to recognize and develop heuristics for solving. One may imagine that by using item times to adapt the test while maintaining a randomized block structure for the sequence of item types, a computer-generated adaptive timed item test could be produced.

Conclusion

Regarding the use of timed items, this chapter has dealt with work in progress, and further work needs to be done to address some key issues. The generality of some of the results reported here needs to be confirmed by applying timed item methods to a broader range of tests. Nevertheless, the results are encouraging in confirming that candidates can cope with responding within a time window and that time-restricted tests yield reliable measures.

A significant issue concerns the way in which the use of time restrictions affect what is being measured. Although the scores obtained from the time-restricted version of the test were strongly correlated with those from the conventional version, the correlation nevertheless fell short of that which would be expected if the two versions were equivalent. There are several alternative explanations for this, and it is important that subsequent work attempts to distinguish between them. One possibility is that scores on the conventional version of the test are contaminated by the candidate's choice of speed–accuracy compromise, as argued by Dennis and Evans (1996). Scores on time-restricted versions of the test would then differ because the contamination has been removed, yielding purer measures of ability.

Another possibility is that having to prepare to respond in a restricted time window takes up attentional resources and that candidates are differentially able to cope with this competing demand. According to this account the nature of the test is changed by the use of time restrictions. All time-restricted tests would partly measure the ability to undertake the additional demands of working within the time limits.

A third alternative is that people differ in their flexibility in being able to operate at different speed–accuracy compromises. By this account, candidates who are less flexible may appear to have lower ability when required to take a version of the test that requires them to respond at a range of times. This raises the possibility that more than one dimension is needed to characterize an individual because people differ in terms of flexibility and ability. However, if this were correct, obtaining estimates of both dimensions may go beyond what it is feasible and necessary in practical testing. What is more important is to have a good understanding of what one is measuring and to measure it efficiently.

The relationship between the characterization of the speed–accuracy trade-off, which is implicit here, and that given by established information-processing accounts warrants some comment. Wickelgren (1977) has argued that there are some features that any reasonable description of the speed–accuracy trade-off needs to have. At short response times, accuracy is at chance and there is some minimum time needed before accuracy starts to rise. Once this minimum time is exceeded, accuracy starts to rise in a negatively accelerated fashion and tends toward a maximum asymptotic accuracy that is approached as response time becomes long. This description suggests that the speed–accuracy trade-off may be characterized in terms of three parameters: the minimum time before accuracy starts to rise, the rate at which accuracy rises as time increases, and the asymptotic accuracy attained at long response times. It is possible, but not easy, with sufficient data from individuals to obtain independent estimates of these three parameters (e.g., Lohman, 1989). For candidates of any given ability, the model used here matches this characterization. Performance remains close to chance as long as t is small. At long response times, accuracy reaches an asymptote that depends on the item type and the ability of the candidate. However, the model used here represents a simplification in characterizing individual differences in terms of only a single parameter. This simplification has the benefit of being applicable in practical testing. How satisfactory and how critical it is will need to be explored on a broader range of tests.

Turning now to psychometric issues, the structured logistic regression models used in this chapter were fitted using the software written in the form of S-Plus functions.

As far as we know, there is no generally available software for fitting these models. (Copies of these S-Plus functions used in this chapter, together with functions for fitting structured logistic IRT models using the EM algorithm, are available for research purposes from the first author.)

Looking toward the future of research in individual differences, the work on psychometrics that brings IRT and factor analysis together in general framework should be highlighted. Apart from one or two notable exceptions (see, e.g., Bartholomew, 1987), IRT and factor analysis have developed as separate strands of research, with IRT being concerned largely with the psychometric properties of items within tests and factor analysis with relationships between scores on different tests. Over the past few years, a number of researchers have attempted to look at factor analysis from an item level rather than a test level. Segall (1996) demonstrated the potential advantage of this in multivariate adaptive testing. Meng and Schilling (1996) described practical ways of fitting multivariate IRT models using MCMC. Sammal, Ryan, and Legler (1997) described an EM approach to fitting models in which the response vector may contain a mixture of binary variables and continuous variables. Applications of these types of models to model item and factor structure have enormous potential for future research on individual differences.

REFERENCES

Albert, J. H. (1992). Bayesian estimation of normal ogive item response curves using Gibbs sampling. *Journal of Educational Statistics, 17,* 251–269.

Bartholomew, D. J. (1987). *Latent variable models and factor analysis.* London: Griffin.

Dempster, A. P., Laird, N. M., & Rubin, D. B. (1977). Maximum likelihood from incomplete data via the EM algorithm (with discussion). *Journal of the Royal Statistical Society B, 39,* 1–38.

Dennis, I., & Evans, J. St. B. T. (1996). The speed–error trade off problem in psychometric testing. *British Journal of Psychology, 87,* 105–129.

Evans, J. St. B. T. (1982). *The psychology of deductive reasoning.* London: Routledge & Kegan Paul.

Evans, J. St. B. T., & Wright, D. E. (1993). *The properties of fixed time tests: A simulation study* (Rep. No. 3-1993). University of Plymouth, Plymouth, United Kingdom.

Gilks, W. R., Richardson, S., & Spiegelhalter, D. J. (1996). Introducing Markov chain Monte Carlo. In W. R. Gilks, S. Richardson, & D. J. Spielgelhalter (Eds.), *Markov chain Monte Carlo in practice* (pp. 1–19). London: Chapman & Hall.

Hambleton, R. K., & Swaminithan, H. (1985). *Item response theory principles and applications.* Norwell, MA: Kluwer Academic.

Lohman, D. F. (1989). Individual differences in errors and latencies on cognitive tasks. *Learning and Individual Differences, 1,* 179–202.

Meng, X. L., & Schilling, S. (1996). Fitting full-information item factor models and an empirical investigation of bridge sampling. *Journal of the American Statistical Association, 91,* 1254–1267.

Mislevy, R. J., Sheehan, K. M., & Wingersky, M. (1993). How to equate tests with little or no data. *Journal of Educational Measurement, 30,* 55–78.

Sammel, L. M., Ryan, L. M., & Legler, J. M. (1997). Latent variable models for mixed discrete and continuous outcomes. *Journal of the Royal Statistical Society B, 59,* 667–678.

Segall, D. O. (1996). Multidimensional adaptive testing. *Psychometrica, 61,* 331–354.

Wickelgren, W. A. (1977). Speed–accuracy trade-off and information processing dynamics. *Acta Psychologica, 41,* 67–85.

Discussion

Extensive discussion of Wright's paper revolved around conceptual and pragmatic difficulties of assessing speed–accuracy trade-off and individual differences. Several discussants raised issues about examining "time" as a factor of assessment and about the pragmatics of implementing the kind of design Wright described in other contexts.

Dr. Widaman: When you had the one picture up there, when you looked at the typically parameterized 44-parameter model and the constrained models, frequently what happens with structural equation or with IRT [item–response theory] models or regression models is that when you add parameters . . . instead of having reasonably constrained parameters, you essentially overfit the model. And it did look like the posterior distributions from the constrained model had smaller confidence intervals around scores. And I was wondering if it was a function of fitting a model that could be well constrained and essentially not fitting error.

Dr. Wright: They were slightly more concentrated, yes. As far as the fitting methodology's concerned, what I've been doing is writing programs in a package called *S Plus* for fitting these models. Which is not a very user-friendly package. It's a bit like MatLab. It took me days to figure out what that program of Albert's was doing in MatLab. It was written on about a half a page of the paper. It was very difficult to read. And S Plus is the same.

Dr. Ackerman: Do you have any sense about whether your speeded test is more-or-less valid in predicting some outcome criteria for those recruits or applicants?

Dr. Wright: None at all, no. I think one of the problems is we keep hitting this G. Time and again people are saying, "This battery measures, G, and very little else." And I think one of the things I'm looking forward to is to try and see a test that gets more separation.

Dr. Ackerman: Yes. But there's some sense about whether the criteria that one wants to predict in the real world are in some ways matching the kinds of predictors that you are developing. So, like your mathematics test, you're not interested in whether or not a person can do a simple addition problem in a half an hour. That the real world involves mathematical computation on the fly in a short period of time. So if that were the case, then the kinds of speeded tests that you're talking about challenge the individual to do something that's much more like what they do in the real world, and one would expect an increase ultimately in valid variance for predicting the criteria.

Dr. Wright: Yes. We haven't had any criterion data.

Dr. Ackerman: But that would also suggest that you wouldn't want to do a history test like this?

Dr. Wright: No.

Dr. Baddeley: What you seem to be doing is taking the control of speed from the subject, so you're changing a self-paced to a paced task.

Dr. Wright: Yes.

Dr. Baddeley: In general, doing that tends to reduce levels of efficiency. So when they first brought out letter-sorting machines over here they used a paced method and there were lots of errors. And in general, you have a situation where you're producing a lot of errors as part of your process. I suppose one question is, Are there very many real-life situations where you're prepared to accept a very high error rate? The second is, in terms of optimal strategy, it may well be that an optimal strategy for dealing with a problem where you don't have enough time is actually an approximation. You use a halo effect or something. So you may actually be picking up something very different. And I think without actually understanding the nature of the task, it's dangerous to simply employ a technique of this sort. So I think the understanding has to come first.

Dr. Wright: I'd agree with you. But I think the reverse is true. I think to just let people sit and dictate their own pace is also a problem. I mean you're just replacing one problem by a different class of problems.

Dr. Baddeley: Well, there is actually a lot of data on reaction times that suggest that what people do is track their error rate, so that they use errors to tell them that they're going too fast. That they can actually self-detect.

Dr. Wright: Yes, but these people don't know they're making errors. The other thing is it's the errors that contain the information about ability. I mean if people maintained accuracy when you closed down the time limits, you wouldn't learn anything about their ability. You know, that's what gives you the differential estimates, the fact that people are making errors.

Dr. Lohman: Back in 1978 when I first stumbled on the business of speed–accuracy trade-off, I had written some harebrained scheme for how I thought we might approach the problem. When Cronbach commented on the draft that I was writing, he scribbled in the margin someplace, "I see pacing as the key." About 15 years later I finally got back to that, and I realized that he might have had more insight into the problem than I realized that he had at the time. But one of the things that they did in the pacing studies was not to pace items but to pace groups of items, which is one of the things that I thought was most promising about the techniques you were using years ago.

We have found in our own work that pacing individual items introduces other factors. For example, anxiety becomes a crucial covariate of performance, and more so as time pressures increase. We've also found that these procedures dramatically disrupt performance for some people. I expect that anxiety is one of the things going on. Have you considered this? And have you followed up the early attempts in your lab to pace not at the level of particular items but rather at the level of groups of items?

Dr. Wright: No. We haven't. The big concern I've got is the one about the stress in people, you know, learning about personality by putting people into stress and making them fail more items than they would normally fail on. I mean that's the problem. I think that's the very weak thing, but I keep coming back to this. The tests now are very imperfect as they stand with people sort of working very slowly and accurately, so it's a trade-off between two classes of problems.

Dr. Kyllonen: There's some data Susan Embretson has, where she administered the Raven Progressive Matrices Tests under three conditions. One condition had no time limits. Another condition had the time limit at the mean of the sample average — or the average response time from the prior study. And the interesting finding there was that under the condition where there was a time limit the Raven's Progressive Matrices Test actually had higher validity with respect to a G-like criterion. The best interpretation is that what happened under conditions of no time limit, people set their own sort of standard or criterion for when to give up on the problem, and people vary dramatically. And so what a time limit is doing is giving a little bit of feedback to get examinees on more or less the same understanding of what it is you want them to do. That's an interesting observation.

The second point is kind of a mundane question. And that is, you said that you're interested in using this sort of an adaptive testing scheme at some point. The question is item selection. And in particular, you replaced a design where you had three or four or five different levels of time envelopes with the function of time. And have you thought about the sort of mechanics of selecting items when you have a scheme that has a function of items rather than discrete items with discrete characteristics?

Dr. Wright: I think if you had a function of time, you could treat time. I mean in principle you could treat time as a continuously variable moderator of difficulty. The problem is that fails because you're going to move outside the range that you've actually got experience of. In my data, I think it was 2 seconds to 5 seconds. I wouldn't want to sort of extrapolate. You could have a system which uses randomized blocks just like it does now involve. But where you allocated the times so that you got maximal information from blocks of items.

Dr. Widaman: I do think one thing that could and should be done is to check out the factorial description of the test under those different conditions. Because they are fairly highly correlated. But if you do think that introducing the time pressure would bring in to the true score that's estimated on the test additional factors in an untimed form, the test may have a very simple factorial nature. When you bring in time constraints, you may be bringing in other factors into the description. But that would lead to sort of basic research to try to understand the factorial description of the tests under different conditions. But when I look at the ASVAB [Armed Services Vocational Aptitude Battery], what I see are quite a number of complex tests. There are very few factor-pure tests. They're complex tests. But in the military, many times what you're trying to predict is complex criteria. And it's possible that the ASVAB works well for prediction precisely because all the tests are complex and you're predicting complex criteria. And so a factor analyst would hate the ASVAB because it's not a factor analyzable battery in any sense. But it may be entirely useful to predict complex criteria. And when you make the task more complex by adding the time pressure, you're bringing in more variance that may be crucial if someone has to react very quickly to something.

Dr. Alexander: But I want to follow that up with what Phil Ackerman was saying and come back to a point that may get lost in the discussion of what we can do methodologically or psychometrically with time as a factor. And that is, theoretically what is the value of adding time or the reason for adding it? And that is, under what conditions do we want this particular task to be timed or not timed? And the other issue that has to be explored is what kind of time seems to make sense theoretically for such a task. Sometimes we can play with these numbers and do some fascinating things, but we lose in the sense of why the heck are we doing this theoretically. And I think that's important.

Dr. Davison: My question had to do with computerized adaptive testing. Usually with computerized adaptive testing, we adjust the difficulty of the test by varying the difficulty of the items. But from the data that you were presenting, it looks like we could use the same items and we could vary the time.

I was wondering if that's what you had in mind. That raises a question about what happens when we vary time, whether we're changing the trait that's measured or we're changing the information function over the trait that's measured.

Dr. Wright: That was one of the strategies to use time to moderate difficulties so you use it in an adaptive testing system. I have grave concerns about adaptive testing. And those concerns just get magnified when I think about using time to manipulate difficulty.

Dr. Ackerman: Well, don't you end up with two dimensions for the test? You have a difficulty dimension, and you have a time dimension. And so you end up with a multivariate situation for dealing with the task.

Dr. Wright: Well, the effect of time is in the difficulty dimension the way that this model's been set up now.

Dr. Ackerman: Yes, but it's not clear that you can make difficulty and time really equivalent. I mean you can make that assumption for your model, but if you have items that are otherwise homogeneous in difficulty and you're changing the time of administration, that's one thing. But if you also have heterogeneous items in terms of difficulty and you're adding the time dimension, then you need to go to a multivariate latent trait model.

Dr. Wright: This is the research really. And, you know, these questions I can't answer because they're more researched questions. The research hasn't been done but — I mean I think you're right. I mean there's a lot of things that need to be done if these methods are going to be pursued any further.

Dr. Matthews: What comes from RT (response time) research is the idea of speed–accuracy operating characteristics (SAOCs). You give the task with different instructions for speed–accuracy trade-off and get a plot of response time against accuracy, the SAOC. The information which you want is in the middle part of that plot. If a person's responding too fast, they're guessing, and perhaps getting time pressured. At the top end you have an error-free zone where the speed is dependent on response criterion. The technique which you've suggested perhaps has a danger that the windows you set aren't going to overlap with those parts of the SAOC which actually have the information you want. So, as an alternative technique, you could have subjects do the task with different instructions. Perhaps the computer can be programmed to keep changing instructions until it's got the information which it needs to get the full SAOC for the subject. So don't have the computer set the times, have the subject set them through instruction.

Dr. Wright: We did do some studies like that where we changed the instructions and told people to work fast but don't worry about accuracy. They all did the same anyway. I mean they didn't seem to take any notice of the instructions.

Dr. Matthews: That would be a problem.

IV

TRAITS

11

Personality and Skill: A Cognitive–Adaptive Framework

GERALD MATTHEWS

Personality traits are important because they make a difference to people's lives. Traits are correlated with proficiency in a variety of acquired real-life skills that contribute to occupational and social success. In the occupational context, meta-analyses have shown that the "Big Five" traits are modestly but robustly associated with job and training proficiency, especially when moderator factors are taken into account (Costa, 1996; Matthews, 1997a). Traits also relate to choice of occupation and vocational interests (Ackerman & Heggestad, 1997; Furnham, 1992). Traits also make a difference in people's personal lives. A variety of personality characteristics are associated with psychopathology, and there is increasing evidence for causal effects of traits (Barnett & Gotlib, 1988; Matthews, Saklofske, Costa, Deary, & Zeidner, 1998). Cognitive models of emotional disorder imply that traits are associated with individual differences in skills for handling stressful life events (Matthews & Deary, 1998; Wells & Matthews, 1994).

In this chapter, I examine frameworks for explaining associations between traits and complex, learned behaviors. I contrast process- and content-oriented explanations. Process-oriented explanations involve basic neural and computational processes that may contribute to individual differences in skill acquisition and performance. Content-oriented explanations are interests and motivations that covary with personality. For example, sociable people may have better social skills simply because they have more experience and interest in social situations. I outline a cognitive–adaptive framework that integrates these two perspectives and demonstrate its application to explaining the behavioral correlates of extraversion and neuroticism.

The cognitive–adaptive framework is based on application of the classical theory of cognitive science (Pylyshyn, 1984) to personality and emotion research (Matthews, 1997b). Three different levels of explanation for personality phenomena

251

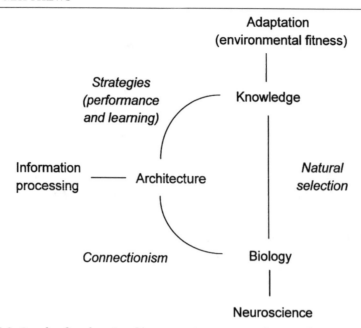

Figure 11.1. Levels of explanation for a cognitive science of personality. From "An Introduction to the Cognitive Science of Personality and Emotion," by G. Matthews, 1997b, in G. Matthews (Ed.), *Cognitive Science Perspectives on Personality and Emotion* (pp. 3–30), Amsterdam: Elsevier. Copyright 1997 by Elsevier. Reprinted with permission of the author.

should be distinguished: those that refer to neuroscience, to the cognitive architecture, and to adaptation to real-world environments, as shown in Figure 11.1. Constructs such as neural nets and strategies bridge the levels. In this chapter I focus on the distinction between explanations in terms of variation of the cognitive architecture with personality and explanations in terms of the person's interests, goals, and choice of activities.

Personality and Information-Processing Models of Skill

The traditional approach to explaining the behavioral expression of traits is psychobiological. Traits are related to individual differences in arousal, or in specified brain structures and circuits (see Zuckerman, 1991, for a review). For example, H. J. Eysenck's (1967) arousal theory attributes extraversion–introversion to individual differences in corticoreticular arousability. Individual differences in arousal affect both learning, via conditioning, and performance, via the Yerkes–Dodson law. The psychobiological approach has two significant advantages: It explains why personality has psychophysiological correlates, and it provides a mechanism for the inheritance of personality traits. Its major and possibly fatal shortcoming is that psychobiological theories simply do not successfully predict individual differences in behavior, especially complex behavior (Matthews, 1992; Matthews & Gilliland, in press). In the context of learning, arousal theory is successful in predicting individual differences in eyeblink conditioning (Levey & Martin, 1981). However, in more complex discrimination learning studies, the predictions fail, and the results appear to become paradigm specific (cf. Corr, Pickering, & Gray, 1995). Likewise, arousal theory cannot explain the way in which personality–performance correlations are moderated by the information-processing demands of the task (Matthews, 1992). Cognitive psychologists, of course, have no difficulty in seeing that conditioning models are inappropriate for explaining skill acquisition.

Recently, studies of individual differences in information processing have become increasingly popular. Perhaps personality relates to parameters of the cognitive architecture, such as the capacity of components of working memory or attentional resource pools. Previously, I have suggested that, like external stress factors, traits may be described in terms of a cognitive patterning (Hockey, 1984), that is, a set of independent processing characteristics associated with the poles of the traits (Matthews, 1992). For example, extraverts seem to have good short-term memory but poor vigilance. The package of processing strengths and weaknesses may then influence the ease with which skills that are based on these cognitive components are acquired. This approach has the advantage of "speaking the same language" as contemporary theories of skill. Take the construct of working memory, for example. On one hand, psychologists can describe individual differences in terms of architectural parameters such as the capacity of individual stores. On the other hand, working memory is linked theoretically and empirically to complex learned behaviors, such as reading and use of language (Gathercole & Baddeley, 1993). In general, the use of information-processing constructs gives more testable theories, and tracing the performance consequences of the cognitive correlates of traits is an essential aspect of personality theory.

Content-Based Approaches to Personality and Skill

Psychobiological and information-processing analyses have a common shortcoming: They neglect the role of the environment. People of different personalities like to pursue different activities in different surroundings. A personality–environment correlation is found more formally in studies of activity and job preference (Furnham, 1992). People's lives differ in their "content," in that they vary in the frequency of behavior such as social interaction, physical activity, and so forth. People differ not only in the frequency with which they execute different skills but also in their knowledge and motivation. Hence, personality differences observed in the laboratory or workplace may be a consequence of these content differences rather than elementary processing components. Why do extraverts make better salespeople than do introverts (cf. Barrick & Mount, 1991)? The content approach offers several possible explanations, assuming that interactions with strangers are a more important aspect of extraverts' than introverts' lives. First, greater practice in social interaction leads to more implicit knowledge or greater proceduralization of interaction (see Snyder, 1992, for a social–cognitive perspective on extraversion and the regulation of social interaction). Second, extraverts' life experiences provide more explicit knowledge, allowing them to adapt their social skills to the needs of the situation strategically. Third, greater interest in social interaction may be associated with more intrinsic motivation, which tends to enhance performance. A specific example is provided by research on associations between test anxiety and impairment of performance in examinations. In some anxious individuals, the anxiety–performance correlation is driven by their lack of preparation for an examination, which influences both variables (Mueller, 1992). Lack of exposure to studying environments drives the performance deficit. Failure to study may be either voluntary (e.g., laziness) or essentially involuntary (e.g., illness).

Clearly, such explanations are incomplete, in that it is far-fetched to attribute the many empirical associations between personality traits and elementary neural and cognitive functions to individual differences in life experiences and interests. However, they do challenge the assumption that personality differences in skilled performance are simply a direct consequence of the cognitive correlates of traits.

A Cognitive–Adaptive Framework for Personality

Thus far, two possible routes for personality–skill associations have been established, neither of which is sufficient in itself. Matthews (1997c, 1997d; Matthews & Dorn, 1995) proposed a cognitive–adaptive framework that attempts to integrate the respective roles of "feed-forward" from essentially fixed characteristics of the cognitive architecture and "feed-back" from the person's interactions with real-world environments. The central proposition is that traits should be identified with adaptations or fitnesses for certain kinds of environments. The term *adaptation* refers to success in achieving personal and socially valued goals, which may or may not reflect an evolved adaptation. Situations may be characterized in terms of the kinds of people who are attracted to them (Schneider, 1987). Hence, a conscientious person is someone who thrives in environments requiring sustained, organized effort; an agreeable person prospers in environments providing opportunities for cooperation with others; and so forth. The overall adaptation has two aspects, loosely described as skills and knowledge, each of which relates to the environments being congruent with the trait.

Skills are learned processing routines for accomplishing specific work or social tasks that are "tuned" to the environments associated with the tasks. *Self-knowledge* refers to representations in long-term memory of the personal significance of environments, which includes preferences, motivations, and beliefs about the efficacy of skills. I also include emotion under knowledge because current cognitive theory emphasizes the role of self-beliefs and self-regulative processing in generating emotional states (Matthews & Wells, in press). Typically, there is some positive feedback between skills and knowledge: People are motivated to do things they are good at and are good at activities that motivate them (cf. Bandura, 1986). The skills/self-knowledge distinction is adaptive rather than architectural. It cuts across processing-level distinctions such as that between controlled and automatic processing. Both skills and self-knowledge are envisaged as having procedural and declarative components that must be distinguished in performance studies.

Figure 11.2 illustrates how the framework incorporates feed-forward and feed-back routes for personality–skill associations. Genes and early learning set neural net parameters, which in turn influence attributes of information processing (i.e., the cognitive architecture) and more diffuse arousal systems. These individual differences in turn feed into skill acquisition. In other words, people have a toolkit of cognitive characteristics that predispose them to acquire some skills and hinder the acquisition of others. Children are preadapted to thrive in some environments but struggle in others. The personality associated with that initial adaptation is then molded through interaction with the environment, as skills and self-knowledge develop and are expressed in actual behavior. To the extent that the individual has a free choice among environments, a stable personality congruent with the person's cognitive characteristics develops. I assume that there is a stabilizing tendency for positive feedback among the three types of constructs — skills, self-knowledge, and adaptive behaviors — that I call the *adaptive triangle*. On the other hand, major life events that influence skills or self-knowledge are likely to perturb personality. The framework resembles investment theories of intelligence, such as Ackerman's (1996) process, personality, interests, and knowledge theory, in that skill acquisition depends on both preexisting cognitive competence and the motivation to apply that competence to specific tasks. However, it differs from Ackerman's theory in relating personality to some aspects of basic processing competence as well as to motivations.

Figure 11.2 shows an outline model that would be hard to test in its entirety. Testable predictions may be developed for its various component parts, however, with respect to specific traits and their correlates. First, the information-processing correlates of a trait should contribute to the skills required for the environments associated with it. Second, there should be congruence between trait-characteristic skills and the various components of self-knowledge, which should be oriented toward the adaptive problems that the skills are designed to solve. Third, over time, there should be reciprocal influences between skills and knowledge on one hand and the measured value of the trait on the other. Next, I apply the framework to two of the most important traits, extraversion–introversion and neuroticism, focusing primarily on studies using objective performance measures as well as on studies of people's subjective reactions to performance environments.

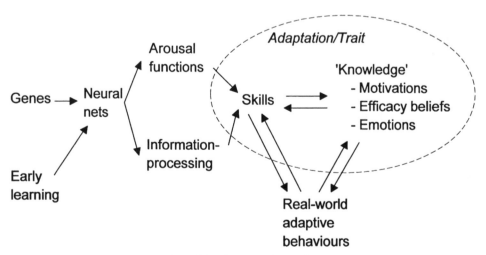

Figure 11.2. A tentative causal model of personality and adaptation. From "Extraversion, Emotion and Performance: A Cognitive–Adaptive Model," by G. Matthews, 1997c, in G. Matthews (Ed.), *Cognitive Science Perspectives on Personality and Emotion* (pp. 399–442), Amsterdam: Elsevier. Copyright 1997 by Elsevier. Reprinted with permission of the author.

Extraversion−Introversion

Environments for Extraverted Skills

The analysis of extraversion begins with an analysis of "extraverted" environments. Extraverts appear to prefer two kinds of environments, as shown by their stated preferences and vocational interests (Matthews & Dorn, 1995). The first are social environments providing frequent and varied interaction, such as parties. Ackerman and Heggestad (1997) found that extraversion was related to social and enterprising occupational interests (i.e., applying verbal and interpersonal skills to supporting or influencing others). The second type of environment imposes high levels of work demands and pressures such as working on oil rigs (Sutherland & Cooper, 1991) or as a financial dealer (Kahn & Cooper, 1993). The common cognitive element in these environments is a tendency for overload of attention. In social interactions, other people tend to deliver multiple verbal and nonverbal signals that are difficult to process fully, as expressed in the "cocktail party" metaphor for attentional overload. Hence, the skills required for these environments include the ability to respond rapidly, to maintain conversation, and to resist distraction by extraneous information and internal stress reactions to overload. Note that rapid response does not necessarily imply rapid or efficient processing; one of the skills appropriate to overload environments is criterion setting (i.e., trading off completeness of analysis for speed of action). Conversely, Matthews (1997d) described how introverts may be adapted to low information-flow environments such as solitude, although this chapter focuses on extraversion.

It seems, too, that extraverts may actually perform better in their preferred environments. Individual differences in objective social behaviors have been neglected, although extraversion has been shown experimentally to influence gross characteristics such as readiness to initiate conversations with strangers (Argyle, Martin, & Crossland, 1989). In the occupational arena, meta-analysis suggests that extraverts excel during training, but not, in general, during operational performance (Barrick & Mount, 1991). One would expect training to be cognitively demanding; Barrick and Mount pointed out that the training programs involved typically required high levels of activity (e.g., assessment centers, police training, and on-the-job sales training). The same review also showed that extraversion was modestly but validly predictive of operational performance among sales personnel and managers, jobs requiring social interaction and the ability to influence others.

Skills for Extraverted Environments

Experimental studies confirm that extraverts have a genuine processing advantage on some demanding tasks. Matthews, Jones, and Chamberlain (1992) conducted a study of the acquisition of keyboard and coding skills required by post office mail sorters that illustrates the performance skills that may be involved. Participants completed a series of 26 self-paced lessons, lasting about 25 hours in total, to learn use of the mail-coding keyboard. Each lesson concluded with a test requiring typing of target characters in a continuous loop of randomly generated characters. The test was demanding because it required the integration of character identification and manual response skills. Figure 11.3 (left panel) shows the speed of performance

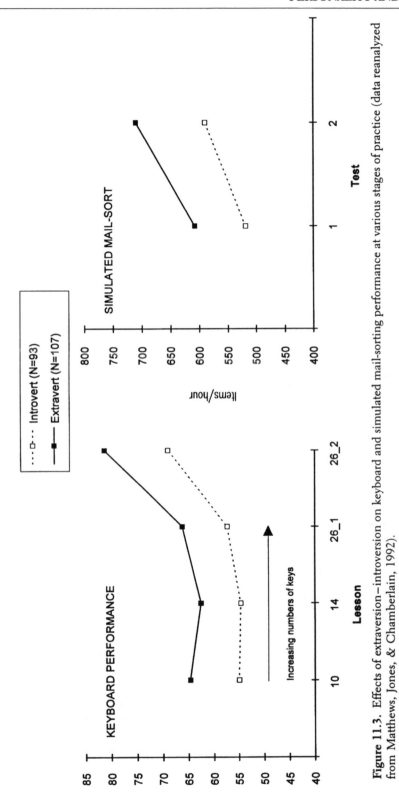

Figure 11.3. Effects of extraversion–introversion on keyboard and simulated mail-sorting performance at various stages of practice (data reanalyzed from Matthews, Jones, & Chamberlain, 1992).

(keystrokes per minute) in extraverted and introverted participants (data reanalyzed). Note that new keys were introduced progressively during the course, so there was no clear practice effect between Lessons 10 and 26_1: growing expertise was related to the use of increasing numbers of keys. In the final 5 hr of training (i.e., Lessons 26_1 to 26_2), participants practiced on the full keyboard, and a practice effect was evident. Participants were also tested on a simulated mail-sorting task requiring integration of keyboard and coding skills on two occasions. The right panel of Figure 11.3 shows that extraverts also had a constant performance advantage over introverts on this task.

Figure 11.3 suggests a general performance advantage for extraverts[1] that was independently significant at each stage of learning (although it is possible that there were differential learning rates in the early stages of practice). A more formal test of whether extraversion relates to individual differences in the *compilation* of proceduralization of skill was provided by Salthouse's (1989) molecular equivalence—molar analysis technique, originally developed for use in studies of aging. Matthews et al. (1992) also had participants perform a battery of processing tasks related to molecular components of the skill, on which extraverts and introverts attained equivalent levels of performance. According to Salthouse (1989), group differences in compilation should be reflected in differences in the strength of association between molecular and molar (i.e., whole-task) performance. Greater compilation (i.e., more proceduralization and automatization) should attenuate molecular—molar correlations. In fact, no group differences were found. For example, by the end of practice, the elementary cognitive tasks predicted 19% of the variance in the speed of keyboard performance in extraverts and 21% in introverts. For mail sorting, the percentages were 23% and 24%, respectively. Hence, in this study at least, extraversion seemed to be related to a general facility for the performance of complex cognitive—motor tasks. In addition, extraversion—performance relationships were not mediated by mood, reinforcing the impression of a fundamental difference in processing competence between extraverts and introverts on the tasks, as opposed to a stress-mediated effect.

Extraversion, Coping, and Self-Knowledge

Extraverts generally show reduced stress vulnerability and use more active, social, and optimistic coping strategies (Costa, Somerfield, & McCrae, 1996). For example, Piedmont and Weinstein (1994) looked at a sample of sales and customer service personnel and found that extraversion was related to supervisor ratings of interpersonal relations, task orientation ("getting things done"), and coping with setbacks. In recent work in Dundee, Scotland, Sian Campbell and I investigated how personality relates to the person's orientation toward demanding performance environments. We developed a comprehensive dimensional model of the affective, motivational, and cognitive states that are experienced in performance settings (Matthews, Joyner, Gilliland, Huggins, & Falconer, in press). In two recent studies of undergraduate samples (Ns = 210 and 304) respondents were asked to complete

---

[1]Analyses reported by Matthews, Jones, and Chamberlain (1992) showed moderating effects of ability on personality–performance correlations (personality was more predictive in more able individuals), but, again, there was no interaction with stage of practice.

TABLE 11.1   Personality Correlates of Measures of States and Coping in Performance
Environments in Two Studies

Correlate	Extraversion		Neuroticism	
	1	2	1	2
State variables				
Energy	27**	18**	−26**	−30**
Tension	−18**	−16**	45**	31**
Hedonic tone	34**	21**	−41**	−31**
Overall motivation	19*	28**	−16*	−14*
Success motivation	15*	—	18*	—
Intrinsic motivation	14*	—	−25**	—
Self-focus of attention	−02	−01	26**	17**
Self-esteem	19**	24**	−54**	−52**
Confidence and control	29**	32**	−35**	−38**
Concentration	15**	15*	−39**	−37**
Worries about the task	03	07	15*	22**
Personal worries	09	01	31*	37**
Coping strategies				
Emotion focus	−01	—	40**	—
Task focus	25**	—	−28**	—
Avoidance	16*	—	11	—
Social support	26**	—	−10	—

Note.   Decimal points have been omitted. Dashes indicate absence of data.
*$p < .05$.   **$p < .01$.

the state items with the instruction to report how they typically felt in mentally
demanding situations requiring concentration or intensive thought.

Personality correlations were highly replicable across samples. The first part of
Table 11.1 shows how extraversion correlates with these "typical state" measures
(neuroticism data are discussed later). Extraverts' reactions were generally more positive, especially so with regard to pleasantness of mood (hedonic tone) and on a
scale for confidence and perceived control. In the first study, participants also completed a short version of Endler and Parker's (1990) coping scales, plus a scale for
coping through social support (Scheier, Weintraub, & Carver, 1989). Extraverts reported greater use of task-focused coping and social support strategies. These more
affectively loaded responses to cognitively demanding environments may also contribute to extraverts' performance advantage through two mechanisms: First, more
positive moods may directly affect the efficiency of elements of the processing architecture; energy seems to relate to attentional resource availability (Matthews &
Davies, 1998). Second, they contribute to more effective strategies for using time at
work, as in taking the initiative rather than waiting on events, for example.

Information-Processing Support for "Extraverted" Skills

The top-down analysis indicates the skills that extraverts require to thrive in their
preferred environments. The next stage is to work from the bottom up, to determine
whether the cognitive correlates of extraversion do in fact match the skills described.
It seems that there is no key process or "Holy Grail" to which extraversion effects

may be attributed. Instead, extraversion–introversion is *distributed* across a set of independent processing functions. Exhibit 11.1 shows the cognitive patterning of extraversion indicated by previous empirical studies (see Matthews, 1992, 1997c, for references). Extraverts are better at a disparate collection of tasks, including short-term memory, especially in interference conditions, divided attention, and resistance to distraction. They also tend to set a lower response criterion. Conversely, introverts excel at maintaining vigilance and at reflective problem solving.

Performance correlates of extraversion may be located at several levels of the cognitive architecture. For example, Matthews and Harley (1993) developed a connectionist simulation of interactive effects of extraversion and arousal on semantic priming that implicates low-level, "automatic processes." By contrast, the effects of extraversion on strategy implicate either individual differences in the architecture supporting high-level executive routines or individual differences in use of the same architecture. Strategy effects also implicate adaptive-level constructs: the participant's beliefs about the task and its personal significance.

Do these cognitive correlates of extraversion facilitate skill learning? Direct evidence is lacking, but a plausible case can be made, as shown in Figure 11.4. Several cognitive characteristics may provide a platform for the acquisition of conversation skills, including good verbal short-term memory for keeping track of the conversation, good divided attention for segregating verbal messages, and fast retrieval from semantic and episodic memory for generating topics of conversation. Divided-attention capabilities may contribute to extraverts' capacity to perform well in more demanding environments. A low response criterion, and a willingness to accept a risky speed–accuracy trade-off, may contribute both to dominating conversation through rapidity of utterance and more generally to fast response.

It is perhaps unsurprising that extraversion relates to behavioral impulsivity and verbal facility. Validating the cognitive–adaptive model requires demonstrations that performance correlates, which are not obviously related to the gross characteristics of extraversion, nevertheless contribute to adaptation in extraverted environments. Such a demonstration is provided by the well-established interactions among extra-

EXHIBIT 11.1   Cognitive Patterning of Extraversion–Introversion: Performance Characteristics of the Extravert

Characteristics of extraversion
Superiority in
Divided attention
Resistance to distraction
Retrieval from memory
Short-term memory
Inferiority in
Vigilance
Reflective problem solving
Long-term memory
Lower response criterion
Little systematic effect on
Attentional selectivity
Reaction time tasks
General intelligence

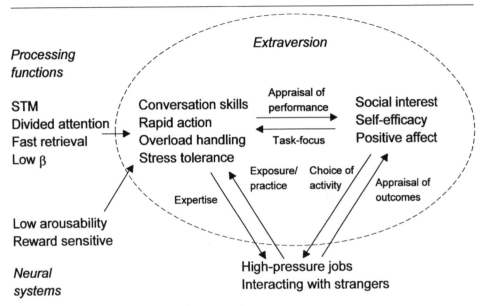

Figure 11.4. A cognitive–adaptive model of extraversion. STM = short-term memory.

version, time of day, and arousal (e.g., Revelle, Humphreys, Simon, & Gilliland, 1980). High arousal facilitates extraverts' performance in the morning but impairs it in the evening, with introverts showing the opposite Arousal × Time of Day interaction. The interaction has been demonstrated both for simple attentional tasks and for intelligence test performance (Matthews, 1992, 1997c). At first glance, this result is puzzling: Extraverts do not turn into introverts at night (Gray, 1981). The adaptive hypothesis offers an explanation. The interaction takes place against a backdrop of circadian variation in subjective energy and alertness, such that people tend to be dearoused early in the morning and during much of the evening (Thayer, 1978). The consequence of the interaction is then to give extraverts a general performance advantage in the evening. This is the time at which social activities generally take place, so the interaction operates to give extraverts a performance advantage in one of their preferred environments. Conversely, introverts have a compensating advantage early in the day. Hence, the strength of the adaptive approach is to bind together the disparate processing correlates of extraversion by demonstrating their common relevance to social and overload environments.

Extraversion and the Adaptive Triangle: Integration of Process and Content Explanations

Figure 11.4 also illustrates how the extraverted skills built on the foundation of the cognitive patterning of extraversion may relate to the other two components of the adaptive triangle. Extraverts are expected to have greater confidence, interest, and positive mood than introverts in environments that provide the opportunity for exercising their characteristic skills, as shown in Table 11.1 (see also Matthews, 1997c), by studies of activity and vocational preferences (e.g., Ackerman & Heggestad, 1997), and objective measures of occupational and social behavior (Matthews, 1997a). At

261

a causal level, process and content explanations are associated with opposite routes around the triangle. The anticlockwise route from skills illustrates the process perspective. Skills support expertise in particular jobs and activities. The person's appraisals of consequent real-world success enhance motivation and confidence, which in turn facilitate the expression of underlying competence in actual skilled performance. Content explanations are demonstrated by the clockwise route. Appraisals of being skilled in particular activities lead to greater motivation and interest (cf. Bandura, 1986), which in turn dictates the choice of real-world activities. Exposure and practice in these real-world settings lead to enhancement of actual skill.

Figure 11.4 shows a dynamic view of extraversion, showing feed-back from exposure to environments as well as feed-forward from stable cognitive and psychobiological characteristics. It thus predicts a reciprocal interaction between skills and extraversion. For example, extraverts have better social skills, but it would be expected that assertiveness or social skills training would increase extraversion. There is a small amount of supportive evidence consistent with the general view that personality and work environments are mutually self-shaping (Semmer & Schallberger, 1996). Extraverts tend to perform better in sales jobs (Barrick & Mount, 1991), but sales training elevates extraversion (Turnbull, 1976): The skills for dealing with customers presumably generalize to other social encounters. Likewise, extraverts have the aptitude for management positions, and a 20-year study of AT&T managers showed that career success was associated with increased impulsivity (Howard & Bray, 1988), a trait contributing to extraversion, but also to other traits such as psychoticism (Eysenck & Eysenck, 1985).

Anxiety and Negative Affectivity

The second major dimension common to virtually all personality models is anxiety, neuroticism, or negative affectivity. This dimension brings together a cluster of positively correlated factors relating to negative emotion, including anxiety and depression. For example, Sian Campbell and I recently found a correlation of .73 between neuroticism on the Eysenck Personality Questionnaire and trait anxiety on the State-Trait Anxiety Inventory, which in turn correlated .80 with trait depression on the latter measure ($N = 210$). I take a broad view of the dimension here, interrelating evidence on traits, the temporary emotional states characteristic of those traits, and related clinical conditions, under the general heading of *anxiety*. There are, of course, important differences between these aspects of affect, but I focus on commonalities. In addition, anxiety factors such as test or driving anxiety may be tuned to specific environments, which more detailed models of these conditions accommodate. (The need to supplement general anxiety measures with environmentally contingent dimensions is another instance of the importance of content.) The analysis here is somewhat tentative because of the lack of evidence on anxiety and skilled performance, which may reflect a tendency for anxiety to affect inner mental life more consistently than it affects observed behavior.

Anxiety: Facilitative and Detrimental Effects on Performance

Like extraversion, anxiety may be characterized in processing terms (e.g., a working memory deficit) or in terms of content through pessimistic evaluations of the world and a tendency to spend time worrying about various real-world threats. Again, the starting point for a cognitive–adaptive analysis of anxiety and neuroticism is to identify the qualities of the environment relative to the traits. Anxiety is often perceived as something of a deficit in personality, but it may be advantageous in some settings. In experimental studies, less anxious individuals tend to have a general performance advantage, especially in environments imposing high cognitive demands or other sources of stress (M. W. Eysenck, 1982; Matthews & Deary, 1998). However, anxiety may be associated with superior performance when the task is easy (M. W. Eysenck, 1981) or when, in test anxiety research, the environment is manipulated to be especially reassuring (Sarason, 1975). Anxious participants are impaired when given failure feedback but appears to learn better than nonanxious participants under success feedback regardless of task difficulty (Weiner & Schneider, 1971; see also M. W. Eysenck, 1981).

In occupational data, the performance advantage for emotionally stable individuals is small: Barrick and Mount (1991) found a mean corrected correlation of .08. Neuroticism also seems to be unrelated to standard dimensions of vocational interests (Ackerman & Heggestad, 1997). However, trait anxiety may relate to performance impairment in particularly stressful contexts such as police work (e.g., Cortina, Doherty, Schmitt, Kaufman, & Smith, 1992) and performance in evaluative contexts such as examinations (Mueller, 1992). As with the laboratory data, there are occasional indications of performance advantage related to anxiety. Mughal, Walsh, and Wilding (1996) found, in two studies, that anxiety was positively correlated with the number of sales closed by insurance sales consultants, although anxious individuals also experienced more subjective stress.

Most data suggest that emotionally stable individuals are at an advantage in stressful environments and, conversely, that trait anxiety may be adaptive when the environment is characterized by a lack of external pressure or by subtle, disguised threats (Matthews & Dorn, 1995) provided that the person is not clinically anxious. However, results such as those of Mughal et al. (1996) indicate that this position is a simplification. The critical moderating variable seems to be the person's level of task motivation. The relationship between anxiety and motivation has been variously described. Much test anxiety research views the anxious individual as motivated to escape the situation, with a corresponding drop in on-task effort (Geen, 1987). By contrast, M. W. Eysenck and Calvo (1992) have linked anxiety to compensatory effort, which may serve to maintain performance effectiveness (but not processing efficiency). Mughal et al. (1996) also found that anxious sales personnel expended more effort by seeing more people and working more hours per month. With regard to academic performance, McKenzie (1989) reviewed evidence that neuroticism is positively related to degree achievement in students selected for high "superego" (i.e., conscientiousness and motivation). Hence, the relationship between anxiety and motivation is unstable and seems to vary with both the coping affordances of the situation and personality factors that may influence coping.

Broadly, the environmental attributes relevant to anxiety may relate to whether the environment tends to elicit task-focused or self-focused coping strategies, such as rumination and self-criticism. Situational qualities such as lack of controllability and severity of threat tend to discourage task focus (Lazarus & Folkman, 1984), but nonanxious participants seem to maintain performance better under such circumstances. Carver, Peterson, Follansbee, and Scheier (1983) showed that test anxiety impaired performance only when self-focus was induced experimentally. Conversely, anxious individuals may do better when pressures are covert rather than overt and clear paths to success or threat avoidance exist (although it may take time and self-reflection to identify them). Anxiety is more often related to a performance deficit than to performance enhancement because appraisal of environmental attributes is itself anxiety biased (Wells & Matthews, 1994). Pessimism and lack of self-efficacy lead anxious participants to interpret demanding situations as requiring self-examination rather than a task-focused response. Anxiety deficits may be clearer in laboratory studies than in real life because experimental tasks are often designed to overload the cognitive architecture, eliciting the appraisal that applying effort to the task is ineffective. Similarly, difficult examinations impose cognitive demands such as requirements for proceduralized intellectual skills that are hard to overcome through effort alone. Consistent with this hypothesis, anxiety has more detrimental effects on intelligence test performance in less able individuals (Spielberger, 1966). In most jobs, however, direct threats are unusual, and people are given at least a partial specification of what to do to succeed. Under these circumstances anxiety may be subjectively unpleasant, but it is not otherwise maladaptive.

Anxiety and Skill in Real Life

Hence, in the case of anxiety, the cognitive–adaptive analysis emphasizes not so much performance skills but skills for evaluating the external world and applying processing effort accordingly. One line of evidence concerns state rather than trait affect measures, but generalization to traits is plausible. Mann (1992) reviewed studies of decision making that characterize the consequences of anxiety and other negative emotions as "cautious and inefficient information processing, selective attention to risks at the expense of benefits, reluctance to choose, and, in many cases, self-defeating choices" (p. 225). Turning this statement around, low-anxious participants may have the advantage in threatening, uncertain situations because they can act decisively without excessive worry or prolonged review of coping options. Under other circumstances, caution and pessimism in decision making may be advantageous. In studies of persuasion, individuals in negative moods process counterattitudinal messages more systematically than those in positive moods (Mackie & Worth, 1991). Results of a variety of other studies suggest that happy people are prone to mental "laziness" in relying on prior beliefs in evaluating stimuli or events, whereas unhappy people are likely to process the information at hand more deeply (Ketelaar & Clore, 1997). Forgas (1995) interpreted the literature as suggesting that, given various antecedent conditions, such as sufficient time for processing, people in negative moods are more likely to use extensive, "substantive" processing strategies, whereas people in positive moods are biased toward using heuristics that require less processing effort. For example, Isen, Means, Patrick, and Nowicki (1982) conducted a study of induced mood effects on the solution of physics problems. When positive mood was induced, participants tended to use intuitive but error-prone strategies. In real life, disasters such as Chernobyl and the *Titanic* have been attributed to neglect of danger signs that a systematic review of possible threats would have detected.

A second line of evidence comes from studies of driver stress (see Matthews & Desmond, 1997; Matthews, Dorn, et al., 1998, for reviews). Drivers' personalities may, in part, be described by a dimension of "dislike of driving." This dimension has many of the formal characteristics of anxiety, including associations with negative emotion and worry states, negative self-beliefs, and objective performance impairment. At the skills level, dislike of driving relates to simulator performance impairment mainly when the task is undemanding, suggesting that the "anxious" driver can cope adaptively with moderate pressure but is vulnerable to distraction when the task is appraised as easy. However, dislike of driving also relates to low levels of risk-taking behavior in simulated driving and fewer speeding convictions in real life. These behavioral correlates are consistent with self-knowledge: Drivers high in dislike of driving have a relatively poor opinion of their competence and safety and tend to use emotion-focused coping to deal with stress. Adaptively, high dislike drivers trade off increased safety through behavioral caution against increased risk due to distractibility.

Anxiety, Coping, and Self-Knowledge

It is well established that anxiety conditions are underpinned by a variety of negative self-beliefs (Wells & Matthews, 1994). The data shown in Table 11.1 illustrate some of the subjective reactions of anxious (high neuroticism) individuals toward performance, including a general negativity of reaction toward demanding environments, bias toward emotion-focus at the expense of task focus, and notably low self-esteem. However, although neuroticism was related to less intrinsic motivation for demanding tasks, Study 2 actually showed a small but significant positive correlation between neuroticism and motivation to succeed on such tasks.

In this analysis I emphasize the role of coping in mediating the effects of self-knowledge and motivation on performance. The efficacy of different coping strategies is contextually dependent (Zeidner & Saklofske, 1996), implying that the coping biases shown by more and less anxious individuals are associated with adaptation to different kinds of environments. The task-focus characteristic of low-anxious individuals is likely to be most beneficial when the situation calls for quick, decisive action, but the self-focus associated with high anxiety may be adaptive when caution or reflection is necessary. Self-focused coping is often emotion focused (e.g., rumination) but does not necessarily imply inaction. One of the characteristics of coping in anxious patients is the use of "safety behaviors" that attempt to forestall anticipated threats; health-anxious individuals may visit the doctor frequently (and unnecessarily), for example. Such behaviors are often maladaptive in patients but may sometimes be advantageous in "normal" anxiety conditions; complacency about health may be dangerous.

Information-Processing Support for Anxiety

Thus far, the argument has been that low-anxious participants are adapted to coping with threats characterized by the need for action in circumstances that mitigate against successful coping. The skills that support the adaptation are primarily those of judgment and decision making: selective attention to positive signals and a willingness to use simple but fast strategies. Conversely, anxious individuals are adapted to situations in which threat is less immediate and coping requires careful reflection, supported by anticipation of danger, attention to threat, and thoroughness in evaluating possible threats and coping strategies.

How are these skills supported by the cognitive correlates of anxiety? Much recent literature identifies one of the principal correlates as bias in selective attention. Anxious, and to some extent depressed, participants are more easily distracted by negative stimulus attributes, as on the emotional Stroop test. In other paradigms, they may show a faster detection of threat (see Wells & Matthews, 1994; Matthews & Wells, in press). The process is best conceptualized as one of active, but not necessarily conscious, vigilance for threat rather than a bias in automatic processing. Matthews and Harley (1996) reported connectionist simulation data suggesting that emotional Stroop inteference is not caused by oversensitivity of network units representing threat but to the top-down activation of threat units initiated by voluntary threat monitoring. Running this strategy as a "background task" in everyday life is likely to cause both pessimism in judgment and decision making and more negative content in self-beliefs. Matthews and Wells (in press) described the effect as being primarily strategic, but there also may be anxiety-related individual differences in the cognitive architecture supporting attentional functions (Derryberry & Reed, 1997). Other cognitive correlates of anxiety and depression are associated with implicit and explicit memory, with several researchers reporting a bias toward negative material, although the data are somewhat inconsistent (Wells & Matthews, 1996). Plausibly, these various cognitive attributes contribute to the acquisition of more complex, high-level processing routines for evaluating the world as negative; for passive or avoidant modes of coping in the face of obvious threat; and for more effortful, compensatory coping when threats are less imminent.

Figure 11.5 shows how the various aspects of anxiety and negative affectivity may be integrated within the general framework. Again, process- and content-oriented outcomes may be distinguished. Processing functions such as bias in selective attention may feed-forward into acquisition of skills for maintaining awareness of danger,

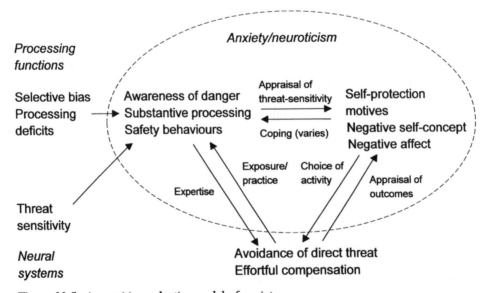

Figure 11.5. A cognitive–adaptive model of anxiety.

application of the skills in real-world environments, and congruent self-knowledge. Conversely, the appraisal of oneself as being forced to deal with a threatening world may lead to negative self-beliefs, emotions, and so on, leading to greater experience in dealing with real-world problems through avoidance, anticipation, or compensation. Studies of clinical depression provide some evidence for reciprocal influences between personality and the negative self-beliefs often seen as a proximal cause of depression. Neuroticism does seem to be a risk factor for depression in prospective studies (Matthews, Saflofske, et al., 1998), but at the same time neuroticism scores rise and fall with pathology: Depression affects neuroticism (Barnett & Gotlib, 1988). In anxiety studies, recovery from anxiety is associated with a reduction in cognitive bias (e.g., Mathews, Mogg, Kentish, & Eysenck, 1995), although a latent predisposition may remain.

Conclusion

The temptation for the cognitive psychologist is to apply a strictly reductionist approach to explaining the personality correlates of skilled performance. Such an approach is only partially correct. Traits may be characterized as qualities of the individual distributed across the cognitive architecture (i.e., a cognitive patterning of processing components) that set predispositions for acquiring specific skills. However, this process-oriented approach has two significant shortcomings. First, even as an information-processing account of skill, it neglects the roles of self-regulative processing and the relationship between personality and strategies for learning and performance. Second, it neglects the adaptive level of explanation (i.e., the role of individual differences in skill in supporting different long-term strategies for life success). The adaptive perspective is required to explain both the interplay between skilled performance and strategies and the interplay between skill and the "content" of the person's life. Cognitive–adaptive models may be developed for both extraversion and anxiety. The model of extraversion identifies the trait with adaptation to attentionally demanding and social environments, supported by skills for managing overload and social interaction, and by self-knowledge that encourages task focus in demanding situations. The model of anxiety relates the trait to adaptation to indirectly threatening environments, supported by skills for anticipation of threat, and a self-concept which emphasizes needs for self-protection and self-scrutiny. The adaptive level of description may be the "natural" level for describing personality traits as integrated constructs. However, generating testable predictions in experimental studies of performance requires the more dissected view of traits provided by descriptions of individual differences in the cognitive architecture.

In this chapter, I have emphasized the Eysenckian extraversion and neuroticism–anxiety traits because of their multifarious performance correlates. However, the cognitive–adaptive framework might also be extended to other traits, such as those of the five-factor model. Agreeableness might relate to skills and interests in environments requiring nurturance or cooperation, as opposed to environments requiring competition or even aggression. Conscientiousness may be linked to environments in which success requires systematic, organized efforts, as opposed to opportunism. Openness is of special importance in scholastic and academic environments, within which this trait relates to both interest and performance on tests of acquired knowledge (Ackerman, 1996). Deciding whether to work with broader or narrower traits is a perennial problem for personality psychology. There may be scope for applying the cognitive–adaptive perspective to narrower traits than those discussed, such as impulsivity, although one of the strengths of the approach is its capacity to illuminate functional links between psychometrically distinct subtraits of broad personality factors.

REFERENCES

Ackerman, P. L. (1996). A theory of adult intellectual development: Process, personality, interests, and knowledge. *Intelligence, 22*, 227–257.

Ackerman, P. L., & Heggestad, E. D. (1997). Intelligence, personality and interests: Evidence for overlapping traits. *Psychological Bulletin, 121*, 219–245.

Amelang, M., & Ullwer, U. (1991). Correlations between psychometric measures and psychophysiological as well as experimental variables in studies on extraversion and neuroticism. In J. Strelau & A. Angleitner (Eds.), *Explorations in temperament*. New York: Plenum.

Argyle, M., Martin, M., & Crossland, J. (1989). Happiness as a function of personality and social encounters. In J. P. Forgas & J. M. Innes (Eds.), *Recent advances in social psychology: An international perspective* (pp. 116–135). Amsterdam: Elsevier.

Bandura, A. (1986). *Social foundations of thought and action: A social cognitive theory*. Englewood Cliffs, NJ: Prentice Hall.

Barnett, P. A., & Gotlib, I. H. (1988). Psychosocial functioning and depression: Distinguishing among antecedents, concomitants, and consequences. *Psychological Bulletin, 104*, 97–126.

Barrick, M. R., & Mount, M. K. (1991). The Big Five personality dimensions and job performance: A meta-analysis. *Personnel Psychology, 44*, 1–26.

Carver, C. S., Peterson, L. M., Follansbee, D. J., & Scheier, M. F. (1983). Effects of self-directed attention and resistance among persons high and low in test-anxiety. *Cognitive Therapy and Research, 7*, 333–354.

Corr, P. J., Pickering, A. D., & Gray, J. A. (1995). Personality and reinforcement in associative and instrumental learning. *Personality and Individual Differences, 19*, 47–72.

Cortina, J. M., Doherty, M. L., Schmitt, N., Kaufman, G., & Smith, R. G. (1992). The "Big Five" personality factors in the IPI and MMPI: Predictors of police performance. *Personnel Psychology, 45*, 119–140.

Costa, P. T., Jr. (1996). Work and personality: Use of the NEO-PI-R in industrial/organisational psychology. *Applied Psychology: An International Journal, 45*, 225–241.

Costa, P. T., Jr., Somerfield, M. R., & McCrae, R. R. (1996). Personality and coping: A reconceptualization. In M. Zeidner & N. S. Endler (Eds.), *Handbook of coping: Theory, research, applications* (pp. 44–61). New York: Wiley.

Derryberry, D., & Reed, M. A. (1997). Motivational and attentional components of personality. In G. Matthews (Ed.), *Cognitive science perspectives on personality and emotion* (pp. 443–474). New York: Elsevier Science.

Endler, N., & Parker, J. (1990). Multidimensional assessment of coping: A critical review. *Journal of Personality and Social Psychology, 58*, 844–854.

Eysenck, H. J. (1967). *The biological basis of personality*. Springfield, IL: Charles C Thomas.

Eysenck, H. J. (1995). Creativity as a product of intelligence and personality. In D. H. Saklofske & M. Zeidner (Eds.), *International handbook of personality and intelligence*. New York: Plenum.

Eysenck, H. J., & Eysenck, M. W. (1985). *Personality and individual differences: A natural science approach*. New York: Plenum.

Eysenck, M. W. (1981). Learning, memory and personality. In H. J. Eysenck (Ed.), *A model for personality* (pp. 169–209). Berlin: Springer-Verlag.

Eysenck, M. W. (1982). *Attention and arousal: Cognition and performance*. New York: Springer.

Eysenck, M. W., & Calvo, M. G. (1992). Anxiety and performance: The processing efficiency theory. *Cognition and Emotion, 6*, 409–434.

Forgas, J. P. (1995). Mood and judgment: The affect infusion model (AIM). *Psychological Bulletin, 117*, 39–66.

Furnham, A. (1992). *Personality at work: The role of individual differences in the workplace.* London: Routledge.

Gathercole, S. E., & Baddeley, A. D. (1993). *Working memory and language.* Hillsdale, NJ: Erlbaum.

Geen, R. G. (1987). Test anxiety and behavioral avoidance. *Journal of Research in Personality, 21,* 481–488.

Gray, J. A. (1981). A critique of Eysenck's theory of personality. In H. J. Eysenck (Ed.), A *model for personality* (pp. 246–276). Berlin: Springer-Verlag.

Hockey, G. R. J. (1986). Varieties of attentional state. In R. Parasuraman & D. R. Davies (Eds.), *Varieties of attention* (pp. 449–483). Orlando, FL: Academic Press.

Howard, A., & Bray, D. W. (1988). *Managerial lives in transition: Advancing age and changing times.* New York: Guilford Press.

Isen, A. M., Means, B., Patrick, R., & Nowicki, G. (1982). Some factors affecting decision making strategy and risk taking. In M. S. Clark & S. T. Fiske (Eds.), *Affect and cognition: The 17th Annual Carnegie Symposium on Cognition* (pp. 243–261). Hillsdale, NJ: Erlbaum.

Kahn, H., & Cooper, C. L. (1993). *Stress in the dealing room: High performers under pressure.* London: Routledge.

Ketelaar, T., & Clore, G. L. (1997). Emotion and reason: The proximate effects and ultimate functions of emotions. In G. Matthews (Ed.), *Cognitive science perspectives on personality and emotion* (pp. 355–396). New York: Elsevier Science.

Lazarus, R. S., & Folkman, S. (1984). *Stress, appraisal, and coping.* New York: Springer.

Levey, A. B., & Martin, I. (1981). Personality and conditioning. In H. J. Eysenck (Ed.), A *model for personality* (pp. 123–168). Berlin: Springer-Verlag.

Mackie, D., & Worth, L. (1991). Feeling good, but not thinking straight: The impact of positive mood on persuasion. In J. P. Forgas (Ed.), *Emotion and social judgments* (pp. 202–220). Elmsford, NY: Pergamon Press.

Mann, L. (1992). Stress, affect, and risk taking. In J. F. Yates (Ed.), *Risk-taking behavior* (pp. 201–230). New York: Wiley.

Mathews, A., Mogg, K., Kentish, J., & Eysenck, M. W. (1995). Effect of psychological treatment on cognitive bias in generalized anxiety disorder. *Behaviour Research and Therapy, 33,* 293–303.

Matthews, G. (1992). Extraversion. In A. P. Smith & D. M. Jones (Eds.), *Handbook of human performance: Vol. 3. State and trait* (pp. 95–126). London: Academic Press.

Matthews, G. (1997a). The Big Five as a framework for personality assessment. In N. Anderson & P. Herriot (Eds.), *International handbook of selection and appraisal* (2nd ed., pp. 175–200). London: Wiley.

Matthews, G. (1997b). An introduction to the cognitive science of personality and emotion. In G. Matthews (Ed.), *Cognitive science perspectives on personality and emotion* (pp. 3–30). Amsterdam: Elsevier.

Matthews, G. (1997c). Extraversion, emotion and performance: A cognitive–adaptive model. In G. Matthews (Ed.), *Cognitive science perspectives on personality and emotion* (pp. 399–442). Amsterdam: Elsevier.

Matthews, G. (1997d). Intelligence, personality and information-processing: An adaptive perspective. In W. Tomic & J. Kingsma (Eds.), *Advances in cognition and educational practice* (Vol. 4, pp. 475–492). Greenwich, CT: JAI Press.

Matthews, G., & Davies, D. R. (1998). Arousal and vigilance: The role of task factors. In R. B. Hoffman, M. F. Sherrick, & J. S. Warm (Eds.), *Integrating perception across psychology: Perspectives on motivation, choice, and individual differences* (pp. 113–144). Washington, DC: American Psychological Association.

Matthews, G., & Deary, I. (1998). *Personality traits.* Cambridge, England: Cambridge University Press.

Matthews, G., & Desmond, P. A. (1997). Underload and performance impairment: Evidence from studies of stress and simulated driving. In D. Harris (Ed.), *Engineering psychology and cognitive ergonomics: Vol. 1. Transportation systems* (pp. 161–167). Aldershot, England: Ashgate Publishing.

Matthews, G., & Dorn, L. (1995). Personality and intelligence: Cognitive and attentional processes. In D. Saklofske & M. Zeidner (Eds.), *International handbook of personality and intelligence* (pp. 367–396). New York: Plenum.

Matthews, G., Dorn, L., Hoyes, T. W., Davies, D. R., Glendon, A. I., & Taylor, R. G. (1998). Driver stress and performance on a driving simulator. *Human Factors, 40,* 136–169.

Matthews, G., & Gilliland, K. (in press). The personality theories of H. J. Eysenck and J. A. Gray: A comparative review. *Personality and Individual Differences.*

269

Matthews, G., & Harley, T. A. (1993). Effects of extraversion and self-report arousal on semantic priming: A connectionist approach. *Journal of Personality and Social Psychology, 65,* 735–756.

Matthews, G., & Harley, T. A. (1996). Connectionist models of emotional distress and attentional bias. *Cognition and Emotion, 10,* 561–600.

Matthews, G., Jones, D. M., & Chamberlain, A. G. (1992). Predictors of individual differences in mail coding skills and their variation with ability level. *Journal of Applied Psychology, 77,* 406–418.

Matthews, G., Joyner, L., Gilliland, K., Huggins, J., & Falconer, S. (in press). Validation of a comprehensive stress state questionnaire: Towards a state "Big Three"? In I. Mervielde, I. J. Deary, F. De Fruyt, & F. Ostendorf (Eds.), *Personality psychology in Europe* (Vol. 7). Tilburg, The Netherlands: Tilburg University Press.

Matthews, G., Saklofske, D. H., Costa, P. T., Jr., Deary, I. J., & Zeidner, M. (1998). Dimensional models of personality: A framework for systematic clinical assessment. *European Journal of Psychological Assessment, 14,* 35–48.

Matthews, G., & Wells, A. (in press). The cognitive science of attention and emotion. In T. Dalgleish & M. Power (Eds.), *Handbook of cognition and emotion.* New York: Wiley.

McKenzie, J. (1989). Neuroticism and academic achievement: The Furneaux factor. *Personality and Individual Differences, 10,* 509–515.

Mueller, J. H. (1992). Anxiety and performance. In A. P. Smith & D. M. Jones (Eds.), *Handbook of human performance: Vol. 3. State and trait* (pp. 127–160). London: Academic Press.

Mughal, S., Walsh, J., & Wilding, J. (1996). Stress and work performance: The role of trait anxiety. *Personality and Individual Differences, 20,* 685–691.

Piedmont, R. L., & Weinstein, H. P. (1994). Predicting supervisor ratings of job performance using the NEO Personality Inventory. *Journal of Psychology, 128,* 255–265.

Pylyshyn, Z. W. (1984). *Computation and cognition: Toward a foundation for cognitive science.* Cambridge, MA: MIT Press.

Revelle, W., Humphreys, M. S., Simon, L., & Gilliland, K. (1980). The interactive effect of personality, time of day and caffeine: A test of the arousal model. *Journal of Experimental Psychology: General, 109,* 1–31.

Salthouse, T. A. (1989). Ageing and skilled performance. In A. M. Colley & J. R. Beech (Eds.), *Acquisition and performance of cognitive skills* (pp. 82–99). New York: Wiley.

Sarason, I. G. (1975). Test-anxiety, attention and the general problem of anxiety. In C. D. Spielberger & I. Sarason (Eds.), *Stress and anxiety* (Vol. 1, pp. 55–70). Washington, DC: Hemisphere.

Scheier, M. F., Weintraub, J. K., & Carver, R. S. (1989). Assessing coping strategies: A theoretically based approach. *Journal of Personality and Social Psychology, 56,* 267–283.

Schneider, B. (1987). The people make the place. *Personnel Psychology, 40,* 437–453.

Semmer, N., & Schallberger, U. (1996). Selection, socialisation, and mutual adaptation: Resolving discrepancies between people and work. *Applied Psychology: An International Journal, 45,* 263–288.

Snyder, M. (1992). Motivational foundations of behavioral confirmation. *Advances in Experimental Social Psychology, 25,* 67–114.

Spielberger, C. D. (1966). The effects of anxiety on complex learning and academic achievement. In C. D. Spielberger (Ed.), *Anxiety and behavior* (pp. 3–20). London: Academic Press.

Sutherland, V. J., & Cooper, C. L. (1991). Personality, stress and accident involvement in the offshore oil and gas industry. *Personality and Individual Differences, 12,* 195–204.

Thayer, R. E. (1978). Toward a psychological theory of multidimensional activation (arousal). *Motivation & Emotion, 2,* 1–34.

Tooby, J., & Cosmides, L. (1992). The psychological foundations of culture. In J. H. Barkow, L. Cosmides, & J. Tooby (Eds.), *The adapted mind: Evolutionary psychology and the generation of culture.* New York: Oxford University Press.

Turnbull, A. (1976). Selling and the salesman: Prediction of success and personality change. *Psychological Reports, 38,* 1175–1180.

Weiner, B., & Schneider, K. (1971). Drive versus cognitive theory: A reply to Boor and Harmon. *Journal of Personality and Social Psychology, 18,* 258–262.

Wells, A., & Matthews, G. (1994). *Attention and emotion: A clinical perspective.* Hillsdale, NJ: Erlbaum.

Wells, A., & Matthews, G. (1996). Anxiety and cognition. *Current Opinion in Psychiatry, 9,* 422–426.

Zeidner, M., & Saklofske, D. (1996). Adaptive and maladaptive coping. In M. Zeidner & N. S. Endler (Eds.), *Handbook of coping: Theory, research, applications* (pp. 505–531). New York: Wiley.

Zuckerman, M. (1991). *Psychobiology of personality.* New York: Cambridge University Press.

Discussion

After Matthews presentation, discussion focused first on his conceptualization of introversion–extraversion, on the stability of personality traits, and then on broader issues of personality and cognition.

Dr. Alexander: You tend to talk about introversion–extraversion as if they are dichotomous. Is it possible that people fall all along some continuum of introversion–extraversion? And how does it affect the model?

Dr. Matthews: It's certainly a continuum; the dichotomy as in an explanatory device. But there is a difference, too, between people at the central part of the continuum, the ambiverts, and people at the two extremes. Presumably an ambivert is a generalist who can function moderately well across a variety of different environments. The introverts and extraverts are specialists with clear preferences for the particular environments associated with those traits.

Dr. Alexander: So in your data have you dichotomized them? I mean, have you gotten rid of the middle people and used the extremes?

Dr. Matthews: It's usually a median split which I take in studies such as the one which I illustrated. And sometimes you can use correlations where you're using the full width of the spectrum.

Dr. Ackerman: It seems to me that by using a broad approach to extraversion as opposed to a narrow one, you sort of lump together the dominance aspects of extraversion with the social closeness aspects of extraversion. So it seems to me that the notion of extraverts just being more highly confident and a higher self-efficacy and so on is more an aspect of dominance than it is people who like to be around other people. Do you have a sense of that?

Dr. Matthews: That's certainly a possibility. Two comments follow, I guess. First

271

of all, there is work on the subtraits which come under the extraversion umbrella, especially on impulsivity and sociability. But the sense which I have is that those data are quite inconsistent (see Amelang & Ullwer, 1991). It's hard to segregate which things go with impulsivity and which things go with sociability, except in very narrowly specified paradigms. And very often the extraversion trait is a more consistent predictor than either subtrait.

The second point is more theoretical. In a sense, personality traits are reflections of properties of the external environment. To the extent that situations require you to be dominant or sociable or whatever, than those environmental properties may be reflected in traits which could be investigated in empirical work. The question then is one of how cleanly the environment is sliced up into these different sub-categories. It may be that there's so much overlap between environments calling for the different attributes of extraversion, that the higher order construct is actually more useful in practice.

Dr. Baddeley: I'm just wondering about stability. What happens to the extravert salesman when he or she loses his or her job? Have people done work on the effect of a major change in environment on that?

Dr. Matthews: There's really rather a shortage of evidence. Work on loss of job has neglected the role of extraversion. There's certainly increased interest in occu-pational psychology on how the person shapes the job and the job shapes the person. Howard and Bray's (1988) study of AT&T executives which showed that as they became more successful they became more impulsive, which is one of the aspects of extraversion. But it's an area which really needs more systematic investigation.

Dr. Woltz: Can anxiety be measured with physiological responses, and if so, how do those correspond to the self-report?

Dr. Matthews: It can be. And some people see physiological anxiety as being one of several systems which come under the broad anxiety heading. However, the im-pression I have is that as far as performance studies are concerned, physiology is largely a red herring in that it's hard to find consistency in psychophysiological correlates of anxiety-like traits in performance settings. And it seems to be the worry element rather than the physiological element of anxiety which is actually predictive of task performance.

Dr. Wagner: If the sales training can increase someone's score in an extraversion worker, do you worry about sort of the method effects? Is there a lot of self-support and personality kinds of things? And how much of the data sort of go beyond this kind of stuff and how frequently? There could be a lot more of these other kinds of things?

Dr. Matthews: There are very few relevant data actually. This whole question of the interplay between the person and occupation requires more systematic investi-gation, as I was saying. There's just the one study showing an increase in extraversion following in sales training (Turnbull, 1976). One would certainly like more behav-ioral data to back that finding up.

Dr. Wittmann: Another face of John B. Carroll's work came to my mind, his model of school learning and all these learning opportunities. What do you think is the causal mechanism in these extraverted environments? Is it simply that an extravert with the same amount of intelligence compared to an introvert just invests more time in that environment and then he gets more knowledge than the introvert?

Or do you think it's simply the kind of extravertedness which improves the knowledge?

Dr. Matthews: I think it's an open question. Laboratory studies identify various processes which may feed into skilled differences between extraverts and introverts, and influence behavior within the 'extraverted' environment. But, equally, personality differences in skill may come out of differences in the content of people's lives, including exposure to environments and time spent practicing skills. The person's general orientation towards that environment, in terms of their interests and motivations may also be important.

Dr. Deary: I think there's an increasing tendency to put things into an adaptive framework these days. Two things are demanded by that. One is that the traits are enmeshed in evolutionarily important things: that they were important in our evolutionary history. And the second is that because there's a continuum it must be an equally adaptive to be on a high or low rank of the continuum. Otherwise one end could have been selected and there would be less variance.

I just wonder if you can demonstrate these two things: that we're talking about evolutionarily important things in our evolutionary history — not just about selling things in the Twentieth Century; and the second is, can you demonstrate there's equal adaptivity at each end of the continuum?

Dr. Matthews: I think the problem with people like Tooby and Cosmides (1992) is that they're conflating two senses of adaptation. The proximal influence on behavior is simply how the person deals with the real-life challenges, which might or might not be controlled by evolutionary systems. So you have to show that evolution has selected for some relevant mechanism or module, and then, as a second step, show how that module is translated into information-processing and behavior. Effects of personality and emotion on cognition and performance are often highly sensitive to contextual and strategic factors, and evolutionary psychology has not provided good explanations for such flexibilities of behavior.

The approach which I'm taking is essentially neutral on the evolutionary questions. It aims to look at behavioral data to try to work out how people of different personality types cope with the central challenges of everyday living. Having said that, it's entirely possible that evolutionary mechanisms are playing some role here, but I'm worried about how you get good evidence for this hypothesis. Next, let me address your second question, concerning the equal adaptivity of each end of the continuum. If that actually is the case, then there should be compensating advantages and disadvantages at each extreme. So in the case of anxiety I try to look for reasons why anxiety might actually be sometimes adaptive rather than just causing of deficits in performance. To take a second example, the third Eysenck dimension of psychoticism (P) looks clearly maladaptive, but it turns out also that high P is related to creativity which may provide a compensating advantage (Eysenck, 1995).

12

Measuring and Understanding G: Experimental and Correlational Approaches

JAN-ERIC GUSTAFSSON

During the first two or three decades of the twentieth century, the general factor held a prominent place in models of the structure of individual differences, and most prominently so in Spearman's (1927) two-factor theory, which was supported by the factor-analytic procedure developed by Spearman (1904). The procedures developed by Binet and Simon (1905, 1908) to measure general intelligence also contributed to the widespread dissemination of the construct. However, when Thurstone (1931) generalized factor analysis to encompass multiple factors, the general factor fell into scientific disrepute. He (e.g., Thurstone, 1938) and other users of multiple-factor analysis demonstrated that models with a multitude of primary mental abilities accounted for the empirical data and that models with a general factor were problematic, both empirically and methodologically. The Thurstonian multiple-factor approach to factor analysis has since become the dominant one, and because this factor-analytic technique does not easily yield a general factor, the G factor was conspicuously absent in models of the structure of cognitive abilities for many decades (e.g., French, Ekstrom, & Price, 1963; Guilford, 1967).

During the 1960s and 1970s, critics pointed out that multiple-factor analysis has an unfortunate tendency to produce many narrow "primary" factors (e.g., Humphreys, 1979, 1985). However, it was not until Cattell (1963), Horn and Cattell (1966), and others extended multiple-factor analysis into higher order realms, by factor-analyzing correlations among lower order factors, that attention shifted from narrow dimensions of ability to broad dimensions of ability (Horn, 1989). The most prominent of these are fluid intelligence (Gf) and crystallized intelligence (Gc), even though other broad factors were also identified, such as general visualization (Gv), general retrieval (Gr), and general auditory ability (Ga). Cattell (1987) and Horn (1988, 1989) interpreted Gf and Gc as separate components, or aspects, of general intelligence, but they (e.g., Horn, 1989) have argued against attempts to identify the general factor as the apex factor of a hierarchy of factors.

Does General Intelligence Exist?

One reason for Cattell's (1987) and Horn's (1988, 1989) reluctance to carry the higher order analysis so far as to yield only a single, general, factor is that this implies that the simple structure criteria cannot be satisfied. These criteria state that any observed variable should be related to as few factors as possible and that each factor should be related only to a subset of the tests. As was demonstrated by Thurstone (1947), these criteria are necessary to ensure factorial invariance. Thus, when a general factor is extracted from a correlation matrix for a battery of tests, the nature of this factor will vary as a function of the composition of the test battery. For example, if there are many verbal, scholastic, tests in the battery, the general factor will be close to Gc; if there are many nonverbal reasoning tests in the battery, the general factor will be close to Gf.

There is, thus, a conflict between the principle of simple structure and the idea of a dimension of individual differences that is broad enough to influence every domain of performance. However, Thurstone (1947) did not admit that multiple-factor analysis is biased against the general factor. In the preface to his 1947 volume *Multiple Factor Analysis*, Thurstone criticized the Spearman tradition of factor analysis as being focused on a restricted set of issues concerning the general factor, and, almost triumphantly, he stated the following:

> Instead of extracting, first, the postulated general factor and then investigating the residuals to determine whether any disturbing group factors must also be admitted, we start with an observation equation in *n* terms which represent as many factors as may be required by the correlations. It becomes, then, a question of fact as to whether one or more of them are general factors and whether one or more of them are positive or bipolar. (Thurstone, 1947, p. vi)

Thurstone (1947) thus ascribed to multiple-factor analysis considerable generality and openness to a variety of different empirical results. He also emphasized the mathematical generality of multiple-factor analysis, embodied in his realization that "the tetrad was merely the expansion of a second-order minor" (p. vi), and he asked the rhetorical question "as to whether multiple-factor analysis would have developed earlier if this interpretation had been stated earlier" (p. vi). Thurstone was, however, not hostile to the idea of a general factor. Somewhat later in the preface, after having discussed objections to the idea of correlated factors, Thurstone pointed out that

> second-order factors which have been determined from the correlated primaries have only recently been introduced, so it is not yet known how fruitful they will be. It seems likely that a second-order general factor, determined from correlated primaries, may turn out to be Spearman's general intellective factor *g*. (pp. vii–viii)

It is easy to understand Thurstone's (1947) enthusiasm over multiple-factor analysis, but it seems that he overestimated the generality and power of the techniques he presented in his book. The conflict between the simple structure principle and the identification of a general factor is thus not resolved by introduction of higher order factors, because when only one factor remains, the simple structure criteria cannot be satisfied.

One way to solve the problem of noninvariance is to bring noncognitive variables into the analysis, to supply what Cattell (e.g., 1987) called "hyperplane stuff." This has been done by Cattell (e.g., 1987) and his collaborators, but it has certainly not been adopted as a general procedure. The most common approach has instead been to disregard the problem of noninvariance of the general factor, and either use principal-factor analysis to extract a general factor (e.g., Jensen, 1987) or continue the higher order modeling approach until a single general factor remains.

The latter approach was adopted by Carroll (1993) in his monumental project of reanalyzing almost 500 matrices of intercorrelations among test scores. Many of the analyses resulted in a general factor, which was assigned to the highest stratum in the resulting *three-stratum model*. Scrutiny of the nature of the G factor in Carroll's reanalyses indicates, however, that the interpretation of this factor is influenced by the composition of the test battery. For example, Carroll (1993, pp. 109–114) reanalyzed a study by Gustafsson (1984), in which the test battery overrepresented visuospatial tests, and he found that the third-order G factor was very highly related to a second-order Gv factor. Carroll's results also showed, however, that the Inductive (I) reasoning factor tended to be the first-order factor most highly related to G.

If the general factor cannot be identified in an invariant fashion, and if its nature is a function of which particular composition of tests is represented in the test battery, then it is not worthy of much attention, because it does not qualify as a useful scientific construct. The problem of noninvariance of the general factor is thus very serious indeed.

It seems, however, that there is a fortuitous empirical circumstance that may be relied on to solve the problem. Gustafsson (1984, 1988; see also Undheim, 1981; Undheim & Gustafsson, 1987) found in higher order confirmatory factor analyses a perfect relationship between a higher order G factor and a lower order Gf factor. This result thus implies that G is equivalent with the nonverbal reasoning factor Gf, which has been identified in numerous studies according to simple-structure criteria. Thus, if this empirical relation can be trusted, an invariant identification of G may be affected just as easily as Gf may be measured.

This line of reasoning relies, however, on the assumption that there is, indeed, such a perfect relationship between G and Gf. As has already been described, the Carroll three-stratum model includes a general factor (G) at the third level. However, even though Carroll's (1993) results indicate that there is a slight tendency for Gf to be the second-stratum factor most highly related to G (see Carroll, 1993, chapter 15), there certainly is no basis for claiming that Carroll's results show a perfect relationship between Gf and G. In a review of Carroll's (1993) work, Spearritt (1996) rather interpreted the evidence as showing that Gc is the factor most highly related to G. There is, thus, an obvious conflict between the results obtained by Carroll and those obtained by Gustafsson. Carroll (1996) said, "In my view it is possible that measures of Gf feature attributes that require specific skills in inductive and deductive reasoning that are not necessarily present in other measures of g" (p. 15).

Gustafsson (1997) argued that one possible explanation for this discrepancy may be that Carroll (1993) has relied on exploratory factor analysis (EFA), whereas Gustafsson has used confirmatory factor analysis (CFA) in the hierarchical analyses. To test this hypothesis, Gustafsson (1997) conducted a reanalysis of the Holzinger and Swineford (1939) study.

The Holzinger and Swineford (1939) study was designed and conducted at a time when it was clearly realized that one general factor does not suffice to describe the structure of cognitive abilities, but before the Thurstonian multiple-factor analysis had been accepted as a de facto standard for factor analysis. Holzinger, who was an American, studied for several years at the University of London with Pearson and Spearman. He developed a special form of factor analysis known as *the bi-factor method* (see Harman, 1967), but he also did a considerable amount of substantive work. Much of that work was conducted with the framework of the so-called Unitary Traits Committee, which was established in 1931 by E. L. Thorndike, under the enthusiastic support of Spearman, who was also a member of the committee.

The last report in a series of technical reports on the Spearman–Holzinger Unitary Trait Study was the Holzinger and Swineford (1939) study, which was titled "A Study in Factor Analysis: The Stability of a Bi-factor Solution." In the preface of this report, the authors stated that the "bi-factor method is essentially an extension of Spearman's two-factor theory to a three-factor theory, where 'two' and 'three' refer to the types of factors assumed. The solutions obtained thus involve a general factor, group factors, and unique factors." Thus, the three-factor model implies an extension of the Spearman two-factor model into a full-fledged hierarchical model.

The test battery comprised 24 tests, and many of these are close to tests still in use. The test battery was designed to measure abilities in five broad areas: spatial, verbal, memory, speed, and mathematical deduction. The bi-factor solution presented by Holzinger and Swineford (1939) supported the hypothesized structure, except that no group factor representing mathematical deduction was found. They pointed out that "while such negative results do not constitute proof, they cast doubt on the existence of a mathematical reasoning factor as distinct from the general factor. Indeed, the general factor may be just such a deductive factor as these tests were expected to measure" (p. 8). On the basis of interpretation of the factor loadings, Holzinger and Swineford also arrived at the conclusion that "the general factor appears to be largely deductive in character — a reasonable assumption in view of the fact that inference and deduction would necessarily be the chief elements in a general factor such as that postulated by Professor Spearman" (p. 27).

In the reanalysis, CFA was used to fit two types of hierarchical models. One type was a higher order model, which included five first-order factors (Gc = verbal, Gv = spatial, Gf = mathematical deductive, Gm = memory, and Gs = speed) and one second-order factor (G). The other type was a so-called nested-factor model (Gustafsson & Balke, 1993), which included a G factor with relations to all 24 tests and residual factors representing Gc, Gv, Gm, and Gs. The higher order models showed beyond any doubt that there is a relation of unity between G and Gf, whereas the relations between G and the other factors were all significantly lower than unity. The nested-factor models also supported the hypothesis of equivalence between G and Gf, because in these models it was not possible to introduce a residual Gf factor, after G was included in the model. This is, of course, because in such a top-down approach the G factor extracts all of the systematic variance associated with Gf.

The reanalysis of the Holzinger and Swineford (1939) data with a modern form of factor analysis thus gave excellent support to the original bi-factor analysis and to the hypothesis of equivalence between G and Gf.

This is, however, not the only reanalysis of the Holzinger and Swineford (1939) data. Probably because of the fact that the technical report presents the scores for each individual student, this has been favorite data material for illustrating newly invented factor-analytic techniques as well as being used as an example in textbooks (e.g., Gorsuch, 1983; Harman, 1967). This implies that there exists a multitude of additional reanalyses of these data (either of all 24 variables or of a subset of 9 variables), in which a wide variety of exploratory factor-analytic techniques has been applied. However, none of these seems to have demonstrated the striking pattern of equivalence between G and Gf present in these data. On the contrary, these re-analyses clearly demonstrate the limitations inherent in EFA: Not only are there uncertainties in the number of factors, and the estimates of factor loadings, but the amount of intercorrelation among the factors in an oblique solution may quite arbitrarily be determined by the researcher by choice of different parameter values in the rotational procedures. Because these correlations determine the relative importance of lower and higher order factors, this makes EFA unsuited for higher order modeling.

The reanalysis of the Holzinger and Swineford (1939) study thus provides further support for the empirical identity between G and Gf, and it also supports the hypothesis that Carroll's (1993) failure to identify this identity was due to his reliance on EFA. For the remainder of the discussion here, it is thus assumed that the G factor may be invariantly identified as Gf. This of course suggests that the proper empirical method of measuring G would be to use a set of nonverbal reasoning tests. It is, however, easy to show that other more traditional techniques of estimating G, such as making a weighted or an unweighted sum of all the tests in the battery, generally provide a good approximation of Gf. Gustafsson (1997) thus showed that the latent Gf factor correlated .88 with a unit-weighted sum of the 24 tests. This also makes it reasonable to assume that empirical studies in which the general factor has been estimated as the first principal factor provide reasonably good approximations of Gf.

Interpretations of G

In spite of the obvious difficulties encountered in attempts to establish noninvariant measures of G, there is in the scientific literature an abundance of interpretations of the nature of general intelligence. During the past decade or so, it seems that interpretations in terms of low-level biological measures and constructs have become popular (see Anderson, 1992; Gustafsson & Undheim, 1996, for overviews). The idea is that individual differences in general intelligence can be accounted for in terms of a set of basic parameters or processes reflecting the efficiency of the neural system. Among the basic processes investigated are simple reaction time (e.g., Jensen, 1982), inspection time (e.g., Deary & Stone, 1996), nerve conductance velocity (Vernon, 1987), and evoked potentials (Eysenck, 1988). In brief summary, it seems that the pattern of findings is such that weak relations are typically found between G and parameters reflecting efficiency of basic neuronal processes, which provides support for the idea that individual differences in G at least to some extent are caused by individual differences in efficiency of a basic processing mechanism (Anderson, 1992).

Other explanations have been formulated in terms of higher level constructs that refer to cognitive process models. The first attempts to interpret G in such terms go back to Spearman (1923, 1927), who may be regarded as the first cognitive psychologist. His theory of G had a qualitative aspect (Spearman, 1923) and a quantitative aspect (Spearman, 1927). The qualitative theory was expressed in terms of the three noegenetic laws, or principles: eduction of relations, eduction of correlates, and apprehension of experience. The two first principles capture basic aspects of reasoning, and the third principle corresponds to what is now called *metacognition*. Spearman's focus on processes of reasoning in interpretations of G indicates that his G (or g) was basically what psychologists now label Gf. This of courses makes the empirical finding that Gf equals G even more compelling and interesting.

Spearman's (1927) quantitative theory of g was formulated in terms of "energy" and the principle of "universal mental competition." The metaphors that Spearman used to express his ideas tend not to ring so many bells in a late twentieth-century mind, but a closer reading of Spearman, as has been documented by Messick (1996), shows his ideas to be ever so modern. As is shown by Messick, Spearman's quantitative theory should be understood as expressing individual differences in limitations on the ability to keep more than a limited number of items in mental focus at the same time. This hypothesis is more or less identical with a current theory that states that G is determined by individual differences in working memory capacity (Kyllonen & Christal, 1990) or capacity to keep in mind, and operate on, a large number of items. There is considerable empirical support for an almost perfect relation between reasoning ability (i.e., Gf) and working memory capacity (e.g., Kyllonen & Christal, 1990).

As was pointed out by Kyllonen (1996), when reflecting on the conclusion that working memory capacity may indeed be essentially Spearman's g, the distinct theoretical and empirical backgrounds of these constructs provide several advantages:

> The working memory system was developed theoretically not as a label for an individual-differences factor, but rather as a construct to explain experimental results in the memory literature. We know how to characterize working memory limitations independently of individual-differences results. We know how to manipulate the working memory requirements of a task without even computing correlations. Unlike the case with other conventional psychometric factors, such as reasoning ability and g, it is possible, in principle, to measure working memory capacity on an absolute rather than relative scale. This property carries with it tremendous potential for, among other things, bridging the individual differences and the cognitive engineering literature. (Kyllonen, 1996, p. 73)

The linking of the concepts of g and working memory capacity thus offers possibilities of a tighter integration of concepts, theories, and approaches of the correlational and the experimental traditions, which may, in turn, be important for the attempts to achieve an understanding of the nature of G.

Experimental and Correlational Approaches

The plea for an integration between the two disciplines of psychology is, of course, not new; it was forcefully made by Cronbach (1957) in his famous presidential address to the American Psychological Association. Much progress has indeed also been made in achieving an integration between the two traditions, and most notably so when in the 1970s researchers (e.g., Hunt, 1978; Sternberg, 1977) started to adopt theories and methods of cognitive psychology in the study of individual differences (Gustafsson & Undheim, 1996; Snow & Lohman, 1989). In several applied fields, such as education and clinical psychology, Cronbach's admonition has also had considerable effect, in the form of research on aptitude–treatment interactions (e.g., Cronbach, 1967; Cronbach & Snow, 1977).

However, in spite of the progress that has been made in joining experimental and correlational psychology, it may be argued, as Eysenck (1995) recently did, that the gulf between experimental and correlational approaches is still too wide. It may also be noted that there still are few examples of studies that actually combine treatment manipulation and randomization, with more sophisticated techniques of measurement and multivariate analysis.

The correlational methods have above all proven useful for taxonomic purposes, and both in the cognitive and noncognitive fields, there is now considerable agreement about the basic taxonomic structures and categories (Gustafsson & Undheim, 1996; Snow, Cormo, & Jackson, 1996). However, during the past couple of decades, the rapid increase in computational power has stimulated development of more powerful tools for the study of individual differences, such as item–response theory and structural equation modeling (SEM). The CFA studies of alternative hierarchical models of the structure of intelligence (referred to previously) thus provide one example of an application of the extremely versatile and powerful SEM technique.

SEM thus allows the researcher to specify a wide variety of hypotheses about different aspects of data, such as patterns of relations between manifest and latent variables. Hypotheses may also be tested about group differences, such as, for example, about differential patterns of relations between manifest and latent variables in different treatment groups. As was argued by Gustafsson (1989), and as is reiterated here, this should make a combination of SEM and experimental manipulation a powerful way of combining the two disciplines of scientific psychology.

In research currently being conducted in Göteborg, Sweden, some researchers are using such an approach to improve understanding both of the nature of G and characteristics of instruments that are good G measures. To make the presentation more concrete, I present one study in somewhat greater detail. A more complete account is given by Carlstedt (1997).

Test Complexity and Measurement of G

The study took a starting point in the observation that there is a relation between the complexity of the task and its amount of relation with G. This hypothesis dates back to Spearman (1927), and it has been expressed and investigated many times. One line of research was started by Guttman (1954), who explicitly formulated the complexity hypothesis. Using multidimensional scaling and hierarchical factor analyses of large-scale test batteries, Marshalek, Lohman, and Snow (1983) demonstrated a relation between task complexity and G loading. The relation has also been observed when the degree of complexity of quite simple tasks has been varied. For example, Frearson and Eysenck (1986) varied the complexity of response rules in choice reaction time tasks and found a higher correlation with intelligence for more complex rules. Similarly, backward memory span has a higher relation with G than forward memory span has (Jensen, 1987).

The complexity hypothesis has also been studied experimentally in several studies. For example, Roberts, Beh, and Stankov (1988) used a competing-task paradigm to vary complexity and found that the amount of relationship between intelligence and performance on a card-sorting task was higher under competing-task than under single-task conditions.

As has already been observed, it is a well-established fact that the highest loadings on G are achieved with complex nonverbal reasoning items, such as the Raven Progressive Matrices Test. The complexities involved in solving the Raven type of items have been analyzed and described by Carpenter, Just, and Schell (1990) on the basis of computer simulations. The simulation indicated the importance of an ability to decompose problems into smaller parts and to manage a hierarchy of goals and subgoals generated by this problem decomposition, with heavy demands on working memory. Other kinds of nonverbal reasoning items have similar cognitive characteristics as the Raven test, and it may be hypothesized that this is why they go together to define an Inductive reasoning factor.

It may be asked, however, if it is possible to define an even higher level of complexity. In an attempt to accomplish this, tests were reconstructed that mix different types of inductive reasoning tasks, under the assumption that heterogenous combinations of items are more complex, because in addition to the complexity offered by each item, this requires switching between different sets of rules and principles. The heterogenous tests have then been compared with the ordinary homogenous subtest designs in fairly large experimental studies, which have been conducted in conjunction with enlistment to military service in Sweden.

Participants and Variables

The study investigated three kinds of items: series, groups, and Bongard, which are internally developed experimental tests. These nonverbal problem-solving tests are described in the following paragraphs.

Groups. Five figures are presented. The task is to find the figure that does not fit thematically (six items).

Series. A sequence of four figures is presented. The task is to select the two figures out of five that will complete the sequence (nine items).

Bongard. Each item contains two separate groups with six squares each, each square framing different figures. The task is to find the feature that unites the figures in one group and that differentiates this group from the other group, in which the figures are united by another feature. Five response alternatives are presented, and the two squares that thematically belong to the two groups should be chosen (seven items).

These items were combined in different ways into two test forms: heterogenous (HET) and homogenous (HOM). In the HOM form, the test items were presented in the following order: groups, series, and Bongard. In the HET form, there was first one groups item, one Bongard item, and then one series item, after which the sequence was repeated. The HET treatment comprised 1,778 participants, and the HOM treatment 363 participants. The experimental tasks were administered along with the regular military enlistment battery, of which three other tests were used: instructions, synonyms, and metal folding. The instructions test presents verbally formulated directives to make markings on an answer sheet. This test has been shown to have a high relation with G (Carlstedt & Mårdberg, 1993). The synonyms test is a multiple-choice vocabulary test. In the items in the metal-folding test, the task is to find the three-dimensional object that corresponds to a two-dimensional drawing of an unfolded piece of metal.

Results

The data were analyzed by fitting confirmatory factor-analysis models within treatment groups and by testing for equality of parameter estimates across groups. In the modeling, the items were divided into half-tests to make it possible to separate systematic item-specific variance from random error, and some models were also fitted to item-level data. Figure 12.1 presents the basic structure of the model.

The model includes a general factor (G), a rather narrowly defined Gc factor with relations to synonyms and instructions, and test-specific factors defined by the half-tests. In the first step, a model was fitted that imposed constraints of equality over the treatment groups on each and every parameter of the model (i.e., factor loadings, factor variances, error variances, and means of latent and manifest variables). The fit of this model was not good, χ^2 (123, N = 2,141) = 228.74, $p < .00$. Further modeling showed that the model fit well within the HOM treatment group, χ^2 (45, N = 363) = 59.61, $p < .07$, but not so well within the HET treatment group, χ^2 (45, N = 1,778) = 98.37, $p < .00$. These results indicate that the differential item sequencing had an effect on the measurement characteristics of the test items.

To investigate more closely the nature of the treatment effect, the constraints of equality were relaxed in several modeling steps, and the improvement in fit of successive models was tested for significance. Relaxing the constraints of equality on the size of the factor loadings for the three experimental tests significantly improved the fit, χ^2 (6, N = 2,141) = 36.11, $p < .00$. However, separate tests of the equality of factor loadings over treatments for each of the three item types showed that series and groups items, but not Bongard items, were affected. Interestingly enough, the pattern of differences was opposite to the hypothesized one, there being a higher relationship between G and performance on series and groups items in the HOM treatment than in the HET treatment.

Further relaxations of constraints over treatments identified a difference between the treatments with respect to the variance of the test-specific factors for series and groups, as well as some other differences. However, the fact that the originally hypothesized model fit well within the HOM treatment, but not within the HET treatment, indicates that not only are there differences between the treatments with

283

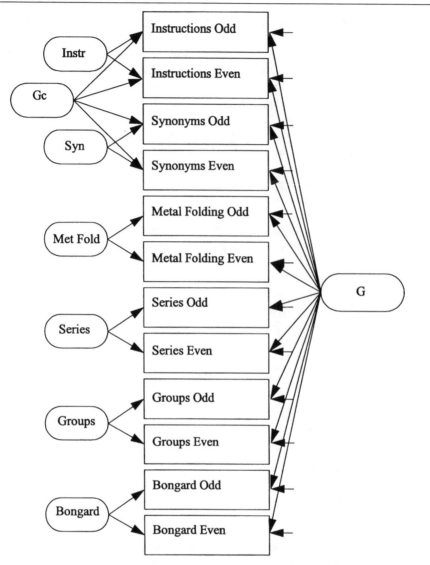

Figure 12.1. The hypothesized model. G = general factor of intelligence; Gc = crystallized intelligence.

respect to the size of parameter estimates but that there is also a structural difference between the models for the two treatments. It may be hypothesized that the HET administration procedure imposed specific demands, such as having to switch between strategies, which affected all of the items in the sequence. If this is the case, it should be possible to identify these effects as a factor specific to the experimental items in the HET treatment. Imposing such a factor (HETSpec) in the HET treatment only did indeed improve the fit of the model, χ^2 (6, N = 1,778) = 50.76, $p <$ .00. After the HETSpec factor was added, the two-treatment model with relaxed constraints had an excellent fit, χ^2 (102, N = 2,141) = 118.63, $p < .12$.

TABLE 12.1   Standardized Loadings of the Tests on the Latent Variables in the Two Treatments

Test	G		Gc		Test spec		HETSpec		Error	
	HET	HOM	HET	HOM	HET	HOM	HET	HOM	HET	HOM
Instructions										
Odd	.81	.81	.26	.26	.36	.36			.39	.39
Even	.81	.81	.28	.28	.36	.36			.38	.38
Synonyms										
Odd	.61	.61	.62	.62					.50	.50
Even	.60	.60	.62	.62					.50	.50
Metal folding										
Odd	.71	.71			.57	.57			.42	.42
Even	.69	.69			.58	.58			.44	.44
Series										
Odd	.61	.71			.25	.31	.22		.72	.63
Even	.56	.67			.27	.32	.11		.77	.67
Groups										
Odd	.55	.57			.25	.35	.22		.76	.74
Even	.47	.58			.24	.29	.22		.82	.76
Bongard										
Odd	.44	.49			.23	.45	.20		.85	.74
Even	.51	.60			.22	.50	.41		.72	.63

Note.   G = general factor of intelligence; GC = crystallized intelligence; HETSpec = factor specific to HET; HOM = homogenous treatment group; HET = heterogenous treatment group.

Table 12.1 presents the standardized parameter estimates for the relations between the latent variables and the tests within the two treatments for this model. As shown, the G loadings tend to be higher in the HOM treatment than in the HET treatment for all of the experimental tests, and particularly so for the series items. These results clearly demonstrate that heterogenous collections of items do not result in better G tests. It may also be noted that the HETSpec factor is quite strongly related to performance on the experimental items in the HET treatment, whereas the test-specific factors are less strongly related to performance in the HET than in the HOM treatment. These results indicate that test-specific components of variance are not only due to characteristics of the different item types but also to contextual and dynamic factors.

Discussion

The results of the study are quite opposed to the predictions made from the complexity hypothesis, but it would of course be rash to conclude that this hypothesis should be rejected. The amount of evidence supporting the hypothesis of a relation between the complexity of a task and its relation with G is too overwhelming to allow such a conclusion. It is equally obvious, however, that the complexity hypothesis cannot account for the strong negative effects of heterogeneity of item sequencing on the amount of relation with G, because the HOM treatment may not be characterized as being more complex than the HET treatment.

An alternative hypothesis could be that the homogenous arrangement allows better possibilities of learning from one item to another; in nonverbal reasoning tests, different principles are typically introduced successively and are combined in the more complex items. In the homogenous arrangement, the high G participants can take advantage of this, but not so easily in the heterogenous arrangement. A closer analysis of the items in the test (see Carlstedt, 1997) gives some support for this line of reasoning. Thus, among the series items, for which the most pronounced effects were found, there were several instances in which later items combined principles encountered in earlier items. The Bongard items, for which no significant effect was found, did not combine principles of solution in a sequential fashion in such an obvious way.

This line of reasoning suggests that within-test dynamic learning effects may be another important factor determining the efficiency of a test as a G measure. Interestingly enough, Raven constructed the Progressive Matrices Test with such dependencies in mind. Raven, Raven, and Court (1995) thus said, "Each problem is the 'mother' or the 'source' of a system of thought and the order in which the problems are presented provides training in the method of working" (p. G42). The Progressive Matrices Test is also described as providing a built-in training program and as being able to measure the ability to learn from experience.

Although the complexity hypothesis cannot account for the results of the present study, it would seem that the hypothesis that G may be accounted for in terms of working memory capacity is compatible with the present results. People with a high working memory capacity may thus be assumed to be more facile in using information encountered in the process of work and in using that to formulate hypotheses about which principles may be induced from the information given in the items. In the heterogenous sequence of items, such a systematic use of previously encountered information may be rendered impossible by the longer distance, so to say, between previously encountered items and the current one and by the intervening work on other types of items. On the other hand, the particular requirements posed by the heterogenous item sequence imply that other abilities may be needed for successful performance. This is, indeed, demonstrated by the emergence of a special factor (i.e., HETSpec), which explains individual differences in level of performance on the heterogeneous sequence of items. There is no further information available about the individuals in the present study, but in further research, it may be of interest to investigate the HETSpec factor more closely. One interesting hypothesis to investigate is that this factor represents conative and stylistic sources of individual differences rather than a cognitive ability in a narrow sense.

Conclusions

Some 100 years ago, Binet introduced the practice of measuring general intellectual ability with a wide range of different tasks. This practice was, furthermore, put on a sound theoretical footing when Spearman (1927) formulated the principle of the "indifference of the indicator." Thus, the basic theoretical and practical principles for measuring G have been known for long, and they have been applied with a respectable degree of success.

However, the mixed collections of tasks have not been widely accepted as measures of G, or even of anything at all. In addition, the conflict among proponents of different factor-analytic schools over the existence of G, which has been raging more or less intensely throughout the century, certainly has not contributed confidence in the G construct. However, the progress made in factor analysis and SEM during the past couple of decades has made it possible to resolve at least some of the doubts concerning the existence of G and to clarify its relations to other ability constructs.

During the past couple of decades, research conducted along experimental lines has contributed greatly to our understanding of the nature of G, both in terms of low-level reductionistic models and in terms of higher level cognitive models. There is, however, still a long way to go until the major individual-differences constructs have been adequately accounted for in theoretical terms. It would seem, however, that an approach combining experimental methodology with multivariate modeling techniques may prove useful in researchers' future attempts to achieve such an understanding.

REFERENCES

Anderson, M. (1992). *Intelligence and development.* Oxford, England: Basil Blackwell.

Binet, A., & Simon, T. (1905). Méthodes nouvelles pour le diagnostic du niveau intellectuel des anormaux [New methods for diagnosing the intellectual level of abnormals]. *L' Année Psychologique, 11*, 191–336.

Binet, A., & Simon, T. (1908). Le développment de l'intelligence chez les enfants [The development of intelligence in children]. *Année Psychologique, 14*, 1–94.

Carlstedt, B. (1997). *Test complexity and measurement of the general factor.* Manuscript submitted for publication.

Carlstedt, B., & Mårdberg, B. (1993). Construct validity of the Swedish Military Enlistment Test. *Scandinavian Journal of Psychology, 34*, 353–362.

Carpenter, P. A., Just, M. A., & Schell, P. (1990). What one intelligence test measures: A theoretical account of the processing in the Raven Progressive Matrices Test. *Psychological Review, 97*, 404–431.

Carroll, J. B. (1993). *Human cognitive abilities.* Cambridge, England: Cambridge University Press.

Carroll, J. B. (1996). A three-stratum theory of intelligence: Spearman's contribution. In I. Dennis & P. Tapsfield (Eds.), *Human abilities: Their nature and measurement* (pp. 1–17). Hillsdale, NJ: Erlbaum.

Cattell, R. B. (1963). Theory of fluid and crystallized intelligence: A critical experiment. *Journal of Educational Psychology, 54*, 1–22.

Cattell, R. B. (1987). *Intelligence: Its structure, growth and action.* Amsterdam: North-Holland.

Cronbach, L. J. (1957). The two disciplines of scientific psychology. *American Psychologist, 12*, 671–684.

Cronbach, L. J. (1967). How can instruction be adapted to individual differences. In R. M. Gagne (Ed.), *Learning and individual differences* (pp. 23–39). Columbus, OH: Charles E. Merrill Books.

Cronbach, L. J., & Snow, R. E. (1977). *Aptitudes and instructional methods.* New York: Irvington.

Deary, I. J., & Stone, C. (1996). Intelligence and inspection time: Achievements, prospects, and problems. *American Psychologist, 51*(6), 599–608.

Eysenck, H. J. (1988). The biological basis of intelligence. In S. H. Irvine & J. W. Berry (Eds.), *Human abilities in cultural context* (pp. 87–104). Cambridge, England: Cambridge University Press.

Eysenck, H. J. (1995). Can we study intelligence using the experimental method? *Intelligence, 20*(3), 217–228.

Frearson, W. M., & Eysenck, H. J. (1986). Intelligence, reaction time (RT) and a new "odd-man-out" RT paradigm. *Personality and Individual Differences, 7*, 807–817.

French, J. W., Ekstrom, R. B., & Price, L. A. (1963). *Manual and kit of reference test for cognitive factors.* Princeton, NJ: Educational Testing Service.

Gorsuch, R. L. (1983). *Factor analysis* (2nd ed.). Hillsdale, NJ: Erlbaum.

Guilford, J. P. (1967). *The nature of human intelligence*. New York: McGraw-Hill.

Gustafsson, J.-E. (1984). A unifying model for the structure of intellectual abilities. *Intelligence, 8*, 179–203.

Gustafsson, J.-E. (1988). Hierarchical models of individual differences in cognitive abilities. In R. J. Sternberg (Ed.), *Advances in the psychology of human intelligence* (Vol. 4, pp. 35–71). Hillsdale, NJ: Lawrence Erlbaum.

Gustafsson, J.-E. (1989). Broad and narrow abilities in research on learning and instruction. In R. Kanfer, P. L. Ackerman, & R. Cudeck (Eds.), *Abilities, motivation, and methodology: The Minnesota symposium on learning and individual differences* (pp. 203–237). Hillsdale, NJ: Erlbaum.

Gustafsson, J.-E. (1997). *On the relation between fluid and general intelligence: A reanalysis of the Holzinger and Swineford (1939) study*. Manuscript submitted for publication.

Gustafsson, J.-E., & Balke, G. (1993). General and specific abilities as predictors of school achievement. *Multivariate Behavioral Research, 28*, 407–434.

Gustafsson, J.-E., & Undheim, J. O. (1996). Individual differences in cognitive functions. In D. Berliner & R. Calfee (Eds.), *Handbook of educational psychology* (pp. 186–248). New York: Macmillan.

Guttman, L. (1954). A new approach to factor analysis: The radex. In P. F. Lazarsfeld (Ed.), *Mathematical thinking in the social sciences* (pp. 216–257). Glencoe, IL: Free Press.

Harman, H. H. (1967). *Modern factor analysis* (2nd ed.). Chicago: University of Chicago Press.

Holzinger, K. J., & Swineford, F. (1939). A study in factor analysis: The stability of a bi-factor solution. *Supplementary Educational Monographs, 48*. Chicago: Department of Education, University of Chicago.

Horn, J. L. (1988). Thinking about human abilities. In J. R. Nesselroade & R. B. Cattell (Eds.), *Handbook of multivariate experimental psychology* (2nd ed., pp. 645–685). New York: Plenum.

Horn, J. L. (1989). Models of intelligence. In R. L. Linn (Ed.), *Intelligence: Measurement theory and public policy* (pp. 29–73). Urbana: University of Illinois Press.

Horn, J. L., & Cattell, R. B. (1966). Refinement and test of the theory of fluid and crystallized intelligence. *Journal of Educational Psychology, 57*, 253–270.

Humphreys, L. G. (1979). The construct of general intelligence. *Intelligence, 3*, 105–120.

Humphreys, L. G. (1985). General intelligence: An integration of factor, test and simplex theory. In B. B. Wolman (Ed.), *Handbook of intelligence: Theories, measurements, and applications* (pp. 201–224). New York: Wiley.

Hunt, E. B. (1978). Mechanisms of verbal ability. *Psychological Review, 85*, 109–130.

Jensen, A. R. (1982). The chronometry of intelligence. In R. J. Sternberg (Ed.), *Advances in the psychology of human intelligence* (Vol. 1, pp. 255–310). Hillsdale, NJ: Erlbaum.

Jensen, A. R. (1987). The g beyond factor analysis. In R. R. Ronning, J. A. Glover, J. C. Conoley, & J. C. Witt (Eds.), *Buros–Nebraska Symposium on Measurement and Testing: The influence of cognitive psychology on testing* (Vol. 3, pp. 87–142). Hillsdale, NJ: Erlbaum.

Kyllonen, P. C. (1996). Is working memory capacity Spearman's g? In I. Dennis & P. Tapsfield (Eds.), *Human abilities: Their nature and measurement* (pp. 77–96). Hillsdale, NJ: Erlbaum.

Kyllonen, P. C., & Christal, R. E. (1990). Reasoning ability is (little more than) working-memory capacity?! *Intelligence, 14*(4), 389–433.

Marshalek, B., Lohman, D. F., & Snow, R. E. (1983). The complexity continuum in the radex and hierarchical models of intelligence. *Intelligence, 7*, 107–128.

Messick, S. (1996). Human abilities and modes of attention: The issue of stylistic consistencies in cognition. In I. Dennis & P. Tapsfield (Eds.), *Human abilities: Their nature and measurement* (pp. 77–96). Erlbaum.

Raven, J., Raven, J. C., & Court, J. H. (1995). *Manual for Raven's Progressive Matrices and Vocabulary Scales: General overview*. Oxford, England: Oxford Psychologists Press.

Roberts, R. D., Beh, H. C., & Stankov, L. (1988). Hick's law, competing-task performance, and intelligence. *Intelligence, 12*, 111–130.

Snow, R. E., Cormo, L., & Jackson, D., III. (1996). Individual differences in conative and affective functions. In D. Berliner & R. Calfee (Eds.), *Handbook of educational psychology* (pp. 243–310). New York: Macmillan.

Snow, R. E., & Lohman, D. F. (1989). Implications of cognitive psychology for educational measurement. In R. Linn (Ed.), *Educational measurement* (3rd ed., pp. 263–331). New York: Macmillan.

Spearman, C. (1904). "General intelligence," objectively determined and measured. *American Journal of Psychology, 15*, 201–293.

Spearman, C. (1923). *The nature of "intelligence" and the principles of cognition*. London: Macmillan.

Spearman, C. (1927). *The abilities of man.* London: Macmillan.

Spearritt, D. (1996). Carroll's model of cognitive abilities: Educational implications. *International Journal of Educational Research, 25* (2), 107–197.

Sternberg, R. J. (1977). Component processes in analogical reasoning. *Psychological Review, 84,* 353–378.

Terman, L. M. (1924). The mental test as a psychological method. *Psychological Review, 31,* 93–117.

Thurstone, L. L. (1931). Multiple factor analysis. *Psychological Review, 38,* 406–427.

Thurstone, L. L. (1938). Primary mental abilities. *Psychometric Monographs,* No. 1.

Thurstone, L. L. (1947). *Multiple factor analysis.* Chicago: University of Chicago Press.

Undheim, J. O. (1981). On intelligence: II. A neo-Spearman model to replace Cattell's theory of fluid and crystallized intelligence. *Scandinavian Journal of Psychology, 22,* 181–187.

Undheim, J. O., & Gustafsson, J. E. (1987). The hierarchical organization of cognitive abilities: Restoring general intelligence through the use of linear structural relations (LISREL). *Multivariate Behavioral Research, 22,* 149–171.

Vernon, P. A. (Ed.). (1987). *Speed of information-processing and intelligence.* Norwood, NJ: Ablex.

Discussion

Discussion of Gustafsson's presentation started with questions about the meaning of the factor of general intelligence. Other issues raised concerned the combinations of experimental and correlational research that were described in Gustafsson's paper and in other presentations.

Dr. Stankov: What I do want to say is related to the link between working memory and intelligence — Gf in particular. What I think is that most of these working memory measures are, in fact, like other tests. And it is hard for me but to think about them as being causal as opposed to being just a part of the battery as it is.

Dr. Gustafsson: I don't think that we need to make any assumptions about a strict causality from working memory to G in order to gain very much from bringing working memory in as a concept. It makes our thinking richer about this, and it gives us more interesting hypotheses to investigate. And I have seen many posters and presentations here which demonstrate that to be true.

Dr. Ackerman: Just one question and one comment. I really enjoyed what you said, but it made me think about what Terman said in 1924 that administering a psychological test really is like an experiment, and we have to think of the whole context. So that's my comment, and I really appreciate your perspective.

My question is, How do you feel about an estimate of general intelligence that's drawn at the limit where you have one question drawn from each test, and so you have as many tests as you have questions? Do you think you're going to get a better estimate of general intelligence or not?

Dr. Gustafsson: If there are correlations among these errors, they will be magnified too when you make the aggregation. It also depends on the representativeness of sampling. The broader your sample, and the more you sample the better it is. But there are problems here, and I think they could be formulated in the following way. Not only relevant variance magnifies in the aggregation but also irrelevant variance. So if you have a common motivational factor influencing all the items, you might get a very good motivational measure. Or if you have a speed component coming into each of these items as systematic but, in terms of G, irrelevant variance, that will also be magnified and it will make your G biased.

There are plenty of examples of this. ASVAB [Armed Services Vocational Battery] is biased towards Gc, and so on. So the problem with the aggregation approach is that it must be guided by some premise. You can't really just make this blindly. That was, of course, the criticism that Spearman had against Binet, who basically did what you're arguing.

Dr. Baddeley: I think I'd like to slightly take issue with the point that actually I made myself that you also made. I'm disagreeing with myself, yes. That experimental cognitive psychology uses experimental techniques but not correlations, and differential psychology does the opposite. That's not actually true. Lots of cognitive psychologists use correlations. They're regarded as rather a weak method, however. Because it is not good for plotting causal relationships. It's part of an armory of methods. And in some ways it's been very flattering and very nice to have a concept that I'm associated with playing a useful role in differential psychology to find how effective, for example, Pat Kyllonen's use of it has been.

But the use within cognitive psychology of an individual-differences method, I think has been on the whole slightly disappointing because what it has tended to do is to produce other tests that can be used, rather than try to understand why they work. And there are exceptions. Randy Engle I think is one. And I think it's very important to not be satisfied because one's got something that will work because ultimately that doesn't lead to any progress. And I think we have to be trying to pull apart why it is that it works, and I think the only effective way to do that is by a combination of experimental and correlational methods.

Dr. Gustafsson: I agree completely. And you could interpret Eysenck as agreeing with you, that there isn't much of true integration.

Dr. Wittmann: Well, the most interesting finding, Jan-Eric, at least in my eyes is that your experimental treatment produced the factor. And this is a really, really interesting thing. You didn't produce the mean differences, but you produced the factor. It means that you influenced the correlations.

Dr. Gustafsson: Exactly.

Dr. Wittmann: And these led to the factor. I guess that must be a differential treatment effect. Some of these people profited differently from that treatment, and this is the most interesting thing we should investigate in the future, that is understanding how to change correlations.

Dr. Gustafsson: I would like to make a final comment which also relates to Dr. Baddeley's presentation about double dissociation and the value of the specifics, the particular profiles, that which doesn't fit into the general pattern. I've been talking about G, but basically I would argue that the conclusion is that given that we identify G with Gf we are also saying that there are many other abilities which are important. All the other broad abilities must be brought into the picture. The first-order abilities must be brought in as well. And there is room for very specific profile differences on particular tasks as well. So if I may make that as a final statement: If you are interested in G, please be interested in the other abilities as well.

13

Individual Differences in Motivation: Traits and Self-Regulatory Skills

RUTH KANFER and ERIC D. HEGGESTAD

In contrast to abilities research, in which nearly everyone agrees with what intelligence is, one of the problems with researching motivation in the context of adult learning and skill acquisition is that people either think that they already know what motivation is or they assert that motivation is an intangible characteristic that defies definition. For us to discuss clearly the concept of motivation, then, it is necessary that we describe our own particular approach to the construct. Thus, we first offer a few of our basic assumptions about motivation. One thing that we attempt to do in this chapter is to delineate motivational *traits*, which are believed to be general and transsituational (such as achievement motivation) from motivational *skills*, which are believed to be more specific and malleable. Along the way, we describe a series of empirical studies and a theory-based taxonomy of motivational traits and skills that provide a "road map" to both the interpretation of the historical literature and a challenge for future research.

Assumptions About Motivation

For adults, motivation can have two qualitatively different representations: it can be represented in terms of *choices*, and it can be represented in terms of a *continuum*. Much of the research during the 1970s and 1980s, especially in industrial/ organizational (I/O) psychology (e.g., see R. Kanfer, 1990, for a review), focused on motivation as choice behavior. Numerous studies have been conducted that demonstrate various trait and situational influences (e.g., goal setting) on the individual's choice of whether to engage a task or choose a particular course of action. F. Kanfer (e.g., see F. Kanfer & Schefft, 1988), Heckhausen (1991), and Gollwitzer (1990),

293

for example, have described this part of the motivational process as *predecisional*; that is, it describes the determinants and the processes that ultimately generate a motivational choice (such as to set a performance goal, quit smoking, lose weight, seek a therapist, and so on).

Our interests, as I/O psychologists, have more often focused on the amount of effort that an individual devotes to a task (or to one of competing tasks). From this perspective, we consider that a decision to engage a task has already been made, but we are interested in how much effort is allocated to a task or how long an individual persists in a task (because in many tasks, a goal can be reached by many different combinations of level of effort and degree of persistence). We have found that the attentional resource metaphor (adapted from Kahneman, 1973), as well as others, provides a reasonable starting point for considering effort as a loosely quantifiable property. However, researchers must all recognize that people differ in the amount of mental effort or attention that they can marshal at any one time — simply put, individual differences in ability in the context of motivation need to be recognized. One way to do this is to merge broad notions of attention as a limited-capacity processing system (e.g., Kahneman, 1973) and notions of individual differences in intelligence as individual differences in attentional capacity, or working-memory capacity, to put this into a more current framework (e.g., see Baddeley, 1986; Kyllonen & Christal, 1990; Zeaman, 1978).

In 1989, with Phillip Ackerman, one of us (Kanfer) proposed that an individual's motivation (as effort) can be thought of as representing a combination of the attentional resource capacity of the individual (e.g., intelligence) and the proportion of the individual's capacity actually engaged (motivational effort; R. Kanfer & Ackerman, 1989). Conceptually, this means that two individuals might devote equal motivational effort (say 80%) but yield different levels of task performance (because of individual differences in relative attentional capacity).

This resource-based approach allowed us (R. Kanfer & Ackerman, 1989) to examine how ability and motivationally inspired interventions (e.g., goal setting) independently and jointly influenced the performance of adult learners in a skill-acquisition paradigm. However, before we describe the results of these studies, it is important to distinguish between two broad classes of motivational influences, namely, *proximal* and *distal* influences.

Distal Motivational Influences

There are numerous distal influences on an individual's current motivational effort on a task. They include not only the kinds of choice briefly described earlier but also motivational traits (more about this later) and an individual's internal calculations of three particular relationships. The first is the relationship between the individual's level of effort and the expected utility of such effort (something we have called the *effort–utility function*, see R. Kanfer, 1987, for an in-depth discussion). That is, some individuals are more prone to conserve their attentional effort, finding it onerous to try hard on a task (and therefore, the effort–utility function is a negative curve, increased levels of effort lead to lower levels of personal utility); see Figure 13.1A for an illustration. Other individuals like a great deal of challenge and thus have an effort–utility function that increases throughout much of the range of in-

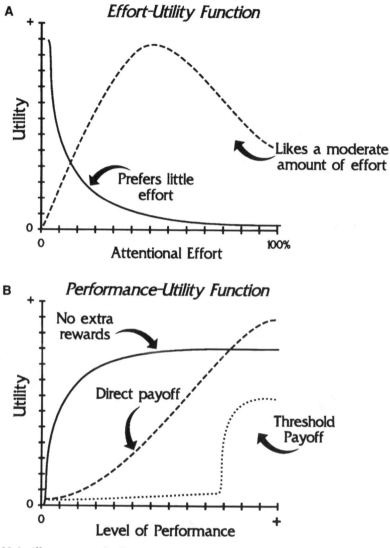

Figure 13.1. Illustrations of effort–utility and performance–utility functions. For effort–utility, two idealized individuals are shown: one who prefers a moderate amount of effort, and one who prefers not to expend effort. For performance utility, three different idealized tasks are shown, one that provides no extra rewards after a minimal level of performance is obtained, one that has a direct payoff increase for every increase in level of performance, and one that provides minimal payoff until a high-performance threshold is crossed. Figure is based on a discussion by Kanfer, 1987.

creased effort. For most people, though, it is likely that the effort–utility function is much like the Yerkes–Dodson curve — an inverse U-shaped function in which a moderate amount of effort has the highest personal utility.

The second relationship is that of a *performance–utility function* (see Figure 13.1B). For many tasks, the performance–utility function is increasing across a broad range of performance (i.e., as performance improves, personal utility increases).

However, some tasks may present the individual with a situation in which higher levels of performance (beyond some threshold) result in no perceptible increase in utility.

The third relationship is the *effort–performance function* (or what Norman & Bobrow, 1975, called the "performance–resource function"). That is, this represents either the objective relationship between the degree of effort devoted to a task and the performance outcome for that task or an individual's "perceived" function between his or her own effort and the expected performance outcome. For example, an individual who perceives that an adequate level of performance (from the performance–utility function) requires more effort than he or she is willing or capable of devoting to a task (from the effort–utility function) may choose not even to engage the task at all (e.g., this is the kind of resistance that researchers often see when new technology is introduced into a work environment). In contrast, an individual who perceives that adequate levels of performance are within a reasonable level of his or her attentional effort, will in turn, choose to engage the task.

Unknown, to date, is whether individuals also take into account the kind of changes in effort–performance functions that occur with task practice (as described by Norman & Bobrow, 1975), so that, with practice, lower levels of effort are associated with equivalent or higher levels of performance. There is a fair amount of controversy in this field. On the one hand, some developmental researchers maintain that some children have a belief system in which abilities and skills are fixed and that other children have a belief system in which abilities and skills are malleable (e.g., Dweck, 1986; Dweck & Leggett, 1988; Nicholls, 1984). On the other hand, there are few researchers who believe that, for young and middle-aged adults, task practice cannot improve performance and in many cases can reduce task-effort demands.

Proximal Motivational Influences

Although distal motivational influences are associated primarily with motivational choice behaviors, proximal motivational processes are ongoing, and are engaged within a task milieu. Proximal processes include self-regulation (e.g., self-monitoring, self-evaluation, and self-reactions). When proximal motivational processes are triggered, they involve an individual's decisions to expend more or less attentional effort to a task, to or away from competing task demands (such as strategy development) or, to or away from off-task activities (such as worry). Such processes may occur naturally as part of internally generated self-regulation, or they may be triggered by external sources (such as goal-setting, self-focus, various kinds of feedback, or specific training). For example, an individual's ongoing decisions about whether to increase effort or whether to give up on a task in the face of frustrations or failure are essentially proximal processes. Clearly, though, the input for an individual's proximal self-regulation processes is made up of both distal influences (e.g., the effort–utility function) and task-specific influences (e.g., feedback and knowledge of results). If an individual changes his or her perceived effort–utility function for a task, that would normally take place as a result of ongoing proximal self-regulatory processes.

Empirical Treatment Studies

In a series of studies, R. Kanfer and Ackerman (1989) examined how abilities (a distal trait) and goal setting (a proximal intervention) induced proximal self-regulation and performance changes during practice on a skill acquisition task (the Kanfer–Ackerman Air Traffic Control [ATC] task). Substantial support for this combined distal and proximal approach was obtained, in that aptitude–treatment interactions were found. Specifically, when lower ability learners were given performance goals (which induces self-regulation and changes the performance–utility function) early in training when the cognitive and working-memory demands outstripped their capacity, they performed more poorly than those without performance goals. In contrast, higher ability learners benefited from the goal induction, in that they had the spare resource capacity to devote to the task when the utility of higher levels of performance was increased.

We (see R. Kanfer, Ackerman, Murtha, Dugdale, & Nelson, 1994, for details) also determined that there is a potential cost to triggering self-regulatory processes through goal setting (i.e., performance goals diverted attention away from the task itself). When we used a goal-setting induction within a massed-practice design (no breaks between task trials), we found impaired performance. However, when we induced the same goals in a spaced-practice design (which provided learners with time to consolidate their conative processes between task trials), performance improved.

Along the way, we (R. Kanfer & Ackerman, 1989) observed many different self-evaluative responses to our goal-setting induction. A series of questionnaires was developed to attempt to understand what kinds of negative and positive motivational processes influenced proximal outcomes. Specifically, we determined that we could classify two broad kinds of proximal motivational processes that occurred during learning and skill acquisition. The processes, which we named after descriptions provided by Kuhl (1985), were identified as *emotion control* and *motivation control*.

Emotion and Motivation Control

During the acquisition of a complex, but consistent and learnable task, effective learners appear to use two different kinds of skills. The first kind of skill, emotion control, involves efforts to minimize performance anxiety, worry, and off-task distractions that occur when the learner confronts initial frustrations and failures during the most difficult and demanding initial phases of skill acquisition. Learners with good emotion-control skills can maintain motivation and resist being sidetracked by self-blame or anticipation of negative consequences for performance failures while in the midst of task practice or training. Learners with poor emotion-control skills, in essence, compound the difficulty of learning a new task by being distracted by worry and anxiety (stress-related processes that effectively reduce the individual's available cognitive resources for the task).

Motivation-control skills appear to be most influential after an adequate level of performance has been reached, typically late in task practice. Learners with good motivation-control skills self-generate goals or find other ways to challenge themselves to improve on performance, even though the task may not actually demand it (e.g., because of a drop-off in the performance–utility function). Such learners often persist at a task, attempting to better their previous performance, or discover ways to compete against other learners, to maintain interest and motivational effort. Learners with poor motivation-control skills typically lower their effort when they reach an "acceptable" level of performance and, thus, may not develop their task skills to the maximum of their capability. We have described these individuals' learning curves as showing an *early asymptote*.

An effort to demonstrate that these processes are trainable skills was made in the context of a part-task training on the Kanfer–Ackerman ATC task (see R. Kanfer & Ackerman, 1990, 1996). We developed a set of training modules for both emotion control (which involved telling the learners not to worry about the performance early on in task practice and not to be distracted by the errors that they made) and motivation control (which involved telling the learners that they should make an additional effort late in practice to reach their own personal maximal performance). After the training, we then subjected the learners to the full ATC task, as a transfer-of-training design. In both cases we were successful. We found that the emotion-control training intervention improved early full-task transfer performance for lower ability trainees and that the motivation-control training improved full-task transfer performance late in transfer practice for higher ability trainees.

Motivational Skills as a Trait

Even though we (Ackerman & Kanfer, 1993) found that we could influence, to a degree, emotion- and motivation-control skills in the laboratory, our learners clearly entered the laboratory with substantial individual differences in these and other motivational skills. In the context of developing a selection battery for air traffic controllers, we attempted to assess the influence of these preexisting individual differences in motivational skills. Given our theoretical perspective of the joint motivational and cognitive ability determinants of skilled performance, though, it was critical to evaluate not just the simple correlational influence of a motivational skills measure but also to place it in the context of individual differences in ability. Toward this goal, we developed a short (18-item) measure of motivational skills, modeled on a broad self-efficacy orientation. The measure assessed the individual's self-confidence in several learning contexts: when memorizing new information, when recalling information for a test, when studying and doing homework, and when faced with a test.

The first thing to note about this measure is that it had low correlations with measures of cognitive ability in samples of university students and air traffic controller trainees (Ackerman & Kanfer, 1993). However, the measure has substantial validity for predicting criterion task performance in the laboratory ($r = .42$, with performance over 15 hours on a high-fidelity ATC task) and in the field ($r = .32$, for success in an $8\frac{1}{2}$ week training and selection program). Moreover, as might be expected from the low correlations with cognitive abilities, the motivational skills measure provided significant incremental validity (over and above the ability test battery) in predicting both the laboratory and the field criterion measures (increments of about 4% to 5% of variance accounted for).

It is also possible to place this motivational skills measure into a larger context. In a subsequent study (Ackerman, Kanfer, & Goff, 1995), we administered the motivational skills questionnaire to a sample of 93 undergraduate students who participated in a large ATC learning study. A battery of other trait measures was also administered, including measures of ability (math, spatial, and perceptual speed), personality (the Big Five), interests (the six themes identified by Holland: (realistic, investigative, artistic, social, enterprising, and conventional), academic self concept, and self-estimates of abilities. A full discussion of the results is beyond the scope of this chapter, but Figure 13.2 illustrates a multidimensional scaling solution of the

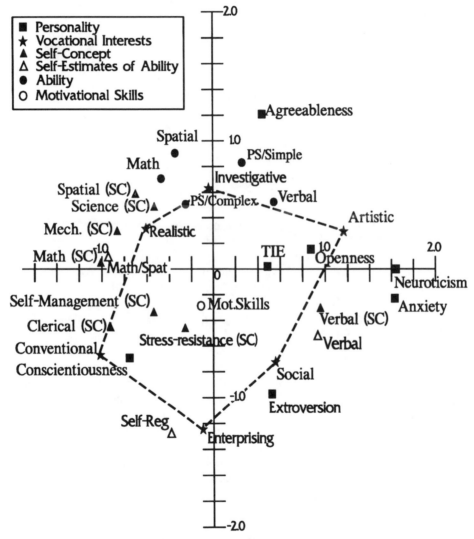

Figure 13.2. Kyst-3 multidimensional scaling solution to a battery of ability, personality, interest, self-concept, self-estimates of ability, and motivational skills measures. From "Cognitive and Noncognitive Determinants and Consequences of Complex Skill Acquisition," by P. L. Ackerman, R. Kanfer, and M. Goff, 1995, *Journal of Experimental Psychology: Applied, 1*, p. 292. Copyright 1995 by the American Psychological Association. Adapted with permission. SC = self-concept; Spat = spatial; PS = Perceptual Speed.

entire battery, including motivational skills. As can be clearly seen, the measure of motivational skills lies at the center of the solution, far removed from most other trait families (but close to a measure of stress resistance self-concept). We therefore believed that we might be assessing something quite different from traditional measures of not only ability but also personality and interests.

However well defined this measure was, at the level of traits, one important question remained for our construct validation: How do motivational skills such as emotion and motivation control relate to self-efficacy? The answer to this question requires that we digress a little into a discussion of what self-efficacy is, as it relates to learning and performance.

Self-Efficacy, Traits, Skills, and Things That Go "Bump" in the Night

Bandura (1986) and others (e.g., Locke & Latham, 1990) have suggested that the self-efficacy construct captures a substantial amount of information about future motivational effort, especially in learning and other change contexts. Thus, one might very well ask whether our conceptualization of motivational skills is simply another way of thinking about self-efficacy. In several studies, we (R. Kanfer, Ackerman, & Heggestad, 1996) have attempted to evaluate this issue, by examining what the determinants of self-efficacy are, as well as by directly relating our measure of motivational skills to a set of task-specific self-efficacy judgments.

In the first series of studies, we (R. Kanfer et al., 1996) examined the influence of four major trait families (ability, personality, interests, and self-concept) as potential determinants of task-specific self-efficacy. The tasks ranged from simple associative learning tasks (e.g., the noun-pair task; see Ackerman & Woltz, 1994, for a discussion), to the low-fidelity ATC task, and to the high-fidelity ATC simulation task (called TRACON [Terminal Radar Approach Control]).

The first issue we (R. Kanfer et al., 1996) investigated was whether any traits predict individual differences in self-efficacy; that is, prior to the individual's first hands-on task trial (but after instruction). In each study, we found that individual differences in cognitive and perceptual abilities accounted for the largest amount of task-specific self-efficacy variance (from 11% to 20% variance accounted for), followed by self-concept (roughly 4% to 5% of variance accounted for), and interests (2% to 6% of variance accounted for). Motivational skills measures (both our own and also motivational skills as measured by the Pintrich, Smith, Garcia, and Mc-Keachie [1993] Motivated Strategies for Learning Questionnaire) significantly correlated with initial-task self-efficacy. However, after entering ability, self-concept, and interests into a prediction equation for initial self-efficacy, motivational skills accounted for a nonsignificant degree of variance in self-efficacy.

In one study, R. Kanfer et al. (1996) administered all three of the tasks mentioned previously to the same group of participants, along with measures of motivational skills, abilities, interests, personality, and self-concept. Figure 13.3 illustrates a path model for predicting self-efficacy for the three tasks (which were given in a fixed sequential order). Two interesting effects should be highlighted here. First, initial self-efficacy (on the TRACON task) was well-predicted by a personality complex of anxiety and by math/science self-concept (which was predicted by objective ability and measures of achievement motivation). Only the associative-learning-task self-efficacy had a significant prediction from motivational skills and self-management

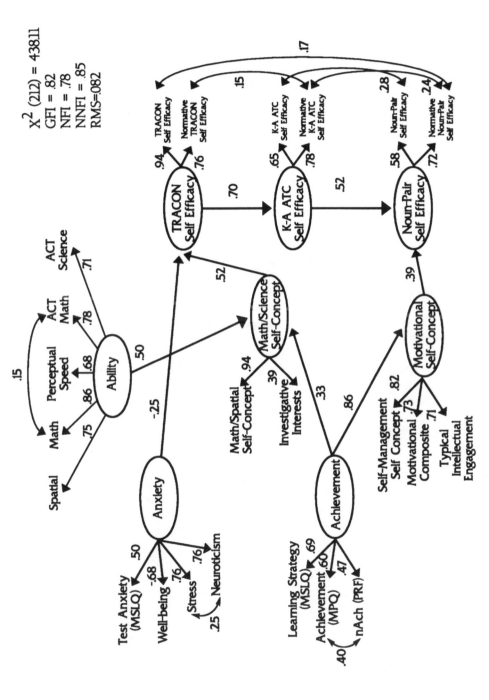

Figure 13.3. LISREL derived structural equation model for ability and nonability trait measures and self-efficacy from TRACON (Terminal Radar Approach Control), K-A ATC (Kanfer–Ackerman Air Traffic Control), and noun-pair tasks. PRF = Personality Research Form; ACT = American College Testing; MPQ = Multidimensional Personality Questionnaire; MSLQ = Motivated Strategies for Learning Questionnaire. From "Motivational Skills and Self-Regulation for Learning: A Trait Perspective," by R. Kanfer, P. L. Ackerman, and E. D. Heggestad, 1996, *Learning and Individual Differences, 8,* p. 204. Copyright 1996 by JAI Press. Reprinted with permission.

self-concept (which we called a "motivational self-concept complex"). Second, and perhaps most interesting for our consideration of motivational skills as a construct, was that three quite divergent tasks had highly correlated self-efficacy scores. That is, far from being task-specific, individuals had transsituational self-efficacy judgments. At least in the kind of learning and skill acquisition environments we (R. Kanfer et al., 1996) have studied, it appears that initial self-efficacy is well determined by traditionally described trait families of aptitudes, personality, and interests. In addition, individual differences in self-efficacy for learning tasks appear to be much more general than would be expected from previous self-efficacy research. Moreover, initial self-efficacy generally fails to predict task performance after substantial task practice.

If much of self-efficacy variance can be accounted for by traditionally assessed individual-differences traits, what accounts for high correlations between self-efficacy and performance? The answer, it turns out, was not motivational skills. Instead, the association between self-efficacy judgments and task performance during practice is wholly accounted for by individual differences in prior task trial performance (e.g., Ackerman et al., 1995). That is, if one computes a correlation between self-efficacy after trial n and task performance on trial $n + 1$, but partials trial n performance out of the equation, the resulting correlation is effectively zero. In less quantitative language, it appears that self-efficacy (after the learner first confronts a new task) is wholly accounted for by prior task performance.

Given the results that many extant traits, such as self-concept, predict initial task self-efficacy, we were left with the conclusion that self-efficacy in the kinds of learning contexts under discussion, rather than being inextricably intertwined with motivational skills, is an epiphenomenon. That is, measures of initial self-efficacy can be replaced with other trait measures to predict initial task performance validly, and measures of self-efficacy taken during task practice simply reflect how well the individual performs the task and add nothing motivational beyond measures of prior task performance.

Summary

At this point, we believe that we have made substantial progress in delineating important aspects of motivation for learning and skill acquisition. First, we determined that two different aspects of motivational processing appear to be important in different phases of skill acquisition. Emotion control is important early in learning, when the cognitive demands of the task are most effort consumptive. Motivation control is important late in learning, when the learner can perform the task adequately, but in which additional effort can lead to subsequent improvement in task performance. Moreover, individual differences in ability interact with the effects of such motivational processing. Lower ability learners benefit most from emotion-control skill training, and higher ability learners benefit most from motivation-control skill training. In addition, the differences in motivational skills that learners bring to a new skill acquisition environment predict later performance differences — in the absence of an explicit motivational skill training program. Finally, self-efficacy appears to provide no additional information in the learning context (over and above other traits of ability, self-concept, etc.) prior to task engagement and no additional information over and above prior task performance, once the learner engages the task. Although we seemed to be getting a good sense of emotion control and motivation control skills at the micro level, two things appeared to be lacking: (a) a nomological network describing how motivational traits and skills related to one another and (b) a better sense of where motivational traits fit within a larger nomolological network of trait classes. The next section describes our efforts at taxonomizing motivational traits and skills, as well as how motivational traits relate to other trait classes.

Revisiting Motivational Traits

Rather than starting off by rediscovering the wheel, we began our taxonomic approach to motivational traits by reviewing two sources of extant literature. The first source was to look at historical conceptual treatments of motivational traits, and the second was to examine assessment batteries and scales that purported to measure motivationally relevant traits. A full discussion of our efforts can be found in Kanfer and Heggestad (1997), but we briefly highlight some of the critical points in the following paragraphs.

Review and Analysis of Extant Literature

Our first pass through the literature indicated that there appear to be two broad classes of motivational traits: those that are *appetitive* (orientation toward expending effort on work tasks), and those that are *aversive* (orientation away from expending effort on work tasks), which we denote as the two broad trait classes of achievement and anxiety. Figure 13.4 shows an illustration of how we see these traits and their components in a larger task–environment milieu. On the basis of work by Murray (1938), Atkinson (1957), and others (e.g., Argyle & Robinson, 1962; Helmreich & Spence, 1978; Nicholls, 1984), we have subdivided the achievement traits into *mastery* (a desire to do well on tasks) and *competitive excellence* (a desire to perform better than others). On the basis of our review of the anxiety literature (Kanfer & Heggestad, 1997), and suggestions by several others (e.g., Alpert & Haber, 1960; Hembree, 1988; Herman, 1990; Morris, Davis, & Hutchings, 1981; Sarason, 1978; Tobias, 1985), the anxiety traits can be subdivided into *general anxiety, test anxiety,* and *fear of failure*. These represent broad, transsituational traits that are believed to be influential across many different tasks and environments.

We also added the motivation- and emotion-control skills (which, as we have shown, also have traitlike characteristics in adult learners) in which the presence of motivation-control skills yields appetitive behaviors (increased effort toward the task at hand), and the lack of emotion-control skills yields aversive behaviors (decreased effort toward the task at hand).

The next step for consideration of this taxonomy was to review assessment batteries and scales to find out whether extant measures were available for assessing the various components of achievement and anxiety motivational traits. The results of the review (R. Kanfer & Heggestad, 1997) were both surprising and challenging. In the domain of achievement, we reviewed the contents of 19 well-known self-report measures of trait differences in achievement (including, for example, the Edwards Personal Preference Schedule [Edwards, 1959], Tellegen's Multidimensional Per-

303

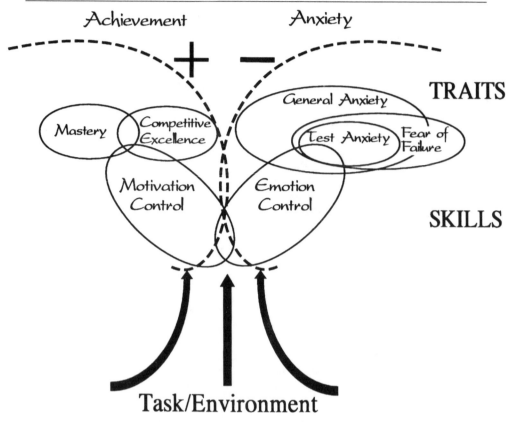

Figure 13.4. Taxonomic framework of motivationally relevant traits and skills. Motivational trait and skill constructs are represented by the solid ovals. The dashed lines indicate the influences of traits, skills, and tasks–environments. From "Motivational Traits and Skills: A Person-Centered Approach to Work Motivation," by R. Kanfer and E. D. Heggestad, 1997, in L. L. Cummings and B. M. Staw, Editors, *Research in Organizational Behavior* (Vol. 19, p. 11). Copyright 1997 by JAI Press. Reprinted with permission.

sonality Questionnaire [MPQ; Tellegen, 1982], the California Psychological Inventory [Gough, 1987], the Jackson Personality Research Form [Jackson, 1984], and Costa and McCrae's NEO–PI–Revised [Costa & McCrae, 1992]), each of which contains an achievement-oriented scale or subscale. Across this wide range of so-called "achievement" measures, fewer than half of the scales (8) include even one item that appears to assess the competitive excellence aspect of achievement. That is, Murray's (1938) notions of competitive excellence had little representation in most measures of achievement traits. Only three measures explicitly separate a mastery motivational achievement trait from a competitive excellence motivation achievement trait (viz., the Nicholls Motivational Orientation Scales [Nicholls, 1989], the Roedel, Schraw, and Plake Goals Inventory [1994], and the Work and Family Orientation Questionnaire [WOFO; Helmreich & Spence, 1978]), none of which is typically considered in a larger framework of other broad personality traits. All of this suggested to us that there was a substantial need for evaluating mastery and competitive excellence in a broader empirical framework.

In the domain of anxiety-related motivational traits, we found substantially more extensive theoretical and empirical research. Much discussion has been offered in the literature about all three traits that make up the anxiety or aversive complex of traits. Our reading of the literature suggested that fear of failure, test anxiety, and general anxiety constructs all have a number of communalities, but they are sufficiently different so that they cannot be easily consolidated in the context of motivation. From a measurement perspective, we found that, at least for general anxiety (and to some degree for test anxiety), by the way in which the constructs were assessed, it was not clear that the traits were sufficiently situationally oriented toward motivational (or task-relevant) behaviors. No extant measures of anxiety delineated the trait in work or task situations from more general anxiety. Conversely, measures of test anxiety were seen as too narrow to provide information about individual differences in aversion to evaluation-oriented task situations. Consistent with previous work about the situationally dependent nature of some broad personality traits (e.g., see discussion in Murtha, Kanfer, & Ackerman, 1996), we conjectured that it might be useful to develop a series of measures that could effectively assess these aversive-oriented traits in a task and work context.

To provide an evaluation of these various issues (e.g., separating mastery and competitive excellence and separating test anxiety from other kinds of motivational anxieties), we set out to create an instrument that would specifically assess each of these hypothesized broad and narrow traits, within a single self-report questionnaire. We could then, in turn, compare these measures with one another and with extant measures of personality, ability, interests, and other relevant traits.

The Motivational Trait Questionnaire

In a series of iterative studies in which items were developed, tried out, and scales revised and the procedure repeated (Heggestad, 1997; Heggestad & Kanfer, 1997), we have explored the structure of motivational traits and the relations between such traits and other trait families. The current version of the Motivational Trait Questionnaire (MTQ) is composed of 157 self-report items. Analyses of the MTQ reveal three well-replicated broad motivational trait factors, identified as *Personal Mastery*, *Competitive Excellence*, and *Motivational Anxiety*. A brief illustration of construct validation results can be seen in Table 13.1, which shows derived correlations between the MTQ factors and several personality and extant motivational measures. Although significant correlations are found between the two appetitive motivational trait factors and scales of the WOFO, and Motivational Anxiety shares variance with several extant general anxiety measures, it is most telling that the Competitive Excellence motivational trait shares little variance with measures of the Big-Five personality factors (e.g., the NEO-Five-Factor Inventory [FFI]) and with Tellegen's MPQ. The only salient correlation with these traditional personality measures is the negative association with Agreeableness on the NEO-FFI (which is probably more illustrative of the fact that competitively oriented individuals are seen as perhaps less agreeable than those who have low orientation to competitive excellence).

Such results provide at least partial support of our approach to motivational traits. On the one hand, it appears that we can augment assessment of appetitive motivational traits by including measures of competitive excellence along with the more traditional measures of mastery. On the other hand, we have found (as others have

305

TABLE 13.1 Correlations Between MTQ Factors and Relevant Personality Measures

Variable	Factor		
	Anxiety	Personal mastery	Competitive excellence
Work and family orientation			
Mastery	−.069	**.569**	.124
Work	.087	**.593**	.022
Competitiveness	.065	−.048	**.759**
Strait–Trait Anxiety Inventory			
(Trait anxiety)	**.568**	−.174	−.069
NEO-Five Factor Inventory			
Neuroticism	**.623**	−.162	−.059
Extroversion	−.125	.159	.163
Openness	−.059	**.338**	−.159
Agreeableness	−.056	.222	−**.345**
Conscientious	.035	**.439**	.030
Typical intellectual engagement	.010	**.602**	−.169
Motivational skills	.010	.253	.000
MPQ			
Control	.282	.297	−.148
Stress reaction	**.709**	−.108	−.009
Absorption	.155	.255	−.189
Traditionalism	**.406**	.115	.002
Harm avoidance	.171	.034	−.073

Note. Salient loadings ($\geq$.3) in boldfaced type. MTQ = Motivational Trait Questionnaire; MPQ = Multidimensional Personality Questionnaire. From *Motivation From a Personality Perspective: The Development of a Measure of Motivational Traits*, by E. D. Heggestad, 1997, unpublished doctoral dissertation, University of Minnesota, Twin Cities. Adapted with permission of the author.

in studying the broad personality trait of anxiety) that the aversive motivational traits (e.g., worry, emotionality, active avoidance, failure affect, and public embarrassment) are not well differentiated from broader anxiety traits. At this relatively early stage of our research program, it is not clear whether such aversive aspects of motivation are essentially the same as a broad personality trait of anxiety or whether we have insufficiently designed our measures to assess the trait complex. Of course, a third possibility is that our college student respondents are insufficiently experienced with the world of work and occupations, such that they do not quite understand the questions. This last possibility is currently being evaluated with a sample of 30–60-year-old respondents.

Summary, Conclusions, and Implications

We started our discussion about motivation with a set of definitions, regarding motivation as a set of processes that lead to choice behaviors and in terms of the degree of attentional effort devoted to a task. Both sources of motivational variance are important to the consideration of individual differences in learning. When a trainee is confronted with a task that requires a greater amount of effort than he or she is willing to expend in the learning environment (or when the perceived utility of performance is insufficiently strong), the trainee may simply abandon the task. Distal traits appear to be influential in determining individual differences in such choice behaviors. Such traits (which include ability, personality, and self-concept factors) generally determine the measures known colloquially as self-efficacy.

Within the learning environment (i.e., after the individual chooses to engage the task), we found two important motivational skills that appear to influence the learner success. The first type of skill we referred to as emotional control — those processes that enable the learner to keep from being distracted by worry and other negative emotions early in task practice. The second type of skill we referred to as motivation control — those processes that spur the learner to increased effort, after a rough level of acceptable performance has been reached. Although such skills can be developed to a degree through instructional interventions, we found that individuals differ in the levels of these kinds of skills that they bring to the learning situation. Such skills capture variance in complex task performance that is not shared with cognitive and intellectual abilities.

We also described the first steps of a research program that attempts to delineate a broad set of motivational traits, including traditional concepts of achievement and anxiety, but also a trait complex of competitive excellence. Our early empirical work in this area suggests that there is much construct overlap with extant measures of personality, for aspects of achievement motivation and motivational aspects of anxiety, but that there is substantially less overlap for measures of competitive excellence.

One of the things that makes the study of motivational traits and skills interesting in the learning context is that motivation represents a qualitatively different class of constructs from intelligence. That is, unlike most intelligence and learning research (in which intelligence is a preexisting trait), we can work with motivation as both a trait and a treatment. At once, however, this aspect of motivation complicates rather than simplifies the picture. If individuals differ in their perceived effort–performance function (with some learners viewing adequate performance as beyond their capabilities, and others perceiving that the effort–performance function will change with task practice), we can either select (for employment) those individuals who have such an incremental view of learning or provide remediation, so that learners more accurately view the task demands (and thus decide to expend effort on the task). We can also provide instruction, so that learners deficient in either emotion- or motivation-control skills can compensate for inherent task characteristics that are "demotivating." Such interventions are believed to have their maximal impact at the level of proximal motivational processes.

However, the trait-level investigations we have completed suggest that there is a number of motivational dimensions along which individuals differ in orientation. Individuals at the high end on aversive motivational traits will seek to avoid task challenge, whereas those at the high end on appetitive motivational traits seek out the same kind of challenge. (Note that those who are at the high end on both aversive and appetitive motivational traits may engage the task but be "high-maintenance" learners — requiring frequent assurance and other kinds of hand-holding — see R. Kanfer & Heggestad, 1997, for a discussion of this issue.)

Ultimately, the best understanding of the roles of motivational traits and skills in the context of learning appears to be through the study of aptitude–treatment interactions. In the final analysis, it seems that motivation in the context of learning is not reducible to a single general trait or a single skill. The future for research in this area is promising, in that there is simply a lot of uncharted territory left to be explored.

REFERENCES

Ackerman, P. L., & Kanfer, R. (1993). Integrating laboratory and field study for improving selection: Development of a battery for predicting Air Traffic Controller success. *Journal of Applied Psychology, 78,* 413–432.

Ackerman, P. L., Kanfer, R., & Goff, M. (1995). Cognitive and non-cognitive determinants of complex skill acquisition. *Journal of Experimental Psychology: Applied, 1,* 270–304.

Ackerman, P. L., & Woltz, D. J. (1994). Determinants of learning and performance in an associative memory/substitution task: Task constraints, individual differences, and volition. *Journal of Educational Psychology, 86,* 487–515.

Alpert, R., & Haber, R. N. (1960). Anxiety in academic situations. *Journal of Abnormal and Social Psychology, 61,* 207–215.

Argyle, M., & Robinson, P. (1962). Two origins of achievement motivation. *British Journal of Social and Clinical Psychology, 1,* 107–120.

Atkinson, J. W. (1957). Motivational determinants of risk taking behavior. *Psychological Review, 64,* 359–372.

Baddeley, A. D. (1986). *Working memory.* London: Oxford University Press.

Baddeley, A. D. (1996). *Human memory,* Oxford, England: Clarendon Press.

Bandura, A. (1986). *Social foundations of thought and action.* Englewood Cliffs, NJ: Prentice Hall.

Costa, P. T., Jr., & McCrae, R. R. (1992). *Revised NEO Personality Inventory and Five-Factor Inventory professional manual.* Odessa, FL: Psychological Assessment Resources.

Dweck, C. S. (1986). Motivational processes affecting learning. *American Psychologist, 41,* 1040–1048.

Dweck, C. S., & Leggett, E. L. (1988). A social–cognitive approach to motivation and personality. *Psychological Review, 95,* 256–273.

Edwards, A. L. (1959). *Edwards Personal Preference Schedule.* New York: Psychological Corporation.

Gollwitzer, P. M. (1990). Action phases and mind-sets. In E. T. Higgins & R. M. Sorrentino (Eds.), *Handbook of motivation and cognition: Foundations of social behavior* (Vol. 2, pp. 53–92). New York: Guilford Press.

Gough, H. G. (1987). *California Psychological Inventory administrators guide.* Palo Alto, CA: Consulting Psychologists Press.

Heckhausen, H. (1991). *Motivation and action.* New York: Springer-Verlag.

Heggestad, E. D. (1997). *Motivation from a personality perspective: The development of a measure of motivational traits.* Unpublished doctoral dissertation, University of Minnesota, Twin Cities.

Heggestad, E. D., & Kanfer, R. (1997). *Assessment of motivational traits: Development and validation of the Motivational Trait Questionnaire.* Unpublished manuscript.

Helmreich, R. L., & Spence, J. T. (1978). The Work and Family Orientation Questionnaire: An objective instrument to assess components of achievement motivation and attitudes toward family and career. *JSAS Catalog of Selected Documents in Psychology, 8,* 35.

Hembree, R. (1988). Correlates, causes, effects, and treatment of test anxiety. *Review of Educational Research, 58,* 47–77.

Herman, W. E. (1990). Fear of failure as a distinctive personality trait measure of test anxiety. *Journal of Research and Development in Education, 23,* 180–185.

Holland, J. L. (1973). *Making vocational choices: A theory of careers.* Englewood Cliffs, NJ: Prentice Hall.

Jackson, D. N. (1984). *Personality Research Form manual* (3rd ed.). Port Huron, MI: Research Psychologists Press.

Kahneman, D. (1973). *Attention and effort.* Englewood Cliffs, NJ: Prentice Hall.

Kanfer, F., & Schefft, B. K. (1988). *Guiding the process of therapeutic change.* Champaign, IL: Research Press.

Kanfer, R. (1987). Task-specific motivation: An integrative approach to issues of measurement, mechanisms, processes, and determinants. *Journal of Social and Clinical Psychology, 5,* 237–264.

Kanfer, R. (1990). Motivation theory and industrial/organizational psychology. In M. D. Dunnette & L. Hough (Eds.), *Handbook of industrial and organizational psychology: Vol. 1. Theory in industrial and organizational psychology* (pp. 75–170). Palo Alto, CA: Consulting Psychologists Press.

Kanfer, R., & Ackerman, P. L. (1989). Motivation and cognitive abilities: An integrative/aptitude–treatment interaction approach to skill acquisition [Monograph]. *Journal of Applied Psychology, 74,* 657–690.

Kanfer, R., & Ackerman, P. L. (1990). *Ability and metacognitive determinants of skill acquisition and transfer.* Air Force Office of Scientific Research Final Report, Minneapolis, MN.

Kanfer, R., & Ackerman, P. L. (1996). A self-regulatory skills perspective to reducing cognitive interference. In I. G. Sarason, B. R. Sarason, & G. R. Pierce (Eds.), *Cognitive interference: Theories, methods, and findings* (pp. 153–171). Mahwah, NJ: Erlbaum.

Kanfer, R., Ackerman, P. L., & Heggestad, E. (1996). Motivational skills and self-regulation for learning: A trait perspective. *Learning and Individual Differences, 8,* 185–209.

Kanfer, R., Ackerman, P. L., Murtha, T. C., Dugdale, B., & Nelson, L. (1994). Goal setting, conditions of practice, and task performance: A resource allocation pespective. *Journal of Applied Psychology, 79,* 826–835.

Kanfer, R., & Heggestad, E. (1997). Motivational traits and skills: A person-centered approach to work motivation. In L. L. Cummings & B. M. Staw (Eds.), *Research in organizational behavior* (Vol. 19, pp. 1–57). Greenwich, CT: JAI Press.

Kuhl, J. (1985). Volitional mediators of cognition–behavior consistency: Self-regulatory processes and action vs. state orientation. In J. Kuhl & J. Beckmann (Eds.), *Action control: From cognition to behavior* (pp. 101–128). New York: Springer-Verlag.

Kyllonen, P. C., & Christal, R. E. (1990). Reasoning ability is (little more than) working-memory capacity?! *Intelligence, 14,* 389–433.

Locke, E., & Latham, G. P. (1990). *A theory of goal setting and task performance.* Englewood Cliffs, NJ: Prentice Hall.

Morris, L. W., Davis, M. A., & Hutchings, C. H. (1981). Cognitive and emotional components of anxiety: Literature review and a revised Worry-Emotionality Scale. *Journal of Educational Psychology, 73,* 541–555.

Murray, H. A. (1938). *Explorations in personality.* New York: Oxford University Press.

Murtha, T. C., Kanfer, R., & Ackerman, P. L. (1996). Towards an interactionist taxonomy of personality and situations. An integrative situational–dispositional representation of personality traits. *Journal of Personality and Social Psychology, 71,* 193–207.

Nicholls, J. G. (1984). Achievement motivation: Conceptions of ability, subjective experience, task choice, and performance. *Psychological Review, 91,* 328–346.

Nicholls, J. G. (1989). *The competitive ethos and democratic education.* Cambridge, MA: Harvard University Press.

Norman, D. A., & Bobrow, D. G. (1975). On data-limited and resource-limited processes. *Cognitive Psychology, 7,* 44–64.

Pintrich, P. R., Smith, D. A. F., Garcia, T., & McKeachie, W. J. (1993). Reliability and predictive validity of the Motivated Strategies for Learning Questionnaire (MSLQ). *Educational and Psychological Measurement, 53,* 801–813.

Roedel, T. D., Schraw, G., & Plake, B. S. (1994). Validation of a measure of learning and performance goal orientations. *Educational and Psychological Measurement, 54,* 1013–1021.

Sarason, I. G. (1978). The test anxiety scale: Concept and research. In I. G. Sarason & C. D. Spielberger (Eds.), *Stress and anxiety* (Vol. 2, pp. 27–44). Washington, DC: Hemisphere.

Tellegen, A. (1982). *Brief manual for the Multidimensional Personality Questionnaire (MPQ).* Minneapolis, MN: Author.

Tobias, S. (1985). Test anxiety: Interference, defective skills, and cognitive capacity. *Educational Psychologist, 20,* 135–142.

Zeaman, D. (1978). Some relations of general intelligence and selective attention. *Intelligence, 2,* 55–73.

Discussion

Several points were raised in the discussion of Kanfer's paper about the status of motivational constructs in relation to other constructs raised in other presentations, such as interests, arousal, and personality. Subsequent discussion centered around the workplace and sports-skills implications of Kanfer's model of motivational traits and skills.

Dr. Wittmann: I thought about asking you for a helping hand for a distinction between motivation and interest. I'm interested in how much time-on-task is invested and that must have something to do with motivation or with interest. Then after awhile you showed that beautiful multidimensional solution with motivation in the middle. And that reminded me, couldn't we interpret that motivation as a total effort, a kind of g of interest? Would you agree with that? That's my first point.

My second point. You referred to these studies with the massed practice and the spaced practice. I was immediately reminded about Dr. Baddeley and working memory. Didn't you produce with these studies a kind of a working memory overload that interfered with the performance of those not having the right amount of working memory capacity and with the spaced practice you reduced that overload?

Dr. Kanfer: Yes.

Dr. Wittmann: And what about the motivation construct in terms of self-efficacy or self-monitoring? Where is self-monitoring? Isn't it possible that somebody who has the right motivation just tailors his or her invested time to the amount of working memory he or she has and then has the best performance. Those who are over-motivated deteriorate and those who are not motivated are worse because they just do nothing and thus we have the Yerkes-Dodson law back again.

Dr. Kanfer: I would argue that motivational skills are distinct from interests and

310

that the interests are determinants of those skills. I see them as skills and as flexible and malleable through training and not as represented as interests alone. Because they're not interests. They are more reasonably thought of as a function of traits. A more complete model would add interest and self-concept as you saw in the LISREL results. All of those things. But I do mean them as skills. I do not mean them as a construct like G.

For the massed and the spaced practice experiment, the answer is yes. The resource allocation model would argue that there are indeed self-regulatory processes that divert attentional resources and that you can have a positive or a negative effect. That is, you can have a facilitating or a debilitating effect by the initiation of a "motivational" intervention. That's what the spaced versus massed experiment results really represent. No time allowed for self-regulation in the massed practice condition. However, in the spaced condition, there is time for the productive use of these self-regulatory processes.

The third point about overarousal is more difficult to deal with. At this point the explanation that you're talking about . . . I'm making no sophisticated assumptions about how these skills work. I'm not saying these are metacognitive. I'm saying these are really rough strategies or skills. You're arguing that there is some correction going on here for moving back if you're overly motivated. And I'm not arguing for those kinds of skills operating here. I'm talking about a repertoire of strategies that people have for coping with situations that involve adjustments and attentional effort that the task does not provide them, or that is contrary to what the task environment in their own skill or their own abilities would lead them to naturally. The role of self-monitoring and self-evaluation and so on, that is part of self-regulation, and when I talk about emotion-control skills, I'm talking about that in an integrated whole. And that was my argument about why we're interested in the *functions* of self-regulatory processes as opposed to the *operations*. So you can show that for people who don't self-monitor, things go wrong and their performance is poor. But then other people show that it depends on what they self-monitor. So I know that self-monitoring, self-evaluation, and self-reactions are all important components of self-regulatory skill. I'm saying it's contained within the emotion-control strategies and motivation-control strategies if that answers that question.

Dr. Baddeley: Really just a thought and a suggestion. It struck me that some of the skills you were talking about would have a very interesting application in the area of neuropsychological rehabilitation, which I think might be a very good test bed for some of your ideas. Because one does get exaggerated differences in the dimensions you talk about and huge interpersonal differences in the extent to which people cope with their problems which are often, almost all orthogonal to how great their problems are. And I wondered if anyone was working in that area.

Dr. Kanfer: I don't know. My actual interest in self-regulation started with depression. And that's where I started with this notion. I don't know in rehabilitation whether or not they have studied these issues. I'm sure there is self-regulation training in rehabilitation situations. Instead, I may have picked the most difficult situation, which is trying to account for performance variance among normals in an ongoing cumulative achievement environment. I guess you would argue that I made it really hard. But I also wanted to make it absolutely clear that such skills play a role and are independent of abilities.

But I agree, and that would be very interesting to look at that and to bring together the literature from the clinical domain. There has been some work by Ann Brown and others on children and there are ability limits on self-regulation training. And to bring that literature together and see what the outside parameters would be and this magnitude of effects would be very interesting.

Dr. Matthews: The motivational skills constructs you talked about seem to be proximal influences on performance in a variety of contexts. But I have a couple of questions about the status of these skills variables as measurement constructs. First of all, to what extent do you see them as transient states rather than stable traits? And secondly, to what extent can you bring them under experimental control? Perhaps some people are so achievement oriented that they are as motivated to perform as they can be, regardless of what you tell them in the experiments.

Dr. Kanfer: I don't think there's a problem. First of all, I don't think they're traits. They're skills. They're not traits. And part of the point about that is because the trait–performance relationships are low, and they should be low. If they were a lot higher, it would be odd. And if they were any lower, it would be odd. And they're low because skills intervene as the most proximal determinants of performance. So they're not traits. As for malleability — I'm arguing that part of it is cumulative and part of it's developmental and part of it is through goal choice, part of it is motivational, part of it is ability.

Now, one way that you could look at this — and I think this question came up in your talk as well — is you can find environments when the political environment changes so dramatically and now initiative was expected, and how quickly people learn motivational control skills to take action in the absence of environmental support. And it's very interesting. (For example, Michael Frese has done this in what was East Germany where he's looked at environments where people traditionally did not take initiative.)

So there are opportunities in nature, in the natural environment, such as organizational downsizing, and we are doing some research on that. Downsizing, when people lose their jobs and are forced to go into training environments that they would never have selected. We would then look at the operation of motivation-control skills and emotion-control skills there. Before we can really do that effectively, of course, we have to be able to have reliable and valid measures, so that's our first order of business.

As a function of individual differences, what brought them into the situation, perhaps historical variables or some data that we're currently looking at that we collected, I showed you the Dwyer extension, but we have some behavioral data as well which shows some childhood history relationships to these trait dimensions as well.

Dr. Hunt: There is another area that's very easy for you to do research in because you get a great deal of cooperation in that field. I'll throw it out because it badly needs some work. And that is the motivational skills of a college athlete. Because what happens is that they come in, every one of them thinking as freshman, that they're going to have a great big professional career in the revenue sports. About three quarters of them find out very quickly that they're not, but they still have another opportunity to do well in college which is something previously they had not been motivated . . .

Dr. Ackerman: Yes. But, Buz, Ruth already mentioned that there's a threshold of ability in order to do self-regulation.

Dr. Hunt: That is the sort of remark that you get from academics who don't actually work with them. Many of these young men and women are, in fact, quite capable, especially at the high-end universities. Places like Stanford where it's harder to get in than it is to succeed.

Dr. Kanfer: Well, what we've studied is our coaches and coaching strategies. Because what we wanted to know is, do they train or implement motivation-control skills, emotion-control skills? Which athletes do they use it for? What's the expertise that makes a great coach? And what kind of skills is he or she using? We have some preliminary data. Coaches do use primarily emotion-control skills — at least that is what they report they use. We don't have observational data. I think the more interesting information on the skills will come from what coaches actually do. It's really the study in a kind of Ericsson-type question of "What do experts supposedly do?" This is what coaches are supposed to do. And then who do they differentially apply it to.

Dr. Hunt: There's a lot of data on that, not for college level but little league coaches. Ron Smith at the University of Washington has very extensive studies on amateur coaches and what they do.

Dr. Kanfer: The first thing that we have done with one of our students, Amy Enrooth, is we've tried to extend the approach to achievement motivation. Almost every item in traditional measures concerns *academic* achievement. So one study we just completed says, let's talk about achievement in three domains. Work, home, and athletic achievement. We wanted to see whether motivation- and emotion-control skills were perceived as needed in the same way in those two domains. I want to make sure that I'm not talking about different things as a function of domain. So you can talk about achievement, and when you talk about achievement in athletics and achievement in academics, mental effort may be very different than physical effort for most people.

14

Mining on the "No Man's Land" Between Intelligence and Personality

LAZAR STANKOV

The aims of this chapter are threefold: First, to review briefly some recent work on self-confidence and emotional intelligence. Second, to call readers' attention to several life-span developmental studies that point to a diminishing role of cognitive abilities in the prediction of individuals' accomplishments. Third, to suggest future research in the area of social attitudes that may elucidate the emerging role of people's outlooks in such prediction. The import of this approach can be better appreciated if one takes into account the social and theoretical background of psychologists' professional activities.

The Context

The development of psychology as a profession in the course of the twentieth century was characterized by a shift away from philosophy and toward a broadly defined area of "social engineering." Medical sciences provided the model. A powerful instrument in that move was the increased use of psychological tests. It is possible to argue that the initial work in individual differences paved the way for societal support for many areas of experimental psychology. The future looked bright at the dawn of this century, and the profession has thrived ever since. What is the outlook for the study of individual differences (and perhaps psychology) at this *fin de siècle*? One concern for all psychologists must be signs of an intended reduction in funding for psychological research by some government agencies.

The causes of possible cuts in funding can be traced, at least in part, to psychologists' own failure to inform the decision makers that the views made vocal by some are not necessarily accepted by all. In my opinion, two views have been particularly damaging. First, there has been an unjustified tendency to overemphasize the role of the general factor at the expense of broad (e.g., Gf [fluid intelligence], Gc [crystallized intelligence], and so forth) and primary factors (Jensen, 1997). A logical conclusion on the part of the decision makers is that research into the usefulness of a variety of tasks is unnecessary — virtually any cognitive task that has satisfactory psychometric properties will do. This is not only an impoverished view of human cognition but is also scientifically dubious because it ignores a large body of contrary evidence. Although the existence of positive manifold among cognitive tests cannot be denied (e.g., Carroll, 1993, reported that the mean of all correlations surveyed in his work was approximately .30), Horn (1997) argued that "positive manifold, and the general factor that can always be calculated on it, does not, in itself, support Spearman's hypothesis of g." A single factor is commonly extracted in studies that place undue emphasis on g. Even if researchers agree with Carroll (1993, p. 624) that "there is abundant evidence for a factor of general intelligence, G, at the highest order of analysis," the spirit of his three stratum theory is lost in the use of a single first-order factor as a proxy. In my own experience, the inclusion of a broad variety of tasks that vary in terms of difficulty and complexity tends to produce a weaker general factor than studies that are based on a narrower sampling of tasks. Thus, when the battery contains both measures of higher order processes and also sensory and psychomotor tasks, the first principal component accounts for only around 20% of the total variance (see Roberts, Stankov, Pallier, & Dolph, 1998).

Second, there is currently a strong tendency to search for biological bases of individual differences. From one point of view, this is natural because the emergence of new technologies (e.g., magnetic resonance imaging and positron–emission tomography) opens the possibility of working at the frontiers of knowledge. It is hard to understand, however, the continuing enthusiasm for this kind of research, given that the outcomes to date have not been very encouraging. Correlations between biological measures and intelligence have remained unimpressive (cf. Stankov & Roberts, 1997) — most are rather low and some have also produced contradictory outcomes. The effects are not any stronger than those achieved through educational interventions. I also think that this simplistic reductionistic agenda has had a stifling influence on explorations of cognitive correlates of intelligence that have been successful in demonstrating a link, for example, between working memory and intelligence (Kyllonen & Christal, 1990; Myors, Stankov, & Oliphant, 1989). While researchers should continue to look through the windows opened by the new technologies, links need to be rekindled with the theoretically fertile area of experimental cognitive psychology. For example, researchers are still far from understanding the notion of complexity in its relationship to intelligence. It is time to move on.

Beyond g and Mindlessness

In this chapter, I outline the directions of some current research in Australia that moves researchers away from g and reductionism. This work pertains to the poorly explored "no man's land" between human abilities and personality. All of this work is in the spirit of the "grand picture" sketched out by Cattell (1971), among others, and enhanced recently by Ackerman (1996). Importantly, most of it is also characterized by the use of new assessment and measurement procedures. Those who criticize "soft-psychology" from the reductionistic position often emphasize the poor measurement properties of the various instruments that have been used. These critics argue that such "land mines" should be avoided to gain scientific credibility. Therefore, I present recent studies that are based on fresh instruments and procedures that may circumvent such problems.

My focus is on (a) the role of metacognitive processes (including self-confidence) when answering cognitive test items and (b) the place of emotional intelligence within the overall structure of abilities and personality. "New" methodologies related to these topics include the measurement of confidence ratings derived from items within cognitive tests and consensual measures of emotional intelligence. Because much recent work has been devoted to studies of self-confidence, in the major part of this chapter I review work in this area. There also appears to be a need to reexamine (a) the relationship between intelligence and interests and outlooks in life and (b) the relationship between intelligence and new measures of social attitudes. An improvement in the measurement of social attitudes can be achieved by using Coombs's (see Michell, 1994) unfolding procedures.

Ten-Up: Prediction of Lifetime Achievements Is Not Restricted to Cognitive Abilities

Intelligence is not the only influence on class structure and achievement in our lives. I illustrate this with three examples.

First, consider a study showing poor predictive validity of an ability test.[1] Concerns over the effects of the defoliant Agent Orange, which was used extensively during the Vietnam War, have prompted the Australian government to support several studies of the well-being of veterans from that war. The most extensive study was initiated in the early 1990s, and close to 20 papers emanating from this material have been written. The project was based on a representative sample of more than 600 people who were given a structured interview that lasted several hours. Information obtained during the veterans's induction process in the 1960s was also available, including participants' scores on the Army Classification Test (ACT). This is an "omnibus" (i.e., it contains a mixture of fluid and crystallized ability items) intelligence test developed in the early 1940s that has been modified somewhat over the years and is still being used for the same purposes today. David Grayson, one of the chief investigators on the Vietnam Veterans project, and I examined the correlations between the ACT and various measures of "success" in life (see Stankov, 1998a, 1998b). We started by looking at the correlation between the current income of the participants and their ACT scores, then moved on to measures of socioeconomic status, mental health and antisocial behavior, marital status, and so forth. The outcome for everything we tried was the same: ACT scores showed low zero-order correlations with these various measures. Consider, for example, a measure of total income, which for the sample in question ranged between A $2,500 and A $200,000, with a mean of about A $38,000. Its correlation with ACT score was .03. These data do not support the findings cited in *The Bell Curve* (Herrnstein & Murray,

---

[1] This subtitle is derived from the title of an excellent British TV series *Seven-Up* that traced the life of a group of young children over a period of several decades, starting when they were age seven.

1994). Needless to say, noncognitive and demographic variables did have predictive validity for various measures of success in life in this data set. For example, the age-left-school variable had a significant ($r = -.18$) correlation with income.

Second, consider an earlier study of Vietnam-era veterans in which the predictors of mortality during midlife were examined (O'Toole & Stankov, 1992). This study compared some 500 veterans who died during the 10-year period following the end of Vietnam War with a sample of some 1,800 of their peers who had survived. The majority of these people (i.e., about 96%) did not go to Vietnam. Multivariate regression analysis indicated that the best predictors of mortality can be divided into two main groups: (a) variables representing transgressions against the Army discipline (AWOL offense, alcohol offense, and motor vehicle offense) and (b) variables related to intellectual achievement and job stability (ACT score, post-secondary school course, and number of jobs). This outcome suggests a significant role for intelligence (ACT) in the prediction — less intelligent people have higher mortality. These findings are perhaps not surprising given that the main causes of death in midlife happen to be motor vehicle accidents and suicides. Importantly, the transgressions against Army discipline are clearly stronger predictors.

Third, and most important, consider a longitudinal study carried out by Hammond (1998) in Melbourne, the results of which will appear in the book *Designing Our Abilities and Outlooks*. In this brief account here, I cannot possibly convey the scope and wealth of data considered in the book itself. The general thrust of the work, however, is very much in keeping with the theme of this chapter. The main body of data for that study was collected from about 400 boys, who were first examined in 1957 when they were 10 years old. Some 340 were examined again at the age of 20, and 310 were available in the mid-1980s when they were 36 years of age. The data were supplemented by information from parents, teachers, and from public records (e.g., the results of all public exams undertaken, offenses against the law, and so on). Hammond's work was influenced by his own ideas about personality. He also found Loevinger's (1976) ideas about ego development levels congenial to his way of thinking. In my opinion, the influence of Cattell's (1971) ideas about the historical effects of interests on the shaping of abilities is also apparent in his approach. Hammond's work was guided by the expectation that the main "foci for personality trait development" (or trait complexes in Ackerman's [1996] terminology) are

> traits of self-regulation such as conformity and tolerance of frustration; traits of social interaction and self-valuation such as social competence, sociability, attachment, and confidence; and traits of mastery to do with task issues such as intellectual competence, dependence, and avoidance.

Much of Hammond's (1998) soon-to-be published book is based on a series of regression analyses in which a 12-point scale of educational achievement at age 36 was used as a criterion. Hammond's interest was mainly in answering the question "Who gets educated?" A surprising finding was the unusually high percentage of variance (70%) of educational achievement at the age of 36 that can be predicted from the variables collected at the age of 10. The variables are descriptive of children as pupils (e.g., competencies drawn from actual educational skills, social role competencies in the classroom and the playground, avoidance of disruptive behavior, and the way that play is used) and of effective parenting in terms of care, control, and stimulation. Hammond also found that, as expected, abilities at age 10 predict a large amount (48%) of variance of education at age 36 (crystallized abilities are somewhat better predictors than fluid abilities). Interestingly, the amount of variance accounted for is raised to 66% by the addition of a couple of "outlook" variables that were apparent at the age of 20 and that become strengthened during the adulthood. The "rational outlook" orientation, as coined by Hammond, is concerned with the individual's motivations and competencies with respect to tasks and values. The Openness or Intellect scale from the Big Five captures this orientation reasonably well. The term "private outlook" orientation was chosen to express a macho siege mentality similar to authoritarian social attitude. People holding this outlook differ from those of a more rational view at age 20 in that they had been employed for some time, were oriented toward building a home or business, and were more concerned with courtship. Private outlook has a substantial negative correlation with educational achievement and with rational outlook. Thus, what the child is like at age 10, and what the person's outlook is at 20 and older, predict a sizable amount of variance in the attained level of education at 36.

It is interesting that in the most recent draft of part of his book, Hammond (1998) decided to develop a scale of work that ranked different jobs people held at the age of 36 into 12 categories in a way similar to categories of education. When this scale was used as a criterion, abilities and rational–private outlooks accounted for only 44% of the variance (instead of 65% for education). On their own, abilities were still important — they accounted for 35% of the variance. Education itself accounted for no more than 59% of the variance, and it took up almost all predictions from abilities and outlooks. In search of possible further predictors of job standings, Hammond focused on the outlook variables and supplemented the rational and private orientations with three additional ones. These orientations were seeking an enterprising role at work, seeking regulation of one's own conduct at work, and wanting an effective social helping role at work. This combination of five outlooks accounted for about 54% of job standings, which is not much different from education (59%) itself. In Hammond's own words, this moves researchers "into the territory of what is coming to be called 'emotional intelligence'!"

Aspects of Hammond's (1998) data seem to be in agreement with the results of the first study of Vietnam veterans previously mentioned. The Vietnam Veterans study was based on somewhat older participants — veterans were close to 50 in the mid-1990s — and the criterion variables Grayson and I used (Stankov, 1998a, 1998b) were closer to Hammond's job status (e.g., income) than to education. Nonetheless, the picture that seems to be emerging is reasonably consistent. Ability scores at age 10 predict educational achievement at age 36 but are less effective in predicting job standing. Similarly, ACT scores are poor predictors of income at age 50. At the same time, from young adulthood onward, noncognitive traits (i.e., outlooks) gain in predictive power of what may be called "life accomplishment."

Hammond (1998) has his own theory that places the individual in context as the object of personality study. He believes that the research issues concerning an individual's personality and ability have been "hopelessly mired in both ideological disputes and administrative conventions". Most current nature-versus-nurture arguments suffer from these problems. Clarification of these issues will only stem from an understanding of how each characteristic develops in the individual. For him, the advantage of follow-up studies resides in the possibility to look at psychological development "as a set of tactical moves as the person and his parents choose their paths and build their strengths at each stage." Hammond sees each person as a "survival machine" and as an "active constructive agent." Therefore, learning is a "motivated building" of knowledge into meaningful blocks. According to Hammond, traits (i.e., abilities, personality characteristics, ambitions, or affections) are "constructed competencies with a history of relevant striving. Each of them has cognitive, motivational, and affective aspects, and each is accessible to the individual for the solution of day to day problems." In his analyses, what happens at age 20 builds on what was available at age 10 and contributes to what will be found at age 36 — prediction from age 10 to 36 cannot be properly understood without the intermediate developments, and material presented in his book provides ample evidence for this ontogenetic process.

It may be concluded that if one of researchers' aims is to understand and predict what happens to people in their lives, intelligence scores on their own are clearly inadequate, and as people grow older they become less important. Noncognitive traits tend to play an increasingly important role. It is therefore necessary to encourage research in this area. The focus should be on the ego-related borderline areas between personality and abilities. New ways of assessing people — methods that do not depend heavily on self-reports — also need to be explored. Our own work has been directed toward the study of self-confidence, emotional intelligence, and social attitudes.

The Trait of Self-Confidence

A person may be described as self-confident by using everyday language, but researchers do not have many empirically based reports in psychology devoted to the study of self-confidence. How can one know that a person is more self-confident than another? One way would be to use self-report measures of the kind used to assess personality traits. For self-confidence, however, a more objective measurement is possible. Thus, researchers can ask participants to carry out a particular task and then state, at its completion, how confident they are that the answer they have provided is correct. The task itself can be short, and a large number of samplings of behavior can be obtained relatively quickly. Cognitive test items are ideal for this purpose. In our work we (Crawford & Stankov, 1996, 1998; Stankov, 1998b, 1998c; Stankov & Crawford, 1996, 1998) have used this procedure utilizing batteries of tests from guidelines provided by the theory of fluid and crystallized intelligence. For all tests, the participants were asked to provide an answer to an item and then to indicate how sure they were that their answer was correct. Two scores were calculated: the typical number-correct score and the average confidence rating score.[2]

---

[2]Because all Stankov and Crawford's (1996) tests were computerized, a measure of time was also routinely available.

The Distinction Between Crystallized Intelligence (Gc) and Broad Visualization (Gv)

The original impetus for Stankov and Crawford's (1996) research in this area came from within the experimental tradition of psychology that suggested a difference in performance between the general knowledge and perceptual tasks. In particular, the relationship between accuracy (i.e., number-correct) scores and confidence ratings is markedly different for these two types of tasks. For the general knowledge tasks, people tend to be overconfident; that is, they frequently act as if they believe that their answer is correct, even though the answer may be wrong. For the perceptual tasks, on the other hand, people tend to be underconfident; that is, they are not quite sure whether a correct answer is really correct.

Within the framework of individual differences, it is important to supplement factor-analytic findings with the results from other areas of psychology. The results that point to the distinction between perceptual and general knowledge processes are consistent with the existence of independent constructs of Gv and Gc abilities. In the process of studying individual differences we, (Stankov & Crawford, 1996, 1997) have examined the effects of some additional experimental manipulations that appeared relevant for the relationship between accuracy and confidence.

Contrary to intuition, our (Stankov & Crawford, 1996, 1997) research showed relatively little difference in confidence ratings for test items presented in the typical simultaneous fashion (i.e., with all alternatives of the multiple-choice items presented on the computer page) as opposed to a successive presentation of the alternatives. Experience with visual and auditory administration of the same test items indicates that even though the level of performance may be the same, participants generally tend to report less confidence in auditorily presented items. Clearly, this low level of confidence with auditory stimuli is not captured by the confidence ratings of successively presented visual items.

We find that if a participant is given feedback about the accuracy (or otherwise) of his or her answer after a confidence rating is registered, the overall effect on performance is relatively small; confidence ratings remain pretty much the same (Stankov & Crawford, 1998). Because the attempted experimental manipulations have minimal effects on confidence ratings, it appears that self-confidence may not be easily modified through changes in experimental task demands.

Correlational Evidence

Although we embarked on this work with a healthy dose of skepticism, our results to date have been encouraging, and it appears that the psychometric properties of confidence ratings are indeed satisfactory. The main findings of these various studies may be summarized as follows:

1. *Reliabilities of confidence ratings.* We found that confidence rating scores have satisfactory reliabilities, comparable to those obtained with accuracy scores (Stankov & Crawford, 1996).
2. *Correlation between confidence ratings and traditional accuracy scores.* An early point of interest was the size of correlation between the actual performance on cognitive tasks and measures derived from confidence ratings. This is crit-

321

ical because high correlation would obviate the use of confidence ratings in individual-differences research. We (Crawford & Stankov, 1998) found that correlations between number-correct scores and measures of self-confidence varied considerably for nine tests derived from the theory of fluid and crystallized intelligence, as listed in Table 14.1. For measures of fluid intelligence, the average raw correlation was .43 and for crystallized intelligence .35. Much lower correlations were obtained between the accuracy scores and self-confidence for short-term memory (.13) and perceptual line length tests (.07). These correlations support the claim that confidence ratings contain something different from the accuracy scores.

3. *Correlations with personality traits, gender, and age.* Our results (Crawford & Stankov, 1996) indicated that scores derived from confidence ratings have low correlations with the personality traits of introversion, neuroticism, and psychoticism, as measured by Eysenck's Personality Questionnaire (EPQ; Eysenck & Eysenck, 1991). These correlations reached zero after partialing out the corresponding accuracy scores. Self-confidence obviously does not capture aspects of these personality traits. Our studies also showed that the difference in confidence ratings between men and women was not significant. Older people show somewhat greater bias (i.e., overconfidence) in their judgments than younger participants. There are frequent references in the literature to certain tendencies, such as thinking carefully before deciding in situations involving uncertainty, being related to wisdom (Baltes & Smith, 1990; Holliday & Chandler, 1986). This often hypothesized link between the concept of wisdom and that aspect of metacognition was highlighted by Meacham (1983) in his article "Wisdom and the Context of Knowledge: Knowing That One Doesn't Know," which, of course, is reminiscent of the classic article in the calibration curves literature by Lichtenstein and Fischhoff (1977), who chose the title "Do Those Who Know More Also Know More About How Much They Know?" Assuming that the concept of wisdom is at least partly captured by good self-monitoring

TABLE 14.1   Factor Analysis (Principal Factors Solution Followed by Oblimin Rotation) of Accuracy and Self-Confidence Scores

Test	Performance scores			Self-confidence scores	
	Gf	Gc	Span	Factor 1	Factor 2
Ravens	78	−15	10	86	−07
Letter series	78	−13	08	48	18
Animals	45	−06	19	22	56
Vocabulary	−19	95	−03	48	24
Proverbs	39	25	13	83	−15
Analogies	14	76	13	46	28
Backward digit span	02	02	75	−04	67
Forward digit span	05	08	78	02	74
Line length	18	08	−07	52	29

Note.   Salient loadings are indicated by boldfaced type. For performance scores, the factor correlations are as follows: Gf and Gc, .22; Gf and Span, .43; Gc and Span, .05. For self-confidence scores, the factor correlations are as follows: Factor 1 and Factor 2, .59. Gf = fluid intelligence; Gc = crystallized intelligence; Factor 1 = broad self-confidence; Factor 2 = span confidence.

ability, the results of Crawford and Stankov's (1996) study imply that older adults are, in fact, less wise than younger adults.[3]

4. *Scores derived from confidence ratings define a strong and replicable factor.* We (Crawford & Stankov, 1996; Stankov, 1998c) found that confidence ratings from a battery of nine measures of three well-known factors from the theory of fluid and crystallized intelligence tend to define a broad factor with loadings from seven measures. It appears that there may be grounds for postulating a broad, perhaps even a general, self-confidence trait. This is supported by the fact that even a measure of perceptual processing, such as the line length test (i.e., state which line from among five 2-cm vertical lines is longer than the rest), has loadings on that factor. Notwithstanding, there is some indication that confidence ratings from the tests of short-term memory may define a different factor (see Table 14.1).

The analyses presented in Table 14.1 were carried out separately for accuracy and confidence-rating scores. The information is not sufficient to deduce what factorial structure would emerge if both accuracy and confidence rating scores were analyzed together. Indeed, given the existence of nonzero correlations between accuracy and confidence scores, mentioned previously in Point 2, it is possible that a clear separation between the accuracy and confidence-ratings factors would not emerge. Nonetheless, in addition to the data presented in Table 14.1, the results of four further studies provide strong evidence for a self-confidence factor that is relatively independent from performance accuracy.

The additional three studies were based on three tasks only: Raven's Progressive Matrices test and perceptual line length test being common to all. A Gc marker test in one study was the synonyms vocabulary test (Stankov & Crawford, 1996, 1998), whereas a geographic knowledge test was used in the second (Kleitman & Stankov, 1998). In both studies, for each test, three scores were calculated: accuracy, average confidence ratings, and the average speed of answering test items. In the second study, two further measures were obtained. The first measure was an estimate of the number of items participants thought that they would solve, given immediately after instruction and practice (i.e., before starting work on test proper), and the second was an estimate of how many items that they thought were answered correctly, which was obtained after completing the test.[4] A remarkable finding stemmed from both studies: Confidence-rating scores from the three tests define a very clear factor. All other scores from the same test (with some exceptions for speed measures) defined the same factor. In other words, three (or five) scores from the Raven's Progressive Matrices defined a Raven factor that was different from vocabulary and line length factors. A recently completed fourth study (Stankov, 1998a, 1998b) confirmed these findings with a new battery of five fluid intelligence markers. This,

---

[3]This link between wisdom and self-confidence derives from the fact that a linear combination (i.e., difference) of accuracy and confidence scores is used in calibration studies to indicate the "realism" of confidence ratings. This linear combination is sometimes referred to as *bias* score. As it turns out, factorial structure of bias scores is very similar to the structure obtained among confidence ratings.

[4]These additional measures were obtained because of the issues raised in studies from experimental cognitive psychology. Pretest estimates of performance are akin to measures of self-efficacy, whereas posttest estimate of performance was postulated by Gigerenzer, Hoffrage, and Kleinbolting (1991) to be a distinct process from that tapped by the item-linked confidence ratings.

together with the results of Table 14.1, provides a strong evidence for the existence of a self-confidence trait. Moreover, given that the tests used in Stankov and Crawford's (1996, 1998) work are so cognitively diverse from the psychometric point of view, a considerable generality of that trait can be assumed.

Self-Confidence Within the Structure of Human Abilities and Personality

Conceptually, what seems to be involved in self-confidence is akin to several existing constructs such as self-efficacy, self-concept, typical-as-opposed-to-maximal performance, practical intelligence, aspects of emotional intelligence, and so forth. Like many of these constructs, self-monitoring, as captured by confidence-rating scores, is neither entirely personality-like nor entirely cognitive in nature. The self-confidence factor may be viewed either as an aspect of metacognition and therefore close to human abilities or as a part of the interface between abilities and personality, an aspect of ego-related motivational effects. The following speculations regarding its placement are presently offered.

Given the low correlations we (Crawford & Stankov, 1996, 1998) have obtained with the personality traits, and nonzero correlations with number-correct scores in our studies, it is tempting to claim that self-confidence is closer to the ability domain than it is to the personality domain. Substantive considerations could lead to the conclusion that this is an aspect of fluid intelligence. The presence of self-confidence in tasks that do not require formal education support this interpretation. Even so, a salient relationship with crystallized intelligence cannot be ruled out because efficient metacognitive processes tapped by confidence ratings may be an essential outcome of a more extensive knowledge base, which indicates greater expertise on any given task.

We believe that self-confidence, as measured in our studies (Stankov, 1998b, 1998c; Stankov & Crawford, 1996, 1997), is an aspect of, or perhaps identical to, what is sometimes called *self-monitoring* — an individual's propensity to appraise (or judge) the degree of accuracy of one's own performance in the course of working through the items of a cognitive test. This trait may be related to test anxiety (see Hembree, 1988). Whether self-confidence will be the only metacognitive factor involved in test taking, or whether there will be others, is difficult to determine at this time. For example, it has been claimed that planning, evaluation, strategic thinking, and the like may represent separate metacognitive skills in addition to self-monitoring (cf. Schraw & Moshman, 1995; Sternberg, 1985).

Psychometric studies carried out in the course of this century have pointed to the importance of metacognitive skills. For example, Spearman's (1927) law of awareness of experience, which states that "A person tends to know himself and items of his own experience," is, in fact, just another name for what is now called *metacognition*. Although it is possible to ascribe a special status to metacognitive abilities within the overall structure of intelligence (e.g., treating these as a super program that directs people's thinking and therefore represents the essence of intelligence), our results indicate that this is an unlikely scenario (Stankov, 1998b, 1998c; Stankov & Crawford, 1996, 1998). Self-confidence is possibly just one of several oligarchic factors.

Self-Confidence Factor on the Borderline Between Personality Traits and Intelligence

Although the placement of self-confidence within the domain of metacognition may be appropriate, it is also possible that its position should be located further away from the realm of human cognitive abilities. Its main role may be to provide a person with the information relevant for an evaluation of his or her strengths and weaknesses and to act as a motivational force that is important for ensuring maximal cognitive effort in that person's areas of strength. The level of self-confidence may be related to feelings of self-esteem and contribute to one's realistic outlook on aspects of achievement and on life in general.

Indeed, factors that are similar to self-confidence may be found in Spearman's (1927) deliberation on human cognition. They are called *oretic* factors and, as such, refer to character (cf. Webb, 1915), desires, emotions, temperaments, and types (or styles), which are distinguished from g and *broad specific* factors such as language, science, retentivity, and speed. Spearman listed three oretic factors that were "first encountered within the sphere of cognition and were only extended to orexis by an afterthought." These are (a) *fluency*, having "pronounced reproductive rather than eductive elements"; (b) *oscillation*, involving fluctuations in mental work (including fatigue); (c) *perseveration*, or inertia, indicating a tendency to be slow to begin doing mental work and slow to cease doing it. Furthermore, Spearman also acknowledged the existence of a prominent factor of character or will. The similarity of these factors to that of self-confidence resides in the fact that their measurement operations are different from those of typical tests of abilities. Subjectivity in scoring measures of these traits is more pronounced. These measures also seem to represent an inclination or a tendency to act in a particular way, rather than arise from an assessment of the accuracy of one's work.

There are other theories of intelligence that contain similar factors that straddle the personality–abilities borderline. For example, the carefulness and persistence factor from the Gf and Gc theory has qualities that seem to be similar to the present self-confidence factor (see Horn, 1988). An even stronger role is ascribed to interests in the theorizing of Cattell's (1971) work. He postulated that crystallized abilities develop from fluid intelligence through the interaction with the interest structures. Initially, these interests are undifferentiated, but in the course of one's life, particular areas gradually gain in importance. Horn (1997) claimed that the evidence to date does not support the historical relationship between Gf and Gc. He did not, however, deny the effects of interest structures on the development of intelligence. Self-confidence may be important in both the initial and the later stages of this development.

The Need for Validation

At present, we have no information about the predictive validity of self-confidence measures for real-life activities. It is conceivable that this trait will be important for any job requiring decision making followed by the appraisal of the decision. Self-confidence may also be important for the initiation of action. It is possible that people exhibiting low self-confidence are prone to procrastination and prolonged deliberation, and highly self-confident individuals may rush into action too precipitously. In other words, high–low self-confidence may be related to Kuhl's (1985) distinction between action and state orientations. Different military and civilian jobs are likely to place demands on one or the other. Our (Stankov, 1998b, 1998c; Stankov & Crawford, 1996, 1998) results suggest that validation studies are warranted. Our results also suggest that the data on self-confidence may be collected relatively easily because (a) they can be obtained from typical ability tests during a routine test administration and (b) a small number of tests can quickly provide a reliable self-monitoring score.

The Elusive Emotional Intelligence

Psychometricians view emotional intelligence with skepticism, although the term was quickly embraced by laypeople a couple of years ago. Even today, the opposition between irrational (i.e., emotional) and rational (i.e., intelligent) thinking appears too contradictory for many psychologists who cannot accept that a combination of these two terms indicates a meaningful construct. Acceptance of this proposition has been somewhat slow in coming. On reflection, however, intelligence refers to adaptive behavior, and perhaps it could be redefined to include "the ability to monitor one's own and others' emotions, to discriminate among them, and to use the information to guide one's thinking and actions" (Salovey & Mayer, 1990, p. 189).[5] Why not? After all, Gardner (1983) has made a similar claim in his descriptions of intrapersonal intelligence.

Although conceptual difficulties can be, in part, resolved through abstract analyses, we (Davies, Stankov, & Roberts, in press) reasoned that empirical data would provide useful information at this stage. Critical, of course, is the availability of suitable measuring instruments. Our search of the published literature and of the Internet uncovered several questionnaires dealing with various aspects of emotional intelligence. Inspection of these self-report measures pointed to considerable similarities between emotional intelligence, personality, and social intelligence. This search also uncovered a paucity of studies on the relationship between traditional tests of intelligence and emotional intelligence. The existence of nonzero correlations (i.e., positive manifold) is crucial if the term *ability* is to be used in the definition of emotional intelligence.

The above-mentioned points were all taken into consideration by Davies et al. (in press), who report the results of three studies. In the first study, a battery of 30 tests was assembled and administered to 100 university students. The tests included (a) 18 putative measures of emotional intelligence, (b) 6 marker tests of Gf and Gc, (c) 2 tests of social intelligence (Hathaway & McKinley, 1967; Hogan, 1969), and (d) the EPQ. The results of a factor analysis of this battery of tests are easy to summarize. First, the two factors of Gf and Gc were clearly defined. Second, three scales of the EPQ — Extraversion, Neuroticism, and Psychoticism — had their highest loadings on three factors. In addition, 7 out of 18 measures of emotional intelligence had their loadings on these three factors as well. These 7 measures cannot

---

[5] A closely related construct, called *alexithymia*, refers to a failure in the regulation of affect. In fact, the Toronto Alexithymia Scale was used in our work on emotional intelligence (Stankov & Crawford, 1996, 1997).

be interpreted as anything else but aspects of the three well-known personality traits, certainly not of emotional intelligence. Social intelligence measures, in particular, are clearly linked to extraversion. Therefore, five out of eight factors are nothing more than traditional ability and personality factors. The second study reported by Davies et al. confirmed the same finding by utilizing a measure of Big-Five personality factors.

The remaining three factors of the first study can, perhaps, be interpreted as emotional intelligence. There are problems, however, because the interpretation of all of these factors is ambiguous. Particularly problematic are the factors we labeled as *Emotional Clarity* (the extent to which individuals both understand and identify their own emotional state) and *Emotional Awareness* (the degree to which individuals think about and express their feelings). The reason for ambiguity lies in the fact that the Neuroticism scale had a low (i.e., around .30) loading on both these factors, indicating that neurotic individuals lack insight into their emotional tone and therefore have no clear notion of certain emotional dynamics (Eysenck & Eysenck, 1991). Thus, although these two factors did not have their highest loadings on the Neuroticism scale, the presence of a low neuroticism component casts doubts on the interpretation of these factors as pure measures of emotional intelligence. Furthermore, the second study reported in Davies et al. (1998) could not replicate these two factors.

The third factor of the first study — *Emotion Perception* — does not appear to have any links with personality or ability traits. It is therefore the most likely candidate for a "pure" measure of emotional intelligence. However, the nonstandard scoring procedure that was used with the measures of this factor makes the interpretation of it as emotional intelligence ambiguous. This factor is defined by four objective tests. The first two tests — Emotion Perception of Faces and Colors — were conceived by Mayer, DiPaulo, and Salovey (1990). The other two tests (Emotion Perception in Musical Excerpts test and Emotion Perception in Sound Intervals test) were developed by ourselves (Davies et al., 1998). In all of these tests, participants were presented with a stimulus (a picture of a face, color, short musical piece, or a sound interval) and a list of six different emotion scales: happiness, sadness, anger, fear, surprise, and disgust. Participants were required to provide ratings (on a scale with responses ranging from 1 to 5) of the extent to which they perceived each emotion to be present in a given stimulus.

The scoring of the Emotion Perception measures can be rather involved. We (Davies et al., 1998) used the procedure suggested by Mayer et al. (1990) to derive a single score representing the degree of accurate emotional perception that a participant exhibited in each content domain. The scores were obtained by summing the number of times the participant agreed with the modal (consensual) response.[6] A consensual response on a given emotion scale was one in which the participant responded within one scale point (either side) of the group's modal re-

---

[6]The method of scoring measures of divergent thinking or fluency is reminiscent of the procedures used with the Emotion Perception tests. With fluency measures, a panel of judges is used to evaluate the quality of responses (e.g., accept the answer as original or not). The difference lies in the fact that in fluency measures, the definition of originality is externally given and the judges know its meaning. In the Emotion Perception measures, the emotion ascribed to the stimulus comes from within the individual judge.

sponse. Although we tried several modifications of this procedure, the essential aspects of the results remained the same.

The use of consensual responses in the way used with the Emotion Perception measures represents an uncommon method of objectifying testing in personality area and might be useful with some other constructs in addition to emotional intelligence. First, however, it will be necessary to ensure that these scores have satisfactory psychometric properties. The examination of some of these properties was the topic of the third study reported by Davies et al. (1998). In that study our aim was to tease out the method and trait aspects of the consensus-based scores we (and others) had used. We wanted to find out if the Emotion Perception factor of the first study was due to consensual scoring or if its appearance was genuinely linked to emotional experience. In the study, the four Emotional Perception tests listed earlier were given together with another four tests in which a consensual answer was required, but the emotional content was minimized (e.g., "What is the most likely profession of the person in this picture?"). We reasoned that if all eight tests were to define the same factor, consensus rather than emotion perception would be the cause of individual differences. A meaningful answer could not be obtained because of the fact that all eight consensually scored tests had dismal internal consistency (i.e., Chronbach's coefficient alpha).[7]

Finally, in our (Davies et al., 1998) data the correlations among all eight factors were low, essentially zero. The Emotion Perception factor in the first study correlated .15 with Gf and .05 with Gc. These correlations were too low for a claim that emotion perception is an ability in the sense in which this term is used with respect to traditional abilities.

On the basis of the data we (Davies et al., 1998) have collected up to now, it appears that emotional intelligence is a much narrower construct than originally claimed by its advocates. Most questionnaire measures of emotional intelligence appear to tap aspects of the well-known personality traits, and emotion perception may yet prove to be the only genuinely new aspect. However, satisfactory reliabilities of the measures of emotion perception ability will need to be demonstrated.

New Generation of Rating Scales for the Measurement of Social Attitudes

This section deals mostly with methodology that may improve on the paucity of substantive data available at this time. My aim is to illustrate a new and improved procedure that can be used profitably to measure social attitudes and personality.[8] This procedure may be particularly useful in gaining a better understanding of what Hammond (1998) called *outlook orientations* that appear to play an increasingly important role in predicting the achievements at a mature age in life.

Consider the set of six statements toward nuclear war that are listed in the top

---

[7] Two of the tests (Faces and Voices) could be scored with respect to the target emotion. Under this scoring procedure, one of the tests (Faces) approaches the lower bound of what may be considered a satisfactory internal consistency (low .70s).

[8] The data presented here were collected by Karon Jannusch for her Honours Empirical Thesis in 1988. Her supervisor was Joel Michell, PhD.

part of Table 14.2. These statements were designed to be unidimensional through the use of the principles described by Michell (1994). The statements were given twice to the same group of participants. In the pair-comparison procedure, participants were given all (i.e., 15) possible pairings of statements and were asked to indicate within each pair the statement they agreed with most (or disagreed with least). In the ratings condition, the participants were given a booklet containing the six statements presented in random order, and immediately below each statement an 11-point rating scale appeared, on which they were instructed to indicate the strength of their agreement with that statement. The administration of the pair-comparison condition is somewhat more time consuming than the use of ratings.

The pair-comparison data allow for the application of the unidimensional unfolding procedures developed by Coombs (see Michell, 1994). If the statements are unidimensional, this procedure can yield information that locates both stimuli (e.g., attitude statements) and individuals on that dimension, and numerical assignments (scores) can be made to both. Furthermore, conjoint measurement can be applied to unidimensional unfolding parameters to test if the attribute under study is quantitative (see Michell, 1994; Stankov & Cregan, 1993). Clearly, these properties are desirable from the measurement point of view. The reason why this approach to attitude scale construction has not been used more frequently in the past is probably because of the rather demanding calculations that need to be carried out—computer programs for unidimensional scaling are not commonly available.

It appears, however, that unidimensional unfolding does not have to be applied to the data from every empirical study, because several of our (Michell, Stankov, & Jannusch, 1998) studies indicate that, for the set of statements that can unfold unidimensionally, ratings procedure tends to provide an equally good ordering of individuals. Consider the correlations between the six statements obtained from the ratings data. These correlations display a simplex pattern, and loadings on the two principal components from that matrix (i.e., Factors 1 and 2), when plotted in a two-dimensional coordinate system, display a semicircular pattern expected from such matrices (see Davison, 1977). Most surprising was the finding that factor scores obtained from this analysis correlated in excess of .90 with the individuals' scores obtained from the application of a laborious unidimensional unfolding procedure.

TABLE 14.2 Correlations and the First Two Principal Components

Statement	1	2	3	4	5	6	Factor 1	Factor 2
1.	—						.819	.464
2.	.75	—					.908	.157
3.	.69	.83	—				.892	.076
4.	.70	.74	.72	—			.891	−.019
5.	.59	.71	.71	.82	—		.869	−.240
6.	.52	.66	.66	.62	.67	—	.791	−.461

Note. Nuclear war attitude statements are as follows: 1. Human nature being what it is, a nuclear war is a certainty. 2. Human nature being what it is, a nuclear war is extremely likely. 3. Human nature being what it is, it is quite likely that the future will bring a nuclear war. 4. Human nature being what it is, it is fairly unlikely that there will be a nuclear war. 5. Human nature being what it is, there will almost certainly not be a nuclear war. 6. Human nature being what it is, nuclear war in the future is an impossibility. $n = 132$

In essence, this means that the initial investment of effort needs to be made to apply both pair comparison and ratings to the same set of statements and, once they are found to be unidimensional, more efficient ratings methods can be used from there on.

In our work (Michell et al., 1998), in addition to the nuclear war statements, we used a set of statements about homosexuality and obtained similar results. Both these items appear in scales of authoritarianism (e.g., authoritarian people endorse negative attitudes toward homosexuals). In one of our studies, we correlated factor scores from both pair-comparisons and ratings data with NEO-Personality Inventory measures of the Big-Five personality factors (Costa & McCrae, 1991). Attitude toward nuclear war had low (about .20) correlations with Neuroticism, Extraversion, and Agreeableness. The Homosexuality scale had a correlation of $-.30$ with Openness and $-.23$ with Agreeableness. People who have highly negative attitude toward homosexuality are less open minded, do not seek intellectually stimulating experiences, and are low on agreeableness. These are the people with private outlooks in Hammond's (1998) work. Furthermore, a measure of crystallized intelligence (vocabulary test) also had medium negative correlation with the attitude toward homosexuality ($-.36$) and positive correlation with the attitude toward nuclear war. This all seems to make good sense.

What I am suggesting here is the construction of a set of six related statements for each item currently used in measures of authoritarianism and other social attitude areas. In addition to having good measurement properties in terms of their quantitative characteristics, such scales are bound to be more reliable as well.

As far as I am aware, there has been little progress in the study of social attitudes since the 1960s, and researchers do not have good measures of the aspects of social life that are now at the top of society's social and political agendas. These include scales for the measurement of attitudes toward work (and welfare), law and order (and drug use), environment (and technological innovations), and gender issues (and sexuality) among others. Such widening of areas of investigation and improvement in measurement is needed to take research programs further into the next century.

Conclusion

It is hard to say whether psychology's predicament is all doom and gloom. The approach that emphasizes a general factor in the cognitive domain at the expense of other broad factors may however take researchers in that direction. There is sufficient evidence in the literature to question this position, but that evidence needs to be made more visible.

The search for physical correlates of intelligence and personality should continue and it may, at some future stage, tell researchers something important about people. However, premature enthusiasm for this area of research has, in my opinion, pushed promising work on cognitive correlates into the background.

The evidence that is based on the follow-up studies reviewed in this chapter points to the importance of noncognitive factors in the prediction of lifetime achievements (i.e., achievements related to one's job and position in society between the ages of 35 and 50). Although some of these factors are captured by the personality traits measured by the existing questionnaires, there are additional promising areas that have not been studied extensively in the past.

It is unlikely that the construct of emotional intelligence will survive closer scrutiny — its status, based on questionnaire measures, is too closely related to personality traits. The Emotion Perception measures that are based on consensual agreement have measurement problems (e.g., poor reliability) that will need to be remedied. These problems are so serious that they render the term *emotional intelligence* theoretically useless for the time being.

The constructs of self-confidence and social attitudes can be assessed by using procedures that have better measurement properties than typical self-report instruments. Empirical studies of self-confidence to date suggest that this is a well-defined trait that can be measured reliably by using the items from the typical tests of abilities. Theoretically, this trait should be located somewhere between personality and intelligence, although predictive validity of self-confidence in the real-life settings is not known at present.

We have done a small amount of empirical work using measures of social attitudes. It is clear, however, that efficient rating scales of such attitudes can be developed by linking them initially to the unidimensional unfolding procedures. Social attitude scales that address the issues of concern in modern society are urgently needed, particularly because they hold promise for the measurement of outlook orientations that seem to be useful in predicting lifetime achievements.

REFERENCES

Ackerman, P. L. (1996). A theory of adult development: Process, personality, interests, and knowledge. *Intelligence, 22,* 227–257.

Baltes, P. B., & Smith, J. (1990). Towards a psychology of wisdom and its ontogenesis. In R. J. Sternberg (Ed.), *Wisdom: Its nature, origin and development* (pp. 87–120). New York: Cambridge University Press.

Carroll, J. B. (1993). *Human cognitive abilities: A survey of factor-analytic studies.* New York: Cambridge University Press.

Cattell, R. B. (1971). *Abilities: Their structure, growth, and action.* Boston: Houghton Mifflin.

Costa, P. T., & McCrae, R. R. (1991). *NEO Five-Factor Inventory.* Odessa, FL: Psychological Assessment Resources.

Crawford, J., & Stankov, L. (1996). Age differences in the realism of confidence judgments: A calibration study using tests of fluid and crystallized intelligence. *Learning and Individual Differences, 6,* 84–103.

Crawford, J., & Stankov, L. (1998). Individual differences in the realism of confidence judgments: Overconfidence in measures of fluid and crystallized intelligence. *Australian Journal of Psychology.* Manuscript submitted for publication.

Davies, M., Stankov, L., & Roberts, R. (1998). Emotional intelligence: In search of an elusive construct. *Journal of Personality and Social Psychology, 75,* 989–1015.

Davison, M. (1977). On a metric, unidimensional unfolding model for attitudinal and developmental data. *Psychometrika, 42,* 523–548.

Eysenck, H. J., & Eysenck, S. B. G. (1991). *Manual of the Eysenck Personality Scales.* London: Hodder & Stoughton.

Gardner, H. (1983). *Frames of mind.* New York: Basic Books.

Gigerenzer, G., Hoffrage, U., & Kleinbolting, H. (1991). Probabilistic mental models: A Brunswikian theory of confidence. *Psychological Review, 98,* 506–528.

Hammond, S. (1998). *Designing our abilities and outlooks.* Manuscript submitted for publication.

Hathaway, S. R., & McKinley, J. C. (1967). *The Minnesota Multiphasic Personality Inventory.* New York: Psychological Corporation.

Hembree, R. (1988). Correlates, causes, effects, and treatment of test anxiety. *Review of Educational Research, 58*, 47–77.

Herrnstein, R. J., & Murray, C. (1994). *The Bell Curve: Intelligence and class structure in American life.* New York: Free Press.

Hogan, R. (1969). Development of an empathy scale. *Journal of Consulting and Clinical Psychology, 33*, 307–316.

Holliday, S. G., & Chandler, M. J. (1986). *Wisdom: Explorations in adult competence.* Basel, Switzerland: Krager.

Horn, J. L. (1988). Thinking about human abilities. In J. R. Nesselroade & R. B. Cattell (Eds.), *Handbook of multivariate experimental psychology* (2nd ed., pp. 645–685). New York: Plenum.

Horn, J. L. (1997). A basis for research on age differences in cognitive capabilities. In J. J. McArdle & R. W. Woodcock (Eds.), *Human cognitive abilities in theory and practice.* Chicago: Riverside Publishing Co.

Jensen, A. R. (1997, July). *Spearman's hypothesis.* Paper presented at the Spearman Seminar, University of Plymouth, England.

Kleitman, S., & Stankov, L. (1998). *Ecological and person-driven aspects of metacognitive processes in test-taking.* Manuscript submitted for publication.

Kuhl, J. (1985). Volitional mediators of cognitive-behavior consistency: Self-regulatory processes and action versus state orientation. In J. Kuhl & J. Beckman (Eds.), *Action control: From cognition to behavior* (pp. 101–128). Berlin: Springer-Verlag.

Kyllonen, P. C., & Christal, R. E. (1990). Reasoning ability is (little more than) working memory capacity?! *Intelligence, 14*, 389–433.

Lichtenstein, S., & Fischhoff, B. (1977). Do those who know more also know more about how much they know? *Organizational Behaviour and Human Performance, 20*, 159–183.

Loevinger, J. (1976). *Ego development: Conceptions and theories.* San Francisco: Jossey-Bass.

Matthews, G., Joyner, L., Gilliland, K., Campbell, S. E., Huggins, J., & Falconer, S. (in press). Validation of a comprehensive stress state questionnaire: Towards a state Big Three? In I. Mervielde, I. J. Deary, F. De Fruyt, & F. Ostendorf (Eds.), *Personality psychology in Europe* (Vol. 7). Tilburg, The Netherlands: Tilburg University Press.

Mayer, J., DiPaulo, M., & Salovey, P. (1990). Perceiving affective content in ambiguous visual stimuli: A component of emotional intelligence. *Journal of Personality Assessment, 54*, 772–781.

Meacham, J. A. (1983). Wisdom and the context of knowledge: Knowing that one doesn't know. In D. Kuhn & J. A. Meacham (Eds.), *On the development of developmental psychology* (pp. 111–134). Basel, Switzerland: Krager.

Michell, J. B. (1994). Measuring dimensions of belief by unidimensional unfolding. *Journal of Mathematical Psychology, 38*, 244–273.

Michell, J. B., Stankov, L., & Jannusch, K. (1998). *Validating ratings via unfolding.* Unpublished manuscript.

Myors, B., Stankov, L., & Oliphant, G. W. (1989). Competing tasks, working memory and intelligence. *Australian Journal of Psychology, 41*(1), 1–16.

O'Toole, B. I., & Stankov, L. (1992). Ultimate validity of psychological tests. *Personality and Individual Differences, 13*, 699–716.

Roberts, R. D., Stankov, L., Pallier, G., & Dolph, B. (1997). Charting the cognitive sphere: Tactile–kinesthetic performance within the structure of intelligence. *Intelligence, 25*, 111–148.

Salovey, P., & Mayer, J. (1990). Emotional intelligence. *Imagination, Cognition and Personality, 9*, 185–211.

Schraw, G., & Moshman, D. (1995). Metacognitive theories. *Educational Psychology Review, 7*, 351–371.

Spearman, C. (1927). *The abilities of man: Their nature and measurement.* New York: Macmillan.

Stankov, L. (1998a). Intelligence arguments and Australian psychology. *Australian Psychologist, 33*, 53–57.

Stankov, L. (1998b). Calibration curves, scatterplots and the distinction between general knowledge and perceptual tests. *Learning and Individual Differences, 8*, 28–51.

Stankov, L. (1998c). *Complexity, metacognition, and fluid intelligence.* Manuscript submitted for publication.

Stankov, L., & Crawford, J. D. (1996). Confidence judgments in studies of individual differences. *Personality and Individual Differences, 21*, 6, 971–986.

Stankov, L., & Crawford, J. (1997). Self-confidence and performance on cognitive tests. *Intelligence*, 25, 93–109.

Stankov, L., & Cregan, A. (1993). Quantitative and qualitative properties of an intelligence test: Series completion. *Learning and Individual Differences*, 5(2), 137–169.

Stankov, L., & Roberts, R. D. (1997). Mental speed is not *the* "basic" process of intelligence. *Personality and Individual Differences*, 22, 1, 69–84.

Sternberg, R. J. (1985). *Beyond IQ: A triarchic theory of human intelligence*. New York: Cambridge University Press.

Webb, E. (1915). Character and intelligence. *British Journal of Psychology Monograph* (Suppl. 3).

Discussion

Discussion of Stankov's paper returned to the issue (raised in the discussion of Hunt's paper) of the relationship between intelligence and income. Other issues raised included cross-cultural concerns, and broader issues about the meaning of intelligence and its correlates.

Dr. Matthews: I have a comment on self-confidence. I think it's an example of how a verbal label can cover what may be several distinct constructs. In the work which my group is doing on the assessment of stress traits, we have a dimension of self-confidence and perceived control, two qualities which seem to go together quite closely (Matthews et al., in press). But our dimension, unlike yours, correlates quite substantially with the EPQ [Eysenck Personality Questionnaire] N scale, and, to a smaller degree, with introversion. I think the difference is that self-confidence in your terms is very much geared to beliefs about the individual responses. But self-confidence, as I've assessed it, is more of a general impression of how you're doing with the task as a whole. It's then an open question how the person's beliefs about individual trials feed into the general impression. It's perhaps at that stage where personality becomes more important.

Dr. Stankov: I completely agree with both the analysis and the interpretation that you're putting on it. And it is my bias I think to go into something that I believe is better measured, if you want, than just a statement. And then there was the opportunity of using it. I was very skeptical when I started working with these measures, and then a series of studies here convinced me that there is something really there. Now, the extent to which this self-confidence is related to self-confidence in the broader context, I do not know. And I think it would be very interesting to measure because I think the very down-to-earth measurement properties of these is interesting and important. And the fact that it exists in such a stable way in our studies points out that it should be used. I also am keen to find out about this predictor variable. I'm very curious whether it can predict anything at all. Or is it just a very narrow sort of thing? I hope not. I think it will go further than that.

Dr. Hunt: You reported rather rapidly about some very low correlations of intelligence test scores of income. Two questions. Was that log income? Because you had a huge range.

Dr. Stankov: It was income, just plain income.

Dr. Hunt: Income, not log income? And in income just the correlations can be very different for those too. And was that after educational achievement had been considered, or was that the raw correlation.

Dr. Stankov: These are the raw correlations. We started looking at it, and we realized how low it is, and we tried then various other things. Well, we just left it at that. It was just very, very low.

Dr. Hunt: But the correlations with educational attainment must have been fairly high?

Dr. Stankov: Between income and educational attainment. It wasn't all that impressive.

Dr. Hunt: That's very interesting because that's contrary to practically every educational survey or every income survey that's been done in North America or Europe.

Dr. Stankov: I would say there's something funny about Australians. Their welfare system is different. Some of the things that are operating in education are different. Many things should be brought to bear on it.

Dr. Alexander: Could it simply be as in the United States — I don't know about the Australian situation — the nature of the population that participated in the Vietnam War was not quite the same kind of cross-section of the individuals who participated in World War II. For example, education was actually an "exempt" status during the Vietnam War. And so could it be something with constrained data set performance?

Dr. Stankov: Yes, we looked at that. It was pointed out to us that people below an IQ of 80 were not selected for the Army in the Australian system. On the other hand, what was interesting in that data is that a lot of people who came back from the Army went on to tertiary education. So there's no distinction on that end. There's a distinction at the bottom end. You cannot apply a restriction of range to a correlation that's virtually zero. It will not do much for you.

Dr. Wittmann: I would be a little bit more interested in what kind of criteria you are looking for where prediction for that new and additional construct pays off. Just trial and error, or what do you think are the most promising ones? If you don't have an answer, I have one for that. What about these old phenomena related to overachievement and underachievement? Shouldn't those overachievers be too confident, and vice versa? Or what do you think about that?

Dr. Stankov: Yeah. Perhaps. I don't know. I haven't looked at it.

Dr. Ackerman: Well, let's not start by bringing back a bad construct though, Werner. I mean we keep trying to throw away underachievement and overachievement as constructs.

Dr. Baddeley: Going back to the beginning of your talk and your measures that seem to correlate with IQ. It reminded me a little bit of a concept that John Duncan has introduced of "goal neglect." And I wondered if you knew about his work and if you'd thought about it. Basically what he does is to give instructions that have several steps but that are very fairly straightforward — then he looks at who can and who can't actually fulfill the instruction. He finds that there is quite a correlation with IQ and also that patients with frontal lobe damage do very poorly. One limitation of John Duncan's work is that it's an effect that only happens during the early stages. But it strikes me that what you may have is a situation where your tasks, particularly the more complex ones, do consistently require holding relatively complex instructions and operating them. I wondered if you'd thought about underlying processes.

Dr. Stankov: Yes, I have thought quite a bit. That is more along my interest. At one stage, as I was preparing for this talk, I wanted to thank Professor Hunt for alerting me to your work in one of his early writings. Your work with Hitch. Very, very influential in my work on complexity. And in fact, on completing tasks in the past. I know Duncan's work, but not that particular aspect of it.

What I believed to be the case behind these particulars — and I think there are two possible explanations in terms of the theory behind it. I'm sure there would be others. But one is the working memory explanation (keeping in mind all those instructions and working through them). That is possible, plausible. I have difficulties with some other aspects of working memory explanations that I have used in the past, but that is a longer story.

What I think the other explanation for this particular set of tasks is — is the lapse in attention. What seems to be happening in these two tasks is — in the Swap's test, for example, what you have to do is swap two letters. Then mentally do that and then swap another two letters and come to the end and then produce the answer. And, the instructions for the Swap's test were left on the screen as the subject is working. So memory load is not present. It is not the case with the triplets. They had to remember. And that was blocked, so they had to remember the rule. We did not let them start on the test until they understood the instructions, and we established that they could produce the rules that they have to work by.

In the Swap's test in particular, there are simple steps that are increased with each one of the additional swaps that lead to the correlation with intelligence. And I think a more reasonable explanation is in terms of the lapses of attention as one goes to these otherwise simple tasks. But as the tasks become too long, occasionally something disappears in the person, that person makes an error. And people with lower IQ perhaps make more of these errors than those with the higher IQ. So both explanations are present. I kind of prefer the second one.

Dr. Baddeley: I don't see them as alternatives. To label something working memory isn't an explanation. It's a description of a problem, if you like. So I would see the second as one instantiation of how it might actually work within a broad working memory concept.

Dr. Süß: Your summary about emotional intelligence response — and emotional intelligence could be tested also by traditional personalities questionnaire. Could it be that this was not shared methods variance? What kind of test did you use to measure emotional intelligence? I think it would be necessary — if you want to measure intelligence, it would be necessary to use performance tests, but I don't know a performance test for emotional intelligence.

Dr. Stankov: Neither do I. All that we did was pick up everything that was on the Internet, and we got in touch with all the people who published in the area and got all their scales. They were very, very helpful, and I think disappointed with the outcome. But they are just questionnaire-type methods. I think I'll leave to somebody else to go on and use performance measures of emotional intelligence in future work. I had enough.

15

Sensory Processes Within the Structure of Human Cognitive Abilities

RICHARD D. ROBERTS, GERRY PALLIER, and
GINGER NELSON GOFF

As a gaggle of Australian expatriates abroad, we are somewhat perplexed at American psychology's current obsession with psychometric *g* (i.e., general intelligence; see Herrnstein & Murray, 1994; Jensen, 1998; Neisser et al., 1996, for recent accounts). Seemingly, it was not all that long ago when almost all introductory psychology textbooks drew a sharp distinction between the American and British approaches to human cognitive abilities. Commenting on this state of affairs at the time of greatest disjunction, Hearnshaw (1951; himself from England, perhaps best known for his biography of Sir Cyril Burt) was moved to suggest:

> While to some extent this divergence of viewpoint is due to differences between British and American methods of factor analysis . . . it is probably to some extent due to the influence of national character. The British view is closed and orderly; the American view less tidy and still adventurous. One would indeed have been more sure of the objectivity of factor studies if British investigators had not discovered an hierarchical society of factors crowned by "*g*," and the Americans a democratic society in which all factors are created equal. In spite of the mathematics it is not certain psychologists have abandoned the political model that Plato was the first to use. (p. 315)

If Hearnshaw is correct, it might be argued that it is modern America's obsession with "all things royal" that accounts for great interest in the ruling general factor. In support of this proposition, the shift in the scientific zeitgeist parallels the rise of

This research was supported by the National Research Council and the Human Effectiveness Division of the U.S. Air Force Research Laboratory at Brooks Air Force Base, Texas. Due acknowledgment is given to each of these respective institutions. We thank Phil Ackerman, Pat Kyllonen, Scott Chaiken, and Lazar Stankov for thoughtful comments on earlier drafts of this chapter.

electronic media and certain political dynasties in the United States during the latter half of the twentieth century. This conjecture is not, however, intended to detract from our appreciation of the enormous and important contributions made by our American colleagues. Indeed, it may even be unfair. Perhaps, instead, the reason for the prominence of g in the current literature is that a paradigm shift of the *utmost* magnitude has occurred in the field of learning and individual differences.

None of the present writers is well qualified to comment on the sociological or philosophical components of this movement in any specific detail. However, we do believe that the data on human cognitive abilities paint a far from incontrovertible picture. We also contend that an overwhelming insistence on psychometric g is stifling to the field of differential psychology. It is stifling because it implies that psychology's map of the intellect (in its broad outlines) is more or less complete. Such a view is surely (to quote again from Hearnshaw, 1951):

> [H]euristically inhibitory and contrary to the exploratory genius of scientific research. The scientist is unlikely to discover anything unless s/he believes that there is something to discover. The history of science, moreover, warns us that even in the more mature physical sciences proclamations of finality, even when apparently most firmly founded, have been falsified by the progress of research. It would therefore be rash to claim anything like finality in the psychologist's map of the intellect unless the arguments are logically overwhelming. (p. 316)

Indeed, were psychometric g a given, there would appear little left for individual-differences psychologists to do but develop more sophisticated instruments for its assessment, rendering each of us working within this field a "master test-maker." Although there is nothing inherently wrong with thinking of psychometric test development as a trade, there is undoubtedly more to the *science* of human cognitive abilities.

We do not wish to expend all of our efforts in this chapter engaging in the often fought controversy as to whether or not it is best to conceive of intelligence as a unitary dimension or a series of relatively independent functional "entities." However, it is important for the major purpose of this chapter to note, at the outset, our preference for an intricate and, at points, still uncharted structural model of human cognitive abilities. We do this because we believe a fruitful source of present (and we hope future) research involves an investigation of individual differences in what we have broadly termed *sensory abilities*. These sensory abilities have, of course, a long and checkered history within individual-differences psychology (e.g., see Galton, 1883). Arguably, were it not for certain historical vagaries and, in particular, overzealous acceptance of methodologically flawed studies (e.g., Wissler, 1901), it is likely the field of individual differences would have given these abilities far greater attention than has, up to now, been the case (Deary, 1994). Although it is possible to give some consideration to sensory processes in relation to psychometric g, a more promising approach posits that they are both structures within, and correlates of, a variety of cognitive ability constructs.

Psychometric g: Empirical Evidence?

Much as a distinction between the British and American approaches to individual differences has allegorically been ascribed to national character, it would seem emblematic of the Australian temperament to always be questioning what the authorities regard as law. Such is the cynicism evidenced in members of a former penal colony! And yet issues of relevance to cognitive ability structure are not merely sociological, nor can they be resolved within the comfort of the philosopher's armchair. If there were overwhelming data in support of both the construct validity and practical utility of psychometric g, then this should be named in honor of it. However, the data, as we see them, very much bring the importance of the first principal factor into question.

In support of this assertion, consideration needs first to be given to Carroll's (1993) monumental attempt to summarize and integrate over 400 studies (i.e., 477 data sets) conducted within the factor-analytic tradition this century. Carroll's careful exploratory factor (re)analysis of each data set led him to a model having three levels (or strata). On Stratum I are located each of the primary mental abilities identified variously in the writings of Thurstone (1938), Guilford (1956), and French and his colleagues (e.g., Ekstrom, French, & Harman, 1976). On Stratum II are a variety of broad cognitive abilities identified by Cattell (1987), Horn (1988, in press), and their associates (e.g., Horn & Noll, 1994; Stankov & Horn, 1980). In addition, on this stratum lie factors Carroll has either redefined to fit more readily into the wider psychological literature (e.g., General Memory and Learning, Gy) or brought to light for the very first time (e.g., Broad Decision Speed, Gp). Finally, on the third stratum is psychometric g (Spearman, 1904, 1927). The hierarchical factor structure comprising this three-stratum model is reproduced in Figure 15.1.

It transpires that this model caters to a great many theories of cognitive ability in one way or another (Carroll, 1993, p. 636ff.). For example, Carroll described how this model is similar to that postulated by Holzinger and Spearman around 1925, the major difference being factors lying on the intermediate level of Stratum II. In a similar vein, Carroll noted correspondence with Cattell and Horn's theory of fluid (Gf) and crystallized (Gc) intelligence, pointing out that Stratum III is so ubiquitous exponents of this theory have erred in not considering it. He also drew favorable analogies to models espoused by Vernon (1950), Thurstone (1938), and a host of others (e.g., Gardner, 1983; Jäger, 1984). Indeed, it would appear the only theory having impact in the intelligence literature this century that cannot simultaneously be encapsulated within the three-stratum framework is Guilford's (1967) Structure-of-Intellect model.

However, as Horn (in press) has recently argued, the most tenuous factor within this three-stratum model is undoubtedly the highest-order construct (i.e., psychometric g). In support of this assertion, Horn noted a number of theoretical and practical difficulties for the Stratum III general factor that have seemingly passed critical attention. For instance, studies specifically designed to test Spearman's model have failed to support the g construct (see Horn, 1988, for a review of this literature). In addition, positive manifold need not mathematically imply g as several commentators (e.g., Jensen, 1985) have erroneously suggested. Further still, a large number of noncognitive variables (e.g., absence of neuroticism, athleticism, absence of psychosis, and openness to experience) each correlates positively with ability tests yet clearly does not represent a functional unity.

Perhaps most damning, however, is Horn's (in press) contention that, of the 33 separate analyses conducted by Carroll (1993) in support of psychometric g, the factor derived from one analysis turns out to be conceptually dissimilar to those of

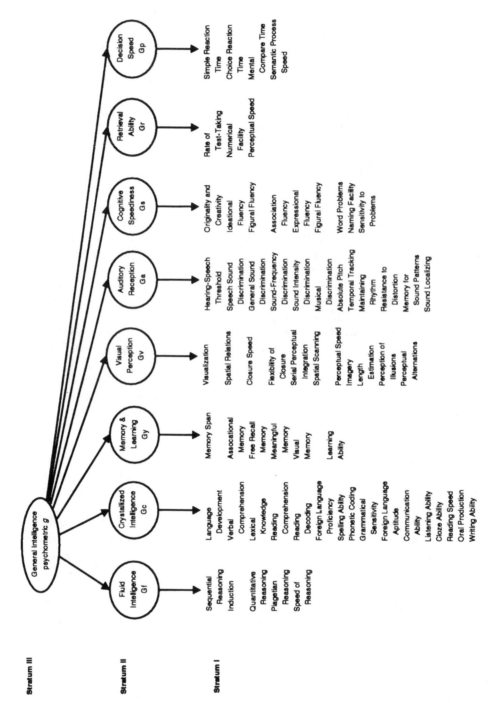

Figure 15.1. Carroll's (1993) three-stratum model of the structure of cognitive abilities. From *Human Cognitive Abilities: A Survey of Factor-Analytic Studies*, by J. B. Carroll, 1993, p. 626. Copyright 1993 by Cambridge University Press. Reprinted with permission.

further analyses. In short, the factors fail to "meet the standards of even the weakest form of factorial invariance namely, configural invariance" (Horn, in press, p. 14 [manuscript page]). Indeed, there is also support for this proposition given the way psychometric g has been conceptualized within the wider scientific literature. Thus, whereas some researchers have suggested that Gf is analogous to the general factor (e.g., Gustafsson, 1984), others have claimed that "verbal/math [i.e., Gc] . . . is frequently considered the avatar of g" (Stauffer, Ree, & Carretta, 1996, p. 199; see also Herrnstein & Murray, 1994; Matarazzo, 1972). In short, the confusion generated by these varying conceptualizations of the g construct seems difficult to reconcile with its reputed sound scientific status.

It is worth noting that while these criticisms and still others may be mounted against the g concept (e.g., Roberts & Stankov, 1998), negative commentary has seldom been directed at the second-order capabilities comprising Carroll's (1993) model. Indeed, even the staunchest supporters of psychometric g are sometimes forced to invoke the "intelligences" distinction implied by this stratum (e.g., Jensen, 1993). Developmental evidence in support of the distinctiveness and importance of broad cognitive abilities may now be considered overwhelming (e.g., see Horn & Noll, 1994). In this respect, readers would be excused if, in undertaking a brief perusal of the aging literature, they assumed that factors lying on Stratum II (rather than g) were paramount. Neurophysiological and genetic studies continue to map differential relationships testifying to the factorial independence of each broad cognitive ability construct (e.g., Thompson, 1985). Perhaps the greatest testament to the utility of factors embellished at this stratum is that many highly regarded contemporary measures of intelligence (e.g., the Woodcock–Johnson Tests of Cognitive Ability, Woodcock & Johnson, 1989) have been designed to assess Stratum II constructs (Daniel, 1997). In fact, even the latest version of the first intelligence scale —the Stanford–Binet IV—has been redesigned to assess three broad cognitive ability constructs: Gf, Gc, and broad memory and learning (see Thorndike, Hagen, & Sattler, 1985). This modification, which clearly diminishes the importance of a single, global measure of IQ, has been well received among many influential psychometricians (see, for example, Anastasi, 1988).

An Empirical Test of Stratum I and Stratum II Constructs

We should emphasize at this point that the structure comprising Carroll's (1993) model was derived from various exploratory factor analyses of a wide range of data sets. However, on average, the sample size of studies that were examined was relatively modest (median = 198; see Carroll, 1993, Table 4.3, p. 118) as was the number of variables used (median = 19.6; see Carroll, 1993, Table 4.7, p. 123). Because of these limitations, many of the structural relations represented in Figure 15.1 are more tenuous than Carroll had presented them, although in fairness he did acknowledge this point (Carroll, 1993, p. 579). Indeed, Carroll was forced to infer certain relationships between first- and second-stratum factors because, even within the expansive range of data sets that he had at his disposal, some constructs remained underrepresented and therefore poorly understood. This problematic feature is no better evidenced than in the case of broad auditory reception (Ga). Here many of the postulated factors turn out to be based on a handful of data sets, none of which offers a completely satisfactory account of the auditory domain (see Carroll, 1993, chapter 9). Of course, this type of shortcoming is through no fault of Carroll. The knowledge so far obtained on human cognitive abilities is constrained by certain practical limitations that are imposed in factorial studies requiring both a large database (i.e., number of tests) and appropriate sample size.

Within this context, it would appear that no investigator has used confirmatory factor-analytic techniques to determine whether there is empirical support for the structure comprising the most salient aspects (i.e., Strata I and II) of Carroll's (1993) model. Neither has there been any attempt to put this theory to the test using a large number of variables. This is no small point, given the enthusiasm in which both theoreticians and practitioners have generally greeted Carroll's model (e.g., see Hammond, 1998; Spearitt, 1996). However, recent advances in structural equation modeling that take into account missing data allow structural issues to be addressed in a particularly compelling manner. Under such conditions, it is possible to devise an experiment in which a certain proportion of participants take a number of tests and others a subset of these measures plus some additional others. By carefully designing the study so that all cells of the covariance matrix are filled (with sufficiently large N, or sample size), it is possible to explore a wider sampling of the cognitive ability domain within one study than has been possible in the past.

Using this rationale, Roberts and Goff (in press; see also Roberts, Goff, & Kyllonen, 1998) reanalyzed data on some 2,879 Air Force enlistees administered various subsets of the Armed Services Vocational Aptitude Battery (ASVAB) and 46 measures from the Kit of Factor-Referenced Cognitive Tests (Ekstrom et al., 1976). Because the general factor is essentially protean, and therefore of questionable scientific merit, Roberts and his coworkers fit this data set according to Stratum I and Stratum II factors of Carroll's (1993) model, with Stratum II factors allowed to correlate freely among themselves. An intermediate Stratum Ia was postulated on the basis of rationale explicated in Carroll (1993, p. 591ff.), whereas primary mental abilities were represented by the sum of at least two tests within each domain.

The results of this solution, which gave a highly adequate fit statistic (root mean square error of approximation [RMSEA] = 0.026), are worth noting in the context of our previous arguments. First, the structure unfolds, predominantly, as Carroll (1993) would have Stratum I and Stratum II constructs. As such, the model resembles that encapsulated by Gf–Gc theory, although we add there are also some differences. In particular, the memory and speed factors of this analysis are broader than that encapsulated by Gf–Gc theory. Second, the ASVAB (which has often been taken as a particularly good indicator of g, e.g., see Herrnstein & Murray, 1994) shares loadings, almost exclusively, on the broad ability factor related to acculturation, Gc. Indeed, despite claims of the ASVAB's predictive validity, Roberts and collaborators found it to underrepresent several broad cognitive ability constructs and overrepresent much narrower others. Finally, if a general factor were to be extracted, it would resemble the Gf factor of Stratum II, although in principle, this construct should reflect much more than the narrow "meaning" this nomenclature invokes (see Roberts & Stankov, 1998).

In short, there is sufficient evidence to suggest that two well-established and often-used tests of cognitive ability give a very different understanding of the intellect if used in a single study and a single construct is derived. This point should not be underemphasized, given that the universe of tests measuring cognitive abilities is large. Plausibly, each test within this universe gives a very different shade of meaning to the general intelligence construct. It is primarily for this reason that we question the efficacy of the construct of psychometric g. In its place we posit a structural model of the type comprising Stratum I and Stratum II of Carroll's (1993) model, which in turn may be seen as an elaboration and extension of the theory of fluid and crystallized intelligence.

Sensory Abilities Within the Structure of Cognitive Abilities

Having freed ourselves of the problematic general factor and demonstrated certain practical and theoretical advantages that might be accrued by using a structural model of intelligence, our attention may be focused on what we see as two fruitful research foci. Notably, these foci serve to enrich (rather than impoverish) the investigation of human individual differences. These areas of interest involve determining (a) those cognitive processes underlying each of the so-called Stratum II (or broad cognitive ability) factors and (b) the range and types of other factors that might be embellished within a still more comprehensive taxonomy. In both instances, our research has led us to consider the influence of psychological constructs tied closely to the human senses.

Mental Speed Within the Structure of Cognitive Abilities: The Role of Sensory Processes

Noting that one of the least well-understood dimensions of Carroll's (1993) three-stratum model was the various broad factors tied to cognitive and decision speed, we initiated a series of studies that examined mental speed constructs from a variety of perspectives (see, for example, Beh, Roberts, & Prichard-Levy, 1994; Roberts, Pallier, & Stankov, 1996; Stankov, Roberts, & Spilsbury, 1994). For example, reaction time (RT) measures derived from the Hick paradigm have generally been correlated with a single measure: number correct on Raven's Progressive Matrices Test (Juhel, 1991, cited in Roberts & Stankov, 1998). There are many issues of relevance given this limitation. For one, it remains uncertain whether the correlation between processing speed derives from a related primary mental ability (e.g., Figural Reasoning) or a second-order construct such as Gf. In a similar vein, the visual processing requirements implicit to Raven's Progressive Matrices Test are high, as are those underlying performance in visual RT tasks (through which most research has been conducted). It remains plausible that shared sensory and perceptual processes account for the substantial correlations that are observed between chronometric and psychometric indexes. Further still, even allowing that such issues are inconsequential, the failure to implement more than one or two RT measures in multivariate studies makes it unclear as to what exactly are the cognitive processes underlying correlation with psychometric markers.

In light of the preceding shortcomings, it became apparent that a carefully conducted research program should be directed at elucidating the nature of mental speed constructs. In perhaps our most important and ambitious attempt to investigate this domain, 179 participants performed 25 psychometric and 11 elementary cognitive tasks (ECTs) over four test sessions, each of approximately 2-hour duration. To eliminate the possibility of shared sensory requirements "driving" correlations, we included a number of psychometric measures of broad auditory (Ga) and broad visualization (Gv) processes in the multivariate design, while also sampling Gf, Gc, and memory factors across different sensory domains. For example, we had participants perform a battery of Gf markers that included tests having strong visual (e.g., Raven's Progressive Matrices Test) or auditory (e.g., Letter Counting Test) components. Similarly, ECTs included constructs that were sampled across diverse sensory modalities. For example, in addition to processing speed being assessed with visual RT tasks, the study included paradigms in which stimuli were presented aurally, and the responses were vocal. A complete description both of these ECTs and psychometric instruments may be found in Roberts (1997, 1998; see also Roberts & Stankov, 1998). These papers point to important features of the microstructure of each ECT used in the investigation, while also reporting cognitive correlates broken down by specific paradigm. Equally important, these papers suggest the number and type of mental speed parameters that are construct valid.

Rather than simply review these papers, we present a reanalysis of the data collected from this multivariate investigation that is in keeping with the main themes of the present chapter. Curiously, although there has been "an explosion of experimental studies into the speed of mental processes" (Eysenck, 1995, p. 225), factor-analytic evidence concerning the status of a range of time-dependent constructs has been either piecemeal or nonexistent. This shortcoming has occurred despite Carroll's (1993) admonition that "If any broad taxonomic classification of cognitive ability were to be formulated, in fact, it might be based on the distinction between level and speed" (p. 644). To redress this imbalance, we report a data set that is one of the first of its kind: a Schmid–Leiman transformation of the 11 ECTs used in the research conducted by Roberts and his associates. The uniqueness of this data set stems from the following two features. First, the number of ECTs used is considerably larger than in any study reported by Carroll (1993, see chapter 11). Second, owing to analyses reported in the papers cited above, only measures of central tendency were used (rather than less reliable or invalid constructs such as slope RT, intraindividual variability in decision time [DT], etc.; Roberts, 1998). In previous applications, such experimental dependence may have made the results of factor analysis equivocal. No such criticism may be leveled at the present data set. The Schmid–Leiman orthogonalized factor matrix of these ECTs (involving three orders of analysis) is given in Table 15.1.

There are several features of this solution that require detailed explication. For instance, there is clear differentiation of DT and movement time (MT) constructs at the first and second order. This outcome is most impressive quite simply for the fact that both MT and DT were obtained (in the vast majority of instances) in the same ECT. Clearly the data speak to separation between psychomotor and processing speed when these measures might easily have loaded together to form task-specific factors. As such, the data support a conceptual distinction between kinesthetic processes captured in the movement phase of these tasks and the DT component that likely includes (as we shall argue shortly) additional functions related to sensory processing.

Significantly, each of the psychomotor factors found at the first order of analysis has empirical antecedents in the literature. Indeed, there is an extensive literature

TABLE 15.1 Factor Loadings of Elementary Cognitive Tasks (ECTs) Obtained From a Schmid–Leiman Orthogonalized Transformation

Variable	O3:F1 t	O2:F2 MT_G	O2:F3 DT_G	O1:F4 MT_{LM}	O1:F5 MT_{MC}	O1:F6 MT_{SA}	O1:F7 DT_{LK}	O1:F8 DT_{PM}	O1:F9 $DT_{S/V}$
Movement Time (MT)									
Fitts's MT	**.32**	**.28**	.04	**.28**	.17	.08	.03	.01	.03
Single-response MT	**.31**	**.30**	.00	**.61**	−.02	.07	−.04	−.00	−.08
Tachistoscopic MT	**.28**	.19	.08	**.36**	.03	.04	.06	.06	−.14
Complex choice MT	**.44**	**.29**	.14	**.47**	.08	.04	.17	.03	.11
Binary reaction MT	**.28**	**.26**	−.00	**.72**	−.02	−.07	−.07	−.02	.12
Cards single MT	**.49**	**.43**	.04	−.02	**.74**	−.03	−.00	−.00	−.03
Cards multitask MT	**.50**	**.43**	.04	−.02	**.70**	.02	.00	.00	−.01
Word single MT	**.38**	**.35**	.01	.04	.06	**.57**	.04	.01	.01
Word multitask MT	**.44**	**.43**	−.01	.01	.02	**.78**	.08	.00	−.00
Decision Time (DT)									
Single response DT	**.24**	.03	**.21**	−.11	.03	−.02	**.80**	.00	.04
Tachistoscopic DT	**.25**	.04	**.20**	.01	.04	−.05	**.39**	.04	.10
Complex choice DT	**.22**	.04	.17	−.04	−.05	.04	**.74**	.01	−.07
Binary reaction DT	**.33**	.11	**.21**	.08	.01	.00	**.76**	.01	.04
Cards single DT	**.67**	−.02	**.66**	.00	.01	.02	.05	**.33**	−.06
Cards multitask DT	**.53**	−.02	**.53**	.02	.02	−.03	.06	**.22**	.19
Word single DT	**.25**	−.03	**.27**	.01	−.02	−.05	.15	−.00	**.78**
Word multitask DT	**.25**	−.06	**.30**	.04	.01	−.15	.06	.04	**.63**
Other									
Joystick reaction time	**.25**	.19	.06	.13	.00	.18	**.37**	−.01	−.02
Lehrl's duration of presence	−.12	−.03	−.08	.02	.00	−.10	.04	−.02	**−.21**
Lehrl's BIP measure	**−.28**	−.17	−.10	−.07	−.12	−.14	.03	−.00	**−.33**

Note. A description of each ECT may be found in Roberts, Pallier, and Stankov (1996). Numbers in boldfaced type represent leadings above .20. Symbols used for factors (or measures) correspond to the following: O and F refer to the order and factor number of each construct, respectively; t = chronometric t (i.e., General Response Speed); MT_G = general movement speed; DT_G = general decision speed; MT_{LM} = speed of limb movement; MT_{MC} = speed of multilimb coordination; MT_{SA} = speed of speech articulation; DT_{LK} = decision time to a light-key stimulus–response code; DT_{PM} = decision time to a pictorial–motor stimulus–response code; $DT_{S/V}$ = decision time to a semantic–verbal stimulus–response code; BIP = basic information processing.

summarizing the dimensions of psychomotor abilities (e.g., Peterson & Bownas, 1982), to which sharp parallels may be drawn with the present data set. For example, Factor 4 (designated MT_{LM} for Speed of Limb Movement) resembles a construct discussed in Peterson and Bownas (1982, pp. 70–72). This ability involves the speed with which discrete movements of the arms or legs are capable of being performed (see Carroll, 1993, p. 533). In similar fashion, the interpretation of Factor 5 (designated MT_{MC} for Multilimb Coordination) is reinforced by a study conducted by Paterson, Elliott, Anderson, Toops, and Heidbreder (1930; cited in Carroll, 1993). This study found psychomotor movements obtained from a card-sorting task (similar to that used in the present investigation) loading substantially on (and hence defining) an analogous factor. Finally, Factor 6 resembles a psychomotor factor identified by Carroll (1993) as Speed of Speech Articulation (hereinafter designated MT_{SA}). This factor appears chiefly in "measures of the speed of performing fast articulations with the speech musculature ... [where] in speech and hearing research, such movements are termed diadochokinetic (from Greek words meaning 'successive movements')" (Carroll, 1993, p. 536).

Each of the findings pertaining to these psychomotor factors is essentially non-controversial. However, this is not true of the DT factors, each of which appears to have been discussed in a rather vague manner in the past. Indeed, we could mount a strong case to suggest that previous interpretations of DT factors have been made within a largely atheoretical framework. For example, in acknowledgment of differential psychology's almost complete ignorance of this domain, Carroll (1993) laments, "it is not possible to derive ... clear evidence for a definite set of speed factors in ECTs" (p. 484).

The question that logically follows is whether there is a model in the experimental–cognitive literature that establishes a rapprochement between theory and the present data set. Elsewhere, Roberts (1998) noted that modeling of stimulus–response (S-R) compatibility effects has provided much of the empirical impetus to the RT literature over the past decade or so. At the same time, much of the cognitive-correlates approach to intelligence has been grounded in paradigms having their origins in the mid-1950s and early 1960s. Might not some of the contemporary research on RT provide a conceptual framework for interpreting DT factors?

The answer to this question is yes. Kornblum, Hasbroucq, and Osman (1990) postulated a conceptual model of S-R compatibility effects that involves the construct of dimensional overlap. Put simply, dimensional overlap is defined as "the degree to which two sets of items have properties or attributes in common, and the degree to which such attributes are similar to one another" (Kornblum, 1992, p. 749). In invoking the notion of congruent and incongruent mapping, the model predicts differences in RT paradigms according to the S-R codes comprising a given RT paradigm. Elsewhere, researchers working within the field of learning and individual differences have suggested that different ECTs implicate differential degrees of cognitive complexity so that "more complex RT tasks show greater correlations with intelligence" (Larson & Saccuzzo, 1989, p. 7). As a corollary, the dimensional-overlap model presently advocated also assuages our discipline's largely atheoretical approach to the construct of cognitive complexity (Roberts & Stankov, 1998).

Under the dimensional-overlap framework, DT factors presented in Table 15.1 may be understood in a compelling (and simple) fashion. Thus, Factor 7 (with

348

loadings deriving from three ECTs involving the same visual stimuli [i.e., lights] may be interpreted as DT to a Light-Key code (hereinafter designated DT_{LK}). Factor 8, on the other hand, may be interpreted as DT to a Pictorial-Motor code (DT_{PM}) because all of the ECTs loading on this trait required manipulation of complex symbolic stimuli that were given in pictorial form. Finally, Factor 9 may be interpreted as DT to a Semantic–Verbal code ($DT_{S/V}$). This factor's interpretation is reinforced by the magnitude and pattern of loadings from tasks presented aurally (i.e., the word-classification task) and tasks in which the stimuli were written words that the individual read aloud (i.e., Lehrl's basic information processing [BIP] measure; see Roberts et al., 1996).

The results presented in Table 15.1 regarding DT components suggest meaningful individual differences in processing speed for specific types of stimuli (in particular, modality and content). Indeed, what might previously have been considered "method variance" appears instead to reflect elementary cognitive abilities tied to specific modalities and symbolic content that correspond to different brain processes.

Because these first-order DT factors find a ready grounding in Kornblum et al. (1990), we may use some of the research conducted within the dimensional-overlap model to address features of our ECTs. Consider, for example, a major biological component of that model. Recently, Riehle, Kornblum, and Requin (1997) demonstrated that sensory-to-motor transformations (implicit in the range of S-R ensembles discussed by Kornblum and his associates that we undoubtedly capitalized on) are continuous processes occurring in the primary motor cortex. In combination with our factor analysis and models of intelligence that stress the importance of cognitive complexity, such findings might also predict that different combinations of S-R mappings would share differential magnitudes of correlation with intelligence measures. In turn, this suggests that our understanding of RT–intelligence correlations need not come from ECTs that are trivially simple (as some biological models accounting for this relationship might adduce).

Having demonstrated the structural properties of the DT and MT constructs in the analysis reported in Table 15.1, we turn our attention briefly, for purposes of completion, to their correlation with broad cognitive abilities. Elsewhere, we report on the derivation (and interpretation) of seven cognitive ability factors from the psychometric portion of the test battery used for this purpose (Roberts, 1997). The correlation of these psychometric factors with the three orders of ECT constructs is given in Table 15.2.

Given our previous interpretation of DT factors within the dimensional-overlap model and our speculations concerning correlation with intelligence measures, it is worth noting that the correlation between these factors and intelligence does indeed vary as a function of differences in S-R compatibility. Thus, the factor defining a particularly compatible dimension ($DT_{S/V}$) shares the lowest correlation with Gf. Furthermore, recall from the start of this section on mental speed that it has remained unclear whether DT factors are linked to intelligence measures because of shared sensory requirements. The relatively small correlations between DT factors and Gv (or in the case of $DT_{S/V}$, Ga) suggest that this account cannot provide a satisfactory explanation for the relationship observed between processing speed and Gf. Nevertheless, Table 15.2 also makes it clear why it is important to focus on broad cognitive abilities (because mental processing speed has been linked previously in almost exclusive fashion with psychometric g). Accordingly, inspection of

TABLE 15.2 Correlations Between the Three Strata of Mental Speed and Second-Order Psychometric Factors

Variable	O3:F1 t	O2:F2 MT_G	O2:F3 DT_G	O1:F4 MT_{LM}	O1:F5 MT_{MC}	O1:F6 MT_{SA}	O1:F7 $DT_{L/K}$	O1:F8 $DT_{P/M}$	O1:F9 $DT_{S/V}$
Fluid intelligence	**-.42**	**-.25**	**-.40**	-.09	-.21	-.21	**-.38**	**-.38**	**-.24**
Crystallized intelligence	-.12	-.03	-.07	-.06	.05	-.10	-.03	-.05	**-.28**
Short-term acquisition	**-.24**	-.16	**-.27**	.02	**-.22**	-.14	-.08	**-.26**	**-.22**
Broad visualization	-.21	-.12	-.17	-.10	-.03	-.14	-.21	-.16	-.08
Broad auditory function	**-.30**	**-.28**	-.12	**-.24**	-.18	**-.22**	-.20	-.09	-.14
Perceptual speed	**.60**	**.46**	**.43**	**.40**	**.29**	**.36**	**.49**	**.40**	.17
Inductive reasoning	**-.24**	-.07	**-.28**	-.03	-.02	-.10	**-.25**	**-.27**	-.16

Note. Numbers in boldfaced type are significant at $p < .01$. See Table 15.1 for definition of factors.

Table 15.2 shows that almost all of the DT factors of the present analysis share no particularly meaningful relationship with an important cognitive ability, Gc. The one exception to this finding (DT$_{S/V}$) is defined by tasks containing a strong verbal component that, despite shared requirements, have very modest correlation.

Support for differentiating between MT and DT is seen in the differing patterns of correlations found between these two general constructs and the seven broad cognitive processes. Nevertheless, all of the constructs have relatively high correlations with the cognitive domain of Clerical Speed. This outcome suggests that this construct may be more complex than extant data have shown, supporting Carroll's (1993, p. 644) previously cited ruminations concerning the primary importance of speed within a comprehensive taxonomy of cognitive abilities. Note also that Carroll (1993, p. 647) made a compelling case that cognitive-correlates approaches will be misleading unless conventional psychometric constructs are referenced to specific strata. The present findings would appear to extend this assertion to mental speed concepts. Consequently, we note that a second-order construct such as broad Decision Speed (DT$_G$) relates to Memory and Reasoning (Gy), whereas broad Psychomotor Speed (MT$_G$) relates to Auditory Function (Ga). The latter correlation is most interesting because it suggests possible links among natural tempo, psychomotor performance, and audition (see Spearman, 1927).

In summary, the hierarchical structure emanating from factor analysis of mental speed constructs provides a number of fresh new possibilities for both empirical research and theory construction that we are in the midst of exploring more fully. It is clear that, in so doing, the role of sensory processes is demonstrated to be pivotal. Nevertheless, it is also apparent that we would *not* have attempted such an undertaking within the restrictive confines of a single factor model of intelligence.

Tactile–Kinesthesia Within the Structure of Cognitive Abilities

Embedded within the original conceptualization of Gf–Gc theory was an inherent possibility that empirical investigations might identify factorially distinct cognitive abilities in addition to those already recognized. There are good reasons to suspect that the modality of stimulus presentation would be a productive area for such research. Thurstone (1948), for example, suggested that "auditory memory is not the same ability as visual memory" (p. 403). In describing his Structure-of-Intellect model, Guilford (1959) postulated that auditory and kinesthetic cognitive abilities existed but required empirical confirmation. Stankov and Horn (1980) undertook such an investigation, and indeed their results provided evidence for the existence of abilities (auditory in this case) that appear to be dependent on the sensory processes involved.

Such experimental support for the structural model underlying Gf–Gc theory poses several interesting questions for psychologists interested in the subdiscipline of learning and individual differences. For instance, if auditory abilities, such as tonal memory, do tap different resources to visual memory, how do these abilities relate to each other? Those subscribing to neo-Spearmanian concepts could presumably tend to disregard such relatively subtle distinctions within any hierarchical structure exhibiting the phenomenon of positive manifold (see Vernon, 1950). The structure of human cognitive abilities highlighted throughout this chapter demands, however, a radically different interpretation. Rather than a hierarchical structure with overtones of "superior" functions, these nascent intimations suggest that consideration of a continuum of abilities, in which each component is complementary, might lead to a more comprehensive taxonomy of intellectual functioning.

Using this conjecture as a starting point, Roberts, Stankov, Pallier, and Dolph (1997) postulated that a tactile–kinesthetic cognitive ability might be discerned by experimental exploration. They attempted to simulate, in tactile form, established marker tests from within the Gf–Gc framework. The underutilization of the tactile sensory modality by psychometricians also led Roberts et al. to use novel tasks suggested by investigators in other psychological disciplines (most especially in neuropsychology and perception). The results of this research project, comparing eight tactile tasks against 18 commonly used psychometric tests (along with latency scores from many of the tests), did indeed suggest the existence of a tactile cognitive ability (hereinafter designated TK for tactile–kinesthesis). However, the exact empirical status of TK is presently uncertain. To highlight the nature of our empirical search for this construct, we now consider the results of that study.

The battery of 26 tests used in the investigation was given to 195 people drawn from a university psychology course and from the Sydney metropolitan population at large. Following a series of suggestions made by Carroll (1995), both exploratory factor analysis (EFA) and confirmatory factor analysis (CFA) were used to analyze the resulting data set. EFA was used first to explore the structure of the data. From these results, a model was hypothesized and tested using CFA methods. Because of the ambiguity of some of the results, another EFA was performed on a slightly reduced number of experimental variables. The results of these analyses suggested the TK factor could not be separated from Gv (at least within this test battery). Table 15.3 presents the factor loadings from a CFA that posited seven factors. The fit of this model is well within accepted values (RMSEA = 0.038).

The interpretation of most of the factors given in Table 15.3 is relatively straightforward. Often-replicated factors, such as Gf and Gc, are clearly well defined. Moreover, as suggested in consideration of the previously reported ECT data, there is evidence for an Elementary Cognitive Speed (ECSp) factor that combines components of DT and MT. The fact that this trait is somewhat distinct from a Test-Taking Speed (TTSp) factor is predicated in Carroll (1993; see also Roberts & Stankov, 1998). Nevertheless, there are some curious features of this solution. In particular, one cannot easily distinguish between the TK and Gv constructs, and the Digit Span Forward (DsF) and Digit Span Backward (DsB) variables (which here combine aspects of both *level* [i.e., accuracy] and *speed*) form two test-specific factors instead of one factor representing Gy (i.e., the broad general memory factor).

CFAs were also performed to examine the structure among these seven first-order factors. Figure 15.2A shows that, at the second order, the highest loadings on the first of three factors comes from TK–Gv and Gf, which again suggests that TK appears as a "link-like" component between these two well-established cognitive ability traits. Figure 15.2B represents a model positing a superordinate "g" factor. The highest loadings on the g factor of this model derive from the TK–Gv and Gf constructs. Although it would be tempting to conclude that this factor merely represents TK–Gv (in a similar manner that Gf has been labeled representative of g), an equally compelling argument could be made that this second-order factor is, in fact, Gf (with a very strong tactile–visualization component). Consistent with this

TABLE 15.3 Confirmatory Factor-Analytic (Standardized) Solution of All Psychometric, Mental Speed, and Tactile–Kinesthetic Measures

| Measure | Level abilities from Gf–Gc theory | | | Mental speed abilities | | Mixed level and speed | | |
	Gc	Gf	TK–Gv	TTSp	ECSp	DsF	DsB	E
Cognitive ability								
Raven's progressive matrices		.856						.516
Letter series	.245	.597						.764
Letter counting			.639					.769
Vocabulary	.818							.575
General information	.701							.713
Esoteric analogies	.660	.344						.668
Digit span forward						.551		.834
Digit span backward							.825	.565
Visual bead memory		.556						.831
Card rotations		.548						.836
Hidden figures	.220	.537						.814
Hidden words	.139	.281		−.197				.906
Number comparison	.170			.328	.203			.927
Mental speed								
Letter series time				.773				.635
Letter counting time				.517				.856
General information time	−.219			.805		.231		.533
Esoteric analogies time				.885		.138		.469
Digit span forward time				.325		.223		.926
Digit span backward time			−.358	.366		−.481	1.035	.283
Hidden words time				.564				.826
Number comparison time				.256				.967
Digit symbol	−.160				.528			.834
Maths classification					.597			.802
Compatibility (M)					.784			.620
Card-sorting decision time				.153	.504			.875
Fitts's movement time					.264			.965
Card-sorting movement time					.409	−.182		.909
Tactual performance								
Finger counting			.519				.170	.789
Tactile texture	.205							.979
Tactile bead memory			.236		.274		.201	.821
Halstead Reitan tactual perform time			1.062		−.457	−.531		.689
Halstead Reitan tactual perform level			.915		−.435	−.345		.800
Tactile shapes			.671					.741
Finger writing[a]			.723					
Gibson's touch[a]			.445					

Note. Gf = fluid intelligence; Gc = crystallized intelligence; TK = tactile–kinesthesis; Gv = broad visualization; TTSp = test-taking speed; ECSp = elementary cognitive speed; DsF = digit span forward; DsB = digit span backward; E = residual error. Data in table are from "Charting the Cognitive Sphere: Tactile–Kinesthetic Performance Within the Structure of Intelligence," by R. D. Roberts, L. Stankov, G. Pallier, and B. Dolph, 1997, *Intelligence, 25,* 111–148. Copyright 1997 by Ablex Publishing. Reprinted with permission.

[a]Given to 108 participants only. These two tests define the TK–Gv factor in that smaller sample of participants. The coefficients for these two tests are not obtained from the sample that provided the data for the overall structural equation modeling solution.

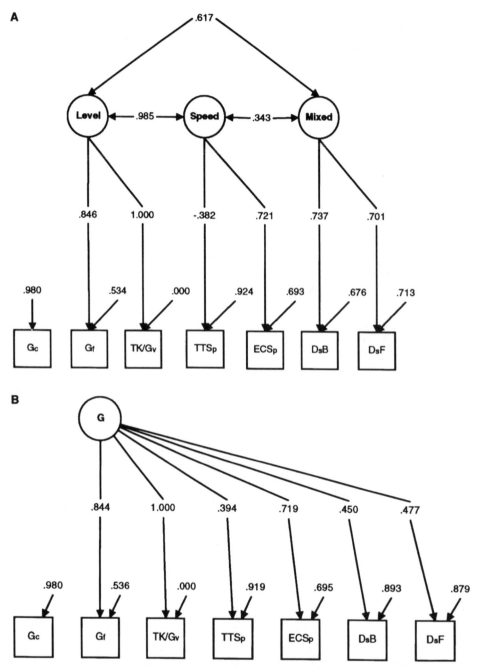

Figure 15.2. Postulated factorial structure involving (a) correlated second-order factors, which in turn produces a satisfactory fit to the data using confirmatory factor-analytic procedures and (b) a higher order general factor, which also produces a satisfactory fit using confirmatory factor analysis. Note, however, crystallized intelligence (Gc) is made largely redundant under this model. Gf = fluid intelligence; TK = tactile–kinesthesis; Gv = broad visualization process; TTSP = test-taking speed factor; ECSp = elementary cognitive speed

proposition, the Gc factor stands apart from the g of this analysis despite being an important part of the universe of cognitive abilities in all extant models of intelligence (Marshalek, Lohman, & Snow, 1983). Of course, this finding is also entirely consistent with propositions outlined at the start of this chapter, in which the utility (and conceptual significance) of a single, general factor in psychometric research was questioned.

This set of experimental results also led Roberts et al. (1997) to conduct an EFA on a set of measures that eliminated all variables that were experimentally dependent. Table 15.4 shows that Gf, Gv, and TK cannot be distinguished from one another in this set of variables and that the two Digit Span tests now anchor a factor representing Gy. The removal of the time-based psychometric scores was expected to result in the general Test-Taking Speed (i.e., TTSp) factor no longer being present, but a "skeleton" factor, defined largely by a single variable, remains in the factor pattern. Gc and ECSp factors (representing a composite of DT and MT constructs because there were insufficient markers of these two domains in the design) remain essentially the same between the two models. In addition, a factor representing Working Memory is found, which has a noteworthy correlation (.46) with the Gf–TK–Gv factor (see Kyllonen & Christal, 1990).

Discrepancies between the memory factors reported in the EFA and CFA solutions call for further examination of the relationship among memory span, tactile processing, and measures of timed performance. It would seem injudicious to favor specific interpretations at this stage. Memory factors do exist in these data sets, but their exact empirical status is unclear. It is worth drawing to the readers' attention that memory and learning factors remain the most poorly understood aspect of Carroll's (1993, chapter 7) model despite the fact that cognitive psychology has provided robust experimental paradigms through which to measure these constructs. It is to be hoped that this shortcoming will be addressed sometime in the future, possibly with some of the sensory paradigms that we allude to later in this chapter (see, for example, Stevenson, Prescott, & Boakes, 1995).

Although the analyses presented here support the inclusion of TK in the overall taxonomy of human cognitive abilities, the boundaries between this ability and other broad cognitive abilities remain somewhat indistinct. It appears that TK shares common variance both with Gf and Gv. Possible interpretations of the location of TK within the overall structure of human cognitive abilities are presented in Figure 15.3. Two options are considered. The first (Figure 15.3A) is whether the TK–Gv factor may be viewed as a broad factor such as Gf, Gv, or Gy. The second option (Figure 15.3B) suggests that TK represents a primary ability much like the Test-Taking Speed factor isolated in the present investigation. If the latter option is true, this construct may constitute a primary mental ability comprising both Gv and Gf simply because of the level of complexity at which tests designed to measure each construct were assessed. Within this context, it must be recalled that commentors have pointed previously to difficulties distinguishing between Gf and Gv when the

factor; DsB = digit span backward variable; DsF = digit span forward variable. From "Charting the Cognitive Sphere: Tactile–Kinesthetic Performance Within the Structure of Intelligence," by R. D. Roberts, L. Stankov, G. Pallier, and B. Dolph, 1997, *Intelligence, 25,* 111–148. Copyright 1997 by Ablex Publishing. Reprinted with permission.

TABLE 15.4 Exploratory Factor-Analytic Solution (Principal Axis Factoring With Oblimin Rotation) of Psychometric, Mental Speed, and Tactile–Kinesthetic Measures Selected to Ensure Experimental Independence

Measure	Gc	Gf–TK–Gv	TTSp	ECSp	Gy	WM	h²
Cognitive ability							
Raven's progressive matrices	.122	.509	-.022	.211	.011	.241	.600
Letter series	.275	.467	-.179	.157	.004	.116	.477
Letter counting	-.097	.333	.137	.155	.309	.135	.424
Vocabulary	.833	-.064	-.110	-.092	.077	-.045	.710
General information	.732	-.008	.119	-.007	-.072	-.029	.530
Esoteric analogies	.657	.190	-.075	.052	.048	.026	.554
Digit-span forward	.039	-.081	-.016	.066	.669	-.085	.436
Digit-span backward	.148	-.020	-.019	-.128	.386	.302	.326
Visual bead memory	.058	.203	-.018	.085	.083	.386	.342
Card rotations	.027	.315	.218	.090	.182	.076	.313
Hidden figures	.165	.590	.151	.149	.151	.201	.513
Hidden words	.147	.142	.098	.005	.084	.075	.141
Mental speed							
Number comparison time	.061	-.088	.716	-.036	-.042	.056	.519
Digit symbol	-.119	.096	.231	.648	.020	-.114	.516
Math classification	.048	.145	-.038	.591	.001	.098	.460
Compatibility (M)	.144	-.076	.074	.732	-.040	.262	.715
Card-sorting decision time + card-sorting movement time	-.018	.050	-.075	.223	-.212	.421	.309
Fitts's movement time	-.034	-.084	-.084	.331	.034	.005	.112
Tactual performance							
Finger counting	-.035	.201	-.046	.048	.285	.351	.386
Tactile texture	-.006	.005	-.036	-.021	-.045	.001	.061
Tactile bead memory	.001	.260	.107	.062	.063	.612	.455
Halstead-Reitan tactual perform level	-.015	.438	.052	-.146	-.023	.157	.261
Tactile shapes	-.109	.442	-.024	.023	.239	.282	.503

Note. Salient loadings are underlined. Gc = crystallized intelligence; Gf = fluid intelligence; TK = tactile–kinesthesis; Gv = broad visualization; TTSp = test-taking speed; ECSp = elementary cognitive speed; Gy = general memory and learning; WM = working memory; h² = communality. Data in table are from "Charting the Cognitive Sphere: Tactile–Kinesthetic Performance Within the Structure of Intelligence," by R. D. Roberts, L. Stankov, G. Pallier, and B. Dolph, 1997, *Intelligence*, 25, 111–148. Copyright 1997 by Ablex Publishing. Reprinted with permission.

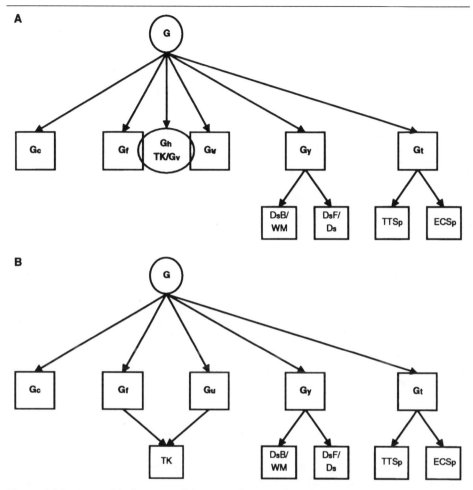

Figure 15.3. A possible location of the (TK) factor within the structure of human cognitive abilities. In this interpretation, a new second-order factor, designated here as general haptic ability (Gh), is postulated that would capture some of the variance of both fluid intelligence (Gf) and visualization processes (Gv). B: An alternative interpretation of the TK factor's position within the structure of human cognitive abilities. In this instance, TK is a primary mental ability that shares loadings on both Gf and Gv. G = general intelligence; Gy = general memory and learning; Gt = general response speed; DsB = digit span backward variable; WM = working memory; Ds = digit span; DsF = digit span forward variable; TTSP = test-taking speed factor; ECSP = elementary cognitive speed factor. From "Charting the Cognitive Sphere: Tactile–Kinesthetic Performance Within the Structure of Intelligence," by R. D. Roberts, L. Stankov, G. Pallier, and B. Dolph, 1997, *Intelligence, 25,* 111–148. Copyright 1997 by Ablex Publishing. Reprinted with permission.

relationships among the visual patterns are not easily manifest (e.g., Humphreys, 1962). Further factorial studies, including those that implement more Gf and Gv marker tests, should improve our understanding of the role of TK in structural models of intellectual functioning. Equally, it would seem judicious to investigate measures of tactual discrimination that are more perceptual in nature. For a series of particularly interesting and valid tactual paradigms appearing in the literature recently, the reader is referred to Turvey (1996).

Although Roberts et al. (1997) considered these results "somewhat pessimistic" (p. 143) for establishing the existence of a distinct tactile factor, the evidence does support these authors' original extrapolations concerning a set of "partially distinct modules" for intellectual abilities. Furthermore, the implications of these results are wide ranging. Using the tactile sensory modality offers additional methods of presenting tasks (especially competing tasks), opens new pathways to psychobiological research, offers the possibility of constructing superior "culture-fair" tests, and gives insight about the autonomy of a type of performance important to comprehensive neuropsychological assessment (see Pallier, Roberts, & Stankov, 1998). Given these set of findings alone, a compelling case can be made that the role of the senses in differential psychology has been undervalued.

Sensory Abilities: Lessons From Other Research

It is apparent that much recent developmental evidence has argued for important concomitants associated with sensory processes (e.g., Lindenberger & Baltes, 1994). For instance, it has been estimated that up to 59% of aging decline in intelligence can be attributed to decrements in auditory and visual information processing (Lindenberger & Baltes, 1997), which in turn affect everyday functioning (Marsiske, Klumb, & Baltes, 1997). These are not the only sensory systems known to be vulnerable to the effects of aging. For example, Cowart (1989) documented age-related declines in absolute gustatory and olfactory sensitivity. Similarly, Stevens and Cruz (1996) used a repeated threshold-testing paradigm to both taste and touch and found significant levels of sensory loss across the life span. The question that needs to be asked is to what extent including additional sensory processes in developmental studies will improve our understanding of decline in cognitive (and everyday) functioning.

It is also worth drawing to the reader's attention that two bastions of conventional approaches to psychological inquiry — each of which have remained relatively "fixed" to specific types of experimental paradigm, that is, (a) learning theory and (b) perception and psychophysics — have invested considerably greater resources in exploring the senses over the past few years. The previously cited study of Stevenson et al. (1995) is perhaps a consummate example, because it demonstrates that associative learning not only plays a major role in acquisition of tastelike properties by odors but also affects modeling (and subsequent understanding) of implicit learning. Equally, Turvey's (1996) summary statement of research examining dynamic touch, wherein he "promoted an image of muscles as smart instruments" (p. 1151), admonished the reader to direct more attention to touch because it has valuable lessons to teach psychology and physiology. All this flurry of research activity is to be compared with Carroll's (1993) cursory treatment of sensory processes in his influential tome, in which a few (rather antiquated) studies receive minor lip service. This shortcoming, in a book that we have had recourse to cite frequently in this chapter, should give the reader a vivid impression of our ignorance concerning sensory constructs within the science of learning and individual differences.

A Sense of the Future

Our exposition of multivariate studies that have at their core the delineation and exploration of sensory constructs, has, of necessity, been both brief and (somewhat) general. However, it is clear from this discussion that, whether we look at ECTs or complex psychometric assessment, sensory processes may constitute a hitherto neglected subject matter (perhaps even a domain) of cognitive ability research. This omission is all the more curious in light of what we believe should constitute the proper frame of reference for methodology in the study of individual differences. Elsewhere, Carroll (1995) argued that the goal of our subdiscipline is the exploration of "the *diversity of intellect* in the people of this planet — the many forms of cognitive processes and operations, mental performances, and creations of knowledge and art" (p. 429). To achieve this end, Carroll suggested that there are untapped domains of mental activity that must be discovered and encapsulated within a comprehensive taxonomic model. Furthermore, the demonstration of the meaning of these concepts and their relevance to real-world activities and problems is critical to progress in the science of individual differences. We concur with these sentiments. Because many creations of knowledge and art (minimally) have at their core aesthetic appreciation of well-honed sensory processes (extending beyond those grounded in either the visual or auditory medium), each surely demands rigorous empirical investigation.

It is equally clear that the psychometric domain cannot be allowed to languish or stagnate (see Horn & Noll, 1994). It is obvious that in recent years the search for a "holy grail," in the form of a basic process underlying intellectual ability, has provided considerable impetus for innovative research. This quest has, however, faltered and, in our opinion, failed to adequately expose a theoretically meaningful, unitary determinate of intelligence (see Stankov & Roberts, 1997).

The time has come to move on to fresh fields of investigation that can explore the increasing complexity revealed by past research. But which direction to take? A number of investigators of both theoretical and empirical bent are presently focusing on the "gray area" between personality and cognitive ability (e.g., Ackerman, 1996; Hammond, 1998; Stankov, 1998). This interface, covering metacognitive functions such as personal confidence, offers insight into life span achievement and why individuals choose particular fields of interest. Other investigators have been exploring, and will continue to explore, the biological basis of intelligence (e.g., see Detterman, 1992). Looking toward the future, these approaches both appear as worthy endeavors (see Matarazzo, 1992).

The approach we advocate, however, is fueled by a reconsideration of the causes behind the direction in which differential psychologists have steered their efforts. Our belief is that this framework will aid the theoretical and pragmatic applications of research. It is clear that assessment procedures have been used by society to both gauge and direct the talents of vast numbers of individuals. Roberts and Goff (in press), for example, noted that the future of over one million people is annually affected by just one instrument (the ASVAB). Deese (1993) was not exaggerating when he remarked on "the awesome responsibility of theorists of human ability on their influence on human affairs" (p. 115). Psychometricians must, therefore, be aware both of moral consequences and of social requirements as technological advances and prevailing sociocultural attitudes alter the individual's worldview. Failure to reexamine the precepts underlying our efforts may cost us dearly. Spearman's

359

(1904) research considered faculties, such as proficiency in Ancient Greek, which would hardly rate a mention in modern research. Yet, in conjunction with Binet and Simon's (1905) assessment procedures, abilities that quickly become outdated still remain as a primary source underlying evaluation of crystallized intelligence.

There can surely be few individuals who would doubt that the societal concepts of intelligent behavior prevailing at the beginning of the century are radically different from those at the *fin de siècle*. We concur with Ackerman (1996) that concepts for the measurement of acculturated abilities are in dire need of revision. The progenitors of differentialism also examined the relationship of sensory processes to intellectual functioning (e.g., Galton, 1883). Unquestioning acceptance of their failure to identify such a relationship has led to almost total disregard of the role of the senses in models of human cognitive ability. However, the methodological inadequacy of this seminal research, compounded by several pioneering researchers' discovery of a correlation between sensory discrimination and intellectual ability, requires a reexamination of this role (see Deary, 1994). This is perhaps even truer as granting agencies demand accountability, and individual-differences psychology is forced to interact more closely with human-factors psychology. Human-factors psychology, after all, ultimately requires that the interaction between machine and the human system (with its disparate sensory channels) be well understood.

As the millenium approaches, technological advances, especially in the "virtual world" offered by computer science and information technology, are placing a greater emphasis on what Galton (1883) called "the avenue of the senses" (p. 27). We may cite, for example, Microsoft's continuing interest in voice recognition (which considerably affects individual differences in the previously elucidated construct of diadochokinetics) as one such instance, tactual feedback from enhanced computer joysticks as another. If psychometricians are to keep abreast of the requirements of society (thus maintaining credibility), avoid intellectual stagnation, and maintain the Baconian precepts of scientific advancement, then due consideration of the senses is essential. The achievement of a more complete taxonomy of intelligence demands such consideration and, because we believe this concept is itself subject to continual variation, will require revision by future generations of differential psychologists.

REFERENCES

Ackerman, P. L. (1996). A theory of adult intellectual development: Process, personality, interests, and knowledge. *Intelligence, 22*, 227–257.

Anastasi, A. (1988). *Psychological testing (6th ed.)*. New York: Macmillan.

Anderson, C., Brown, C. P., & Tallal, P. (1993). Developmental language disorders: Evidence for a basic processing deficit. *Current Opinion in Neurology and Neurosurgery, 6*, 98–106.

Beh, H. C., Roberts, R. D., & Prichard-Levy, A. (1994). The relationship between intelligence and choice reaction time within the framework of an extended model of Hick's Law: A preliminary report. *Personality and Individual Differences, 16*, 891–897.

Binet, A., & Simon, T. (1905). Méthodes nouvelles pour le diagnostic du niveau intellectuel des anormaux [New methods for diagnosing the intellectual level of abnormals]. *Anneé Psychologique, 11*, 191–336.

Carroll, J. B. (1993). *Human cognitive abilities: A survey of factor-analytic studies*. New York: Cambridge University Press.

Carroll, J. B. (1995). On methodology in the study of cognitive abilities. *Multivariate Behavioral Research, 30*, 429–452.

Cattell, R. B. (1987). *Intelligence: Its structure, growth and action.* Amsterdam: North Holland.

Cowart, B. J. (1989). Relationships between taste and smell across the adult life span. *Annals of the New York Academy of Sciences, 561,* 39–55.

Daniel, M. H. (1997). Intellectual testing: Status and trends. *American Psychologist, 52,* 1038–1045.

Deary, I. J. (1994). Sensory discrimination and intelligence: Postmortem or resurrection? *American Journal of Psychology, 107,* 95–115.

Deese, J. (1993). Human abilities versus intelligence. *Intelligence, 17,* 107–116.

Detterman, D. K. (Ed.). (1992). Biology and intelligence [Special issue]. *Intelligence, 16,* 257–427.

Ekstrom, R. B., French, J. W., & Harman, H. H. (1976). *Manual for Kit of Factor-Referenced Cognitive Tests, 1976.* Princeton, NJ: Educational Testing Service.

Eysenck, H. J. (1995). Can we study intelligence using experimental method? *Intelligence, 20,* 217–228.

Galton, F. (1883). *Inquiries into human faculty and its development.* New York: Macmillan.

Gardner, H. (1983). *Frames of mind: The theory of multiple intelligences.* New York: Basic Books.

Guilford, J. P. (1956). The structure of intellect. *Psychological Bulletin, 53,* 267–293.

Guilford, J. P. (1959). Three faces of intellect. *American Psychologist, 14,* 469–479.

Guilford, J. P. (1967). *The nature of human intelligence.* New York: McGraw-Hill.

Gustafsson, J.-E. (1984). A unifying model for the structure of intellectual abilities. *Intelligence, 8,* 179–203.

Hammond, S. (1998). *Designing our abilities and outlooks.* Unpublished manuscript.

Hearnshaw, L. S. (1951). Exploring the intellect. *British Journal of Psychology, 42,* 315–321.

Herrnstein, R. J., & Murray, C. (1994). *The bell curve: Intelligence and class structure in American life.* New York: Free Press.

Horn, J. L. (1988). Thinking about human abilities. In J. R. Nesselroade & R. B. Cattell (Eds.), *Handbook of multivariate experimental psychology* (2nd ed., pp. 645–685). New York: Plenum.

Horn, J. L. (in press). A basis for research on age differences in cognitive capabilities. In J. J. McArdle & R. W. Woodcock (Eds.), *Human cognitive abilities in theory and practice.* Chicago: Riverside.

Horn, J. L., & Noll, L. (1994). System for understanding cognitive capabilities: A theory and the evidence on which it is based. In D. K. Detterman (Ed.), *Current topics in human intelligence* (Vol. 4, pp. 151–203). Norwood, NJ: Ablex.

Humphreys, L. G. (1962). The organization of human abilities. *American Psychologist, 17,* 475–483.

Jäger, A. O. (1984). Intelligenszstruckturforschung: Konkurrierende Modelle, neu Entwicklungen, Perspectiven [Research on intelligence structure: Competing models, new developments, perspectives]. *Psychologische Rundschau, 35,* 21–35.

Jensen, A. R. (1985). The nature of black–white differences on various psychometric tests: Spearman's hypothesis. *Behavioral and Brain Sciences, 8,* 193–263.

Jensen, A. R. (1993). Why is reaction time correlated with psychometric *g? Current Directions in Psychological Science, 2,* 53–56.

Jensen, A. R. (1998). *The g factor: The science of mental ability.* Westport, CT: Praeger.

Kornblum, S. (1992). Dimensional overlap and dimensional relevance in stimulus–response and stimulus–stimulus compatibility. In G. E. Stelmach & J. Requin (Eds.), *Tutorials in motor behavior II* (pp. 747–777). Amsterdam: North-Holland.

Kornblum, S., Hasbroucq, T., & Osman, A. (1990). Dimensional overlap: Cognitive basis for stimulus–response compatibility — a model and taxonomy. *Psychological Review, 97,* 253–270.

Kyllonen, P. C., & Christal, R. E. (1990). Reasoning ability is (little more than) working memory capacity?! *Intelligence, 14,* 389–433.

Larson, G. E., & Saccuzzo, D. P. (1989). Cognitive correlates of general intelligence: Toward a process theory of *g. Intelligence, 13,* 5–31.

Lindenberger, U., & Baltes, P. B. (1994). Sensory functioning and intelligence in old age: A strong connection. *Psychology and Aging, 9,* 339–355.

Lindenberger, U., & Baltes, P. B. (1997). Intellectual functioning in old and very old age: Cross sectional results from the Berlin Aging Study. *Psychology and Aging, 12,* 410–432.

Marshalek, B., Lohman, D. F., & Snow, R. E. (1983). The complexity continuum in the radex and hierarchical models of intelligence. *Intelligence, 7,* 107–127.

Marsiske, M., Klumb, P., & Baltes, M. M. (1997). Everyday activity patterns and sensory functioning in old age. *Psychology and Aging, 12,* 444–457.

Matarazzo, J. D. (1972). *Wechsler's measurement and appraisal of adult intelligence* (5th ed.). Baltimore: Williams & Wilkins.

Matarazzo, J. D. (1992). Psychological testing and assessment in the 21st century. *American Psychologist,* 47, 1007–1018.

Mowbray, G. H., & Rhoades, M. V. (1959). On the reduction of choice reaction time with practice. *Quarterly Journal of Experimental Psychology,* 11, 16–23.

Neisser, U., Boodoo, G., Bouchard, T. J., Jr., Boykin, A. W., Brody, N., Ceci, S. J., Halpern, D. F., Loehlin, J. C., Perloff, R., Sternberg, R. J., & Urbina, S. (1996). Intelligence: Knowns and unknowns. *American Psychologist,* 51, 77–101.

Pallier, G., Roberts, R. D., & Stankov, L. (1998). *Biological vs. psychometric intelligence: Halstead's (1947) distinction re-evaluated.* Manuscript submitted for publication.

Peterson, N. G., & Bownas, D. A. (1982). Skill, task structure, and performance acquisition. In M. D. Dunnette & E. A. Fleishman (Eds.), *Human performance and productivity: Vol. I. Human capability assessment* (pp. 49–105). Hillsdale, NJ: Erlbaum.

Riehle, A., Kornblum, S., & Requin, J. (1997). Neuronal correlates of sensorimotor association in stimulus–response compatibility. *Journal of Experimental Psychology: Human Perception and Performance,* 23, 1708–1726.

Roberts, R. D. (1997). Fitts' law, movement time and intelligence. *Personality and Individual Differences,* 23, 227–246.

Roberts, R. D. (1998). *Individual differences in performance on elementary cognitive tasks (ECTs): Lawful vs. problematic parameters.* Manuscript submitted for publication.

Roberts, R. D., & Goff, G. N. (in press). ASVAB: Little more than acculturated learning? In *Proceedings of the 39th Annual Conference of the International Military Testing Association.* San Antonio, TX: Air Force Research Laboratory.

Roberts, R. D., Goff, G. N., & Kyllonen, P. C. (1998). *Stalking the ghost that is psychometric g.* Unpublished manuscript.

Roberts, R. D., Pallier, G., & Stankov, L. (1996). The basic information processing (BIP) unit, mental speed and human cognitive abilities: Setting the BIP to RIP? *Intelligence,* 23, 133–155.

Roberts, R. D., & Stankov, L. (1998). *Individual differences in speed of mental processing and human cognitive abilities: Towards a taxonomic model.* Manuscript submitted for publication.

Roberts, R. D., Stankov, L., Pallier, G., & Dolph, B. (1997). Charting the cognitive sphere: Tactile–kinesthetic performance within the structure of intelligence. *Intelligence,* 25, 111–148.

Spearitt, D. (1996). Carroll's model of cognitive abilities: Educational implications. *International Journal of Educational Research,* 25, 107–198.

Spearman, C. (1904). "General intelligence," objectively determined and measured. *American Journal of Psychology,* 15, 201–292.

Spearman, C. (1927). *The abilities of man.* New York: Macmillan.

Stankov, L. (1998). Mining on the "no man's land" between intelligence and personality. In P. L. Ackerman, P. C. Kyllonen, & R. D. Roberts (Eds.), *Learning and individual differences: Process, trait, and content determinants* (pp. 315–337). Washington, DC: American Psychological Association.

Stankov, L., & Horn, J. L. (1980). Human abilities revealed through auditory tests. *Journal of Educational Psychology,* 72, 19–42.

Stankov, L., & Roberts, R. D. (1997). Mental speed is not *the* "basic" process of intelligence. *Personality and Individual Differences,* 22, 69–85.

Stankov, L., Roberts, R. D., & Spilsbury, G. (1994). Attention and speed of test-taking in intelligence and aging. *Personality and Individual Differences,* 17, 273–284.

Stauffer, J. M., Ree, M. J., & Carretta, T. R. (1996). Cognitive-components tests are not much more than g: An extension of Kyllonen's analyses. *Journal of General Psychology,* 123, 193–205.

Stevens, J. C., & Cruz, A. L. (1996). Spatial acuity of touching: Ubiquitous decline with aging revealed by repeated threshold testing. *Somatosensory and Motor Research,* 13, 1–10.

Stevenson, R. J., Prescott, J., & Boakes, R. A. (1995). The acquisition of taste properties by odors. *Learning and Motivation,* 26, 433–455.

Thompson, R. F. (1985). *The brain: An introduction to neuroscience.* New York: Freeman.

Thorndike, R. L., Hagen, E. P., & Sattler, J. M. (1985). *Stanford–Binet Intelligence Scale* (4th ed.). Chicago: Riverside.

Thurstone, L. L. (1938). *Primary mental abilities.* Chicago: University of Chicago Press.

Thurstone, L. L. (1948). Psychological implications of factor analysis. *American Psychologist,* 3, 402–408.

Turvey, M. T. (1996). Dynamic touch. *American Psychologist,* 51, 1134–1152.

Vernon, P. E. (1950). *The structure of human abilities*. London: Methuen.

Watson, B. U. (1991). Some relationships between intelligence and auditory capabilities. *Journal of Speech and Hearing Research, 34,* 621–627.

Wissler, C. (1901). The correlation of mental and physical tests. *Psychological Review Monograph, 8*(Suppl. 3), 1–62.

Woodcock, R. W., & Johnson, M. B. (1989). *Woodcock–Johnson Tests of Cognitive Ability: Standard and supplemental batteries*. Chicago: Riverside.

Discussion

After Roberts's presentation, several discussants provided additional information about previous investigations of sensory abilities. Other comments related to the difficulties in establishing strong associations between low-level process measures and higher level measures of intellectual abilities.

Dr. Deary: I would like to make a few comments. One is, first of all, in the tactile sense, I'd like to remind you to look at Cyril Burt's original study in 1909 in the *British Journal of Psychology* when he looked at sensory abilities in schoolchildren. I believe he actually did this study!; he examined visual, auditory and tactile, and higher order abilities. And like Spearman, he was arguing that, whereas vision and audition related to higher order abilities, tactile didn't. He had an evolutionary theory about that. So it might be interesting for you to go and have a look at that.

Also, the person who is the most multimodal that I've read is, in fact, in the area of dyslexia that I was asked about earlier, and that's Paula Tallal (e.g., Anderson, Brown, & Tallal, 1993). She very strongly argues that there is a sort of central processing speed that covers right across vision, audition, and touch. And in fact, Ted Nettelbeck did, in fact, try to do some tactile inspection time research. And we built a device that I still have, but all it did was actually make people's fingers numb, so we didn't develop it any further.

I have a couple of questions. One is whether you've looked into the individual differences research that has been done by Chuck and Betty Watson on the Tests of Basic Auditory Capabilities. They've taken a more psychophysical approach to audition. There is a kit of different auditory abilities that's available on digital audiotape. They've already published data on that, on the association between mental ability levels and auditory capabilities (Watson, B. U., 1991).

And the last point is that Ulman Lindenberger and Paul Baltes (1994), when they looked at senses and ability, they're working within a deficit model. And what they're actually arguing is not that speed of processing is decreased. These are actually acuity measures they're using. And, of course, as you probably know, their argument is "common cause." Lots of things that happen in old age might have common underlying causes and that the senses are just one marker. So they're not quite using these in the same sense that I think you are.

Dr. Roberts: I think you've said some very nice things in terms of directions that one can pursue.

Dr. Baddeley: I like your final result because it seems to fit very nicely into the visuospatial sketchpad — and in particular, the high correlation with G, it's not inevitable, but on the whole it's much harder to get visuospatial tasks that don't depend, in our terminology, on a central executive.

Secondly, a standard way of interfering with the sketchpad with visual imaginary is motor activity. I think where maybe I slightly take issue is in referring to them as visual and kinesthetic and hoping that maybe if you move to auditory information you'll avoid the bottleneck. Because another way of conceptualizing it is if you think of the sketchpad as a multimodal representational system so that you will get an interference with visuospatial representation with auditory presentation if that auditory presentation is spatial in nature. So if you give someone, while they're tracking a task that involves spatial visualization like trying to imagine a football game while you're steering a car, then you'll get interference. So I like your results.

Dr. Roberts: I think these are interesting research questions with important theoretical implications. However, it is still very early days in our research examining the tactile modality. For example, Carroll's (1993) review of the psychometric domain isolated only four studies, none of which were very much concerned with tactile–kinesthesis per se. Dr. Stankov and I have, however, recently collected some additional data. We hope to gain a clearer picture of the tactile domain with this new data set, although there is clearly room for still further research.

Dr. Hunt: How much time did your participants have to learn how to do mainly the tactile–kinesthesis tasks.

Dr. Roberts: We spent some time with them going through the various procedures and quite a few practice trials. Specifically, the number of such trials varied anywhere from 2 to 10, depending on the apparatus.

Dr. Hunt: That's not really an awful lot.

Dr. Roberts: No, but this is similar to other tasks in the literature.

Dr. Hunt: With the perceptual motor task, over training periods, you actually get a movement in different brain areas that are involved in exactly the same task. I am really seriously concerned that what you're doing is measuring the participant's ability to understand the task and develop a strategy for it.

Dr. Ackerman: But if that's the case, Buz, then his results are even stronger than what he presented because he's showing that they don't correlate very highly with the top stratum of abilities (with general intelligence). So you're expecting that with more practice the correlations with general intelligence will decline.

Dr. Hunt: No. I'm looking at those tasks, and I'm looking at the correlation with Gf, the Gf which is fairly high, and also with the visual representation which also has a strategic component. You have to sort of decide how you're going to envision these tasks.

And I'm quite serious about this because there's a great deal of learning that goes into a psychomotor task. And before it becomes a pure tactile or kinesthetic task, the strategy has really got to be developed quite well. And I really think that what you may be doing in a very strong point is tapping learning abilities.

Dr. Stankov: Can I comment? That is possible. But what you should keep also in mind is that some of these tasks come from the neurological test batteries like Reitan's memory task. It hasn't been all that often used in the larger battery of tests as we have done here. And when neurologists talk about it, they clearly are trying to say that there's something measured by the WAIS [Wechsler Adult Intelligence Scale], for example, and there's something else biological they say sometimes. Biologically intelligence is measured by this particular task. And we follow the procedures that they have used, and it doesn't come as a surprise to me that . . .

Dr. Hunt: Okay. Yes, I see what you mean, Lazar. And this is an important point I think looking at neuropsychology and cognitive tasks. And let me give you an analogy with orthopedics and athletics. That the number of legs you have is not a very good individual-differences variable for a decathlon athlete, but it's really quite good in orthopedics. The Reitan battery was developed to check for brain injury and to check on minor brain injury for evaluation of brain injury after surgery. And it's very useful for major deficits. So that it is quite sensitive within the range in which it was intended. But that doesn't mean that it's going to be a particularly good task to pick up individual-differences variables in other levels of ability.

Dr. Ackerman: Buz, let's just focus in on that because I think that was an important point that Rich made in his talk. And I want to try to put a few more stronger words in your mouth. When you use the ASVAB [Armed Services Vocational Aptitude Battery] and the ETS [Educational Testing Service] kit, the first thing I said is the same thing that you did, these are really lousy tests if we want to understand the basics of human abilities. Of course, I have a belief that the Raven is a particularly lousy test too. Would it be fair to characterize what you're saying formally as that one of the problems and one of the reasons why we end up thinking about G, per se, is because we have lousy tools as psychometricians, as individual-differences psychologists?

Dr. Roberts: Phil, I concur wholeheartedly with this sentiment.

Dr. Ackerman: Except for the CAM-4 [Cognitive Abilities Measurement, Version 4] battery; right, Pat?

Dr. Roberts: Yeah. That would be lovely if we could get the CAM-4 battery up and running, but the point is that a lot of those tactile–kinesthesis measures very closely parallel the results in the literature for all sorts of normal populations with the different tasks. We did get very close correspondence.

Dr. Hunt: Oh, there is no question. And in typically in those cases, not with the work with brain injury, but in those cases very little practice is allowed. My question is basically to what extent are these actually tactile discriminatory tasks.

Dr. Roberts: And it turns out that's probably true too of a lot of processing-speed research, but I mean—I know now Mowbray and Rhoades (1959) did 45,000 trials to get the Hick's law to disappear. When do you say "enough's enough?" I mean practically or theoretically. I mean at that point no one would become very interested in Hick's law anymore.

Dr. Hunt: I do think that concern for whether or not you had reached stable performance level is an issue and that it makes things very difficult because it makes things very expensive.

Dr. Pisoni: But, Buz, I wanted to make a related comment and maybe the flip side of what you said. Do you worry a little bit about the stand of cognitive psychology experiment that's done nowadays, which is basically an hour experiment with an undergraduate freshman or sophomore. When in a lot of domains the kind of learning that we're really looking at takes place over very long periods of time. But much of the theorizing and modeling that goes on are these categorization studies or attention, whatever it might be.

Dr. Hunt: I don't think I've done a study like that in a number of years.

Dr. Pisoni: You haven't.

Dr. Hunt: Within a 50-minute hour because I do think that is a very serious concern. I think there's a great desire especially in individual-differences research to want to pack in lots and lots variables so we have a great big matrix and not take all that much concern for what the quality of the data points are going into those matrices.

Dr. Pisoni: It's not only the quality I think of the data that's being collected, but it's the kind of task where, you know, it's a one-hour experiment. What about a set of abilities that emerge over time that might be 1 year or 2 years? No graduate student or postdoc in anybody's lab here, maybe excepting the Air Force lab, but in any of the academic labs, no graduate student or postdoc is going to take on a project that takes 1 year or 2 years.

Dr. Hunt: You have never heard of Warner Schaie's PhD dissertation, which is still ongoing.

Dr. Ackerman: Right. But I think that's a good example though, Buz, is that Schaie's work was started in the 1950s and continues today, and it's stuck using Thurstonian measures of abilities. So, you know, in 1950 something — you know, popularized tests of fluid and crystallized intelligence come out, and he's still doing, you know, Thurstonian factor analysis.

Dr. Hunt: Well, you're right. And I don't want to do a critique with Roberts here of Shaie's work. He wasn't necessarily stuck in that.

Dr. Alexander: I'm going to flip a bit more to the philosophical–psychological end of this. I find the issue of the tactile–kinesthetic fascinating indeed. And you're right, I think many of us do not think about it. And as someone who spends most of the time studying the phenomenon of learning and individual differences in the messy thing we call a classroom, I want to explore an issue with you. It seems that many of the tasks that you, of course, have used very sensibly so, put this tactile kinesthetic to the forefront. Whether it's in the laboratory experiment or it with the pilots or aviators. As I watch learning in classrooms, particularly after the early childhood periods, much of what emerges as the nature of schooling or the demands on learning have very few correlates to the tactile–kinesthetic. How would that play out at all theoretically . . .

Dr. Roberts: Yes. I know certainly of laypeople who say I liked the "hands-on approach" to this or that phenomenon.

Dr. Alexander: Yeah, right.

Dr. Lohman: I had a similar response, and I believe it was also congruent with Dr. Baddeley's concern. I was not so much concerned with the modality of input as with the demands on spatial ability. I was particularly interested in those rela-

367

tionships because some theorists have hypothesized that spatial procedural knowledge is formed by the internalizing physical interactions with the world. Piaget claimed that this sort of learning was particularly important early in development. Therefore, I would like to see more work on this in terms of its implications for the development of spatial abilities.

Dr. Roberts: Sure. This is the early days, and I think you're all making excellent points quite frankly.

Dr. Wittmann: I found this work very interesting especially from the perspective of Germany. A German expression for understanding literally means "put your hands on it." Do you have any data because I think that is really important for the technical and vocational schools? Maybe that expression is related to the German tradition in manufacturing things and all that stuff. And I think this should be a real promising construct. What do you think goes on? Is that what you are going to use tactile abilities for?

Dr. Roberts: I have no idea at this stage. I think these are early days, and I think that you'd really have to get into that literature. I mentioned the Turvey (1996) work, which looks at torque and there is a whole physics model built into it. And I think that might be a very nice way of going to it. Looking to see where you can get an individual-differences application across to that.

V

CONTENT

16

Searching for Determinants of Performance in Complex Domains

RICHARD K. WAGNER

It is fortunate that the field of psychology has accumulated over a century of research on relations between measures of ability and performance in a variety of settings. Library shelves are stuffed with volumes of psychology and education journals that contain countless reports of validity coefficients between IQ tests and a wide variety of criterion tasks. The vast majority of these studies are small scale, with sample sizes under 100, and the results are inconsistent. IQ test scores predicted performance in some studies but not others, even when the IQ tests and measures of criterion performance are the same or similar. This led some to argue that the validity of cognitive ability tests was situation specific. However, the development of meta-analysis changed this view. By making it possible to combine the results of small studies quantitatively into a quasi massive-scale study, strong evidence emerged of remarkably general validity for IQ tests across a wide variety of educational and employment-related contexts (Hunter & Schmidt, 1983). More recent large-scale studies of military personnel and others confirmed this finding (e.g., McHenry, Hough, Toquam, Hanson, & Ashworth, 1990).

Of course, IQ and related tasks do not measure ability directly. Rather, the tests sample knowledge and skill that individuals have been exposed to over recent years. Some IQ subtests sample existing knowledge and skill directly by asking examinees to provide factual information outright, as in defining words on a vocabulary test. Others reflect existing knowledge and skill more indirectly, as in a digit-span test for which performance depends on language-based phonological processing as well as strategies such as rehearsal. Inferences are made about individual differences in ability using a logic that rests on several assumptions. Assuming equal exposure to the material to be tested and equivalent experience with the tasks on the test, the inference is made that individuals who have learned the most have the most learning ability or aptitude (Anastasi, 1958; Carroll, 1982).

The content of tasks found on IQ-type tests represents a sample of material that often has been learned incidentally. Were it the case that a person had advanced knowledge of which 30 words he or she would be asked to define on a vocabulary subtest and an opportunity to look up and memorize their meanings, his or her performance obviously would skyrocket. Similarly, the tasks themselves are not tasks that are practiced in everyday life. Although it commonly is assumed that providing training that consists of repeated practice on the kinds of tasks found on IQ tests would result in modest, at best, improvements in performance, dramatic improvements in performance on tasks measuring "basic" abilities are possible if training results in the development of a more efficient strategy for performing the task.

Consider the case of digit span, a task common to individually administered IQ tests. Strings of digits are presented, and the examinee's task is to recall the strings in order. If the examinee listens to a string of digits such as "8-3-7-9-1-6-2" for the purpose of recalling them, he or she is most likely to code the digits for temporary storage by their names, as opposed to visualizing the string of figures represented by the digits. As such, the task is believed to measure relatively short-term phonological memory. The memory assessed is (a) short term in that the person soon will forget the individual digit strings presented and (b) phonological (derived from the Greek *phone*, which means sound or voice) in that it is the sounds of the digit names that are held in temporary storage.

For years, no one thought to see what would happen if individuals were given practice at the task.[1] The assumption was that any increase in performance would be minimal. Surprisingly, dramatic improvements in digit span have been achieved by a few highly motivated individuals merely by providing repeated practice at the task over a period of months. Untrained college students can recall strings of somewhat under 10 digits in length. After several months of practice, skilled individuals have recorded digit spans in excess of 100. Adopting the standard estimates of 7 plus or minus 2 for mean and standard deviation, respectively, a digit span of 100 would correspond to an SAT score of approximately 5,300. (Throw in a Kaplan's SAT preparation course and the score might be bumped up to 5,350!) The participants had adopted a strategy of coding the digits in meaningful sequences such as plausible running times, thereby changing the fundamental nature of what the task measured.

The characteristic of assessing relatively untrained performance applies not only to IQ-test-type tasks but also to the measures of criterion performance used to validate them. Criterion measures used for the vast majority of these studies have been individual differences in initial status (i.e., differences in rank order of performance) or rates of skill acquisition during initial phases of learning. I noted earlier that training can have a profound effect on performance on some measures of basic skill by changing the nature of the task. Is there evidence of a comparable shift in the nature of criterion performance as individuals move from initial to more advanced levels of performance?

A meta-analysis of validity coefficients by Hulin, Henry, and Noon (1990) bears

---

[1]Although the effects of practice had not been investigated for the digit-span task, such effects had been studied previously for other tasks, including the pioneering study of mental multiplication by Thorndike (1908). See Ackerman (1987) for a review.

on this question. The specific focus of their study was the effect on the size of validity coefficient of the time interval between the test and criterion performance. The predictors included in the study ranged from IQ test scores to measures of physical coordination. The domains from which criterion variables were available ranged from grades in college and graduate school, athletic performance, and job performance. The main result of interest was that from initial performance to final performance, the average change in validity coefficient was a decrement of .6, after correction for range restriction and unreliability. In other words, IQ test scores and other predictors of initial levels of performance were substantially less predictive of later levels of performance (however, see Barrett, Alexander, & Doverspike, 1992, for a critique of this view).

What accounts for the decline in predictive validity from initial to higher levels of performance is unclear. Part of the answer may be that, with learning, task performance changes from an initial resource-dependent, controlled processing to an increasingly resource-independent, automatic processing (Ackerman, 1987; Anderson, 1982; Salthouse, 1991). Part of the answer may be that the decline of validity coefficients reflects variability in training and practice undergone by individuals over time.

The meta-analysis of Hulin et al. (1990) extended measures of criterion performance beyond initial levels of performance but did not extend to the development of superior or even world-class levels of performance. Understanding the acquisition of superior levels of performance is of interest for both theoretical and practical reasons. Theoretical interest centers on the question of the extent to which knowledge about the mechanisms responsible for the acquisition of extraordinary levels of performance has implications for the more common acquisition of ordinary levels of performance. The practical importance of the study of superior performance derives from the fact that in domains for which performance is not artificially constrained and high levels of performance are rewarding (either extrinsically or in the satisfaction of intrinsic motivational needs and desires), a relatively small proportion of superior performers accounts for a majority of the output. Thus, in science, for example, the distribution of citation rates is highly skewed. The overwhelming majority of scientists have citation rates near zero, with a minority having citation rates in excess of 100. A rule of thumb that has emerged from study of productivity in a wide variety of domains is that the top 20% of producers account for about 80% of the total output (Simonton, 1995).

The rest of this chapter is divided into four major parts. In the first part, I review the development of expert levels of performance. In the second part, I consider limitations in the design of existing studies and present the acquisition of reading skills over a period of years as an example of the widespread attainment of a superior level of performance in a complex domain. In the third part, I discuss issues concerning the analysis of multiple waves of data and present an example of growth curve modeling applied to the case of reading acquisition. Finally, I draw some conclusions.

Lessons From Legendary Performers

The programmatic study of world-class performers across a diverse variety of pursuits including chess, various sports, and music has begun to pay off in a big way. Despite popular folk accounts to the contrary, Simon and Chase's (1973) observation that no one attains the level of grandmaster in chess with less than a decade of intense preparation appears to be true for chess and for other domains of expertise. Bobby Fischer, regarded as perhaps the best example of a modern chess prodigy, required at least 9 years of preparation before becoming a grandmaster (Krogius, 1976). Eminent composers who produced distinguished work as young as their early 20s had begun training in music roughly 15 years previously. Similar results have been reported from the study of performance musicians, scientists, businessmen, tennis players, and runners (Bloom, 1985; Ericsson, Krampe, & Tesch-Romer, 1993).

The fact that at least a decade of intense, sustained training is required for world-class levels of performance has implications that extend well beyond the study of expert performance per se. Were it the case that world-class performers were freaks of nature whose achievements shortly after birth surpassed what 99% of us could hope to accomplish in our lifetime, there would seem to be few, if any, implications for the acquisition of more ordinary levels of performance. But it appears to be the case that experts require years of hard work involving a more intense and sustained application of the identical mechanisms of acquisition that result in the attainment of more ordinary levels of performance (Wagner & Stanovich, 1996).

That the attainment of expert performance requires a sustained period of intense effort certainly is not a new observation. Consider the following observation of Plato:

> What I assert is that every man who is going to be good at any pursuit must practice that special pursuit from infancy, by using all the implements of his pursuit both in his play and in his work. For example, the man who is to make a good builder must play at building houses, and to make a good farmer he must play at tilling land; and those who are rearing them must provide each child with toy tools modeled on real ones. Besides this, they ought to have elementary instruction in all the necessary subjects — the carpenter, for instance, being taught in play the use of the rule and measure, the soldier being taught riding or some similar accomplishment. So, by means of their games, we should endeavor to turn the tastes and desires of the children in the direction of that object which forms their ultimate goal. (*The Laws*; cited in Wagner & Oliver, 1996, p. 89)

Several principles of the acquisition of expert performance appear to apply regardless of domain:

1. *All practice is not equally profitable.* If all that was required for the achievement of world-class performance was merely a decade of experience, I would have been playing tennis in the U.S. Open as opposed to having (sigh) just lost in the second round of a local tournament. If experience is not enough, what kind of practice is required? Typically, it is a coached regime of intense and effortful practice activities that have been selected with the goal of improving current level of performance (Ericsson et al., 1993). A live coach may be optional for some domains provided an alternative means of getting feedback about the effects of one's training activities on one's performance is available (Charness, Krampe, & Mayr, 1996).

2. *Expertise is not acquired cheaply.* World-class performers typically begin their training in childhood, supported and encouraged by parents. The expenses are con-

siderable, involving paying for a coach and transporting children to regional and perhaps national competitions. It may ultimately be necessary to relocate to be in close proximity with the best coaches and the highest level of competition. In addition to money, the acquisition of expertise is costly in terms of time required. People may dream of attaining a world-class level of performance in some domain, but few will be able to add the several hours of daily intense training required to already crowded days.

3. *Motivation.* Ackerman (1988) provided a compelling account of the changing roles of cognitive abilities and information processing as participants acquired skill in tasks such as category word search, choice reaction-time tasks, and a simulated air-traffic-controller task. The amounts of training provided were under 10 hours provided across multiple sessions. Ackerman addressed the generalization of the results to situations involving longer training periods:

> For logistic (and theoretical) reasons, highly complex tasks were not considered here. The logistic reasons pertained to the need for training times within the time allowed for subject samples. Generalizations to tasks that, for example, require 20 hr or more for a transition between skill-acquisition phases to occur should be straightforward, though other variables may have obscuring effects. Prominent among these is motivation. When tasks are simple and training time is short, the demands for perseveration are relatively small. Longer training times will surely exacerbate different allocations to performanced improvement and maintenance, especially under attention-intensive controlled-processing conditions. (Ackerman, 1988, p. 311)

If motivation is likely to become important to accounting for skill acquisition over the course of the training regimes described by Ackerman (1988), imagine its role in a training regime spanning a decade. Because the kind of practice required to achieve expertise is effortful, intensive, and directed toward the goal of improving level of performance, it often is not enjoyable. Players training to high-level competitive tennis spend hours performing footwork drills, developing their physical conditioning, and practicing individual strokes such as the serve for hundreds of repetitions. None of these activities are as potentially enjoyable as the actual competition. For every individual who endures, countless others will burn out and cease training.

4. *Domain specificity.* Development of expert levels of performance requires the acquisition of a phenomenal amount of knowledge and skill, the overwhelming majority of which is specific to the particular domain.

The evidence is overwhelming that a decade of intense preparation is necessary for expert levels of performance. But is it sufficient? If we were switched at birth with Bobby Fisher and experienced the instruction and practice at chess he experienced, how close would we come to achieving his level of performance?

Galton (1869/1979) argued that eminence was attributable to inherited natural ability. The development of this ability was analogous to the development of physical strength.

> So long as he is a novice, he perhaps flatters himself there is hardly an assignable limit to the education of his muscles, but the daily gain is soon discovered to

diminish, and at last it vanishes altogether. His maximum performance becomes a rigidly determinate quantity. (cited in Wagner & Oliver, 1996, p. 89)

In contrast, Ericsson et al. (1993) argued that the acquisition of expert levels of performance is not determined by individual differences in talent or basic abilities but rather determined by cumulative amount of effortful practice. Although expert performers demonstrate faster reactions, more accurate perceptions, and better memory for tasks in their domain of expertise, their enhanced performance does not extend to other domains (Ericsson, 1996). For example, elite athletes show no advantage in basic perceptual abilities or reaction time over control subjects (Abernathy, 1987; Starkes, 1987). In general, the magnitude of individual differences found among untrained performers is small compared with the magnitude of differences that result from differential levels of training. Consequently, initial levels of performance on ability measures provide less information about the probability of achieving extraordinary levels of performance than is provided by measures of training (Ericsson et al., 1993).

However, even small initial differences can have large consequences if the differences cumulate over time. Abelson (1985) demonstrated that the percentage of variance in batting performance attributable to differences in skill level among major league players can be calculated statistically. The percentage of variance in any single at bat explained by batting skill is .00317, about one third of 1%. This result seems paradoxical in that one of the most important determinants of having a winning record is the batting averages of players in the lineup. What resolves the paradox is that the differences cumulate. There indeed is virtually no difference in the probability of getting a hit for a single at bat between a player with a batting average of .320 compared with a player with a batting average of .220. With regard to the probability of getting a hit at a single at bat, a manager might as well pick at random from the roster. But over a season of 500 at bats, the player with the higher average will make 50 more hits. This cumulative difference is in turn cumulative over players on the team. The end result is that team batting averages largely determine the season yet matter little on any given at bat.

Unfortunately, intractable limitations in existing data make attempts to answer the question of the sufficiency of such preparation speculative. The problem is that it is impractical to do a prospective, developmental study of 50 million individuals to obtain an ultimate sample of 50 individuals whose level of performance is 1 in a million. Therefore, studies of expert performers begin with identifying experts and then either working backward through retrospective, correlational studies or laterally by comparing expert performance with that of novices. The problem with such studies is potential selection bias. Those who do well in the early phase of training may self-select, or be selected by the sports establishment that controls entry into elite training and performance opportunities. Most individuals drop out of training before reaching expert levels of performance. If individuals at increasingly advanced levels of training and performance represent an increasingly selective sample, it becomes problematic to make inferences about determinants of their success.[2]

---

[2]For an analysis of other problems associated with attempts to predict the performance of individuals whose unusual characteristics make them rare in the population, see Meehl and Rosen (1955).

Developing Expertise in Reading

With perhaps a little suspension of critical disbelief, one can view schooling as providing the natural developmental study previously described (Wagner & Stanovich, 1996). In fact, millions of children undergo more than a decade of preparation to master academic subjects and master skills such as reading. Consequently, studies of skill acquisition of academic subjects such as reading to the level of performance attained by most adults are relevant to theories of the development of expert levels of performance. However, this assertion would appear to be valid for some definitions of expertise but not for others. Therefore, before considering the development of expertise in reading, I need to address an important preliminary issue, specifically, an appropriate definition of expertise.

Defining Expertise

In most domains, expertise has been defined with reference to individual differences. For example, an expert might be defined as someone who falls in the top 5% of performers in a domain. Experts are those whose achievements stand out from the majority. The study of expertise then becomes one of seeking to "understand and account for what distinguishes outstanding individuals in a domain from less outstanding individuals in that domain, as well as from people in general" (Ericsson & Smith, 1991, p. 2).

A working definition of expertise that is based on individual differences is sensible in the context of some assumptions about the acquisition and distribution of expertise but not to others. For example, such a definition makes sense if expertise is largely inherited rather than acquired, and if the distribution of these inherited traits is limited as opposed to widespread. A working definition of expertise that is based on individual differences also is sensible if expertise is largely acquired, but access to the environmental conditions or training opportunities necessary for the development of expertise is limited rather than widespread. For each case, a small percentage of individuals is expected to stand out from the majority. The characteristics that make them stand out from the majority are central to understanding their expertise.

But consider the problems for a working definition of expertise that is based on individual differences posed by a situation in which expertise is largely acquired but nearly everyone has access to the training opportunities required to develop expert levels of performance. Or, alternatively, what if expertise is largely inherited but with a widespread rather than narrow distribution?

Expertise demonstrated by the majority of individuals, as opposed to a small minority, is precluded by working definitions of expertise that is based on individual differences. But if expertise is largely acquired, and one were to provide widespread access to the requisite training opportunities, there is no reason to expect that a small percentage of individuals would stand out from the majority for any reason other than random error.

Realistically, the resources required to develop expert levels of performance are so great that society would be bankrupt if it attempted to develop all of its members to the point of playing a scratch game of golf. But basic skills such as literacy are highly valued in modern societies, to the point that 13 or more years of free public school instruction are made available to nearly everyone in a number of countries.

Other equally acceptable approaches to defining expertise would not preclude expertise being demonstrated by the majority of individuals in a society. For example, expert performance could be defined in reference to developmental as opposed to individual differences. Thus, expert performance could be defined as performance at a level that is 5 (or 10 or 15) standard deviations above the mean performance shown by individuals with a year of training. Alternatively, for some domains it might be possible to define expertise in terms of mastery of performance-based criteria. Neither of these approaches would preclude expert levels of performance attained by a majority of participants in a domain.

Acquisition of Word-Level Reading

Studies of the acquisition of word-level reading skill indicate that children begin reading instruction differentially prepared to profit from it. This appears to largely be attributable to individual differences in prerequisite language abilities. These differences play a role in differential early success at learning to read.

The prerequisite language abilities of most importance to reading are collectively referred to as *phonological processing*, that is, using the phonological or sound structure of oral language when processing oral and written language (Wagner & Torgesen, 1987). Spoken words represent combinations of basic sounds or *phonemes*. All of the words in spoken English can be produced as combinations of about 40 basic phonemes. Of the nearly infinite number of possible combinations of phonemes, only a relatively small number actually occur, and most combinations of phonemes occur in multiple words. Thus, *bat* and *cat* each contains three phonemes, the latter two of which are shared. This fact is represented by their spellings, which have different initial letters and identical medial and final letters, because the spellings in alphabetic orthographies such as English represent sound as well as meaning.

Developmental and individual differences in phonological processing abilities appear to be causally related to the acquisition of reading skills, although the direction, magnitudes, and underlying mechanisms responsible for such causal relations have yet to be established (Wagner & Torgesen, 1987).

My colleagues and I (Wagner et al., 1997) investigated causal relations between individual differences in phonological processing abilities and word-level reading skills in a longitudinal correlational study of 216 children. Three kinds of phonological processing abilities were assessed: phonological awareness (i.e., one's awareness and access to the phonological structure of oral language), phonological naming (i.e., retrieving and producing pronunciations for common stimuli), and phonological memory (i.e., phonological coding of information for brief storage). The three kinds of phonological processing abilities, word-level reading skills, and vocabulary were assessed annually from kindergarten through fourth grade, as the children developed from nonreaders to beginning readers and finally to fluent readers.

Individual differences in phonological processing abilities were remarkably stable from kindergarten through fourth grade. Structural equation models were constructed to assess the causal influences of individual differences in phonological processing abilities on subsequent individual differences in word-level reading for the time periods kindergarten to second grade, first grade to third grade, and second grade to fourth grade.

The results of primary interest are the structure coefficients presented in Table 16.1. The structure coefficient for a given exogenous causal variable represents the predicted change in word-level reading associated with a one-unit change in the causal variable, when the values of the other causal variables in the model are constant. In other words, structure coefficients provide estimates of the unique causal influence of each exogenous cause. The proportion of variance accounted for indicates the proportion of total variance in word-level reading accounted for by the set of exogenous variables. The structural equation models included all of the exogenous causes listed in Table 16.1 as simultaneous predictors.

There were four main results of interest. First, for every time period, individual differences in phonological awareness exerted a causal influence on subsequent individual differences in word-level reading. Second, individual differences in naming and vocabulary exerted independent causal influences on subsequent individual differences in word-level reading initially. But with development, these influences faded in the face of the increasing stability of individual differences in word-level reading (i.e., the increasing autoregressive effect of prior word-level reading on subsequent word-level reading). Third, individual differences in phonological memory did not exert an independent causal influence on subsequent individual differences in word-level reading for any time period. Fourth, the proportion of total variance in word-level reading accounted for by the phonological processing and control

TABLE 16.1 Causal Influences of Individual Differences in Phonological Processing Abilities, Vocabulary, and the Autoregressive Effect of Prior Reading on Subsequent Individual Differences in Word-Level Reading

	Time period		
Exogenous causes	K to 2nd grade	1st to 3rd grade	2nd to 4th grade
Phonological processing variables			
Awareness	.37**	.29*	.27**
Memory	.12	−.03	.07
Naming	.25*	.21*	.07
Control variables			
Vocabulary	.10	.22**	−.01
Autoregressor	.02	.27*	.57**
Portion of variance accounted for	.48	.64	.77

Note. Prior reading included the time period kindergarten (K), first, and second grades; word-level reading included the time period second, third, and fourth grades. Adapted from "Changing Relations Between Phonological Processing Abilities and Word-Level Reading as Children Develop From Beginning to Skilled Readers: A 5-Year Longitudinal Study," by R. K. Wagner, J. K. Torgesen, C. A. Rashotte, S. A. Hecht, T. A. Barker, S. R. Burgess, J. Donahue, and T. Garon, 1997, *Developmental Psychology,* 33, p. 476. Copyright 1997 by the American Psychological Association.
*$p < .05$.   **$p < .001$.

379

variables was considerable for each time period, and it increased as children developed from beginning to fluent readers.

Growth Curve Modeling

Fully capturing the acquisition of performance in a domain over a considerable period of time requires a relatively large number of repeated observations. Unfortunately, structural equation models of the sort just described become unwieldy with more than about three observations. The number of parameters to be estimated increases dramatically and invariably leads to unstable solutions as a consequence of approaching or reaching one or more linear dependencies in the modeled parameters.

Fortunately, growth curve modeling (also known as multilevel analysis or hierarchical linear modeling) provides another way to analyze longitudinal data. Unlike structural equation modeling, growth curve modeling becomes more feasible and flexible as the number of repeated observations exceeds three.

Traditionally, attempts to quantify and analyze growth have relied on only two measurement points (i.e., pretest and posttest), with growth represented by a difference score or a residual change score. Although such scores provide unbiased estimates of growth, they often suffer from poor reliability for individual-difference analyses and provide little information about the nature of growth (Rogosa, Brandt, & Zimowski, 1982; Willett, 1988), both of which are detrimental to understanding the acquisition of expert performance.

Growth curve modeling has proved to be a powerful new method for quantifying and analyzing growth that largely overcomes the problems associated with difference scores and residual change scores (Bryk & Raudenbush, 1987; Rogosa et al., 1982; Willett, 1988; Willett & Sayer, 1994). Instead of having only two measurement points, multiple waves of data are collected. Three or more waves are sufficient for fitting linear growth curve models; four or more waves are sufficient for fitting nonlinear models.

Just as variability in observed scores obtained on a single occasion can be divided into true score variance and measurement error, growth in observed performance can be divided into true growth (i.e., true score change) and measurement error. Estimates of true growth parameters, their variances, and their reliabilities can be obtained.

Conceptually, growth curve modeling involves two levels of analysis. At the within-person level, growth parameters are calculated for each participant by regressing performance on an algebraic function of time, training trials, or some other relevant index. At the between-persons level, individual differences in growth parameters over participants are analyzed, and attempts are made to account for these individual differences by examining potential correlates of growth. Computationally, both levels of analysis proceed simultaneously, yielding more reliable estimates of growth parameters than would be obtained by performing separate ordinary least-squared regressions to solve within-person and between-persons models.

Growth curve modeling has proved to be a powerful new tool in developmental studies of the acquisition of reading skill. An example of the application of growth curve modeling applied to the development of word-level reading skills is provided by the longitudinal study of 216 children from kindergarten through fourth grade described previously. Five waves of annual assessment data were available. One reading variable of particular interest is decoding nonwords, which assesses children's mastery of the alphabetic code that links letters and sounds in alphabetic languages such as English.

The results of growth curve modeling of children's development of nonword reading are presented in Table 16.2. The values in the parameter estimate column are the growth curve parameters. The intercept parameter is the true status (level of nonword reading) when time is equal to zero. In many studies, there is no actual origin of time, so the researcher can define time zero at some interesting or convenient point of the study. In the present analyses, time zero represents the midpoint of the study (i.e., performance in second grade), at which point the data indicate that students got about 12 items correct. The linear growth rate parameter represents the average yearly linear increase in true score, which is between 6 and 7 items per year, and the quadratic growth rate parameter represents yearly nonlinear change in true score, which is about 1 item per year on average. The values in the parameter variance column represent the amount of true variance in growth curve parameters across participants. This represents variance that might be accounted for by predictors representing characteristics of the children and their reading instruction. The results suggest substantial variability in both status and linear growth. The values in the reliability column represent the reliability of the growth curve parameters. Reliabilities are substantial for the intercept and linear growth but not for quadratic growth. The reliability for linear growth is higher than the typical reliabilities for difference scores, showing the advantage of multiple waves of data collection.

My colleagues and I are carrying out additional analyses to determine what accounts for individual differences in growth curve parameters. For present purposes, I present results for two predictors obtained in kindergarten: phonological awareness (a phoneme elision task in which children listen to a word and then say it after deleting a target phoneme) and, for control purposes, verbal aptitude (Stanford–Binet Vocabulary score). I used these variables to predict individual differences in the two reliable growth curve parameters — intercept and linear growth. Variability in the intercept was predicted by both initial levels of phonological awareness (.857, $p < .001$) and verbal aptitude (.438, $p < .01$), with both variables being used in a simultaneous regression model. Thus, the effects of initial level of phonological awareness on second-grade status in nonword decoding were independent of those of verbal aptitude. Variability in linear growth also was predicted by both variables (.232, $p < .01$, and .192, $p < .05$, respectively).

TABLE 16.2   Growth Curve Analysis for Nonword Decoding (Longitudinal Sample)

Measure	Parameter estimate		Parameter variance		Reliability
	Value	SE	Value	SE	
Intercept	11.99	0.42	33.08	1.07	.93
Linear growth	6.65	0.17	6.29	0.13	.72
Quadratic growth	0.99	0.09	0.59	0.00	.20

Note.   For all parameters estimates and variances, $p < .001$.

Conclusion

Beginning the search for determinants of the acquisition of superior performance in complex domains is likely to involve efforts directed at several fronts. These include expanding the set of predictor variables, expanding the time frame of performance assessment, and investing in training research (Wagner, 1997).

Expanding the Set of Predictors

After decades of research that include major efforts in the 1980s and 1990s, it is unlikely that refinements in cognitive ability tests will result in substantial gains in validity (Schmidt, 1994) for most domains.[3] However, expanding the set of predictor variables to include variables relevant to the long-term acquisition of superior levels of performance is likely to be fruitful. What are the most promising new predictors to consider? Several contenders have emerged from recent studies.

The first includes personality, temperament, interests, and motivation. Project A, the Army's Selection and Classification Project, represents a massive $25 million effort over 7 years to expand and refine predictors of performance in the military, as well as to expand and refine measures of job performance. Efforts to improve cognitive ability-related predictors in relation to the existing Armed Services Vocational Aptitude Battery resulted in only minimal gains in prediction. However, measures of personality, temperament, interests, and motivation contributed substantial gains to prediction provided by cognitive ability for three of the five job performance factors evaluated. Especially important are likely to be motivational variables that predict who will persevere in rigorous, long-term training regimes.

The second includes measures of the ability to acquire implicit knowledge from experience. It is not possible to train every aspect of performance, particularly in complex domains. Successful individuals are able to profit from their own experience as well as from their observations of the experiences of others. These types of skills are not represented on traditional IQ tests but have been the focus of efforts to develop and measure the construct of practical intelligence or common sense. Neisser (1976) was one of the first modern psychologists to call attention to a distinction between the "academic intelligence" type of tasks found in the classroom and on IQ tests and the type of tasks found in the everyday world that require a more practical kind of intelligence (see also McClelland, 1973). In the past decade, practical intelligence has been the focus of a growing number of studies carried out in a wide range of settings and cultures. Summaries of various parts of this literature have been provided by Ceci (1990), Rogoff and Lave (1984), Sternberg (1985), Sternberg and Frensch (1991), Sternberg and Wagner (1986, 1994), Sternberg, Wagner, and Okagaki (1991), and Voss, Perkins, and Segal (1991). However, see Jensen (1993), Ree and Earles (1993), and Schmidt and Hunter (1993) for critiques of the view that practical intelligence is a construct independent of either general cognitive ability or job knowledge. Measures of practical intelligence relevant to areas such as business management and sales appear to predict job performance independently of general cognitive ability and common personality inventories (Sternberg, Wagner, Williams, & Horvath, 1995; Wagner, 1987).

---

[3]For an exception to this conclusion for the selection of air-traffic controllers, see Ackerman (1994).

Expanding the Time Frame of Performance Assessment

Despite 60 years of effort, the "criterion problem" of deciding how best to measure performance remains among the most pernicious problems facing psychologists (Gottfredson, 1991). At issue are the method or format of the assessment and the content of what is assessed. It is clear that a top priority is expanding the time frame of the assessment of performance. In the domain of job performance, the majority of data in selection studies over the years has been provided by individuals with 5 or fewer years of job experience on average. There is a paucity of well-designed studies, particularly longitudinal ones, that extend beyond this time period.

Investing in Training Research

Although important issues remain to be studied in the area of selection, a greater payoff is likely from advances in the understanding of training. In the domains of employment and education, few individuals receive frequent feedback and training activities designed to improve their performance. In employment, most individuals receive only yearly performance reviews, the majority of which are exceedingly general. Most of the learning that results in improved performance happens informally in the form of learning from one's own experience (Wagner, 1991). In education, an astonishingly small amount of time is actually spent in instruction in which one-on-one feedback is provided to children while they are practicing basic skill development, as in reading instruction.

REFERENCES

Abelson, R. P. (1985). A variance explanation paradox: When a little is a lot. *Psychological Bulletin, 97,* 129–133.

Abernathy, B. (1987). Selection attention in fast ball sports: II. Expert–novice differences. *Australian Journal of Science and Medicine in Sports, 19,* 7–16.

Ackerman, P. L. (1987). Individual differences in skill learning: An integration of psychometric and information processing perspectives. *Psychological Bulletin, 102,* 3–27.

Ackerman, P. L. (1988). Determinants of individual differences during skill acquisition: Cognitive abilities and information processing. *Journal of Experimental Psychology: General, 117,* 288–318.

Ackerman, P. L. (1994, July). *Theory and application of individual differences in skill acquisition: Writing the new textbook for selection.* Paper presented at the International Congress of Applied Psychology, Madrid, Spain.

Anastasi, A. (1958). *Differential psychology: Individual and group differences in behavior* (3rd ed.). New York: Macmillan.

Anderson, J. R. (1982). Acquisition of cognitive skill. *Psychological Review, 89,* 369–406.

Barrett, G. V., Alexander, R. A., & Doverspike, D. (1992). The implications for personnel selection of apparent declines in predictive validity over time: A critique of Hulin, Henry, and Noon. *Personnel Psychology, 45,* 601.

Bloom, B. S. (1985). Generalizations about talent development. In B. S. Bloom (Ed.), *Developing talent in young people* (pp. 507–549). New York: Ballantine.

Bryk, A. S., & Raudenbush, S. W. (1987). Application of hierarchical linear models to assessing change. *Psychological Bulletin, 101,* 147–158.

Carroll, J. B. (1982). The measurement of intelligence. In R. J. Sternberg (Ed.), *Handbook of human intelligence* (pp. 29–120). New York: Cambridge University Press.

Ceci, S. J. (1990). *On intelligence . . . more or less: A bio-ecological treatise on intellectual development.* Englewood Cliffs, NJ: Prentice Hall.

Charness, N., Krampe, R. T., & Mayr, U. (1996). The role of practice and coaching in entrepreneurial skill domains: An international comparison of life-span chess skill acquisition. In K. A. Ericsson (Ed.), *The road to excellence: The acquisition of expert performance in the arts and sciences, sports, and games* (pp. 51–80). Mahwah, NJ: Erlbaum.

Ericsson, K. A. (Ed.). (1996). *The road to excellence: The acquisition of expert performance in the arts and sciences, sports and games.* Mahwah, NJ: Erlbaum.

Ericsson, K. A., Krampe, R., & Tesch-Romer, C. (1993). The role of deliberate practice in the acquisition of expert performance. *Psychological Review, 100,* 363–406.

Ericsson, K. A., & Smith, J. (Eds.). (1991). *Toward a general theory of expertise: Prospects and limits.* Cambridge, England: Cambridge University Press.

Galton, F., Sir. (1979). *Hereditary genius: An inquiry into its laws and consequences.* London: Julian Friedman. (Original work published 1869)

Gottfredson, L. S. (1991). The evaluation of alternative measures of job performance. In A. K. Wigdor & B. F. Green, Jr. (Eds.), *Performance assessment in the workplace* (Vol. 1, pp. 75–126). Washington, DC: National Academy Press.

Hulin, C. L., Henry, R. A., & Noon, S. Z. (1990). Adding a dimension: Time as a factor in the generalizability of predictive relationships. *Psychological Bulletin, 107,* 328–340.

Hunter, J. E., & Schmidt, F. L. (1983). Quantifying the effects of psychological interventions on employee job performance and work-force productivity. *American Psychologist, 38,* 473–478.

Jensen, A. R. (1993). Test validity: g versus "tacit knowledge." *Current Directions in Psychological Science, 1,* 9–10.

Krogius, N. (1976). *Psychology in chess.* New York: RHM Press.

McClelland, D. C. (1973). Testing for competence rather than for "intelligence." *American Psychologist, 28,* 1–14.

McHenry, J. J., Hough, L. M., Toquam, J. L., Hanson, M. L., & Ashworth, S. (1990). Project A validity results: The relationship between predictor and criterion domains. *Personnel Psychology, 43,* 335–354.

Meehl, P. E., & Rosen, A. (1955). Antecedent probability and the efficiency of psychometric signs, patterns, or cutting scores. *Psychological Bulletin, 52,* 194–216.

Neisser, U. (1976). General, academic, and artificial intelligence. In L. Resnick (Ed.), *Human intelligence: Perspectives on its theory and measurement* (pp. 179–189). Norwood, NJ: Ablex.

Ree, M. J., & Earles, J. A. (1993). g is to psychology what carbon is to chemistry: Reply to Sternberg and Wagner, McClelland, and Calfee. *Current Directions in Psychological Science, 1,* 11–12.

Rogoff, B., & Lave, J. (Eds.). (1984). *Everyday cognition: Its developmental and social context.* New York: Cambridge University Press.

Rogosa, D. R., Brandt, D., & Zimowski, M. (1982). A growth curve approach to measurement of change. *Psychological Bulletin, 90,* 726–748.

Salthouse, T. A. (1991). Expertise as the circumvention of human processing limitations. In K. A. Ericsson & J. Smith (Eds.), *Toward a general theory of expertise: Prospects and limits* (pp. 286–300). Cambridge, UK: Cambridge University Press.

Schmidt, F. L. (1994). The future of personnel selection in the U.S. Army. In M. Rumsey, C. Walker, & J. Harris (Eds.), *Personnel selection and classification* (pp. 333–350). Hillsdale, NJ: Erlbaum.

Schmidt, F. L., & Hunter, J. E. (1993). Tacit knowledge, practical intelligence, general mental ability, and job knowledge. *Current Directions in Psychological Science, 1,* 8–9.

Simon, H. A., & Chase, W. G. (1973). Skill in chess. *American Scientist, 61,* 394–403.

Simonton, D. K. (1995). *Creative expertise.* Paper presented at the conference on the Acquisition of Expert Performance, Wakulla Springs, FL.

Starkes, J. L. (1987). Skill in field hockey: The nature of the cognitive advantage. *Journal of Sport Psychology, 9,* 146–160.

Sternberg, R. J. (1985). *Beyond IQ: A triarchic theory of human intelligence.* New York: Cambridge University Press.

Sternberg, R. J., & Frensch, P. (Eds.). (1991). *Complex problem solving: Principles and mechanisms.* Hillsdale, NJ: Erlbaum.

Sternberg, R. J., & Wagner, R. K. (Eds.). (1986). *Practical intelligence: Nature and origins of competence in the everyday world.* New York: Cambridge University Press.

Sternberg, R. J., & Wagner, R. K. (Eds.). (1994). *The mind in context.* New York: Cambridge University Press.

Sternberg, R. J., Wagner, R. K., & Okagaki, L. (1991). Practical intelligence: The nature and role of tacit knowledge in work and at school. In H. W. Reese & J. M. Puckett (Eds.), *Mechanisms of everyday cognition* (pp. 205–227). Hillsdale, NJ: Erlbaum.

Sternberg, R. J., Wagner, R. K., Williams, W. M., & Horvath, J. A. (1995). Testing common sense. *American Psychologist, 50,* 912–927.

Thorndike, E. L. (1908). The effect of practice in the case of a purely intellectual function. *American Journal of Psychology, 19,* 374–384.

Voss, J. F., Perkins, D. N., & Segal, J. W. (Eds.). (1991). *Informal reasoning and education.* Hillsdale, NJ: Erlbaum.

Wagner, R. K. (1987). Tacit knowledge in everyday intelligent behavior. *Journal of Personality and Social Psychology, 52,* 1236–1247.

Wagner, R. K. (1991). Managerial problem-solving. In R. J. Sternberg & P. Frensch (Eds.), *Complex problem solving: Principles and mechanisms* (pp. 159–183). Hillsdale, NJ: Erlbaum.

Wagner, R. K. (1997). Intelligence, training, and employment. *American Psychologist, 52,* 1059–1069.

Wagner, R. K., & Oliver, W. L. (1996). How to get to Carnegie Hall: Implications of exceptional performance for understanding environmental influences on intelligence. In D. K. Detterman (Ed.), *Current topics in human intelligence* (Vol. 5, pp. 87–102). Norwood, NJ: Ablex.

Wagner, R. K., & Stanovich, K. E. (1996). Expertise in reading. In K. A. Ericsson (Ed.), *The road to excellence: The acquisition of expert performance in the arts and sciences, sports, and games* (pp. 189–225). Mahwah, NJ: Erlbaum.

Wagner, R. K., & Torgesen, J. K. (1987). The nature of phonological processing and its causal role in the acquisition of reading skills. *Psychological Bulletin, 101,* 192–212.

Wagner, R. K., Torgesen, J. K., & Rashotte, C. A. (1994). Development of reading-related phonological processing abilities: New evidence of bidirectional causality from a latent variable longitudinal study. *Developmental Psychology, 30,* 73–87.

Wagner, R. K., Torgesen, J. K., Rashotte, C. A., Hecht, S. A., Barker, T. A., Burgess, S. R., Donahue, J., & Garon, T. (1997). Changing relations between phonological processing abilities and word-level reading as children develop from beginning to skilled readers: A 5-year longitudinal study. *Developmental Psychology, 33,* 468–479.

Willett, J. B. (1988). Questions and answers in the measurement of change. In E. Z. Rothkopf (Ed.), *Review of research in education* (Vol. 15, pp. 345–422). Washington, DC: American Educational Research Association.

Willett, J. B., & Sayer, A. G. (1994). Using covariance structure analysis to detect correlates and predictors of individual change over time. *Psychological Bulletin, 116,* 363–381.

Discussion

A lively exchange about the utility of studying experts started the discussion of Wagner's paper. Participants discussed whether an analysis of expertise can fit into traditional approaches to the study of individual differences in learning and the broader implications of the study of expertise.

Dr. Ackerman: I find your advocacy of studying experts to be interesting and certainly worthwhile. But my question is, Where do you go from that, in terms of addressing issues that are more general? In other words, if you're identifying characteristics that are common to people who spend 10 years acquiring a special skill, how does that relate to the other 4,999,500 people?

Dr. Wagner: I would argue that sort of the mechanisms that we're going to be looking at are going to be pretty much the same. We'll see them in their extreme form if we study the experts. But realistically what I think we need to do is move beyond 1 year or 2. You know, nearly all the studies don't go beyond initial acquisition of performance in most domains. And the predictive validity studies again don't go beyond 1 year or 2. I don't think we should only focus on expert performance. I think we need to start filling in the gap between those two end points.

Dr. Wittmann: I'm always interested in long-term prediction. I think it's very important. But what strikes me most is that you use as examples, single items. It strikes me that you make the same case as when we accuse others using single cases, which is really not bad, but we should pay attention not to falsely generalize from a single case to the whole population or with single items to a broad construct. The example which you have given, has Donald Campbell's terms no *external* or *construct validity*. In Cronbach's terms you falsely generalize from such a small item to a broad nomothetic construct. In Susan Embretson's term your single item lacks "nomothetic span."

Dr. Wagner: Like the garbage-can example that you're talking about? I would agree with that. I mean, I sort of tried to provide an example or two to illustrate the construct. I didn't feel I had time here to talk about the work I've done in practical intelligence, but we actually do work with instruments that involve multiple items and relate them to interesting constructs.

Unidentified: Have you any results about the stability of the practical intelligence if you use a broad battery?

Dr. Wagner: In terms of temporal stability? Test–retest? No, I don't. I'm interested in sort of pursuing developmental studies of sort of practical abilities, but I haven't done that yet. But that's on the agenda.

Dr. Alexander: Yeah, just two questions fairly quickly. First, do you, therefore, believe that everyone can become an expert? That's the first question to you. And the second question related to that: Could I, therefore, train someone to become an expert? Is that your implication?

Dr. Wagner: We don't know the answer to that question. The two contrasting views are that on the one side training is everything and that anyone can become an expert if they're willing to endure a decade of intense preparation. That's one view. The other view is that it's all talent. That you'll quickly reach a maximum and that talent is the key thing. There are two camps in the area. And in fact, we do not have the data to know which of those in use is more accurate. I would be remarkably surprised if it didn't turn out that people who would undergo a decade of intense training would do remarkably better. I mean their performance would improve dramatically. But there have to be individual differences in the trajectories in their response to that decade of training.

My prediction would be that after 10 years of training people would be dramatically better, but that's not going to be sufficient to make you one of the top 2% or necessarily world-class levels of performance. But the key thing is we don't know because of the data. The data don't exist to answer that question yet.

Dr. Alexander: But your own position? I mean you don't have a theoretical premise going into it as to what you expect at all?

Dr. Wagner: What I would expect to happen is that there would be individual differences in response to those trainings, and there would be dramatic mean gains, but there would be variability. But, it depends on how we define expertise or an expert. If we rely on the individual-differences definition, it's impossible to. Because we say that an expert is somebody who's in the top 2% of performance in a domain. But what I think is interesting is that common definition is, in fact, at odds with at least one theoretical camp as to how expertise is developed. Because it would only be consistent with a sort of a skill acquisition or a training point of view if, in fact, we restricted opportunities to access that 10 years of training. And in fact, that happens routinely now. But in the case of schooling — if we relax our critical disbelief a bit, we can argue that, in fact, that's a situation where at least we provide lots of people with a fair amount of training. And when you do that, what do you see? You see substantial gains in performance over the years, but also remarkable individual differences in response to that training. And I suspect that's what we'd see in the expertise literature were the data available.

Dr. Ackerman: But, Rick, that points out a fundamental flaw in the Ericsson et al. and the expert–novice AI [artificial intelligence] approach, which is the idea that you can train anybody to do anything. Nobody in the AI or the Ericsson camp has taken a child with an IQ of 60 and devoted even a year of training to see whether they would fall on a trajectory to be an expert physicist or an expert chess player. I mean it's simply not a realistic account of what we all know that individual differences in intelligence are.

Dr. Wagner: I agree with that. And there's even a better example. If level of performance is determined by accumulative amounts of deliberate practice, you can only get better. You'd see no tail off as people age. And clearly people do tail off as they age. So clearly, within-subject processes matter in terms of what's going on.

Dr. Hunt: Well, there are areas in which we have quite a lot of data for expertise. In our culture it's in psychomotor performance, athletic performance where training starts earlier and earlier. In tennis your champions now hit at 10, but they start training at 6. You get the champions in their teens and their late 20s and start training at 6. It used to be you didn't start training in tennis until you were 13 or 14, and the champions appeared in their mid-20s. Now, I think that quite a lot of data could be looked at there in our culture. For some reason nobody's ever looked strongly at some of the Asian nations where you do have frightening amount — by our standards frightening — number of hours that a student spends in school or school-related topics. It's much higher in Japan and Taiwan and South Korea than it is in our culture. And the high school performance is substantially higher as well. Now, I think there you could look at this. And then these are fairly recent developments, so that goes to some of your question of expertise. The interesting thing to me is that these countries do not maintain the advantage into the college years.

Dr. Wagner: And what's real interesting about the Asian education example relative to the U.S. tennis example is that with the tennis we have the dropout problem. In that lots of kids start tennis pretty early, but the number that actually stick with it, that doesn't burn out is remarkably small, and so the selection bias, I think really limits the conclusion we can draw from that example.

Dr. Baddeley: I suppose it makes two points. One is that in certain areas of experimental psychology people do use correlations. And secondly, it's a very weak design. That on the whole, replicating it 57 times with 57 different professions still doesn't unconfound amount of practice–talent–motivation. And the only way to unconfound it is by some form of experimental design, and I think your school example is halfway there. But the fact that you're at school for this amount of time doesn't, of course, mean that you're getting the same amount of practice.

So I think one has to give two instances where training is limited, where people who have been trained are keen. Maybe learning to fly, for example. Maybe learning a keyboard skill in a culture where keyboards are not common. Because I don't think continually looking in the real world and doing correlations is ever going to answer the question. Although it might be fascinating to know about violinists and chess players.

Dr. Wagner: I agree totally. But I think we're ready for a major investment in long-term training research. We need to do the expensive prospective studies, and we don't need to follow them out for 10 years. If we follow them out well for 5 years with good predictor sets using growth curve modeling, I think we'd know an awful lot more than we know now.

17

Individual Differences in Reasoning and the Heuristics and Biases Debate

KEITH E. STANOVICH and RICHARD F. WEST

A substantial research literature — one comprising literally hundreds of empirical studies conducted over nearly three decades — has firmly established that people's responses often deviate from the performance considered normative on many reasoning tasks. For example, people assess probabilities incorrectly, display confirmation bias, test hypotheses inefficiently, violate the axioms of utility theory, do not properly calibrate degrees of belief, and display numerous other information-processing biases (for summaries of the large literature, see Baron, 1994; Evans & Over, 1996; Kahneman & Tversky, 1996; Osherson, 1995; Shafir & Tversky, 1995). Indeed, demonstrating that descriptive accounts of human behavior diverged from normative models was a main theme of the so-called heuristics and biases literature of the 1970s and early 1980s (see Kahneman, Slovic, & Tversky, 1982).

The interpretation of the gap between the descriptive and the normative in the human reasoning and decision-making literature has been the subject of contentious debate for almost two decades now (for summaries, see Cohen, 1981; Evans & Over, 1996; Gigerenzer, 1996; Kahneman & Tversky, 1996; Stanovich, in press; Stein, 1996). The debate has arisen because some investigators wished to interpret the gap between the descriptive and the normative as indicating that human cognition was characterized by systematic irrationalities. Disputing this contention were numerous investigators who argued that there were other reasons why instances of actual reasoning performance might not accord with the normative theory (see Cohen, 1981, and Stein, 1996, for extensive discussions of the various possibilities). First, perfor-

This research was supported by a grant from the Social Sciences and Humanities Research Council of Canada to Keith E. Stanovich and a James Madison University Program Faculty Assistance Grant to Richard F. West. We thank Penny Chiappe, Alexandra Gottardo, Walter Sa, Robin Sidhu, and Ron Stringer for their assistance in data coding.

mance may depart from normative standards because of performance errors: temporary lapses of attention, memory deactivation, and other sporadic information-processing mishaps. Second, there may be computational limitations that prevent the normative response (Cherniak, 1986; Oaksford & Chater, 1993, 1995). Third, in interpreting performance, researchers might be applying the wrong normative model to the task. Alternatively, the correct normative model may be applied to the problem as set, but the participant might have construed the problem differently and may have provided the normatively appropriate answer to a different problem (Adler, 1984; Hilton, 1995; Schwarz, 1996).

One aspect of performance that has been neglected by all parties in these disputes has been individual differences. What has largely been ignored is that although the average person in these experiments might well display an overconfidence effect, underutilize base rates, choose P and Q in the selection task, commit the conjunction fallacy, and so forth, on each of these tasks, some people give the standard normative response. In a series of studies, our research group has been exploring the possibility that these individual differences and their patterns of covariance might have implications for explanations of why human behavior often departs from normative models. In this chapter, we illustrate how we have explored these implications.

Performance Errors and Patterns of Individual Differences

Theorists who argue that discrepancies between actual responses and those dictated by normative models are not indicative of human irrationality (e.g., Cohen, 1981) sometimes attribute the discrepancies to performance errors (see Stein, 1996, pp. 8–9). Borrowing the idea of a competence–performance distinction from linguists, these theorists view performance errors as the failure to apply a rule, strategy, or algorithm that is part of a person's competence because of a momentary and fairly random lapse in ancillary processes necessary to execute the strategy (e.g., lack of attention, temporary memory deactivation, and distraction).

This notion of a performance error as a momentary attention, memory, or processing lapse that causes responses to appear nonnormative, even when competence is fully normative, has implications for patterns of individual differences across reasoning tasks. For example, the strongest possible form of this view is that *all* discrepancies from normative responses are due to performance errors. This strong form has the implication that there should be virtually no correlations among performance on disparate reasoning tasks. If each departure from normative responding represents a momentary processing lapse that is due to distraction, carelessness, or temporary confusion, then there is no reason to expect covariance in performance across various indices of rational thinking. In contrast, positive manifold among disparate rational thinking tasks would call into question the notion that all variability in responding can be attributable to performance errors.

We have found very little evidence for the performance error view. With virtually all of the tasks from the heuristics and biases literature that we have examined, there is considerable internal consistency. Furthermore, at least for certain classes of task, there are significant cross-task correlations. The direction of these correlations is almost always the same — participants giving the normative response on one task are

TABLE 17.1   Intercorrelations Among Several
Reasoning Tasks

Variable	1	2	3
1. Syllogisms	—		
2. Selection task	.363***	—	
3. Statistical reasoning	.334***	.258***	—
4. Argument evaluation	.340***	.310***	.117

Note. ns = 188–195.
***p < .001, two-tailed.

usually significantly more likely to give it on another. A typical set of results (see Stanovich & West, 1998) is displayed in Table 17.1. The tasks shown here included a syllogistic reasoning task in which the believability of the conclusion contradicted logical validity. Next were five abstract selection task problems (Newstead & Evans, 1995; Wason, 1966). The third task was derived from the literature on statistical reasoning and was inspired by the work of Nisbett and Ross (1980). The fourth task was an argument evaluation task (Stanovich & West, 1997) that taps reasoning skills of the type studied in the informal reasoning literature (Baron, 1995; Klaczynski & Gordon, 1996; Klaczynski, Gordon, & Fauth, 1997; Kuhn, 1993).

The correlations among the four rational thinking tasks are displayed in Table 17.1. Five of the six correlations were significant at the .001 level. The significant relationships among most of the rational thinking tasks (which derive from very different reasoning domains) suggest that departures from normative responding on each of them were due to systematic factors and not to nonsystematic performance errors. On an individual task basis, however, most of the correlations were of a modest magnitude. Nevertheless, it should also be emphasized that many of the relationships might be underestimated due to modest reliability. Due to the logistical constraints of a multivariate investigation involving so many different tasks, scores on some of these measures were based on a few number of trials.

Implications of Individual Differences for Prescriptive Models: Algorithmic-Level Limitations

Patterns of individual differences might have implications that extend beyond testing the view that discrepancies between descriptive models and normative models arise entirely from performance errors. Additionally, judgments about the rationality of actions and beliefs must take into account the resource-limited nature of the human cognitive apparatus (Baron, 1985; Cherniak, 1986; Goldman, 1978; Harman, 1995; Oaksford & Chater, 1993, 1995; Stich, 1990). The idea of computational limitations is best discussed by first making a distinction, popular in cognitive theory, between the algorithmic level of analysis (concerning the computational processes necessary to carry out a task) and the rational level of analysis that encompasses the goals of the system, the beliefs relevant to those goals, and the choice of action that is rational, given the system's goals and beliefs (see Anderson, 1990; Marr, 1982; Newell, 1982, 1990).

The important point for the present discussion is that even if all humans were optimally adapted to their environments at the rational level of analysis, there may still be computational limitations at the algorithmic level that prevent the normative response. Thus, the magnitude of the correlation between performance on a reasoning task and cognitive capacity provides an empirical clue about the importance of algorithmic limitations in creating discrepancies between descriptive and normative models. A strong correlation suggests important algorithmic limitations that might make the normative response not prescriptive for those of lower cognitive capacity. In contrast, the absence of a correlation between the normative response and cognitive capacity suggests no computational limitation and thus no reason why the normative response should not be considered prescriptive (see Baron, 1985; Bell, Raiffa, & Tversky, 1988).

In our studies, we have operationalized cognitive capacity in terms of well-known cognitive ability and academic aptitude tasks such as the Scholastic Aptitude Test (SAT). All are known to load highly on psychometric g (Carpenter, Just, & Shell, 1990; Carroll, 1993; Matarazzo, 1972), and such measures have been linked to neurophysiological and information-processing indicators of efficient cognitive computation (Deary & Stough, 1996; Detterman, 1994; Hunt, 1987; Stankov & Dunn, 1993; Vernon, 1991, 1993).

The top half of Table 17.2 indicates the magnitude of the correlation between SAT total scores and the four reasoning tasks discussed previously. SAT scores were significantly correlated with performance on all four rational thinking tasks. The

TABLE 17.2   Correlations Between the Reasoning Tasks and SAT Total Score

Task	Correlation
Syllogisms	.470***
Selection task	.394***
Statistical reasoning	.347***
Argument evaluation	.358***
Replication and extension	
Syllogisms	.410***
Statistical reasoning	.376***
Argument evaluation task	.371***
Covariation detection	.239***
Hypothesis testing bias	−.223***
Outcome bias	−.172***
If/only thinking	−.208***
RT1 composite	.530***
RT2 composite	.383***
RT composite (all tasks)	.547***

Note. For replication and extension, sample size ranged from 527 to 529. SAT = Scholastic Aptitude Test; RT1 composite = standard score composite of performance on argument evaluation task, syllogisms, and statistical reasoning; RT2 composite = standard score composite of performance on covariation judgment, hypothesis testing task, if/only thinking, and outcome bias; RT composite (all tasks) = rational thinking composite score of performance on all seven tasks in the replication and extension experiment.
***$p < .001$, two-tailed.

correlation with syllogistic reasoning was the highest (.470), and the other three correlations were roughly equal in magnitude (.347 to .394). All were statistically significant ($p < .001$).

The remaining correlations in the table are the results from a replication and extension experiment (see Stanovich & West, 1998). Three of the four tasks from the previous experiment were carried over (all but the selection task), and added to this multivariate battery was a covariation detection task. Three new tasks assessing cognitive biases were also added to this multivariate battery of tests. The first was a hypothesis testing task modeled on Tschirgi (1980) in which the score on the task was the number of times participants attempted to test a hypothesis in a manner that did not unconfound variables. Outcome biases was measured by using tasks introduced by Baron and Hershey (1988). This bias is demonstrated when participants rate a decision with a positive outcome superior to a decision with a negative outcome, even when the information available to the decision maker was the same in both cases. Finally, *if/only bias* refers to the tendency for people to have differential responses to outcomes on the basis of the differences in counterfactual alternative outcomes that might have occurred (Epstein, Lipson, Holstein, & Huh, 1992). The bias is demonstrated when participants rate a decision leading to a negative outcome as worse than a control condition when the former makes it easier to imagine a positive outcome occurring.

The bottom half of Table 17.2 indicates that the correlations involving the syllogistic reasoning task, statistical reasoning task, and argument evaluation task were similar in magnitude to those obtained in the previous experiment. The correlations involving the four new tasks were also all statistically significant. The sign on the hypothesis testing, outcome bias, and if/only thinking tasks was negative because high scores on these tasks reflect susceptibility to nonnormative cognitive biases. However, it must again be emphasized that the logistical constraints dictated that the scores on some of the new tasks were based on an extremely small sample of behavior. The outcome bias score was based on only a single comparison, and the if/only thinking score was based on only two items.

The remaining correlations in the table concern composite variables. The first composite involved the three tasks that were carried over from the previous experiment: the syllogistic reasoning, statistical reasoning, and argument evaluation tasks. The scores on each of these three tasks were standardized and summed to yield a composite score. The composite's correlation with SAT scores was .530. A second rational thinking composite was formed by summing the standard scores of the remaining four tasks: covariation judgment, hypothesis testing, if/only thinking, outcome bias (the latter three scores are reflected so that higher scores represent more normatively correct reasoning). SAT total scores displayed a correlation of .383 with this composite. Finally, both of the rational thinking composites were combined into a composite variable reflecting performance on all seven tasks, and this composite displayed a correlation of .547 with SAT scores. It thus appears that, to a considerable extent, discrepancies between actual performance and normative models can be accounted for by variation in capacity limitations at the algorithmic level — at least with respect to the tasks investigated in this experiment. However, in the following experiments presented we examine individual differences in situations in which the interpretation of the gap between the descriptive and the normative is much more contentious.

Applying the Right Normative Model

In addition to performance errors and algorithmic limitations, there are further reasons why observed performance might depart from normative prescriptions. For example, psychologists have traditionally appealed to the normative models of other disciplines (e.g., statistics, logic, mathematics, and decision science) to interpret the responses on various tasks. There is a danger in this procedure. The danger arises because there is a lack of consensus on the status of the normative models in many of the disciplines from which psychologists borrow. Heavy reliance on a normative model that is in dispute often engenders the claim that the gap between the descriptive and normative occurs because the psychologist is applying the wrong normative model to the situation; in short, the problem is with the experimenter and not with the participant (see Cosmides & Tooby, 1996; Levi, 1983; Lopes, 1981; Macdonald, 1986). For example, Birnbaum (1983) demonstrated that conceptualizing the well-known taxicab base-rate problem (see Bar-Hillel, 1980; Tversky & Kahneman, 1982) within a signal-detection framework can lead to different, normatively correct conclusions than those assumed by the less flexible Bayesian model that is usually applied. Likewise, Dawes (1989, 1990) and Hoch (1987) argued that social psychologists have too hastily applied an overly simplified normative model in labeling performance in opinion prediction experiments as displaying a so-called false consensus (see also Krueger & Clement, 1994; Krueger & Zeiger, 1993).

One way to test indirectly the claim that the wrong normative model is being applied is to investigate how responses on reasoning tasks correlate with measures of cognitive capacity. If that correlation is positive, it would seem to justify the use of the normative model being used to evaluate performance; whereas negative correlations might indicate that an inappropriate normative model is being applied to the situation. This would seem to follow from the arguments of the optimization theorists, who emphasize the adaptiveness of human cognition (Anderson, 1990, 1991; Cosmides & Tooby, 1994, 1996; Oaksford & Chater, 1993, 1994, 1995; Payne, Bettman, & Johnson, 1993; Schoemaker, 1991; Shanks, 1995). The responses of organisms with fewer algorithmic limitations would be assumed to be closer to the response that a rational analysis (Anderson, 1991) would reveal as optimal. For example, the optimal strategy might be computationally more complex, and only those with the requisite computational power might be able to compute it. Under standard assumptions about the adaptive allocation of cognitive resources (Anderson, 1991; Payne et al., 1993; Schoemaker, 1991), the additional computational complexity would only be worth dealing with if the strategy were indeed more efficacious. Alternatively, the optimal strategy might not be more computationally complex. It might simply be more efficient and more readily recognized as such by more intelligent organisms. Thus, negative correlations with the response considered normative might call into question the appropriateness of the normative model being applied.

With these arguments in mind, it is thus interesting to note that the direction of all of the correlations displayed in Table 17.2 (as well as in Table 17.1) is consistent with the standard normative models used by psychologists when interpreting tasks in the reasoning and decision-making literature. This is not always the case, however. We examine here a case of a task in which the normative model to be applied has been the subject of enormous dispute and in which our analysis of individual differences suggests that the model traditionally applied in the heuristics and biases literature may be questionable.

The statistical reasoning problems utilized in the experiments discussed so far (those derived from Fong, Krantz, & Nisbett, 1986) have a less controversial history because they involve causal aggregate information, analogous to the causal base rates discussed by Ajzen (1977) and Bar-Hillel (1980, 1990); that is, base rates that had a causal relationship to the criterion behavior. In contrast, noncausal base rates — those bearing no obvious causal relationship to the criterion behavior — have been the subject of over a decade's worth of contentious dispute (Bar-Hillel, 1990; Cohen, 1981, 1986; Cosmides & Tooby, 1996; Gigerenzer & Hoffrage, 1995; Kahneman & Tversky, 1996; Koehler, 1996; Levi, 1983). In several experiments (see Stanovich & West, 1998) we have included some of these noncausal base-rate problems that are notorious for provoking philosophical dispute. One was an AIDS testing problem modeled on Casscells, Schoenberger, and Graboys (1978):

> Imagine that AIDS occurs in one in every 1,000 people. Imagine also there is a test to diagnose the disease that always gives a positive result when a person has AIDS. Finally, imagine that the test has a false positive rate of 5 percent. This means that the test wrongly indicates that AIDS is present in 5 percent of the cases where the person does not have AIDS. Imagine that we choose a person randomly, administer the test, and that it yields a positive result (indicates that the person has AIDS). What is the probability that the individual actually has AIDS, assuming that we know nothing else about the individual's personal or medical history?

The Bayesian posterior probability for this problem is slightly less than .02. Thus, responses of less than 10% were interpreted as indicating Bayesian amalgamation, responses of over 90% were scored as indicating strong reliance on indicant information, and responses between 10% and 90% were scored as intermediate. Using this classification scheme, we classified 107 participants as strongly reliant on indicant information, 50 as intermediate, and 40 as approximately Bayesian.

As indicated in Table 17.3, the three groups displayed a significant difference in their mean total SAT scores. The mean SAT score of the participants strongly reliant on indicant information (1,115) was higher than the mean score of the Bayesian participants (1,071) whose mean was higher than that of the group showing moderate reliance on indicant information (1,061). Significant differences were also observed on the Raven Progressive Matrices Test (Raven, 1962), Nelson–Denny Comprehension Test (Brown, Bennett, & Hanna, 1981), and a syllogistic reasoning task. In each case, the indicant participants outperformed the other two groups. No significant differences were obtained on the selection task, statistical reasoning task, and argument evaluation task, although the differences tended in the same direction.

Exactly the same trends were apparent in a replication experiment displayed at the bottom of Table 17.3. The mean SAT score of the participants strongly reliant on indicant information (1,153) was significantly higher than the mean score of either the Bayesian participants (1,103) or the intermediate participants (1,109). There was a statistically significant difference in the group mean scores on the composite score for the causal aggregate statistical reasoning problems. Most interesting, however, was the direction of the differences. The highest mean score was achieved by the group highly reliant on the indicant information in the AIDS problem, followed by the mean of the group showing moderate reliance on indicant

TABLE 17.3   Mean Task Performance for the Groups Classified as Indicant, Intermediate, and Bayesian on the AIDS Problem

Task	Indicant (n = 107)	Intermediate (n = 50)	Bayesian (n = 40)	dfs	F
SAT total	1,115$_a$	1,061$_b$	1,071	2, 181	4.26
Raven Matrices	10.09$_a$	8.56$_b$	9.40	2, 194	4.82**
Nelson–Denny	20.23	19.52	19.05	2, 194	3.09*
Syllogisms	4.79$_a$	3.66$_b$	4.21	2, 192	4.65
Selection task	1.61	1.46	1.11	2, 188	0.48
Statistical reasoning	0.421	−0.472	−0.537	2, 194	2.42
Argument evaluation	0.345	0.322	0.351	2, 191	0.30
		Replication			
	(n = 118)	(n = 57)	(n = 36)		
SAT total	1,153$_a$	1,109$_b$	1,103$_b$	2, 198	4.60
Raven Matrices	9.49	9.04	8.64	2, 189	0.89
Nelson–Denny	20.47	20.08	19.47	2, 194	1.95
Syllogisms	5.40	4.93	4.92	2, 208	1.32
Statistical reasoning	0.726$_a$	−0.840$_b$	−1.051$_b$	2, 208	7.24**

Note.   Means with different subscripts are significantly different (Scheffé). SAT = Scholastic Aptitude Test.
*$p < .05$.   **$p < .01$.

information. The participants giving the Bayesian answer on the AIDS problem were *least* reliant on the aggregate information in the causal statistical reasoning problems.

The results from both of these experiments indicate that the noncausal base-rate problems display patterns of individual differences quite unlike those shown on the causal aggregate problems. On the latter, participants giving the statistical response (choosing the aggregate rather than the case or indicant information) scored consistently higher on measures of cognitive ability and were disproportionately likely to give the standard normative response on other rational thinking tasks (see Tables 17.1 and 17.2). This pattern did not hold for the AIDS problem in which the significant differences were in the opposite direction: participants strongly reliant on the indicant information scored higher on measures of cognitive ability and were more likely to give the standard normative response on other rational thinking tasks, including other base-rate problems (of the causal variety, see Bar-Hillel, 1980, 1990). Interestingly, the AIDS problem (or close variants of it) has been the focus of intense debate in the literature, and several authors have argued against making the automatic assumption that the indicant response is nonnormative in the version that we had utilized.

Which Task Construals Are Associated With Differences in Cognitive Capacity?

Theorists who resist attributing irrational cognition as a cause of the gap between normative and descriptive models have one more strategy in addition to those described previously. It is the argument that researchers may well be applying the correct normative model to the problem as set but that the participant might have construed the problem differently and be providing the normatively appropriate answer to a different problem (Adler, 1984, 1991; Hilton, 1995; Levinson, 1995; Margolis, 1987; Schwarz, 1996). Such an argument is somewhat different from any of the critiques that have been mentioned so far. It is not the equivalent of positing that a performance error has been made, because performance errors (e.g., attention lapses and temporary memory lapse) would not be expected to recur in exactly the same way in a readministration of the same task. In contrast, if the participant has truly misunderstood the task, he or she would be expected to do so again on an identical readministration of the task.

Correspondingly, this criticism is quite different from the argument that the task exceeds the computational capacity of the participant. The latter explanation puts the onus of the suboptimal performance on the participant. In contrast, the alternative task construal argument places the blame at least somewhat on the shoulders of the experimenter for failing to realize that there were task features that might lead participants to frame the problem in a manner different from that intended. In locating the problem with the experimenter, it is similar to the wrong norm explanation. However, it is different in that in the latter, it is assumed that the participant is interpreting the task as the experimenter intended, but the experimenter is not using the right criteria to evaluate performance. In contrast, the alternative task construal argument is that the experimenter may be applying the correct normative model to the problem the experimenter intends the participant to solve, but the participant might have construed the problem in some other way and be providing a normatively appropriate answer to a *different* problem.

An example of the alternative task construal interpretation is provided by one of the most famous problems in the heuristics and biases literature, the so-called Linda Problem (Tversky & Kahneman, 1983):

> Linda is 31 years old, single, outspoken, and very bright. She majored in philosophy. As a student, she was deeply concerned with issues of discrimination and social justice, and also participated in anti-nuclear demonstrations. Please rank the following statements by their probability, using 1 for the most probable and 8 for the least probable.
>
> a. Linda is a teacher in an elementary school
> b. Linda works in a bookstore and takes Yoga classes
> c. Linda is active in the feminist movement
> d. Linda is a psychiatric social worker
> e. Linda is a member of the League of Women Voters
> f. Linda is a bank teller
> g. Linda is an insurance salesperson
> h. Linda is a bank teller and is active in the feminist movement

Because Alternative h is the conjunction of Alternatives c and f, the probability of h cannot be higher than that of either Alternative c or Alternative f, yet 85% of the participants in Tversky and Kahneman's (1983) study rated Alternative h as more probable than Alternative f. What concerns us here is the argument that there are subtle linguistic and pragmatic features of the problem that lead the participant to evaluate alternatives different than those listed. For example, Hilton (1995) argued that under the assumption that the detailed information given about the target means that the experimenter knows a considerable amount about Linda, then it is reasonable to think that the phrase "Linda is a bank teller" does not contain the phrase "and is not active in the feminist movement" because the experimenter already knows this to be the case. If "Linda is a bank teller" is interpreted in this way, then rating Alternative h as more probable than Alternative f no longer represents a conjunction fallacy. Several other investigators have suggested that pragmatic inferences lead to seeming violations of the logic of probability theory in the Linda Problem (see Adler, 1991; Dulany & Hilton, 1991; Politzer & Noveck, 1991). These criticisms all share the implication that actually displaying the conjunction fallacy is a rational response to an alternative construal of the different statements to be ranked.

In a recent study (Stanovich & West, in press-b), we have examined the question of whether the different construals of the task are associated with differences in cognitive ability. That is, assuming that those displaying the so-called conjunction fallacy are making a nonextensional interpretation and that those avoiding the so-called fallacy are making the extensional interpretation that the investigators intended, we asked whether the participants making the nonextensional, pragmatic interpretation were participants who were disproportionately the participants of higher cognitive ability. Because this group is in fact the majority in most studies — and because the use of such pragmatic cues and background knowledge is often interpreted as reflecting adaptive information processing (e.g., Hilton, 1995) — optimization models of human cognition (e.g., Anderson, 1990) might be thought to predict that they would be the participants of higher computational capacity.

In our study, we examined the performance of 150 participants on the Linda Problem presented previously. Consistent with the results of previous experiments on this problem (Tversky & Kahneman, 1983), 80.7% of our sample (121 participants) displayed the conjunction effect — they rated the feminist bank teller alternative as more probable than the bank teller alternative. However, the individuals who displayed the conjunction effect had mean SAT scores 82 points below the mean of the individuals who did not display the effect (1,080 vs. 1,162), $t(148) = 3.58$, $p < .001$. This difference is sizable — translating into an effect size of .746, which Rosenthal and Rosnow (1991, p. 446) classified as "large."

Another problem that has spawned many arguments about alternative construals is Wason's (1966) selection task, mentioned briefly earlier (see Stanovich & West, in press-a). The participant is shown four cards lying on a table showing two letters and two numbers (A, D, 3, 7). They are told that each card has a number on one side and a letter on the other and that the experimenter has the following rule (of the if P, then Q type) in mind with respect to the four cards: "If there is an A on one side, then there is a 3 on the other." The participant is then told that he or she must turn over whichever cards are necessary to determine whether the experimenter's rule is true or false.

Performance on such abstract versions of the selection task is extremely low. Typically, less than 10% of participants make the correct selections of the A card (P) and 7 card (not Q). The most common incorrect choices made by participants are the A card and the 3 card (P and Q) or the selection of the A card only (P). The preponderance of P and Q responses has most often been attributed to a so-called matching bias that is automatically triggered by surface-level relevance cues (Evans,

1996; Evans, Newstead, & Byrne, 1993), but some investigators have championed an explanation that is based on an alternative task construal. For example, Oaksford and Chater (1994, 1996; see also Nickerson, 1996) argued that rather than interpreting the task as one of deductive reasoning (as the experimenter intends), many participants interpret it as an inductive problem of probabilistic hypothesis testing. They showed that the P and Q response is then dictated under a formal Bayesian analysis that assumes such an interpretation.

Table 17.4 presents the mean SAT scores of participants giving a variety of response combinations to a selection task problem (see Stanovich & West, in press-a). Respondents giving the deductively correct P and not-Q response had the highest SAT scores followed by the participants choosing the P card only. All other responses, including the modal P and Q response, were given by participants having SAT scores some 100 points lower than those giving the correct response under a deductive construal.

One possible interpretation of the individual differences displayed on the Linda Problem and on the selection task is in terms of two-process theories of reasoning (Epstein, 1994; Evans, 1984, 1996; Evans & Over, 1996; Sloman, 1996). For example, Sloman distinguished an associative processing system with computational mechanisms that reflect similarity and temporal contiguity and a rule-based system that operates on symbolic structures having logical content. According to Sloman, the associative system responds to the similarity in the Linda Problem ("representativeness," in the terminology of Tversky & Kahneman, 1983); whereas the rule-based system engages extensional probabilistic concepts that dictate that the bank teller alternative is more probable.

We conjecture here that large differences in cognitive ability will be found only in problems that strongly engage both reasoning systems and that cue opposite responses. This is because the two systems are identified with different types of intelligence. Clearly, the rule-based system embodies analytic intelligence of the type measured on SAT tests (Carpenter et al., 1990; Carroll, 1993). The associative system, in contrast, might be better identified with what Levinson (1995; see also Cummins, 1996) termed *interactional intelligence*. He speculated that evolutionary pressures were focused more on negotiating cooperative mutual intersubjectivity than on understanding the natural world. Having as its goals the ability to model other minds to read intention and to make rapid interactional moves on the basis of those modeled intentions, interactional intelligence is composed of pragmatic heuristics that operate to facilitate intention attribution.

TABLE 17.4   Mean SAT Total Scores as a Function of Response
Given on the Selection Task

Response	Score	n
Correct	1,190	24
P	1,150	38
All	1,101	21
P, Q	1,095	144
P, Q, NQ	1,084	14
Other	1,070	53

Note.   SAT = Scholastic Aptitude Test.

If the two systems cue opposite responses in a particular task, the rule-based system will tend to cue differentially those of high analytic intelligence, and this tendency will not be diluted by the associative system nondifferentially drawing participants to the same response (because the associative system is unrelated to analytic intelligence; see Reber, 1993). The Linda Problem maximizes the tendency for the associative and rule-based systems to prime different responses, and this problem displayed a large difference in cognitive ability. The selection task might likewise maximize the tendency for the associative and rule-based systems to prime different responses.

Thinking Dispositions and Individual Differences in Rational Thought

In several studies in our research program (see Stanovich & West, 1997, 1998), we have examined one other critical issue — whether there is reliable variance in performance on rational thinking tasks after differences in computational power have been accounted for and whether this residual variation is associated with cognitive strategies, styles, propensities, or dispositions. The conceptual basis for this aspect of our research resides in models of thinking that distinguish between cognitive capacities and thinking dispositions (e.g., Baron, 1985, 1994; Klaczynski et al., 1997; Norris, 1992; Sternberg & Ruzgis, 1994). For example, it is possible that these two constructs (cognitive ability and thinking dispositions) are actually at different levels of analysis in a cognitive theory and that they do separate explanatory work. Variation in cognitive ability refers to individual differences in the efficiency of processing at the algorithmic level. In contrast, thinking dispositions of the type studied in this investigation elucidate individual differences at the rational level. They are telling us about the individual's goals and epistemic values (see Kruglanski, 1989; Kruglanski & Webster, 1996).

With regard to thinking dispositions, we focused on those most relevant to epistemic rationality — processes leading to more accurate belief formation and to more consistent belief–desire networks (Harman, 1995; Stanovich, 1994, in press; Stanovich & West, 1997; Thagard, 1992). We attempted to tap the following dimensions: epistemological absolutism, willingness to perspective switch, willingness to decontextualize, and tendency to consider alternative opinions and evidence.

In the case of many of the individual tasks examined in our research program, thinking dispositions of this type do in fact predict residual variance. In lieu of displaying all of these analyses (see Stanovich & West, 1997, 1998), we present an analysis that is based on composite variables. The variance partitioning is displayed in Table 17.5 in the form of a commonality analysis. The criterion variable was the first rational thinking composite score discussed earlier, reflecting combined performance on the argument evaluation, statistical reasoning, and syllogistic reasoning tasks. SAT total scores and the thinking dispositions composite score attained a multiple R with this criterion variable of .600, $F(2, 526) = 148.15$, $p < .001$. Thus, a substantial amount of variance (36%) on these rational thinking tasks is jointly explained by these two predictors. SAT total was a significant unique predictor (partial correlation = .478, unique variance explained = .190), $F(1, 526) = 156.17$, $p < .001$, as was the thinking dispositions composite score (partial correlation =

TABLE 17.5 Commonality Analysis on Rational Thinking
Composite Score

		Total	
Variable	Unique	Common	Variance explained
SAT	.190***	.091***	
TDC composite	.079***	.091***	
			.360

Note. SAT = Scholastic Aptitude Test; TDC = thinking dispositions composite.
***$p < .001$, two-tailed.

.332, unique variance explained = .079), $F(1, 526) = 65.03$, $p < .001$. Correlations and partial correlations involving these variables are presented in Table 17.6.

In several other analyses structurally similar to this one, dispositions toward open-minded and counterfactual thinking, and the lack of dogmatic and absolutist thinking, were associated with superior performance on rational thinking tasks, even after the variance accounted for by several measures of general cognitive ability had been partialled out. These results support the distinction between thinking dispositions and cognitive capacities that is championed by some investigators (e.g., Baron, 1985) and validate the increasing attention that is being given to processes that are at the borderline of cognitive psychology and personality research (Ackerman & Heggestad, 1997; Goff & Ackerman, 1992; Klaczynski & Gordon, 1996; Sternberg, 1997; Sternberg & Ruzgis, 1994). Thinking dispositions of the type we have examined may provide information about epistemic goals at the rational level of analysis (see Anderson, 1990). What such a result may be telling researchers is that to understand variation in reasoning in such tasks, they need to examine more than just differences at the algorithmic level (computational capacity). In addition, the epistemic goals of the reasoners must also be examined.

The importance of thinking styles in discussions of human rationality has perhaps not received sufficient attention because of the heavy reliance on the competence–performance distinction in philosophical treatments of rational thought in which all of the important psychological mechanisms are allocated to the competence side of the dichotomy. Cohen (1982), for example, argued that there are really only two

TABLE 17.6 Correlations and Partial Correlations

Variable	1	2	3
1. SAT		.53***	.27***
2. RT1 composite	.48***		.41***
3. TDC composite	.06	.33***	

Note. Zero-order correlations are shown above the diagonal, and partial correlations are shown below the diagonal. SAT = Scholastic Aptitude Test; RT1 composite = standard score composite of performance on argument evaluation task, syllogisms, and statistical reasoning; TDC = thinking dispositions composite score.
***$p < .001$, two-tailed.

factors affecting performance on rational thinking tasks: "normatively correct mechanisms on the one side, and adventitious causes of error on the other" (p. 252). Not surprising, given such a conceptualization, the processes contributing to error ("adventitious causes") are of little interest to Cohen (1981, 1982). There is nothing in such a view that would motivate any interest in patterns of errors or individual differences in such errors.

In contrast, Johnson-Laird and Byrne (1993) articulated a view of rational thought that parses the competence–performance distinction much differently from that of Cohen (1981, 1982, 1986) and that simultaneously leaves room for cognitive styles to play an important role in determining responses when people face situations in which problem solving or decision making is required. At the heart of the rational competence that Johnson-Laird and Byrne (1993) attributed to humans is only one metaprinciple: People are programmed to accept inferences as valid provided that they have constructed no mental model of the premises that contradict the inference. Inferences are categorized as false when a mental model is discovered that is contradictory. However, the search for contradictory models is "not governed by any systematic or comprehensive principles" (Johnson-Laird & Byrne, 1993, p. 178). In this passage, Johnson-Laird and Byrne seem to be arguing that there are no systematic control features of the search process. However, epistemically related cognitive dispositions may in fact be reflecting just such control features. Individual differences in the extensiveness of the search for contradictory models could arise from a variety of cognitive factors that, although they may not be completely systematic, may be far from adventitious — factors such as dispositions toward premature closure, cognitive confidence, reflectivity, dispositions toward confirmation bias, ideational generativity, and so forth.

Conclusions

In our research program, we have attempted to demonstrate that a consideration of individual differences in the heuristics and biases literature may have implications for debates about theories of the gap between normative models and descriptive models of actual performance. In reply to Cohen's (1981) well-known critique of the heuristics and biases literature — surely the most often cited of such critiques — Jepson, Krantz, and Nisbett (1983) argued that "Cohen postulates far too broad a communality in the reasoning processes of the 'untutored' adult" (p. 495). Jepson et al., we argue, were right on the mark, but their argument has largely been ignored in more recent debates about human rationality and the tasks that we use to assess it (for exceptions, see Slugoski, Shields, & Dawson, 1993; Stankov & Crawford, 1996; Yates, Lee, & Shinotsuka, 1996). For example, philosopher Nicholas Rescher (1988) argued that

> to construe the data of these interesting experimental studies [of probabilistic reasoning] to mean that people are systematically programmed to fallacious processes of reasoning — rather than merely that they are inclined to a variety of (occasionally questionable) substantive suppositions — is a very questionable step. (p. 196)

There are two parts to Rescher's (1988) point here: the "systematically programmed" part and the "inclination toward questionable suppositions" part. Rescher's focus — like that of many who have dealt with the philosophical implications of the idea of human irrationality — is on the issue of how humans are systematically programmed. Inclinations toward questionable suppositions are of interest only to those in the philosophical debates as mechanisms that allow one to drive a wedge between competence and performance (Cohen, 1981, 1982; Rescher, 1988), thus maintaining a theory of near-optimal human rational competence in the face of a host of responses that seemingly defy explanation in terms of standard normative models (Baron, 1994; Piattelli-Palmarini, 1994; Shafir, 1994; Shafir & Tversky, 1995; Wagenaar, 1988).

One of the purposes of the present research program was to reverse the figure and ground in this dispute, which has tended to be dominated by the particular way that philosophers frame the competence–performance distinction. Specifically, from a psychological standpoint, there may be important implications in precisely the aspects of performance that have been backgrounded in the controversy about basic reasoning competence. That is, whatever the outcome of the disputes about how humans are "systematically programmed" (Cosmides, 1989; Johnson-Laird & Byrne, 1991, 1993; Oaksford & Chater, 1993, 1994; Rips, 1994), variation in the "inclination toward questionable suppositions" is of psychological interest as a topic of study in its own right. The experiments reported here indicate that, at least for certain subsets of tasks, the "inclination toward questionable suppositions" has some degree of domain generality, it is in some cases linked to computational limitations, and it is sometimes predicted by thinking dispositions that can be related to the epistemic and pragmatic goals of rational thought.

REFERENCES

Ackerman, P. L., & Heggestad, E. D. (1997). Intelligence, personality, and interests: Evidence for overlapping traits. *Psychological Bulletin, 121,* 219–245.

Adler, J. E. (1984). Abstraction is uncooperative. *Journal for the Theory of Social Behaviour, 14,* 165–181.

Adler, J. E. (1991). An optimist's pessimism: Conversation and conjunctions. In E. Eells & T. Maruszewski (Eds.), *Probability and rationality: Studies on L. Jonathan Cohen's philosophy of science* (pp. 251–282). Amsterdam: Editions Rodopi.

Ajzen, I. (1977). Intuitive theories of events and the effects of base-rate information on prediction. *Journal of Personality and Social Psychology, 35,* 303–314.

Anderson, J. R. (1990). *The adaptive character of thought.* Hillsdale, NJ: Erlbaum.

Anderson, J. R. (1991). Is human cognition adaptive? *Behavioral and Brain Sciences, 14,* 471–517.

Bar-Hillel, M. (1980). The base-rate fallacy in probability judgments. *Acta Psychologica, 44,* 211–233.

Bar-Hillel, M. (1990). Back to base rates. In R. M. Hogarth (Ed.), *Insights into decision making: A tribute to Hillel J. Einhorn* (pp. 200–216). Chicago: University of Chicago Press.

Baron, J. (1985). *Rationality and intelligence.* Cambridge, England: Cambridge University Press.

Baron, J. (1994). *Thinking and deciding* (2nd ed.). Cambridge, England: Cambridge University Press.

Baron, J. (1995). Myside bias in thinking about abortion. *Thinking and Reasoning, 1,* 221–235.

Baron, J., & Hershey, J. C. (1988). Outcome bias in decision evaluation. *Journal of Personality and Social Psychology, 54,* 569–579.

Bell, D., Raiffa, H., & Tversky, A. (Eds.). (1988). *Decision making: Descriptive, normative, and prescriptive interactions.* Cambridge, England: Cambridge University Press.

Birnbaum, M. H. (1983). Base rates in Bayesian inference: Signal detection analysis of the cab problem. *American Journal of Psychology, 96,* 85–94.

Brown, J., Bennett, J., & Hanna, G. (1981). *The Nelson–Denny Reading Test.* Lombard, IL: Riverside Publishing Co.

Carpenter, P. A., Just, M. A., & Shell, P. (1990). What one intelligence test measures: A theoretical account of the processing in the Raven Progressive Matrices Test. *Psychological Review, 97,* 404–431.

Carroll, J. B. (1993). *Human cognitive abilities: A survey of factor-analytic studies.* Cambridge, England: Cambridge University Press.

Casscells, W., Schoenberger, A., & Graboys, T. (1978). Interpretation by physicians of clinical laboratory results. *New England Journal of Medicine, 299,* 999–1001.

Cherniak, C. (1986). *Minimal rationality.* Cambridge, MA: MIT Press.

Cohen, L. J. (1981). Can human irrationality be experimentally demonstrated? *Behavioral and Brain Sciences, 4,* 317–370.

Cohen, L. J. (1982). Are people programmed to commit fallacies? *Journal for the Theory of Social Behavior, 12,* 251–274.

Cohen, L. J. (1986). *The dialogue of reason.* London: Oxford University Press.

Cosmides, L. (1989). The logic of social exchange: Has natural selection shaped how humans reason? Studies with the Watson selection task. *Cognition, 31,* 187–276.

Cosmides, L., & Tooby, J. (1994). Beyond intuition and instinct blindness: Toward an evolutionarily rigorous cognitive science. *Cognition, 50,* 41–77.

Cosmides, L., & Tooby, J. (1996). Are humans good intuitive statisticians after all? Rethinking some conclusions from the literature on judgment under uncertainty. *Cognition, 58,* 1–73.

Cummins, D. D. (1996). Evidence for innateness of deontic reasoning. *Mind and Language, 11,* 160–190.

Dawes, R. M. (1989). Statistical criteria for establishing a truly false consensus effect. *Journal of Experimental Social Psychology, 25,* 1–17.

Dawes, R. M. (1990). The potential nonfalsity of the false consensus effect. In R. M. Hogarth (Ed.), *Insights into decision making* (pp. 179–199). Chicago: University of Chicago Press.

Deary, I. J., & Stough, C. (1996). Intelligence and inspection time. *American Psychology, 51,* 599–608.

Detterman, D. K. (1994). Intelligence and the brain. In P. A. Vernon (Ed.), *The neuropsychology of individual differences* (pp. 35–57). San Diego, CA: Academic Press.

Dulany, D. E., & Hilton, D. J. (1991). Conversational implicature, conscious representation, and the conjunction fallacy. *Social Cognition, 9,* 85–110.

Epstein, S. (1994). Integration of the cognitive and the psychodynamic unconscious. *American Psychologist, 49,* 709–724.

Epstein, S., Lipson, A., Holstein, C., & Huh, E. (1992). Irrational reactions to negative outcomes: Evidence for two conceptual systems. *Journal of Personality and Social Psychology, 62,* 328–339.

Evans, J. St. B. T. (1984). Heuristic and analytic processes in reasoning. *British Journal of Psychology, 75,* 451–468.

Evans, J. St. B. T. (1996). Deciding before you think: Relevance and reasoning in the selection task. *British Journal of Psychology, 87,* 223–240.

Evans, J. St. B. T., Newstead, S. E., & Byrne, R. M. J. (1993). *Human reasoning: The psychology of deduction.* Hove, England: Erlbaum.

Evans, J. St. B. T., & Over, D. E. (1996). *Rationality and reasoning.* Hove, England: Psychology Press.

Fong, G. T., Krantz, D. H., & Nisbett, R. E. (1986). The effects of statistical training on thinking about everyday problems. *Cognitive Psychology, 18,* 253–292.

Gigerenzer, G. (1996). On narrow norms and vague heuristics: A reply to Kahneman and Tversky (1996). *Psychological Review, 103,* 592–596.

Gigerenzer, G., & Hoffrage, U. (1995). How to improve Bayesian reasoning without instruction: Frequency formats. *Psychological Review, 102,* 684–704.

Goff, M., & Ackerman, P. L. (1992). Personality–intelligence relations: Assessment of typical intellectual engagement. *Journal of Educational Psychology, 84,* 537–552.

Goldman, A. I. (1978). Epistemics: The regulative theory of cognition. *Journal of Philosophy, 55,* 509–523.

Harman, G. (1995). Rationality. In E. E. Smith & D. N. Osherson (Eds.), *Thinking* (Vol. 3, pp. 175–211). Cambridge, MA: MIT Press.

Hilton, D. J. (1995). The social context of reasoning: Conversational inference and rational judgment. *Psychological Bulletin, 118,* 248–271.

Hoch, S. J. (1987). Perceived consensus and predictive accuracy: The pros and cons of projection. *Journal of Personality and Social Psychology, 53,* 221–234.

Hunt, E. (1987). The next word on verbal ability. In P. A. Vernon (Ed.), *Speed of information-processing and intelligence* (pp. 347–392). Norwood, NJ: Ablex.

Jepson, C., Krantz, D., & Nisbett, R. (1983). Inductive reasoning: Competence or skill? *Behavioral and Brain Sciences, 6,* 494–501.

Johnson-Laird, P. N., & Byrne, R. M. J. (1991). *Deduction.* Hillsdale, NJ: Erlbaum.

Johnson-Laird, P. N., & Byrne, R. M. J. (1993). Models and deductive rationality. In K. Manktelow & D. Over (Eds.), *Rationality: Psychological and philosophical perspectives* (pp. 177–210). London: Routledge & Kegan Paul.

Kahneman, D., Slovic, P., & Tversky, A. (Eds.). (1982). *Judgment under uncertainty: Heuristics and biases.* Cambridge, England: Cambridge University Press.

Kahneman, D., & Tversky, A. (1996). On the reality of cognitive illusions. *Psychological Review, 103,* 582–591.

Klaczynski, P. A., & Gordon, D. H. (1996). Self-serving influences on adolescents' evaluations of belief-relevant evidence. *Journal of Experimental Child Psychology, 62,* 317–339.

Klaczynski, P. A., Gordon, D. H., & Fauth, J. (1997). Goal-oriented critical reasoning and individual differences in critical reasoning biases. *Journal of Educational Psychology, 89,* 470–485.

Koehler, J. J. (1996). The base rate fallacy reconsidered: Descriptive, normative and methodological challenges. *Behavioral and Brain Sciences, 19,* 1–53.

Krueger, J., & Clement, R. (1994). The truly false consensus effect: An ineradicable and egocentric bias in social perception. *Journal of Personality and Social Psychology, 65,* 596–610.

Krueger, J., & Zeiger, J. (1993). Social categorization and the truly false consensus effect. *Journal of Personality and Social Psychology, 65,* 670–680.

Kruglanski, A. W. (1989). *Lay epistemics and human knowledge: Cognitive and motivational bases.* New York: Plenum Press.

Kruglanski, A. W., & Webster, D. M. (1996). Motivated closing the mind: "Seizing" and "freezing." *Psychological Review, 103,* 263–283.

Kuhn, D. (1993). Connecting scientific and informal reasoning. *Merrill-Palmer Quarterly, 38,* 74–103.

Levi, I. (1983). Who commits the base rate fallacy? *Behavioral and Brain Sciences, 6,* 502–506.

Levinson, S. C. (1995). Interactional biases in human thinking. In E. Goody (Ed.), *Social intelligence and interaction* (pp. 221–260). Cambridge, England: Cambridge University Press.

Lopes, L. L. (1981). Performing competently. *Behavioral and Brain Sciences, 4,* 343–344.

Macdonald, R. (1986). Credible conceptions and implausible probabilities. *British Journal of Mathematical and Statistical Psychology, 39,* 15–27.

Margolis, H. (1987). *Patterns, thinking, and cognition.* Chicago: University of Chicago Press.

Marr, D. (1982). *Vision.* San Francisco: Freeman.

Matarazzo, J. D. (1972). *Wechsler's measurement and appraisal of adult intelligence* (5th ed.). Baltimore, MD: Williams & Wilkins.

Newell, A. (1982). The knowledge level. *Artificial Intelligence, 18,* 87–127.

Newell, A. (1990). *Unified theories of cognition.* Cambridge, MA: Harvard University Press.

Newstead, S. E., & Evans, J. St. B. T. (Eds.). (1995). *Perspectives on thinking and reasoning.* Hove, England: Erlbaum.

Nickerson, R. S. (1996). Hempel's paradox and Wason's selection task: Logical and psychological puzzles of confirmation. *Thinking and Reasoning, 2,* 1–31.

Nisbett, L., & Ross, L. (1980). *Human inference: Strategies and shortcomings of social judgment.* Englewood Cliffs, NJ: Prentice Hall.

Norris, S. P. (1992). Testing for the disposition to think critically. *Informal Logic, 14,* 157–164.

Oaksford, M., & Chater, N. (1993). Reasoning theories and bounded rationality. In K. Manktelow & D. Over (Eds.), *Rationality: Psychological and philosophical perspectives* (pp. 31–60). London: Routledge & Kegan Paul.

Oaksford, M., & Chater, N. (1994). A rational analysis of the selection task as optimal data selection. *Psychological Review, 101,* 608–631.

Oaksford, M., & Chater, N. (1995). Theories of reasoning and the computational explanation of everyday inference. *Thinking and Reasoning, 1,* 121–152.

Osherson, D. N. (1995). Probability judgment. In E. E. Smith & D. N. Osherson (Eds.), *Thinking* (Vol. 3, pp. 35–75). Cambridge, MA: MIT Press.

Payne, J. W., Bettman, J. R., & Johnson, E. (1993). *The adaptive decision maker*. Cambridge, England: Cambridge University Press.

Piattelli-Palmarini, M. (1994). *Inevitable illusions: How mistakes of reason rule our minds*. New York: Wiley.

Politzer, G., & Noveck, I. A. (1991). Are conjunction rule violations the result of conversational rule violations? *Journal of Psycholinguistic Research, 20,* 83–103.

Raven, J. C. (1962). *Advanced progressive matrices (Set II)*. London: H. K. Lewis.

Reber, A. S. (1993). *Implicit learning and tacit knowledge*. New York: Oxford University Press.

Rescher, N. (1988). *Rationality: A philosophical inquiry into the nature and rationale of reason*. New York: Oxford University Press.

Rips, L. J. (1994). *The psychology of proof*. Cambridge, MA: MIT Press.

Rosenthal, R., & Rosnow, R. L. (1991). *Essentials of behavioral research: Methods and data analysis* (2nd ed.). New York: McGraw-Hill.

Schoemaker, P. (1991). The quest for optimality: A positive heuristic of science? *Behavioral and Brain Sciences, 14,* 205–245.

Schwarz, N. (1996). *Cognition and communication: Judgmental biases, research methods, and the logic of conversation*. Mahweh, NJ: Erlbaum.

Shafir, E. (1994). Uncertainty and the difficulty of thinking through disjunctions. *Cognition, 50,* 403–430.

Shafir, E., & Tversky, A. (1995). Decision making. In E. E. Smith & D. N. Osherson (Eds.), *Thinking* (Vol. 3, pp. 77–100). Cambridge, MA: MIT Press.

Shanks, D. R. (1995). Is human learning rational? *Quarterly Journal of Experimental Psychology, 48A,* 257–279.

Sloman, S. A. (1996). The empirical case for two systems of reasoning. *Psychological Review, 119,* 3–22.

Slugoski, B. R., Shields, H. A., & Dawson, K. A. (1993). Relation of conditional reasoning to heuristic processing. *Personality and Social Psychology Bulletin, 19,* 158–166.

Stankov, L., & Crawford, J. D. (1996). Confidence judgments in studies of individual differences. *Personality and Individual Differences, 21,* 971–986.

Stankov, L., & Dunn, S. (1993). Physical substrata of mental energy: Brain capacity and efficiency of cerebral metabolism. *Learning and Individual Differences, 5,* 241–257.

Stanovich, K. E. (1994). Reconceptualizing intelligence: Dysrationalia as an intuition pump. *Educational Researcher, 23*(4), 11–22.

Stanovich, K. E. (in press). *Who is rational? Studies of individual differences in reasoning*. Mahwah, NJ: Erlbaum.

Stanovich, K. E., & West, R. F. (1997). Reasoning independently of prior belief and individual differences in actively open-minded thinking. *Journal of Educational Psychology, 89,* 342–357.

Stanovich, K. E., & West, R. F. (1998). Individual differences in rational thought. *Journal of Experimental Psychology: General, 127,* 161–188.

Stanovich, K. E., & West, R. F. (in press-a). Cognitive ability and variation in selection task performance. *Thinking and Reasoning*.

Stanovich, K. E., & West, R. F. (in press-b). Individual differences in framing and conjunction effects. *Thinking and Reasoning*.

Stein, E. (1996). *Without good reason: The rationality debate in philosophy and cognitive science*. London: Oxford University Press.

Sternberg, R. J. (1997). *Thinking styles*. Cambridge, England: Cambridge University Press.

Sternberg, R. J., & Ruzgis, P. (Eds.). (1994). *Personality and intelligence*. Cambridge, England: Cambridge University Press.

Stich, S. (1990). *The fragmentation of reason*. Cambridge, MA: MIT Press.

Thagard, P. (1992). *Conceptual revolutions*. Princeton, NJ: Princeton University Press.

Tschirgi, J. E. (1980). Sensible reasoning: A hypothesis about hypotheses. *Child Development, 51,* 1–10.

Tversky, A., & Kahneman, D. (1982). Evidential impact of base rates. In D. Kahneman, P. Slovic, & A. Tversky (Eds.), *Judgment under uncertainty: Heuristics and biases* (pp. 153–160). Cambridge, England: Cambridge University Press.

Tversky, A., & Kahneman, D. (1983). Extensional versus intuitive reasoning: The conjunction fallacy in probability judgment. *Psychological Review, 90,* 293–315.

Vernon, P. A. (1991). The use of biological measures to estimate behavioral intelligence. *Educational Psychologist, 25,* 293–304.

Vernon, P. A. (1993). *Biological approaches to the study of human intelligence.* Norwood, NJ: Ablex.

Wagenaar, W. A. (1988). *Paradoxes of gambling behavior.* Hove, England: Erlbaum.

Wason, P. C. (1966). Reasoning. In B. Foss (Ed.), *New horizons in psychology* (pp. 135–151). Harmonsworth, England: Penguin.

Yates, J. F., Lee, J., & Shinotsuka, H. (1996). Beliefs about overconfidence, including its cross-national variation. *Organizational Behavior and Human Decision Processes, 65,* 138–147.

Discussion

After the Stanovich presentation, discussion focused on how heuristic reasoning and problem-solving performance relate to individual differences in traditional measures of intellectual abilities. The issue of contextualized versus decontextualized thinking was extensively considered.

Dr. Wittmann: I thought about where there could be some flaws in that approach. What comes in my mind are the victims of group think. How can you avoid that argument in your analysis? Say that the majority votes what is normatively correct or the best vote available, what is the normative correct answer? And if you look in the group think literature, that was in the end not the correct answer.

Dr. Stanovich: Right. But it's exactly that type of linkage that we've tried to break with this work. The philosophers — and I'm thinking of people like Cohen and Wetherick and the psychologists who've relied on their work — have tended to focus on the modal response. The group think that you're talking about. Well, why is this? Because the philosophers view untutored human intuition as the sine qua non of normativity. And they've been at pains to justify that response. I mean they're the ones that are victims of the group think. I've tried to disassociate the individual-differences characteristics from the modal response.

So, for instance, a typical critique of Kahneman and Tversky asks, "Why do Tversky and Kahneman differ from the rest of the world in the answers to their problems?" (Macdonald, 1986, p. 15). Well, in fact, they don't differ from the rest of the world. This tends to be framed in terms of the elitist versus populist view to go back to your group think idea with the philosophers on the populism side and the nasty psychologists who design these problems as being on the elitist side. Those philosophers siding with human intuition now have taken on the mantle of the person in the street. But in fact it doesn't break down that way. It's not Kahneman and Tversky versus the rest of the world. In fact, the more competently capable individuals on some problems line up with Kahneman and Tversky.

What I'm doing is agreeing with you, but saying I'm trying to go in exactly that direction. That is, getting away from trying to model only the modal response. The philosophers use the modal response as something that primes their intuitions on what is normative. There would be no dispute. There would have been no dispute if people had answered these problems in the way that the psychologists originally thought they would. The philosophers wouldn't be raking Kahneman over the coals. The empirical fact that the modal response departed from the normative model that had been applied to the task has primed the intuitions of critics of the heuristics and biases literature about what must be normative. But I'm saying there are other empirical facts that might prime our intuitions about normativity. So I'm agreeing with you maybe in a roundabout way.

Dr. Hunt: A couple of points. One is that I think that individuals who score well on the SAT [Scholastic Aptitude Test] and the sort of measures you use, require decontextualized thinking. And that the issue of taking a perspective may not be all that bad. Let me give you an example of some work we've been doing with the statistics department on views, facets, and beliefs. You say from a urn containing 500 balls and an urn containing 3,500. And to estimate a frequency. And they correctly say you have to have the sample size the same to get equal accuracy, which is true. You ask them — and the way we frame the question is for Seattle University and the University of Washington, and it's a survey about whether you feel safe at night. Now, students don't easily put themselves in the position of a ball in an urn. But University of Washington is about five times bigger than Seattle University. They will say that you have to have a five times larger sample at the University of Washington. And when pressed, they will argue, reasoning from the perspective not of the statistician but of the person being sampled, that "Do I have a chance to get my opinion registered in this sample." In which cases we indeed do have to have a larger sample in a larger population. I think that there's lot to that. The Waisson task, where the issue comes up do you ask the person to be completely decontextualized or do you provide a context within which they can reasonably project themselves. And it's not clear to me what the right thing to do is in that situation.

Dr. Stanovich: Two responses, Buz. The first is a straightforward empirical response on the SAT that their responses do generalize across other measures like a crystallized measure or something. So that doesn't necessarily involve as much decontextualization. So that's just a little empirical point.

But I think the most important point about contextualization — the point is well taken. I mean you can push performance around on all of these tasks. And, of course, the selection task is the classical example with the drinking age problem that everyone can solve or almost everyone can solve. But I think therein lies the problem with the contextualist–decontextualized positions. That is, when you contextualize the task, you vastly constrict individual differences. That is, almost everyone can do it. That certainly happens on the selection task. You can easily invoke manipulations where virtually all people will chose P and not Q.

For those of you not familiar with this literature, which has taken on a life of its own, you know, the drinking age problem is where the subject evaluates the rule "If a person is drinking beer, they must be over 21 years of age." There's an analogous problem called the "Sears problem," where the subject says if the customers get a gift, then they must have purchased over $35. Now, that pushes the modal performance way up on the selection task. But it simultaneously wipes out cognitive ability differences. And so that's the problem I have, Buz, that when you go into these contextualized situations — virtually everyone does it. I mean there's nothing interesting to analyze from an individual-differences point of view.

Dr. Hunt: The question I am raising here is whether there's sort of an implication in all these things that contextualizing not so good, you shouldn't do contextualizing. And we see this again also in studying physics where students that contextualize a problem and have a terrible time with Newton's laws. They'd actually be rational if you organized for action. To have lots of little contextualized rules that can be activated quickly as opposed to doing these complicated inferential rules that work everywhere but are very difficult to deal with.

Dr. Stanovich: Again that's very true. And, of course, that's been one of the main points of the Gigerenzer group that has led the critique of the heuristics and biases tradition. But, you know, I think we're in a problem again that's come up at this conference before about differences in mean levels and differences in variability. That is something can be adaptive for everyone but maybe not a source of individual differences in the environment in which we operate. I mean you yourself have written about transformations in the modern industrialized society. And we're called on to make more and more decontextualized types of decisions and decontextualized types of reasoning. When I go down to the bank, for a loan. And there's a good example. Fifty years ago you went into a highly contextualized situation. Now you fill out the forms and you get an if–then wrong and you're turn down for your mortgage.

Dr. Hunt: Right. And the result is that one person has to be capable of decontextualized reasoning. The person who wrote the computer program. And all those bank managers merely have to see that the form is filled out, which is a contextualized act.

Dr. Stanovich: That's true, but it recycles back again to the ideas in your book. That if one wants to be one of the — one of Robert Reich's symbol manipulators — then you better know how to operate in both modes. You better know how to operate in the contextualized mode and the decontextualized mode because Robert Reich's symbol manipulators have to do decontextualized things all the time. Yes, but the point's well taken.

Dr. Ackerman: Keith, let me follow up on something that you said in response to Buz. Am I correct in presuming that you've correlated the scores on these tests to your cultural literacy measures?

Dr. Stanovich: Yes. And the result is that they predict significantly, but they're not as good as cognitive ability measures. Okay. It was very disappointing. In fact, I have a paper I haven't published yet. But I published a paper a few years ago with the title — you know, "Does Reading Make You Smarter?" And after some of this work I have another title which is, "Reading Does Make You Smarter, But It May Not Make You Wiser." The correlations are there, but they're small.

Dr. Ackerman: So then let's think about this kind of Bayesian or normative reasoning. Do you see it as something fundamentally the same as other forms of inductive and deductive reasoning? Or do you see them as somehow different? Part of the whole normative discussion, at least that I've seen in the literature is, maybe a radiologist needs to be a normative thinker, but maybe a pig farmer doesn't. And so the question is, "Is that something fundamentally different kind of reasoning, or do you see it as all fitting together in one large sort of form of that kind of reasoning?"

Dr. Stanovich: Well, it's somewhat different in the empirical sense. In that the last few relationships that I showed, the relationships with thinking dispositions and cognitive styles are much more strongly related to these belief bias or decontextualized tasks than they are to just a pure inductive reasoning or a pure syllogistic reasoning. So I think I'm tapping into something else with these types of tasks that pit prior belief directly against a logical validity. They have a much higher dispositional component than any series completion test. So in that sense I think they're different.

Dr. Ackerman: So do you think a better form of a reasoning test would be a series of these kinds of questions rather than a syllogistic reasoning test?

Dr. Stanovich: I think for certain purposes, yes. And in fact, we have been trying to show for some of these processing styles, whether they had any domain generality, and so we had demonstrated at least modest domain generality for some notion of the ability to avoid belief bias in inefficacious situations and to use prior belief when it's efficacious.

Dr. Baddeley: You've been looking at differences across individuals in capacity. If you look within individual differences by giving a concurrent load, is it conceivable that different strategies might be differentially resistant to a load? And from a survival point of view, that might actually be an important variable.

Dr. Stanovich: Yes. I don't know if you were the reviewer who asked us exactly that, asked us to take the cognitive ability analyses within an individual and push a cognitive load around. And not exactly in your sense, but I think I see the direction you're going. And so we've already been pushed in that direction and are making some tentative steps. I don't have anything to show.

Dr. Wright: I was thinking about that statistics problem. If you think about the people that get that problem right, they might comprise two groups. The people who sort of get the naive wrong answer and just kind of guess that answer and the people who actually know quite a bit of statistics, and they get it right because they know how to solve it properly. I mean so you've got this mixture of people getting it right. There's people who get it right because they know how to get it right, and there's the people who get it right because they almost guess it right. And so you get a bigger variation in that group. And you've got very weak people in that group, which accounts for the low average score. Then you've got these more advanced statistical people who get it right because they know how to solve that problem.

Dr. Stanovich: Right. We've looked at that a little bit. It's not bimodal. I mean we looked for bimodality among that group, and we don't get it. We've done a couple of other little analyses. Actually, I have maybe stronger hypotheses about the other group — the high-ability group who is sticking with the indicant response. I think that, as some critics have pointed out, the high-ability people may be having problems with the base rate because of lack of reference class specificity. So I've looked more at the that end of the distribution. On the other group, all I can say is that they're not bimodal.

411

18

Learner Profiles: Valuing Individual Differences Within Classroom Communities

PATRICIA A. ALEXANDER and P. KAREN MURPHY

Among the dominant trends in the educational literature is the practice of characterizing the teachers and students who populate classrooms as learning communities (e.g., A. L. Brown & Campione, 1990; Cognition and Technology Group at Vanderbilt, 1996; Wade, in press) and thinking in terms of the collective more than the individual (e.g., J. S. Brown, Collins, & Duguid, 1989; Christensen, 1991; Resnick, 1991). Within this orientation, a focus on differences between individual students may be cast as counterproductive to efforts to build communities that work together for the educational good (Damon, 1991). The individual as the centerpiece of theory, research, and practice is thus supplanted with discussions of *distributed cognition* or *shared cognition* and *social learning* (Pea, 1989; Resnick, Levine, & Teasley, 1991; Rogoff & Chavajay, 1996; Salomon, 1993). What some holding to this perspective appear to seek are the elements that lead to internal cohesion among group members, with limited regard for the conditions that contribute to community disaggregation, to whatever degree. Conversely, there are those, as seen in the literature on special populations (e.g., special, gifted, or multicultural education), whose interests understandably lie in grasping the circumstances that distinguish one chosen group over others.

Yet, concern for individual differences need not be discounted or, worse, vilified in efforts to acknowledge or embrace the social or cultural forces at work in classrooms. We view this increased attention to group dynamics and sociocultural forces as a positive direction within the educational literature (Alexander, 1996; Alexander, in press; Murphy & Woods, 1996), provided that it does not obscure the essential merits of the person in situ. As we hope to convey, research on individual differences can reinforce and complement inquiry into distributed, shared, or social processes (Alexander, 1997a). It certainly need not be cast as antithetical to such stances.

413

Thus, the position we posit in this chapter is that the understanding of cognitive and motivational differences among individual community members can only serve to promote learning and instruction for the whole. That is, within any community of learners, there will be subcommunities who share similar cognitive and motivational patterns. By uncovering these various subcommunities, educators may have a greater likelihood of orchestrating learning environments that serve not only the collective but also the individual. From a statistical standpoint, it certainly is critical to appreciate that communities are not uniform or unidimensional in their character. Rather, as educators have frequently attested (Jetton & Alexander, 1997), classrooms can and do differ, even for the same teacher, same content, or within the same school. Such diversity has to do, in part, with the specific configuration of individuals who populate these classrooms, individuals who differ in their knowledge, interests, and strategic capabilities. In essence, the nature of each classroom community is shaded and shaped by such individual distinctions. Accordingly, the more educational researchers and practitioners understand about the cognitive and motivational attributes of individuals, the more they can appreciate about the nature of the collective (Alexander, in press; Damon, 1991).

In our program of research, we have found cluster analysis to be a theoretically valid and practically sound technique for reasserting the value of individual differences within social models of learning and instruction. For this reason, we explore what cluster analysis is and what it has to offer in the study of individual differences. We then attempt to validate these claims by describing two cluster-analytic investigations that profiled cognitive and motivational distinctions among college-aged learners. These investigations represented two varied domains of learning as well as individuals of different backgrounds and career orientations. Yet, as we show, there were striking similarities in the cognitive and motivational profiles that arose in these studies. These consistencies, along with the intriguing nature of the resulting profiles, give rise to significant implications, not only for educational research, but also for instructional practice.

Cluster Analysis: What It Is and What It Has to Offer

Methods for categorizing and classifying similar objects can be found throughout the annals of history. For instance, Aristotle developed an elaborate system for categorizing animals into groups on the basis of whether they had red blood. He further classified these two groups on the basis of how their young were produced. Like Aristotle, educational researchers find it necessary, as well as useful, to categorize the objects and people around them into groups in an effort to arrange, simplify, and perhaps better understand them (Aldenerfer & Blashfield, 1984). In essence, a categorization or classification system represents a pragmatic way to organize data so that they can be interpreted efficiently and effectively (Everitt, 1993). There are several statistical techniques that researchers might use to reduce data into manageable or interpretable units. Among those techniques are multidimensional scaling, exploratory and confirmatory factor analyses, and cluster analysis.

When considering these various sorting techniques, researchers must have some clear purpose in mind because each provides a unique way of classifying objects or people. For instance, multidimensional scaling can be used to produce a geometrical or spatial representation of data in multidimensional space on the basis of similarities between the objects under investigation. Multidimensional scaling, however, is best suited to the examination of variables that can be represented in three or fewer dimensions (Everitt & Dunn, 1991). By comparison, exploratory and confirmatory factor analyses allow researchers to investigate the degree to which one or more observed variables reflect some unobservable variable or construct (Bollen, 1989). Yet, these techniques do not readily allow close examination of an individual's performance compared with that of the larger group. Cattell's (1952) "Q" factor analysis is one exception to this general pattern. Finally, the family of clustering techniques allows researchers to contrast the multidimensional and multifactorial nature of individual learner performance with the performance of the classroom community.

In essence, cluster analysis gives researchers the ability to explore the dynamic interplay between n cases (i.e., the number of respondents) and p variables (e.g., domain knowledge, interest, or strategic processing). Further, this technique searches for similarities and differences between the performances of individuals within the data set (Anderberg, 1973). Thus, cluster analysis enables educational researchers to explore the learning profiles of the subcommunities within classrooms, formed on the basis of both internal cohesion and external isolation (Cormack, 1971; Gordan, 1980).

For our research program, we used a hierarchical cluster analysis. In a *hierarchical analysis*, the classification takes place in a series of steps that may run from n clusters, each containing a single individual (i.e., divisive method), to a single cluster containing all individuals (i.e., agglomerative method). The goal of both of these methods is to find the step or point at which the clusters are optimally comprised of those individuals whose profiles, or response vectors, are most similar and, at the same time, separated from those individuals whose response vectors are most different. Hierarchical cluster-analytic techniques have several advantages over other cluster techniques (Du Toit, Steyn, & Stumpf, 1986). First, no assumptions are made about the probability distribution of the population from which the sample was obtained. That is, unlike other multivariate analytic techniques (e.g., confirmatory factor analysis), hierarchical cluster analysis does not require that the sample come from a multivariate normal distribution. Further, the calculations used to determine the clusters are relatively simple and acceptable from a mathematical perspective. Finally, as opposed to other procedures, such as regression analysis, the order in which individuals or variables are entered has no effect on the outcomes.

One disadvantage of this procedure, however, is that two or more clusters may be mistakenly linked by one isolated observation. Such an event is referred to as a *chain effect* and is usually associated with single-link forms of hierarchical clustering. One way to avoid this problem is not to use the single-link method and another is to conduct exploratory graphing techniques (du Toit et al., 1986). Graphing techniques, such as cluster maps and dendrograms, allow investigators to examine the emerging clusters visually. Within our research, we chose Ward's minimum variance hierarchical clustering procedure because it is considered to be particularly effective in recovering the underlying structure of a given data set (e.g., Atlas & Overall, 1994). When using Ward's minimum variance clustering technique, as with all clustering techniques, several steps or procedures should be followed as a way of substantiating the emerging clusters (Everitt, 1993). First, the use of an exploratory technique like Ward's must be rooted in a strong theoretical foundation. This allows

415

researchers to make predictions concerning the number of expected clusters given a particular data set. For example, our investigations into the interplay between knowledge, interest, and strategic processing were based on the *Model of Domain Learning* (MDL; Alexander, 1997b). Second, researchers should conduct a thorough review of literature in search of other studies that investigated similar variables using cluster analysis. Knowledge of similar studies will help confirm predictions relative to resulting clusters.

From a statistical standpoint, several procedures can be used to substantiate the emerging clusters. First, Milligan and Cooper (1985) recommended a technique in which one variable, an external criterion variable, is used to validate the differences among resulting profiles. The variable chosen to serve as the external criterion variable should be able to function well as an independent indicator of cluster-group differences. In effect, the relationship between the cluster profiles and the external criterion variable operates as a measure of convergent validity. Further, a multivariate analysis of variance can be used to test for statistically significant differences between the resulting clusters using cluster group as the independent variable and the grouping variables as dependent variables. This omnibus test can be followed with univariate analysis of variance tests for the dependent variables and the external criterion variable to pinpoint the source of the differences (e.g., knowledge or interest) between the various clusters.

Discriminant function analysis can also be used to validate the presumed multidimensional character of the clusters (Stevens, 1996), in which the number of resulting functions should be one less than the number of emerging clusters. In effect, this procedure provides support for the notion that the emerging clusters arose from an interplay of multiple variables and could not be ascribed to one variable. Further, Cohen's kappa can be used to determine the percentage of individuals who were correctly classified over and above what would be expected due to chance. Finally, as noted, a dendrogram (i.e., a two-dimensional diagram that illustrates the fusions or divisions made at each step of the cluster analysis) can aid in interpreting the resulting cluster profiles (Everitt, 1993). In these dendrograms, the number of meaningful clusters is based on an identification of the largest distances between cluster groups.

Profiling Cognitive and Motivational Differences in Academic Development: Two Cluster-Analytic Investigations

Recently, Alexander (1997b) articulated the MDL, which attempts to capture the nature of individuals' development within an academic field (e.g., mathematics, history, or physics). Because the cluster-analytic studies to be overviewed were specifically designed to test the underlying assumptions of the MDL, we think a brief description of the model is warranted.

The Model of Domain Learning

In the MDL, academic development progresses through three stages: acclimation, competence, and proficiency or expertise. Each of these stages can be captured in terms of quantitative and qualitative transformations in three primary dimensions and their resulting interactions: subject-matter knowledge, interest, and strategic processing. Subject-matter knowledge is conceptualized in two corresponding forms, domain and topic knowledge. *Domain knowledge*, which was the primary form of subject-matter knowledge examined in these cluster studies, is an individual's breadth of understanding within a specified field. As such, domain knowledge encompasses all the declarative, procedural, and conditional knowledge a person has relative to that specified academic field, whether that information is explicitly or tacitly known. *Topic knowledge*, by comparison, is an individual's depth of understanding of particular concepts or topics pertinent to the identified domain. For example, a student with a relatively strong base of human biology and human immunology knowledge may demonstrate a variable understanding of such topics as viral nucleic acids, the Krebs cycle, or bacteriophages.

Interest, as with subject-matter knowledge, also takes two forms. On the one hand, there is the short-lived or fleeting interest that a learner can display at any given moment in time. *Situational interest*, as it has been termed (Hidi, 1990; Schiefele, 1991), tends to be context or situation dependent and therefore, difficult to track developmentally (Alexander, Kulikowich, & Schulze, 1994). When people's attention and thoughts are momentarily drawn to a certain image or message, they are showing situational interest. On the other hand, there is a more enduring form of interest, *personal* or *individual interest* (Hidi, 1990; Schiefele, 1991), that is linked to one's vocational and avocational pursuits. It is this form of abiding interest that was targeted in these two cluster-analytic studies.

The final dimension within the MDL is *strategic processing*. Within the MDL, strategic processing pertains to the general cognitive and metacognitive procedures that individuals purposefully and consciously use when confronted with performance problems or nonoptimal learning (e.g., Garner, 1987; Pressley et al., 1992; Weinstein & Mayer, 1986). Various strategies are considered more simplistic in form because they appear to demand less cognitive effort or rely on surface features of the problem. Such procedures can be thought of as lower level strategies (Alexander, Graham, & Harris, 1998), as when students reread segments of text or underline words or phrases. Other strategies, however, are more demanding in that they require significant manipulations or transformations of given information. Examples of these higher level strategies in the processing of text would be building mental models or creating alternative graphic or linguistic representations of the content (Alexander et al., 1998). Although domain-specific strategies are frequently studied relative to the development of competence or expertise (e.g., Chi, Glaser, & Farr, 1988; Glaser, 1984), this class of strategies is incorporated in the subject-matter knowledge component of the MDL.

As stated, these dimensions of subject-matter knowledge, interest, and strategic processing are expected to undergo change as students progress from acclimated to competent or proficient learners. In effect, as individuals move from acclimation into competence, their knowledge of the domain should increase markedly and become more cohesive and more principled (Alexander, 1998; Gelman & Greeno, 1989). Proficient or expert learners, by comparison, not only have vast stores of domain knowledge, which are tightly organized around fundamental principles, but they also contribute new knowledge to that domain. Individual interest should also manifest a concomitant rise from acclimation to competence and, again, from competence to proficiency. The pattern of change is somewhat different for learners' strategic processing. Specifically, acclimated learners are expected to rely heavily on general strategies, including lower level strategies that are necessary for building an initial base of domain knowledge. Competent learners, however, should display a decrease in general strategy use, especially of lower level strategies, as certain processes and problems associated with the domain become somewhat routinized. As more complex problems are encountered in competence and proficiency, an increase in the use of deeper level strategies should be anticipated.

Explorations of Human Immunology and Education Psychology

Because the MDL posits particular configurations of cognitive and motivational variables at each developmental juncture, cluster analysis was an appropriate procedure for documenting the Knowledge × Interest × Strategy configurations that might form within and between particular communities of learners. Therefore, to provide a more effective gauge of the model, Alexander and colleagues (Alexander, Jetton, & Kulikowich, 1995; Alexander & Murphy, in press) planned two cluster-analytic investigations with somewhat heterogeneous participants and within two seemingly dissimilar domains.

The first investigation (Alexander et al., 1995) involved 30 premedical students and 17 graduate students in educational psychology (Experiment 1), along with 78 undergraduate education majors (Experiment 2). For both Experiments 1 and 2, the principal domain of study was human immunology, although physics was included so that cross-domain performance could be explored. Participants in the second investigation (Alexander & Murphy, in press) were 329 undergraduates enrolled in an introductory course in educational psychology, the target domain. For both of these investigations, the variables focused on students' subject-matter knowledge (i.e., domain or topic), individual interest, and strategic processing (i.e., their recall of demanding domain-specific exposition or documented strategy use during studying). A measure of domain knowledge was chosen as the external criterion variable in this first investigation, whereas a domain-specific analogy task served that function in the second.

Profiles in human immunology.   In light of these various predictions from the MDL, it made sense to turn to cluster analysis. For example, it would be expected that students with higher levels of domain knowledge would likewise be those with more reported interest. Students fitting this profile should also be those who demonstrated more effective and efficient use of strategies when presented with a text-processing task. Thus, in Experiment 1, Alexander et al. (1995) focused on premedical students and graduate students who had well-defined career paths that would be associated with differential training in the target domain of human immunology. This selection was expected to magnify differences in students' knowledge and interest, contributing to distinct clusters. Interest, in this case, was marked by students' ratings of interest in domain passages.

Because participants in Experiment 2 were enrolled in an unrelated undergraduate course, it was assumed that levels of human immunology knowledge, interest, and strategic processing would be more restricted than in Experiment 1. In this experiment, a measure of topic knowledge was added to the clustering variables, along with a global interest rating for the domain. However, it was expected that distinctions in these variables would exist nonetheless and that similar patterns in knowledge, interest, and strategic processing would emerge. Overall, what Alexander et al. (1995) found was that patterns in knowledge, interest, and strategic processing were well matched to the MDL predictions. Further, these patterns generally held even when the participating group changed from advanced students with well-honed career paths relevant to the target domain to undergraduate students with limited background knowledge and reported interest.

As can be seen in Table 18.1, three distinct clusters captured the data in Experiment 1. Cluster 1, which was composed almost entirely of premedical students, had the highest reported level of interest and recalled the most from the demanding exposition. Along with Cluster 2, this group of students demonstrated significantly higher levels of domain knowledge than Cluster 3, which was dominated by the educational psychology graduate students. What was intriguing about Cluster 2 was their relatively moderate levels of interest and recall in spite of a strong body of domain knowledge. This interplay of knowledge, interest, and strategic processing within Cluster 2 was not consistent with the predictions of the MDL. The profile of Cluster 3, however, with its lowest levels of knowledge, interest, and strategic processing, did conform to model expectations.

When the analysis centered on more acclimated students enrolled in educational psychology (Experiment 2), four clusters emerged (see Table 18.2). Clusters 1 and 4 were most distinct in terms of the model dimensions. Specifically, students in Cluster 1 had the descriptively highest levels of domain knowledge and one of the statistically higher scores on the topic knowledge test. In addition, these students were most interested in what they read and recalled the most from the domain texts. Inversely, Cluster 4 students had limited domain and topic knowledge and were the lowest in interest and recall. Clusters 2 and 3 demonstrated an adequate-to-strong base of subject-matter knowledge. Cluster 2 students evidenced significantly higher interest in the domain passages than their counterparts in Cluster 3. In effect, this group appeared to consist of students who not only found texts interesting, but who also seemed strategically effective at learning from difficult exposition. Cluster 3 students, on the other hand, resembled students who had acquired some relevant knowledge of the domain but who seemingly disliked studying expository texts.

Profiles in educational psychology. As in Experiment 2 of the Alexander et al. (1995) study, undergraduates enrolled in an introductory educational psychology course served as participants in the Alexander and Murphy (in press) investigation. In this instance, however, the target domain was educational psychology, and student profiles were constructed at the outset and conclusion of the semester. We were interested in determining whether profiles comparable to those in the Alexander et al. (1995) study would emerge despite a focus on a domain that was considered to be less well structured than human immunology (e.g., Alexander, 1992; Spiro, Feltovich, Jacobson, & Coulson, 1992; Spiro & Jehng, 1990). Additionally, we had the opportunity to track participants across the semester and to monitor changes in their profiles during this learning period.

As can be seen in Table 18.3, three clusters statistically described the pretest data, which included the clustering variables of domain knowledge, ratings of interest in important domain concepts, a strategy-use inventory, and a measure of recall. Clus-

TABLE 18.1 Means and Standard Deviations for the Knowledge, Interest, and Recall Measures for the Three Clusters in Alexander, Jetton, and Kulikowich's (1995) Experiment 1

	Cluster groups					
	Cluster 1 (n = 17)		Cluster 2 (n = 13)		Cluster 3 (n = 17)	
Variable	M	SD	M	SD	M	SD
Immunology knowledge (max. = 25)	17.41_a	1.87	17.46_a	3.02	15.17_b	3.09
Bacteriophage interest (max. = 10)	7.94_a	1.34	6.15_b	1.91	4.00_c	2.65
Bacteriophage recall (max. = 29)	50.82_a	11.83	38.00_b	14.09	17.12_c	7.36
Viral nucleic acids interest (max. = 10)	8.18_a	1.01	6.46_b	2.63	5.35_b	2.87
Viral nucleic acid recall (max. = 28)	58.11_a	9.16	36.00_b	6.65	16.18_c	6.27

Note. Subscript letters that differ in each row denote which cluster means are significantly different from one another ($\alpha = .05$). max. = maximum. Data in table are from "Interrelationship of Knowledge, Interest, and Recall: Assessing a Model of Domain Learning," by P. A. Alexander, T. L. Jetton, and J. M. Kulikowich, 1995, *Journal of Educational Psychology, 87,* 559–575. Copyright 1995 by the American Psychological Association. Adapted with permission of the authors.

TABLE 18.2 Means and Standard Deviations for the Knowledge, Interest, and Recall Measures for the Four Clusters in Alexander, Jetton, and Kulikowich's (1995) Experiment 2

| | Cluster groups | | | | | | | |
| Variable | Cluster 1 ($n = 13$) | | Cluster 2 ($n = 22$) | | Cluster 3 ($n = 22$) | | Cluster 4 ($n = 21$) | |
	M	SD	M	SD	M	SD	M	SD
Domain knowledge (max. = 25)	19.38	2.79	17.59	4.07	18.09	3.08	16.67	2.61
Topic knowledge (max. = 10)	6.93_a	1.66	6.13_a	1.86	7.05_a	1.43	4.76_b	1.14
Bacteriophage interest (max. = 10)	8.15_a	0.80	5.50_b	1.34	2.82_c	1.40	2.14_c	1.49
Bacteriophage recall (max. = 29)	33.69_a	19.77	34.64_a	22.16	28.52_a	12.28	13.63_b	9.50
Viral nucleic acids interest (max. = 10)	7.46_a	1.05	4.73_b	1.16	2.59_c	1.65	1.43_d	1.08
Viral nucleic acids recall (max. = 28)	43.68_a	28.24	33.28_b	19.72	25.49	16.65	17.52_c	12.05

Note. Subscript letters that differ in each row denote which cluster means are significantly different from one another ($\alpha = .05$). max. = maximum. Data in table are from "Interrelationship of Knowledge, Interest, and Recall: Assessing a Model of Domain Learning," by P. A. Alexander, T. L. Jetton, and J. M. Kulikowich, 1995, *Journal of Educational Psychology, 87*, 559–575. Copyright 1995 by the American Psychological Association. Adapted with permission of the authors.

TABLE 18.3 Means and Standard Deviations for the Analogical Reasoning, Knowledge, Interest, Strategic Use, and Recall Tasks for the Three Pretest Clusters in Alexander and Murphy (in press)

| | Cluster groups | | | | | |
| | Learning Oriented (n = 108) | | Strong Knowledge (n = 68) | | Low Profile (n = 153) | |
Variable	M	SD	M	SD	M	SD
Analogical reasoning (max. = 56)	20.64_a	7.99	20.53_a	8.21	18.03_b	7.45
Domain knowledge (max. = 24)	12.82_b	1.90	14.84_a	1.78	11.58_c	1.94
Individual interest (max. = 182)	135.85_a	20.66	111.92_c	10.97	126.76_b	19.11
Strategic use (max. = 30)	10.42_a	3.99	7.49_b	2.88	6.09_c	2.64
Recall (max. = 85 of 93)	5.40_a	3.13	4.21_b	1.80	2.67_c	1.64

Note. Subscript letters that differ in each row denote which cluster means are significantly different from one another ($\alpha = .05$). max. = maximum. Data in table are from "Profiling Differences in Students' Knowledge, Interest, and Strategic Processing," by P. A. Alexander and P. K. Murphy, 1998, *Journal of Educational Psychology, 90*, p. 440. Copyright 1998 by the American Psychological Association. Adapted with permission of the authors.

ter 1, which was labeled the *Learning-Oriented group*, had a moderate level of domain knowledge combined with a high reported interest. These students also documented the most strategy use, recalled the most from the domain passages they read, and did the best on the analogy task. Cluster 2, the *Strong Knowledge group*, began the semester with the highest level of domain knowledge but with the lowest level of interest in the domain. These students' strategy use and their passage recalls, by comparison, were only moderate. The final group, the *Low-Profile group*, consisted of students with only moderate domain interest, the least domain knowledge, the lowest reported strategy use, and the worst performance on the recall task. With the exception of the Strong Knowledge cluster, student profiles at pretest tended to confirm predictions of the MDL and closely paralleled the three clusters described by Alexander et al. (1995) in Experiment 1.

By the conclusion of the semester, however, the three initial clusters gave way to four (see Table 18.4), a condition that corresponds to the fan-spread effect evidenced in developmental studies (Bryk & Weisberg, 1977). Such a developmental spread is also consistent with the within-individual transformations anticipated by the MDL. Two profiles, Learning Oriented and Strong Knowledge, were retained from pretest to posttest with one difference. After 15 weeks of instruction, those in the Learning-Oriented group had also achieved one of the highest levels of domain knowledge. Further, by the end of the term, no student retained the low knowledge, low interest, and low strategy characterization observed in the Low-Profile cluster at pretest. Instead, this single cluster was replaced with two groups that bore certain similarities to Clusters 2 and 3 in Experiment 2 of Alexander et al. (1995). The first of these was the *Effortful Processor cluster*, so called because the students in this group reported the highest level of strategy use in studying the lengthy and demanding domain passages. Yet, students in this group were the least successful in building their base of domain knowledge over the course of the semester. The final cluster consisted of students who exerted the least amount of strategic effort in their text processing and, not surprisingly, recalled the least from these passages. Because of this, the group was labeled the *Nonstrategic Reader cluster*. What remained unclear was whether the limited strategy use and low recall were attributable to an inability or an unwillingness to engage in strategic processing.

What These Profiles Reveal

Our overarching goal in this discussion was to promote the value of cluster analysis as a statistical procedure that allows for both an individual and group perspective within classroom communities. Toward that end, we revisit the various profiles that emerged in the aforementioned investigations and consider what they have to tell about the various subcommunities that exist within the whole. For one, the intraindividual interplay of knowledge, interest, and strategic processing variables results in distinct student profiles that are associated with differential success within the classroom. Classroom communities certainly are not homogeneous, and the combination of cognitive and motivational factors offers promise in teasing out the clusters of students who reside there.

Moreover, these profiles display certain consistencies across varied domains and populations. Whether the participants were advanced premedical or graduate students performing in human immunology or undergraduate students taking part in

423

TABLE 18.4 Means and Standard Deviations for the Analogical Reasoning, Knowledge, Interest, Strategic Use, and Recall Tasks for the Four Posttest Clusters in Alexander and Murphy (in press)

	Cluster groups							
	Learning Oriented (n = 94)		Strong Knowledge (n = 39)		Effortful Processors (n = 76)		Nonstrategic Readers (n = 120)	
Variable	M	SD	M	SD	M	SD	M	SD
Analogical reasoning (max. = 56)	45.49	4.76[a]	45.46	4.75[a]	43.55	4.79[b]	43.28	5.12[b]
Domain knowledge (max. = 24)	18.17	2.28[a]	18.82	2.46[a]	15.96	1.94[c]	16.65	2.23[b]
Individual interest (max. = 182)	156.52	12.36[a]	113.38	17.72[c]	145.67	14.66[b]	148.43	11.61[b]
Strategic use (max. = 30)	9.78	3.30[b]	7.77	3.13[c]	12.66	3.61[a]	6.67	2.22[d]
Recall (max. = 85 of 93)	11.79	2.99[a]	8.54	3.87[b]	8.36	2.48[b]	6.22	2.66[c]

Note. Superscript letters that differ in each row denote which cluster means are significantly different from one another ($\alpha = .05$). max. = maximum. Data in table are from "Profiling Differences in Students' Knowledge, Interest, and Strategic Processing," by P. A. Alexander and P. K. Murphy, in press, *Journal of Educational Psychology.* Copyright 1998 by American Psychological Association. Adapted with permission of the authors.

an introductory class in educational psychology, the elements of successful or un-successful performance were remarkably similar. Further, optimal performance did not rest on one single factor, even domain knowledge. Specifically, although back-ground knowledge has long been recognized as a powerful predictor of academic success (Alexander & Murphy, 1998), it was not knowledge alone that was indicative of the most successful learners in these studies. Rather, what distinguished the "most" successful from the "relatively" successful students in both investigations (i.e., Clusters 1 vs. 2 in Experiment 1, and Clusters 1 vs. 3 in Experiment 2, Alexander et al., 1995; Learning Oriented vs. Strong Knowledge clusters, Alexander & Murphy, in press) was their strong interest and apparent willingness to exert effort toward understanding.

According to the MDL, such a combination of knowledge, interest, and strategic ability is essential if students hope to attain higher levels of competence or profi-ciency in any academic domain (Alexander, 1998). Others have documented similar distinctions in the profiles of generally successful students. Renkl (1997), for in-stance, used the phrase "principle-based explainers" to signify those learners who had only moderate levels of subject-matter knowledge but whose efforts helped to propel them to success. Renkl contrasted these students with the *anticipative rea-soners*, who, like the Strong Knowledge cluster in Alexander and Murphy's (in press) study, appeared to rely on the body of relevant knowledge they had managed to accumulate to that point.

Even though there were several pathways to success within these investigations, it was clear that the combination of low knowledge, low interest, and limited stra-tegic ability was directly aligned with poor performance. The Low-Profile group in Alexander and Murphy's (in press) study was prototypical of such acclimated stu-dents. However, at pretest, there was no way to ascribe cause for this configuration or to determine what might become of these low-knowledge, low-interest, and low-strategy students. On one hand, some of these Low-Profile learners may merely lack the experiences they need to alter their current situation. On the other hand, prob-lems of skill or will may force others in this cluster to remain relatively unsuccessful in their journey toward competence.

After a semester of instruction intended to alter students' knowledge, interest, and strategic processing, less successful students formed two clusters. First, there were Effortful Processors, who seemed to care about their learning, who did fairly well when learning from text, but who struggled unsuccessfully to acquire a strong base of domain knowledge. Then there were the Nonstrategic Readers, who could not or would not perform well when faced with demanding exposition. Others have used such adjectives as "superficial" or "passive" to describe this student profile (e.g., Chi, Bassok, Lewis, Reimann, & Glaser, 1989; de Jong & Ferguson-Hessler, 1986, 1991; Recker & Pirolli, 1995; Renkl, 1997). Collectively, these two profiles give rise to particular questions and concerns.

In the case of the Effortful Processors, there is the unsettling possibility that some students enrolled in higher education have learned to compensate for limited domain-specific ability by virtue of the time and energy they invest in studying. Perhaps with even more time to acclimate, these individuals would eventually ac-quire the breadth or depth of subject-matter knowledge requisite for continued ac-ademic development. Yet, it is conceivable that these students may never have an-other occasion to become knowledgeable in this domain. Whether for this or other reasons, it could be that members of this subcommunity will never acquire the principled body of subject-matter knowledge they need to advance into competence or proficiency.

The profile of the Nonstrategic Reader gives even more cause for concern. This was the largest contingent of students at posttest in Alexander and Murphy's (in press) investigation. The literature is replete with studies suggesting that younger and older students alike are frequently unwilling or unable to learn from demanding exposition (e.g., Garner, 1987; Pressley, Johnson, Symons, McGoldrick, & Kurita, 1989; Weinstein, Goetz, & Alexander, 1988). This was certainly the case in our exploration of learner profiles. Of course, we must acknowledge the possibility that a number of students within the Nonstrategic Reader cluster had the necessary text-processing skills but merely elected not to use them. Nonetheless, because text remains the primary mechanism of information transmission within American schools (Alexander & Knight, 1993; Yore, 1991), this situation deserves serious attention.

As stated, we were not able to disentangle the influences of skill or will within the Low-Profile and Nonstrategic Reader subcommunities. Maybe one key to unlocking the differences in these two varied groups are the goals these students bring into the learning environment. Do some of these Low-Profile students or Nonstrategic Readers profess a desire to master the content (i.e., learning goal)? Alternatively, is their aim merely to get an acceptable grade, look smart to others, or, even worse, to avoid demanding academic work (e.g., Dweck & Leggett, 1988; Meece & Holt, 1993)? By soliciting goal statements from students at the outset and conclusion of these learning experiences, we hope to make finer discriminations in these perplexing profiles. In effect, these additional data may aid us in predicting the pathways that these students eventually follow in their academic development during the semester.

Implications for Theory, Research, and Practice

1. *Theoretical orientations that focus on classrooms as social entities would be informed by recognizing the individual differences in cognition and motivation that contribute to the character of the whole community.* Individuals are undoubtedly influenced by the nature of the communities to which they belong (Bronfenbrenner, 1989). Likewise, each community is colored or shaped by the character of its individual members (Alexander, in press). Given that groups and individuals affect one another reciprocally, studies of individual differences would seem complementary to research on learning communities. The point is that studies of individual differences need not be cast as antithetical to educational theories that center on the collective. Rather, when suitably applied and appropriately interpreted, investigations of the variability between students can help to conceptualize the attributes of such instructional communities. For example, using cluster analysis, we have attempted to capture something of the cognitive and motivational subgroups that reside within classrooms. Because the resulting profiles were built on information about each and every member of the classroom community, we feel that a cluster-analytic approach has the potential to address individual and group dimensions simultaneously.

2. *There appears to be a good measure of consistency in the learner profiles reported in various investigations that encompassed not only diverse domains but also varied student populations.* From an instructional standpoint, we believe that the measure of consistency in learner profiles documented in the literature augments their practical value. That is, we have a relatively good sense that classroom communities will often contain a clustering of students who report some interest in what they are learning and who have at least some moderate base of subject-matter knowledge. Should these characteristics be combined with an ability to engage in strategic processing, these students are apt to do well over the course of the learning period. There was support for this contention in studies ranging from physics (de Jong & Ferguson-Hessler, 1986) to computer programming (Pirolli & Recker, 1994) in both novices and experts (Chi et al., 1989; de Jong & Ferguson-Hessler, 1986). It might even be posited that students with these three attributes (i.e., moderate knowledge, high interest, and strong strategic ability) would likely be successful in a wide range of classroom contexts.

At the other end, however, there are those students who enter a learning environment with little or no interest in the subject, a piecemeal knowledge of the domain, or limited strategic capability. The academic future for such students would seem more precarious. Moreover, the probability of achieving competence or proficiency is dramatically affected when students operate under multiple constraints (e.g., low knowledge, low interest, and low strategic ability). The task for teachers is far more complex under these circumstances. We hope that effective instructors can begin to provide these students with the beginnings of principled knowledge, help them see the personal relevance of the subject matter, and give them guidance in developing their strategic repertoires (Alexander, Murphy, & Woods, 1996). We are aware of instructional programs that seem to be achieving these desired ends (e.g., Schools for Thought, Cognitive and Technology Group at Vanderbilt, 1996; CORI program, Guthrie, McGough, Bennett, & Rice, 1996) and that may prove effective in fostering the academic development of acclimated students.

3. *When appropriately applied and precautionary steps taken, cluster analysis is a viable procedure for investigating individual differences.* The individual differences of learners can be explored with a variety of statistical procedures ranging from multidimensional scaling or confirmatory factor analysis to cluster analysis. Choosing from among these various techniques depends on the users' knowledge of the procedure itself as well as on the dimensions (e.g., the number of participants or variables) and purpose of one's study. Each of these procedures provides information about individual differences that is distinct from the others. In addition, each statistical procedure is based on slightly different assumptions about the population from which the sample is taken. On the basis of our interest in subcommunities of learners within classrooms and the interplay of cognitive and noncognitive factors associated with formal learning, we chose to use cluster analysis.

The proper application of cluster analysis depends on a strong theoretical framework, combined with additional statistical safeguards, that serve to validate the emerging clusters. In essence, because cluster analysis is an exploratory data-analytic technique, researchers must be equipped with the theoretical orientation and statistical skills necessary to interpret the multitude of possible outcomes. Specifically, the complexity of cluster analysis lies in deciding how many clusters are necessary to accurately describe a particular sample. In our research, we have used the MDL

427

and relevant cluster-analytic studies to formulate predictions and inform decisions about the learner profiles. Also, we used additional procedures, such as discriminant function analysis, a multivariate analysis of variance, and an analysis of variance, as a way of cross-validating the resulting clusters. By taking precautionary steps, we have found cluster analysis to be an informative and effective technique for exploring individual differences within classrooms.

4. *Research on individual differences that is multidimensional and acknowledges the influence of motivational factors, as well as cognitive forces, seems more in keeping with the complexity of formal learning.* The quality of the profiles researchers construct by means of cluster analysis, or related techniques, certainly depends on the validity and utility of the data on which they are based. When efforts are directed at portraying individual differences associated with learning, two considerations become evident: First, academic learning is a complex and dynamic phenomenon that is best represented multidimensionally. Regardless of how powerful a single factor may prove to be (e.g., knowledge), it will likely prove inadequate in differentiating between those who are more or less successful at academic learning. In the MDL, we have found it essential to frame this developmental process in terms of three components: subject-matter knowledge, interest, and general strategic ability. Second, we have become increasingly more convinced that the key to reaching competence or proficiency in any demanding academic domain lies in the motivations that students bring into the instructional environment. Therefore, we would hold that motivational variables (e.g., interest, goals, or self-beliefs) should be wedded to cognitive dimensions in explorations of formal learning.

5. *Researchers still know little about the changes in knowledge, interest, and strategic ability that students should manifest during the course of their academic development.* In this cluster-analytic exploration of learner profiles, we were guided by the MDL. This particular model offers a multidimensional picture of the prospective changes that should ensue as learners progress from acclimation through competence to proficiency in an academic domain. Yet, even when one considers the support for this particular model in these investigations and elsewhere (e.g., Alexander et al., 1994; Alexander, Murphy, Woods, Duhon, and Parker, 1997), it is apparent that little is known about the nature of academic development. Part of the problem is the time required to witness a transformation from acclimation to competence or from competence to proficiency. Without question, one semester or even one year of data may afford us only a glimpse of such a conversion. Consequently, what is needed is a longitudinal examination of students' academic growth that encompasses several years of instructional engagement. Further, this longitudinal exploration should target several seemingly diverse subject-matter areas to ensure that the observed patterns are generalizable across domains. Only in this way can we begin to profile more fully and accurately the role that students' knowledge, interest, and strategic processing play in their own learning and in the character of the classroom communities to which they belong.

REFERENCES

Aldenerfer, M. S., & Blashfield, R. K. (1984). *Cluster analysis.* Newbury Park, CA: Sage.

Aiexander, P. A. (1992). Domain knowledge: Evolving themes and emerging concerns. *Educational Psychologist, 27,* 33–51.

Alexander, P. A. (1996, August). *Wedding domain knowledge to motivation and strategic processing: Connubial bliss or conceptual blunder?* Paper presented at the 104th Annual Convention of the American Psychological Association, Toronto, Ontario, Canada.

Alexander, P. A. (1997a). Knowledge-seeking and self-schema: A case for the motivational dimensions of exposition. *Educational Psychologist, 32*(2), 83–94.

Alexander, P. A. (1997b). Mapping the multidimensional nature of domain learning: The interplay of cognitive, motivational, and strategic forces. In M. L. Maehr & P. R. Pintrich (Eds.), *Advances in motivation and achievement* (Vol. 10, pp. 213–250). Greenwich, CT: JAI Press.

Alexander, P. A. (1998). Positioning conceptual change within a model of domain literacy. In B. Guzzetti & C. Hynd (Eds.), *Theoretical perspectives on conceptual change* (pp. 55–76). Mahwah, NJ: Erlbaum.

Alexander, P. A. (in press). *Cognition and multicultural education: Contributing to the goals of knowledge construction and prejudice reduction.* New York: Carnegie Foundation.

Alexander, P. A., Graham, S., & Harris, K. (1998). A perspective on strategy research: Progress and prospects. *Educational Psychology Review, 10,* 129–154.

Alexander, P. A., Jetton, T. L., & Kulikowich, J. M. (1995). Interrelationship of knowledge, interest, and recall: Assessing a model of domain learning. *Journal of Educational Psychology, 87,* 559–575.

Alexander, P. A., & Knight, S. L. (1993). Dimensions of the interplay between learning and teaching. *Educational Forum, 57,* 232–245.

Alexander, P. A., Kulikowich, J. M., & Schulze, S. K. (1994). How subject-matter knowledge affects recall and interest on the comprehension of scientific exposition. *American Educational Research Journal, 31,* 313–337.

Alexander, P. A., & Murphy, P. K. (1998). The research base for APA's learner-centered principles. In N. M. Lambert & B. L. McCombs (Eds.), *How student's learn: Reforming schools through learner-centered education* (pp. 25–60). Washington, DC: American Psychological Association.

Alexander, P. A., & Murphy, P. K. (in press). Profiling differences in students' knowledge, interest, and strategic processing. *Journal of Educational Psychology.*

Alexander, P. A., Murphy, P. K., & Woods, B. S. (1996). Of squalls and fathoms: Navigating the seas of educational innovation. *Educational Researcher, 25*(3), 31–36, 39.

Alexander, P. A., Murphy, P. K., Woods, B. S., Duhon, K., & Parker, D. (1997). College instruction and concomitant changes in students' knowledge, interest, and strategy use: A study of domain learning. *Contemporary Educational Psychology, 22,* 243–249.

Anderberg, M. R. (1973). *Cluster analysis for applications.* New York: Academic Press.

Atlas, R. S., & Overall, J. E. (1994). Comparative evaluation of two stopping rules for hierarchical cluster analysis. *Psychometrika, 59,* 581–591.

Bollen, K. A. (1989). *Structural equations with latent variables.* New York: Wiley.

Bronfenbrenner, J. (1989). Ecological systems theory. In R. Vasta (Ed.), *Annals of child development* (Vol. 16, pp. 187–251). Greenwich, CT: JAI Press.

Brown, A. L., & Campione, J. S. (1990). Communities of learning and thinking, or a context by any other name. *Contributions to Human Development, 21,* 108–126.

Brown, J. S., Collins, A., & Duguid, P. (1989). Situated cognition and the culture of learning. *Educational Researcher, 18*(1), 32–42.

Bryk, A. S., & Weisberg, H. I. (1977). Use of the nonequivalent control group design when subjects are growing. *Psychological Bulletin, 85,* 950–962.

Cattell, R. B. (1952). *Factor analysis.* New York: Harper.

Chi, M. T. H., Bassok, M., Lewis, M. W., Reimann, P., & Glaser, R. (1989). Self-explanations: How students study and use examples in learning to solve problems. *Cognitive Science, 18,* 145–182.

Chi, M. T. H., Glaser, R., & Farr, M. J. (1988). *The nature of expertise.* Hillsdale, NJ: Erlbaum.

Christensen, C. R. (1991). Premises and practices of discussion teaching. In C. R. Christensen, D. Garvin, & A. Sweet (Eds.), *Education for judgment: The artistry of discussion leadership* (pp. 15–34). Boston: Harvard Business School Press.

Cognition and Technology Group at Vanderbilt. (1996). Looking at technology in context: A framework for understanding technology and education research. In D. C. Berliner & R. C. Calfee (Eds.), *Handbook of educational psychology* (pp. 807–840). New York: Macmillan.

Cormack, R. M. (1971). A review of classification. *Journal of the Royal Statistical Society, 134,* 321–367.

Damon, W. (1991). Problems of direction in socially shared cognition. In L. B. Resnick, J. M. Levine,

429

& S. D. Teasley (Eds.), *Perspectives on socially shared cognition* (pp. 384–397). Washington, DC: American Psychological Association.

de Jong, T., & Ferguson-Hessler, M. G. M. (1986). Cognitive structure of good and poor novice problem solvers in physics. *Journal of Educational Psychology, 78,* 279–288.

de Jong, T., & Ferguson-Hessler, M. G. M. (1991). Knowledge of problem situations in physics: A comparison of good and poor novice problem solvers. *Learning and Instruction, 1,* 289–302.

Du Toit, S. H. C., Steyn, A. G. W., & Stumpf, R. H. (1986). *Graphical exploratory data analysis.* New York: Springer-Verlag.

Dweck, C. S., & Leggett, E. L. (1988). A social–cognitive approach to motivation and personality. *Psychological Review, 95,* 256–273.

Everitt, B. S. (1993). *Cluster analysis* (3rd ed.). New York: Arnold.

Everitt, B. S., & Dunn, G. (1991). *Applied multivariate data analysis.* New York: Arnold.

Garner, R. (1987). *Metacognition and reading comprehension.* Norwood, NJ: Ablex.

Gelman, R., & Greeno, J. G. (1989). On the nature of competence: Principles for understanding in a domain. In L. B. Resnick (Ed.), *Knowing, learning, and instruction: Essays in honor of Robert Glaser* (pp. 125–186). Hillsdale, NJ: Erlbaum.

Glaser, R. (1984). Education and thinking: The role of knowledge. *American Psychologist, 39,* 93–104.

Gordan, A. D. (1980). *Classification.* London: Chapman & Hall.

Guthrie, J. T., McGough, K., Bennett, L., & Rice, M. E. (1996). Concept-oriented reading instruction: An integrated curriculum to develop motivations and strategies for reading. In L. Baker, P. Afflerbach, & D. Reinking (Eds.), *Developing engaged readers in school and home communities* (pp. 165–190). Mahwah, NJ: Erlbaum.

Hidi, S. (1990). Interest and its contribution as a mental resource for learning. *Review of Educational Research, 60,* 549–571.

Jetton, T. L., & Alexander, P. A. (1997). Instructional importance: What teachers value and what students learn. *Reading Research Quarterly, 32,* 290–308.

Meece, J. L., & Holt, K. (1993). A pattern analysis of students achievement goals. *Journal of Educational Psychology, 85,* 582–590.

Milligan, G. W., & Cooper, M. C. (1985). An examination of procedures for determining the number of clusters in a data set. *Psychometrika, 45,* 159–179.

Murphy, P. K., & Woods, B. S. (1996). Situating knowledge in learning and instruction. *Educational Psychologist, 31*(2), 141–145.

Pea, R. D. (1989). Socializing the knowledge transfer problem. *International Journal of Educational Research, 2,* 639–663.

Pirolli, P., & Recker, M. (1994). Learning strategies and transfer in the domain of programming. *Cognition and Instruction, 12,* 235–275.

Pressley, M., Johnson, C. J., Symons, S., McGoldrick, J. A., & Kurita, J. A. (1989). Strategies that improve children's comprehension of text. *Elementary School Journal, 90,* 3–32.

Pressley, M., Wood, E., Woloshyn, V. E., Martin, V., King, A., & Menke, D. (1992). Encouraging mindful use of prior knowledge: Attempting to construct explanatory answers facilitates learning. *Educational Psychologist, 27,* 91–109.

Recker, M. M., & Pirolli, P. (1995). Modeling individual differences in students' learning strategies. *Journal of the Learning Sciences, 4,* 1–38.

Renkl, A. (1997). Learning from worked-out examples: A study on individual differences. *Cognitive Science, 21,* 1–29.

Resnick, L. B. (1991). Shared cognition: Thinking as social practice. In L. B. Resnick, J. M. Levine, & S. D. Teasley (Eds.), *Perspectives on socially shared cognition* (pp. 1–20). Washington, DC: American Psychological Association.

Resnick, L. B., Levine, J. M., & Teasley, S. D. (1991). (Eds.). *Perspectives on socially shared cognition.* Washington, DC: American Psychological Association.

Rogoff, B., & Chavajay, P. (1996). Cognitive processes are culture-dependent: Intellectual development of children is shaped by their actual activities, which vary by culture. *American Psychologist, 50,* 859–877.

Salomon, G. (1993). *Distributed cognition: Psychological and educational considerations.* Cambridge, England: Cambridge University Press.

Schiefele, U. (1991). Interest, learning, and motivation. *Educational Psychologist, 26,* 229–323.

Spiro, R. J., Feltovich, P. J., Jacobson, M. J., & Coulson, R. L. (1992). Cognitive flexibility, constructivism, and hypertext: Random access instruction for advanced knowledge acquisition in ill-structured domains. In T. M. Duffy & D. H. Jonassen (Eds.), *Constructivism and the technology of instruction* (pp. 57–75). Cambridge, England: Cambridge University Press.

Spiro, R. J., & Jehng, J. C. (1990). Cognitive flexibility and hypertext: Theory and technology for the nonlinear and multidimensional traversal of complex subject matter. In D. Nix & R. J. Spiro (Eds.), *Cognition, education, and multimedia* (pp. 163–205). Hillsdale, NJ: Erlbaum.

Stevens, J. (1996). *Applied multivariate statistics for the social sciences* (3rd ed.). Mahwah, NJ: Erlbaum.

Wade, S. E. (in press). *Preparing teachers for inclusive education: Case pedagogies and curricula for teacher educators*. Mahwah, NJ: Erlbaum.

Weinstein, C. E., Goetz, E. T., & Alexander, P. A. (Eds.). (1988). *Learning and study strategies: Issues in assessment, instruction, and evaluation*. San Diego, CA: Academic Press.

Weinstein, C. E., & Mayer, R. E. (1986). The teaching of learning strategies. In M. C. Wittrock (Ed.), *Handbook of research on teaching* (3rd ed., pp. 315–327). New York: Macmillan.

Yore, L. D. (1991). Secondary science teachers' attitudes toward and beliefs about reading and science textbooks. *Journal of Research in Science Teaching, 28,* 55–72.

431

Discussion

The discussion of Alexander's paper started with questions about the stability and generality of the clusters of learners she identified. Further discussion focused on more general discrepancies between the student and teacher perspectives on the purpose of education and on the importance of knowledge acquisition in education.

Dr. Ackerman: I have a qualitative question about these clusters and as it pertains to the developmental process. Do you expect the students to change what cluster they are in over time, or do you think this is a style of learner that you have?

Dr. Alexander: That's the question I want to know, and I think that is the one to answer next. Let me answer it by first telling you something I've done. I've started out by asking students what they think should change as a result of their own schooling. "Undergraduates, what do you think should happen to you as a result of schooling?" What they report is very little.

Dr. Ackerman: And it is true for them; right?

Dr. Alexander: But it is true. But I'd ask the teachers or people who are practicing individuals what they think education or the classroom experience does to the students, and they say it "markedly changes them." So we are actually in an interesting epistemological conflict here because I think students don't change a lot... I don't even know that they expect to change. I think part of it is that the students don't necessarily go through our schooling experience with the notion of garnering a principled body of knowledge or suddenly becoming deeply interested in it. I think they go through a lot of the schooling process to get through it, so to speak.

But back to what I believe because I'm the teacher. I believe that I should be able to change my students. Part of it is when students are functioning within an acclimated domain, when they're first exposed to something, like educational psychology, they don't have any idea what the subject is. My hope is, if nothing else, I can through a combination of both situational and personally relevant information spark some of them to define some reason to become interested beyond the grades. I think a lot of it is they're so concerned with getting grades, to score so well that the knowledge becomes almost a secondary notion to them along the way.

Dr. Stanovich: I'm following up on that. I mean you mentioned in answering Phil the issue of epistemological orientation. Have you ever given these people anything like Marlene Schommer's instrument...

Dr. Alexander: I don't like Marlene's measure for what we are doing. I find it too narrow in its view of epistemological beliefs.

Dr. Stanovich: Or anybody else's then?

Dr. Alexander: Yes. Actually, we're developing one now. I do ask them a series of epistemological questions about what they think about knowledge and the role of education. I think it's important to ask questions about what people think about *knowledge* in academic settings. But I think epistemological frameworks are much broader than that. What they value, what matters to them.

Eric Rolfhus and I had a great talk the other day about how do personal interests even develop. And I think when you talk about issues like value systems, I think that plays into what people are drawn to, as interests. Along with this, somebody said this morning you tend to be drawn to things you look good in, or you may do well in. I think that's part of it. But I do believe epistemological frameworks is an area that must be looked at. And the instrumentation out there to look at them is not very good at this point.

Dr. Hunt: What about simply demographic variables? How many of them are working their way through school? How many are in fraternities and sororities? I'm kind of a fan of Steinberg's belief that the issue is not the person, it's the competing demands on them, say in high school.

Dr. Alexander: Well, I was going to say in the fifth grade, the third graders, and fourth graders that we've studied, no. But as they go up, the competing issues become big in their lives, and one of the things again to try to get it. These notions go back to what Keith Stanovich was saying. I mean, we asked them general questions like, "What is it you're striving for?" "Why are you in school?" "What does education mean to you?" Part of what you get is not exactly what you're talking about in a way. But what they're in it for is social. They are not in it for the education per se. They'll say this very honestly (about 80% of them). It's for a profession that brings them money. They don't even care if they're interested in it. How does that translate? It means they spend a lot of time — at the three institutions where we gathered these data, in much more social ventures than in academic pursuits.

Dr. Hunt: I would expect that your medical students didn't. Anybody who works with them knows that serious medical students are the most incredibly focused individuals...

Dr. Alexander: They're premed students, and it was a preparatory course for minority students. What factor that may have held, I'm not sure. But you could see they did well. I mean they're the ones who demonstrated the highest levels of interest and knowledge. So I think you're absolutely right. I knew when I paid for my undergraduate schooling that it mattered a lot to me. I was not very happy when I found a professor wasn't giving me what I wanted from that situation. But most of the students — I'm not sure why — if you ask them why they're there, it's not for knowledge. It's not for academics. They'll tell you that very openly.

Dr. Pisoni: There's a book by Murray Sperber. He had one book on college sports, but recently he's published another book on what he calls the college experience. And 50% of the kids that are in Big Ten schools, according to his research, are there for the college experience. Another 20% are there to get a job. That's all they go to college for.

Dr. Alexander: Yes, but when they translate getting a job and my students tell me about this book, it's getting the degree, because I'm going to learn what I need to learn on the job. Is it similar to that? Is it the degree?

Dr. Pisoni: Yes, get the degree to get a job. And then the interesting thing is that only 10% of these kids are actually really interested in the intellectual aspect of college. His point is, of course, that the universities are not oriented toward the elitist professors who think that the most important thing is studying individual differences or Sternberg's scanning or automatic control. That's a small minority of what college is really all about. It's the sororities and fraternities and Golden Gopher Basketball and Bobby Knight and that kind of stuff.

Dr. Alexander: Oh, that's true. But let me tell you what's even more perplexing. We asked elementary school teachers what they thought the purpose of education was. And knowledge or building knowledge was one of the lower, if mentioned, factors. It was nurturing. So at what point does the realization come on board — and maybe it never does — that maybe what schools are about is building people to be able to have principled bodies of knowledge that they can use in some other point in their life. It seems to me that the fact that knowledge was a low ranked, or a low stated issue, even among elementary school teachers, worries me. It perplexes me in part.

Dr. Wittmann: Yes. I wondered about that interesting factor, the low lows. I thought about where might they be behind, and I suggest they might be behind on emotional intelligence. What I found very interesting is whether we have the right methodology to map what happens with changes in classes and things like that? I'm not very well prepared to answer such a question.

Dr. Alexander: You mean from a moral sense...

Dr. Wittmann: Just from a psychometric standpoint. What does it mean to implement changes in class teaching and things like that? And the other point is, did you think about that aptitude–treatment interaction paradigm? Take for example the cluster [of students] which already has high knowledge, they should not go to your lecture.

Dr. Alexander: Except that when I say "high knowledge," I kept saying it's relative. This is high introductory knowledge, which is not high against our knowledge base by any stretch.

Dr. Wittmann: You were the teacher. Maybe the question is a little bit embarrassing. What about the quality of teaching?

Dr. Alexander: Oh, it's great.

Dr. Wittmann: How would you change your teaching with that knowledge of the clusters you now have?

Dr. Alexander: I think what I would do, if I could do some preidentification, I would at least have some sense of the students who came in with some base of knowledge and draw them in more. I would use their knowledge as a way to help to stimulate perhaps. That could be one of them. But let me go back to your other point about how would I do it. Right now I'm struggling with that issue. If I do the 5-year study, I'm going to have to do cases for sure. I want them in broad-base testing. But within that I want to focus down while I have the big picture, I want to do some focused studies as well.

Dr. Widaman: It was interesting that you came up with three clusters at one point in time and four in the other. Did you look at how stable people were across time?

Dr. Alexander: Yes, I did. Actually, I tracked every one of them. The learning-oriented people by far were the most stable. The ones who came in with that goal orientation were those that seemed to be driven for most part to do what they needed to do.

Dr. Widaman: This was by and large the same individuals in the cluster at Time 1 and Time 2?

Dr. Alexander: Yes, exactly. As I said, the other pattern was that in tracking them, that those who initially were in the low profile typically went to one of the two lower rungs. They either became the effortful processors or they became the non-strategic readers. So yes, we did that. We followed them along.

Dr. Widaman: The second question has to do with the outcomes. Did you have any measures of course outcomes?

Dr. Alexander: Yes, but — you know, can I tell you — and I'm going to say this quietly, but there's not much variability in grades in introductory courses these days. With grade inflation, it doesn't do much. It just doesn't pan out very well. I'm sorry that I had to say that, but it's true.

Dr. Widaman: Are your tests too easy?

Dr. Alexander: I'm just too good of a teacher.

Dr. Widaman: There was a professor at my university who didn't care for teaching evaluations. So what he did was in the first day of class he gave all the students the final exam, and then at the end of the course he gave them the final exam again, and he turned those into the faculty committee saying here are my teaching evaluations. Look at the changes of scores. You give the final exam the first day of class, the final exam the last day of class, and there are huge increases. I must be doing something. What I was wondering was, even if you only have the posttest, the grades in the class, scores on the set of tests across the course, did you have those there?

Dr. Alexander: That's what the pretest and posttest were. They took that test the first day of class, and I used it to frame the instruction. They took the same test. That's what they took. That was their final exam.

Dr. Ackerman: One of the things I really like about your orientation — and I don't mean to put words in your mouth at this point — but it seems to me that what you're arguing for is the notion of education as building knowledge and building content as opposed to building abilities.

Dr. Alexander: And interest.

Dr. Ackerman: In a sense that we're not developing critical problem-solving skills, but, instead focusing on knowledge and what it is that people are learning as far as content is concerned. But doesn't that really put you at odds with teachers. . .

Dr. Alexander: With a lot of the community?

Dr. Ackerman: Yes.

Dr. Alexander: Yes. And I would say you and I share something similar in that.

What I will tell you is the most powerful linkage to even interest and to strategies is the knowledge base. The knowledge base is the doorway. So the attempts that are going on right now in a lot of the public school arena and with a lot of our colleagues, this notion that you build the interest or you build problem-solving strategies isolated from knowledge — makes no sense to me whatsoever in the face of the kind of data pattern we get. The knowledge is a key, it is a key to competence.

19

Traits and Knowledge as Determinants of Learning and Individual Differences: Putting It All Together

PHILLIP L. ACKERMAN

There is an old joke about the different parts of the body getting into an argument about which is the most important part. For readers who have not heard the joke, I will skip the scatological details. However, this book is an attempt to avoid the historical parallel in the field of learning and individual-differences research. That is, does process, traits, or content have primacy in determining individual differences in learning? In case readers think that this is hyperbole, I provide an example from experimental psychology. The Stroop effect (Stroop, 1935) is a phenomenon that has had enduring interest to many psychological researchers.[1] At various times in this century, the work has been devoted to finding the process determinants of performance or trait determinants of performance. Of the hundreds of investigations of the Stroop effect, few studies have been conducted that grappled with the obvious dominant determinant of the conflict: *literacy* in (or knowledge of) the language of the words in the conflict condition. That is, if the participant cannot make sense of the letters or words, it is obvious that there will be little or no conflict effect in the color–word condition. Thus, content — or the participant's language knowledge and reading skill — critically determines how the task is performed (e.g., see MacLeod, 1991). In this case, content is the most important determinant of performance; it is only the fact that the typical experimental study of the Stroop effect includes only literate participants that obscures this obvious point.

---

[1]The Stroop effect is obtained by subtracting the speed of naming the colors of a set of colored Xs on a page from the time to name the colors of a set of color words on a page (where the color words are printed in colored ink that is incompatible with the words).

Background

The history of intelligence assessment has had some interesting turns about such issues, with *process* having primacy in the late 1800s (e.g., Galton and James McKeen Cattell) and *traits* having primacy from the 1910s to the mid-1970s (e.g., Terman, Thurstone). However, processes had a rediscovery through the context of information processing and cognitive psychology in the 1970s to the 1990s (e.g., Hunt, Sternberg, etc.). I will leave it to others to decide whether research on process determinants of learning and individual differences is waxing or waning.

Content (or knowledge), however, has traditionally had a "poor cousin" relationship with the traditional approaches to abilities and individual differences (at least outside of educational psychology, where "knowledge tests" are primarily referred to as "achievement tests"). Although knowledge is both explicitly incorporated into other assessments of some abilities (e.g., verbal ability, general information) and implicitly incorporated into assessments of ability (e.g., nearly all group tests of abilities require reading skills), there has been a tendency for many investigators to attempt to limit the inclusion of knowledge into the assessment of individual differences in abilities. One source of such attempts comes from the traditional process approach of experimental (now called *cognitive*) psychology, where the elusive search continues for the fundamental building blocks for determining individual differences in intelligence (e.g., simple reaction time, inspection time, neural conduction speed, etc.). From the trait side of the equation, attempts to eliminate knowledge from consideration of the traitlike aspects of intelligence have come from investigators who have embraced so-called "fluid intelligence tests" (e.g., abstract reasoning tests such as Raven's Progressive Matrices or the Culture-Fair Intelligence Test).

When I first started investigating learning and individual differences, I attempted to bridge the first two of these determinants, namely processes and traits. Specifically, I was interested in predicting performance on tasks that were designated as either requiring controlled information processing or tasks that allowed automatic information processing to develop after substantial task practice (e.g., see Ackerman, 1984, 1986). Because controlled processing was thought to be used when a participant deals with novelty or learns and unlearns information, it seemed clear to me that the logical prediction was that individual differences in controlled information processing were determined by individual differences in *fluid intelligence* (Gf).[2] Conversely, automatic processing was thought to be attained only after a participant had learned a set of invariant stimulus–response associations. Therefore, practiced performance on a consistent task should have been well predicted by individual differences in *crystallized intelligence* (Gc).

Although all these predictions sounded reasonable to me before the study was completed, the data that were obtained told a story that was, in many ways, less than satisfying for three reasons:

1. It was difficult to obtain a good assessment of Gc in a sample of high school seniors and college students based on common standardized ability tests (such

---

[2]This is where "fluid" intelligence was generally concordant with the operational descriptions provided by Cattell and Horn (Horn, 1965, 1968; Horn & Cattell, 1966). I was (and am still) agnostic about Cattell and Horn's claims about the "physiological" basis for fluid intelligence.

438

as those found in the Educational Testing Service's Kit of Factor-Referenced Cognitive Tests, namely Vocabulary, Controlled Associations, and Verbal Analogies). I return to this point later.

2. When there was underlying common "content" for two criterion tasks (such as two verbal information-processing tasks or two spatial information-processing tasks), individual differences in content ability traits (e.g., verbal, spatial ability) turned out to be *more* influential in predicting performance across learning trials than process-oriented measures. That is, learners did not appear to have "controlled processing abilities" or "automatic processing abilities." When there is some dominant content for the task, performance tends more to depend on the respective content ability, such as spatial, verbal, or numerical abilities.

3. Although this dawned on me much later, it appears that the whole information-processing approach to individual differences in learning may be founded on a poor strategic judgment (one that has its counterpart in the abstract reasoning movement in intelligence theory and research). That is, this whole approach to understanding learning and individual differences was predicated on a narrow analysis of information-processing tasks that are either devoid of cultural material or made up of extremely common stimuli, so that nearly all participants are familiar with them.

The problem with linking the information-processing approach to learning and individual-differences phenomena (especially for adults) is that it simply is the wrong level of analysis for the applied task at hand. An engineer does not worry about quantum physics when there is a bridge to be built, and a psychologist, by analogy, should not be concerned about individual differences in simple reaction time when trying to teach a student about science, math, literature, history, or even how to drive a truck or fly a plane. It turns out that individual differences in simple information-processing tasks provide relatively poorer predictions of learning task performance when the task to be learned requires knowledge, effort, and persistence over time.

It may be that process theorists and researchers have identified the fundamental building blocks for individual differences in abilities, which in turn determine individual differences in learning (just like the physicists have worked out the details on quarks and charm). My point is that both the engineer and the applied psychologist can pretty well be advised to ignore the lowest level information in nearly all applied systems.

Furthermore, tasks that depend only on extremely common stimuli are similarly poorer predictors of real-world learning task performance, most simply because such tasks obscure the substantial effects that individual differences in *knowledge* have on learning and performance. Such a consideration suggests that the most promising source of uncharted territory for understanding and predicting individual differences in learning is in the domain of the knowledge that the learners bring to the learning environment to begin with.

Process, Traits, and Knowledge

Trying to conceptualize the contrasts among process, traits, and content (knowledge) is a little difficult, especially across predictor and criterion spaces. Figure 19.1 is an

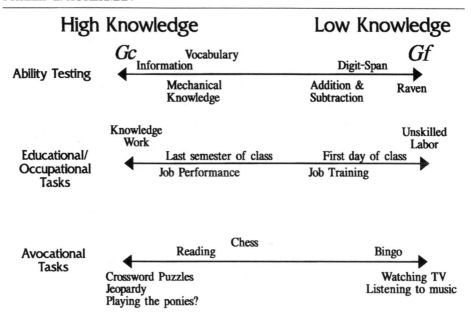

Figure 19.1. High knowledge and low knowledge across three different domains: Ability testing, educational/occupational tasks, and avocational tasks.

illustration of three parallel continua that may help illuminate the current conceptualization. The figure shows three constructs: assessment, educational and occupational tasks, and avocational tasks. For each construct, the line indicates a continuum between "low knowledge" and "high knowledge."

For assessment, one can consider both "process" assessments and "trait" assessments. Low-knowledge process measures include simple reaction time, memory tests with common words, digit span, and so on. Such assessments depend on either highly familiar or highly simple stimuli for presentation. Low-knowledge trait measures generally include abstract reasoning tests (e.g., the ever-popular Raven's Progressive Matrices) or measures that have highly familiar stimuli (e.g., a simple computational arithmetic test). In the past 20 years of research, there has been an empirical wave of new and interesting measures of both processes and traits that have reduced-knowledge demands. However, the information-processing approach to individual differences in learning has neglected high-knowledge tasks (especially those studies that incorporate a cognitive-correlates research methodology). Although there are numerous ability measures that demand high knowledge, there is uncertainty in the literature about whether high-knowledge tests are assessments of traits per se or assessments of attainment or skills. Calling a high-knowledge test an "achievement test," though, perhaps obscures the traitlike status of such person characteristics. Indeed, if Hebb (1942, 1949), Cattell (1943, 1957, 1971/1987), and others are correct, knowledge-based traits are likely to have greater permanence across the adult life span than low-knowledge-based traits, such as speeded reasoning or working memory capacity.

Parallel to the assessment instruments are low-knowledge/high-knowledge dimensions for learning and performance on educational and occupational tasks and avocational tasks. Drawing on these parallels, one sees that both the first day of class and the first day on the job are situations in which the learner has relatively low knowledge. As such, it is reasonable to consider Gf, memory, and abstract reasoning assessments as providing good measures for predicting learning and performance (as indeed they do; see the discussion by Ackerman, 1994, and data from Humphreys & Taber, 1973). It similarly follows that, after training or on-the-job experience, relevant assessments of high-knowledge traits will provide a better prediction of job or task performance (e.g., see Ackerman, 1994). Although this follows from the analysis, it remains to be seen how valid this prediction is. Several analyses from diverse places support this assertion, but there are too few empirical investigations that have assessed knowledge beyond a limited sampling of Gc or a test of specific job knowledge. Some of the work that my colleague Eric Rolfhus and I have been doing will yield a test of these assertions, but this is a long-range work in progress.

Ironically, if the world is actually organized as it is conceptualized in Figure 19.1, Gf measures will be most important in predicting individual differences in learning and performance in highly complex (but novel) situations *and* in situations in which knowledge simply has a very small role in performance (e.g., performance in un-skilled tasks). By contrast, Gf will have an attenuated prediction of performance when long investments of knowledge acquisition are needed to achieve job or task skills. Outside the educational and occupational systems, an individual's propensity to engage in low-knowledge hobbies or avocational activities may be a result of low Gf or a lack of investment in obtaining the knowledge necessary to successfully engage in any high-knowledge activities such as crossword puzzles, bridge or chess, and so on.

Content, Knowledge, and Gc

The analysis provided earlier, along with a series of empirical studies (e.g., Acker-man, 1988, 1992; Ackerman & Kanfer, 1993), seem to indicate that if the goal is to predict the early acquisition of real-world knowledge or skills, especially when researchers are working with novice learners, the focus should be on obtaining predictors from the Gf/process side of the continuum. By now, researchers are fa-miliar with the utility of using such measures in a wide range of these kinds of situations (e.g., see Schmidt & Hunter, 1993; Stauffer, Ree, & Carretta, 1996). However, if researchers are interested in predicting performance after training, and after time on the job, Gf and process measures simply are not the optimal predictors. Instead, researchers need to focus on content, knowledge, and Gc.

Before continuing, I want to return to that observation from my early attempts to use Gc to predict individual differences in automatized information-processing per-formance. Notwithstanding the low-knowledge task that I was trying to predict (a word category search task with high-frequency exemplars), the bottom line was that the traditional measures of Gc did not adequately sample the construct[3] and, as such, did not meet the potential of Gc/trait predictions of learning and performance.

The reason for the inadequacy of traditional Gc measures is that, as Cattell (1971/1987) suggested, Gc becomes highly specialized for individuals as they make the transition from a common school curriculum (usually in secondary school) to col-

---

[3]That is, especially in a sample of participants who are relatively homogeneous in age (in contrast to Horn's, 1965, empirical investigation, in which the participant ages ranged from 14 to 61 years).

lege or university education or to occupational and avocational adult experiences. Specifically, Cattell suggested that for adults, one had a choice between assessing Gc by constructing as many tests as there are kinds of knowledge or by sampling "historical" Gc, namely what one learned in high school, when the curriculum was nearly universal. Fundamentally, this is the kind of justification used for Graduate Record Examinations to focus on algebra and geometry when testing college students, for the Wechsler Adult Intelligence Scale to ask about common cultural knowledge, and so on. The creators of intelligence and broad aptitude tests for adults have attempted to eliminate occupationally-specific questions in favor of the kind of information that one learns in high school or through broad cultural exposure, even though that specific occupational and avocational knowledge may represent a far greater portion of what individuals bring to a job or a hobby than does what they learned in high school.

The solution to this problem of assessing adult Gc turns out to be difficult: It involves developing a large number of knowledge measures (to include the kinds of knowledge that are not common to the entire dominant culture but are present in varying degrees for different individuals) that allow for the development of a knowledge structure profile for each individual. However, I am getting ahead of myself. Below is one attempt to put many of the insights gained from investigating processes and traits into a comprehensive approach for adult intellect.

Putting It All Together: A Theory of Adult Intellect and Development

To encompass the wide range of literature on the relations among personality, interests, and intellectual development, I created an integrated theoretical representation of adult intelligence (Ackerman, 1996). The proposed theory draws heavily on the general framework of Cattell's investment theory (Cattell 1971/1987) but provides several departures. To capture the four major components of this theory, it is called *PPIK*, for intelligence as Process, Personality, Interests, and intelligence as Knowledge. The theory is illustrated in Figure 19.2 (although it shows only academic knowledge domains) and has the following properties:

- General intelligence (g) is represented as two broad factors (i.e., process and knowledge), rather than Gf and Gc (from Cattell, 1971/1987), but it is closer to Hebb's (1949) notions of Intelligence A (physiological) and Intelligence B (educational, cultural).
- To the degree possible, as revealed by meta-analysis and recent research, explicit representation is provided for a small set of personality factors and interest factors as related to intelligence and adult intellectual development (Ackerman, 1996; Ackerman & Heggestad, 1997; Rolfhus & Ackerman, 1996).
- There is representation of adult intellectual knowledge and skill as "aptitude complexes" (after Snow, 1989), for which different individuals may demonstrate little overlap (e.g., the knowledge structures of a physicist may have little in common with the knowledge structures of a historian).

The core PPIK components of adult intellect are described in turn.

442

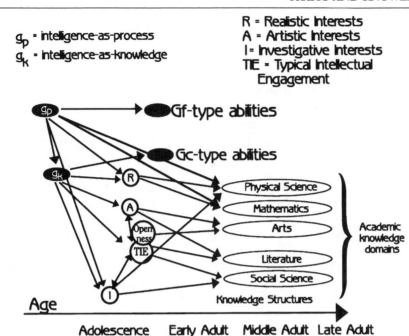

Figure 19.2. Illustration of the PPIK theory, outlining the influences of intelligence as Process, Personality, Interests, and intelligence as Knowledge during adult development, covering academic and occupational knowledge. Solid arrows represent correlational influences (supported by significant correlations from the data collected by Rolfhus & Ackerman, 1996). Gp = intelligence as process; Gk = intelligence as knowledge; Gf = Cattell's fluid intelligence; Gc = Cattell's crystallized intelligence; R = realistic interests; I = investigative interests; TIE = typical intellectual engagement. From "A Theory of Adult Intellectual Development: Process, Personality, Interests, and Knowledge," by P. L. Ackerman, 1996, *Intelligence*, 22, p. 238. Copyright 1996 by Ablex Publishing. Reprinted with permission.

1. *Intelligence as process.* There is an inherent danger in segregating process from knowledge, just as has been demonstrated in the attempts by Cattell and his followers to separate Gf from Gc. That is, for Cattell's theory, some tests will load on Gf in one sample (e.g., children) but load on Gc in another sample (e.g., adults). Similarly, it is impossible to eliminate all content from ability tests. That is, even familiarity with the testing environment (see Detterman & Andrist, 1990) or practice on simple reaction time tasks (Ackerman, 1990) results in changes in correlations between simple, Gf-type tests and a general factor of intelligence.

Nonetheless, when one integrates the physiological literature (e.g., Hebb, 1949) and the more recent information-processing literature, such as the componential work by Sternberg (1977, 1985b; Sternberg & Berg, 1987) and the empirical work on age-related differences in perception and memory (e.g., Rogers, Fisk, & Hertzog, 1994), it is clear that the speeded aspects of intelligence that decline during normal adult development (at least up to age 65 or so) are well encompassed within a "process" categorization. These information-processing components include reasoning, memory span (short-term, or working memory), perceptual speed, and spatial rotation (for an extensive review, see Carroll, 1993; also see Baltes & Schaie,

1976; Horn & Donaldson, 1976; Salthouse, 1996; Schaie, 1970, 1974). When a cognitive-components approach (Sternberg, 1985a) is taken to intelligence tests, the information-processing components (as opposed to the content, or knowledge components) appear to be those that show peak performance at young adult ages.

Whether process components of intelligence are more or less influential in the acquisition and retention of new knowledge and skills for adults remains to be demonstrated. The cognitive science literature is rife with examples of how knowledge structures appear to be more important to development of skilled memory than process components (e.g., see Chase & Ericsson's, 1981, study of skilled memory span; Chase & Simon's, 1973, study for chess; and Charness's, 1987, study for bridge, etc.). Thus, a direct causal link from intelligence as process to adult intelligence as knowledge is tentative, and it requires additional empirical evaluation.

2. *Personality.*   The personality domains that relate to intelligence appear to be of two types, as related to process and content, respectively. Intelligence as process correlates weakly with most broad personality factors, except for those that are associated with neuroticism and test anxiety. Another major exception to this generalization is the meta-analytic finding by Signorella and Jamison (1986) that individual differences in masculinity–femininity show significant correlations with math and spatial content abilities.

For intelligence as knowledge, two related personality factors appear to be instrumental (Rolfhus & Ackerman, 1996). The first is the personality trait of openness (also called intellectence, intelligence, culture, etc.), and the second is typical intellectual engagement (TIE; Ackerman & Goff, 1994; Goff & Ackerman, 1992; Rocklin, 1994). The construct of intelligence as typical performance was proposed by Ackerman (1994) to develop a parallel ability construction to the maximal versus typical distinction Cronbach established for ability versus personality measures. That is, Ackerman suggested that one reason why intelligence tests do not highly correlate with measures of advanced academic performance or occupational performance is that intelligence is measured within a "maximal" paradigm and that long-term academic and occupational performance takes place in a "typical" environment.

The theory states that a measure of intelligence as typical performance would be more highly associated with crystallized abilities (knowledge), whereas intelligence as maximal performance would be more highly related to fluid abilities (process). The theory has been generally supported via a self-report measure (for details, see Goff & Ackerman, 1992). Indeed, additional data and reviews show that both openness and TIE are related to intelligence (Ackerman, Kanfer, & Goff, 1995), especially in the verbal and crystallized ability domain (see also Ackerman & Goff, 1994; Rocklin, 1994). Such traits have been shown to be generally uncorrelated with intelligence-as-process measures.

3. *Interests.*   Using a framework based on Holland's (1959, 1973) hexagonal model of vocational interests (the six interest themes are realistic, artistic, investigative, social, enterprising, and conventional; see Holland, 1973), Ackerman and Heggestad (1997) reviewed the literature that evaluates correlations between interests and intellectual abilities. From this review, and from our own investigations, we identified three domains of interests that are linked to intelligence (and to the personality factors that are also related to intelligence): realistic, investigative, and artistic interests. According to Holland (1959, 1973), individuals who express realistic interests (also called *motoric interests*) "enjoy activities requiring physical strength,

aggressive action, motor coordination and skill" (Holland, 1959, p. 36). Individuals expressing investigative interest (also called *intellectual interests*) are "task-oriented people who generally prefer to 'think through,' rather than 'act out,' problems. They have marked needs to organize and understand the world" (p. 36). Individuals who express artistic interests (also called *esthetic interests*) "prefer indirect relations with others. They prefer dealing with environmental problems through self expression in artistic media.... They resemble persons with an intellectual orientation in their intraceptiveness and lack of sociability" (p. 37).

From the review and empirical research (e.g., Rolfhus & Ackerman, 1996, see also Lowman, Williams, & Leeman, 1985), one can see that the degree of realistic and investigative interests shows substantial correlations with intelligence-as-process factors (e.g., reasoning, math, spatial) as well as substantial correlations with abilities that are close to the process–knowledge boundary (e.g., mechanical knowledge). Individual differences in artistic interests are the most closely aligned with intelligence as knowledge (e.g., verbal and crystallized abilities), but investigative interests also show substantial correlations with verbal and crystallized abilities.

Although some studies have shown positive correlations between conventional interests and clerical and perceptual speed abilities, the associations are generally small, and leaving them out of the equation allows one to focus on the major influences across domains.

4. *Intelligence as knowledge.* The conceptualization of intelligence as knowledge has its roots in the early developments of modern intelligence testing. Even the Binet–Simon tests include explicit knowledge tests (e.g., Information). The basis for including intelligence as knowledge as a central ingredient of adult intellect is scattered but impressive. It comes from the high predictive validities of the Advanced/Subject tests of the Graduate Record Examinations for predicting graduate school and professional success (e.g., see Willingham, 1974), from the importance of job knowledge in predicting job performance (Hunter, 1983), and from the documentation of the sources of expert–novice differences pertaining mainly to knowledge structures and their acquisition (e.g., Alexander, Kulikowich, & Schulze, 1994; Baldwin, Peleg-Bruckner, & McClintock, 1985; Chi, Glaser, & Rees, 1982). The nature of intelligence as knowledge matches the first description of Gc provided by Cattell (1987) in his investment theory (but is much broader than common assessment techniques for Gc). That is, there are probably as many domains of knowledge as there are occupations (and nonoccupational pursuits as well). A test of intellect as knowledge must be contextual (just as was proposed by Colvin, cited in Whipple, 1922), in that any one individual's pursuit of knowledge may be idiosyncratic.

There are, for most intents and purposes, a finite and generally workable number of domains that would require assessment for all but specific occupational knowledge held by members of particular specializations. That is, knowledge about various humanities and the arts, the sciences, and so on has some common elements across occupational domains. Most physicists, psychologists, accountants, and so on, have some core knowledge that is common to the broad professions, and knowledge outside these domains need not be probed as deeply as knowledge within the profession. To get a first-order representation of an adult's intelligence as knowledge, one would have to provide for two types of tests: a deep test of professional knowledge and a broad array of more shallow tests outside the profession.

The pattern of development among different aspects of intelligence is loosely

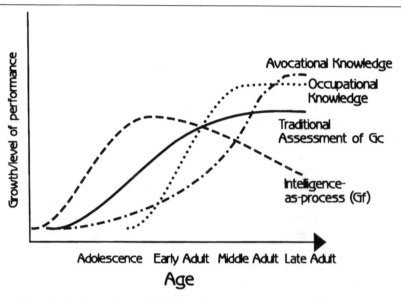

Figure 19.3. Hypothetical growth level of performance curves across the adult life span for intelligence as process, traditional measures of crystallized intelligence (Gc), occupational knowledge, and avocational knowledge. (Intelligence as process [Gf] and Gc are modeled after Horn [1965].) From "A Theory of Adult Intellectual Development: Process, Personality, Interests, and Knowledge," by P. L. Ackerman, 1996, *Intelligence*, 22, p. 242. Copyright 1996 by Ablex Publishing. Reprinted with permission.

illustrated in Figure 19.3. Using Horn's (1965) model of the development of Gf to represent intelligence as process, and his model of the development of Gc to provide a comparison against other knowledge domains, estimates of average occupational knowledge level (which develops mostly in early adulthood and is presumed to have diminishing returns in middle age) have been added, along with avocational knowledge (e.g., current events, hobbies), which is presumed to continue in growth up to late adulthood. The hypothesized growth curves are qualitative but are supported by data from the Terman Study of the Gifted (Holahan & Sears, with Cronbach, 1995). Those authors reported that the pursuit of avocational activities (e.g., intellectual [reading nonfiction books], cultural [playing a musical instrument], social [community service], active recreation [traveling], and passive recreation [reading newspapers]) show both substantial continuity from middle adulthood on to late adulthood, and persistence into late ages (70+). By contrast, occupational knowledge for most individuals is presumed to level off as they move through a transition from full-time work to retirement.

On the basis of the proposal that intelligence as knowledge is generally monotonically increasing throughout most of adulthood, it is indeed possible to arrive at an approach to assessing adult intellect that is age or experience based, much as the Binet–Simon scales are age based on content. Also, knowledge scales may be directly content referenced. Rather than using normative scores, ratio scales of knowledge, or at least interval scales with meaningful zero points, which correspond to a complete lack of knowledge about a domain, can be derived. Such a feature removes one large impediment to evaluating interindividual and intraindividual differences in adult intellect.

Some Early Results

Eric Rolfhus and I have recently conducted a pilot "proof-of-concept" study of adult knowledge structures, ability, and nonability traits (Ackerman & Rolfhus, 1998a, 1998b; Rolfhus, 1998; Rolfhus & Ackerman, 1998). For the first time, we used a series of objective knowledge tests in evaluating the PPIK theory. I now provide a brief description of the design and preliminary analysis of the results.

Ability battery. Tests were selected to assess the following abilities or factors. For verbal and verbal reasoning, we used the Verbal Analogies, Controlled Associations, and Extended Range Vocabulary Test. For math and numerical problem solving, we used Math Knowledge, Problem Solving, and Number Series. For spatial abilities, we used Paper Folding, the Verbal Test of Spatial Abilities, and Spatial Orientation. For mechanical knowledge, we used the Mechanical Knowledge test.

Self-report battery. To measure personality, we used the 60-item inventory (the NEO Five-Factor Inventory) to assess five traits: neuroticism, extraversion, openness, conscientiousness, and agreeableness. Additional measures of personality traits were also used. To assess interests, we used six interest themes identified by Holland (1973; 90 items from the Unisex Edition of the ACT Interest Inventory [ACT = American College Testing]): realistic, investigative, artistic, social, enterprising, and conventional. Self-concepts for competencies and aptitudes in several specific areas were assessed with a 30-item self-report questionnaire. For self-ratings of ability, a 21-item questionnaire was used. Participants were instructed to respond with a self-evaluation relative to other persons their age. Participants also completed a biographical questionnaire (not discussed here). Twenty tests of knowledge were constructed, sampling from six broad taxonomic categories: natural, physical sciences, and statistics (astronomy, biology, chemistry, physics, and statistics); social sciences and law/business (business/management, economics, geography, law, and psychology); history and western or American civilization (American government, American history, and western civilization); arts and literature (American literature, art, music, and world literature); and technology and tools (electronics, technology, tools/shop).

Participants. Two samples of participants were drawn for this study. One sample ("younger") was sampled from a large undergraduate introductory psychology course at the University of Minnesota (mean age = 19 years, SD = 1.2). The second sample ("older") was drawn from the larger university community. The participants were required to be at least 30 years of age and younger than 60 years of age and to be either a university student or graduate (mean age = 40 years, SD = 7.2). The results were based on 141 younger participants and 135 older participants. (This is admittedly a sample of convenience; no efforts were made to match younger and older age groups on education, socioeconomic status, or any other variable. Tests were conducted to assess the comparability of the 30- to 59-year-old age group on education and gender [by age decade: 30s, 40s, and 50s]. No significant differences for education or gender were found.)

447

Abilities. The first set of results is a standard cross-sectional comparison between the older and younger adults, done to evaluate the general representativeness of the samples. Based on the literature, our a priori expectations were that the older group would show higher scores on the verbal tests and equivalent or lower scores on the math and spatial tests. Two sets of comparisons were computed: mean differences between the younger and older groups and within-groups correlations between test scores and chronological age for the older participants. These results are shown in Table 19.1.

Clearly, the older sample performed substantially better than the younger sample on the verbal ability tests and the Mechanical Knowledge test, less well on the numerical ability tests (except for the word-problem test), and mixed on the spatial ability tests. Moreover, significant negative age correlations were found for the spatial ability tests and two of the numerical ability tests for the 30- to 59-year-old group. Such results suggest that these groups are not unusual with respect to the kinds of cross-sectional comparisons that are found in the ability and aging literature.

Knowledge scales. The next set of preliminary results, shown in Table 19.2, is particularly illuminating and further indicates the promise of the research program. In reviewing Table 19.2, it is important to refer back to Table 19.1, which shows that the older adult group, although performing better than the younger group on verbal abilities, performed more poorly on the numerical abilities, as would be expected. However, in all but 2 of the 20 tested knowledge domains shown in Table 19.2 (chemistry and statistics), the older adult group performed significantly better than the younger adult group. In addition, only one of the tests showed a significant correlation with age for the older group (tools/shop showed an increase with age). Group differences, with the areas of greatest advantage to the older group, are as follows:

1. Arts and literature mean z-score difference = 1.42 SD units
2. Technology and tools mean z-score difference = 1.04 SD units
3. History and western/American civilization mean z-score difference = 0.99 SD units
4. Social sciences and law/business mean z-score difference = 0.97 SD units
5. Natural, physical sciences, and statistics mean z-score difference = 0.35 SD units

These results provide additional support for the theory, in that the older adult group had higher mean performance in all of the knowledge categories that were assessed, although the largest differences between older–younger groups were found in the arts and literature domain, and the smallest differences in knowledge were on the natural and physical sciences. One potential interpretation here is that the older adult sample excelled in domains that are traditionally "electives" in post-secondary curricula and that the younger sample came closest to staying even with the older adults on the physical science topics (e.g., chemistry and physics) that are more traditionally "required" high school and college courses. (Informal reflection would further support this point by suggesting that many fewer continuing-education students take courses in physics or chemistry than take courses in art or literature.)

TABLE 19.1 Ability Tests: Data for Older Group Age Correlations

Ability area and measure	Younger (18–27)		Older (30–59)		t (274)	Older (30–59) correlation with age
	M	SD	M	SD		
Verbal ability						
Verbal Analogies	26.76	5.71	32.68	5.58	8.71***	−.01
Controlled Associates	23.34	7.67	29.61	9.47	6.06****	−.01
Extended Range Vocabulary	15.29	6.70	31.62	7.58	18.98****	.15
Spatial ability						
Paper Folding	12.48	5.06	10.09	4.87	−4.01***	−.28**
Verbal Test of Spatial	11.52	4.33	12.08	4.90	1.01	−.19*
Spatial Orientation	7.28	3.85	7.21	3.83	−0.15	−.30**
Numerical ability						
Math Knowledge	17.45	6.31	9.69	5.69	−10.71***	−.21*
Problem Solving	4.34	2.27	4.56	2.19	0.83	−.11
Number Series	10.30	2.78	8.81	3.21	−4.10	−.18*
Mechanical knowledge						
Mechanical Knowledge	7.02	3.94	8.87	3.83	3.95***	.01

Note. ns = 141 (younger) and 135 (older). For the correlations, the degrees of freedom were 133.
*p < .05. **p < .01. ***p < .001.

TABLE 19.2 Knowledge Scales (Number Correct): Data for Older Group Age Correlations

Knowledge area	Younger (18–27)		Older (30–59)		t (274)	Older (30–59) correlation with age
	M	SD	M	SD		
Natural, physical sciences, and statistics						
Astronomy	16.47	10.12	19.49	12.82	2.00*	.17
Biology	16.32	10.92	22.75	12.63	4.44***	−.09
Chemistry	16.05	8.86	15.88	9.41	0.15	−.12
Physics	12.96	6.39	15.67	6.12	3.57***	−.06
Statistics	7.45	4.58	8.70	5.54	1.94	−.13
Social sciences and law business						
Business/management	13.35	7.59	23.67	9.26	10.12***	.00
Economics	18.17	13.43	27.78	14.18	5.72***	−.11
Geography	21.04	12.13	29.52	13.35	5.12***	−.06
Law	17.94	10.35	30.49	10.75	9.84***	−.06
Psychology	14.03	7.56	19.71	7.98	6.06***	.01
History and western/American civilization						
American government	24.41	13.54	39.05	14.02	8.73***	−.03
American history	39.33	20.12	58.94	24.00	6.84***	.03
Western civilization	23.04	12.59	34.10	16.21	6.24***	.04
Arts and literature						
American literature	34.25	14.40	55.41	17.12	11.09***	.11
Art	12.21	6.03	19.41	4.74	9.68***	−.09
Music	20.02	10.16	33.44	10.25	10.20***	.13
World literature	31.14	13.97	53.40	19.24	11.02***	.05
Technology and tools						
Electronics	10.61	5.90	18.16	7.46	8.58***	.14
Technology	19.05	10.99	30.68	12.58	7.37***	−.03
Tools/shop	16.29	6.16	20.98	7.40	5.55***	.19*

Note. The maximum sample sizes were 141 (younger) and 135 (older). The degrees of freedom for the correlation were 133.
*p < .05. ***p < .001.

Ability Correlates of Knowledge

To many researchers interested in adult intelligence, the most important results of this investigation will be captured in the associations between traditional ability factors and knowledge scale performance. Although a review of individual ability test–knowledge scale correlations is illuminating, an attempt has been made to provide a means toward summarizing the noteworthy associations between the battery of ability tests and the battery of knowledge scales. The first pass with these data included a hierarchical factor analysis of the ability tests (using the procedure described by Schmid & Leiman, 1957), so that an oblique first-order factor solution can be recast as an orthogonalized factor matrix of two orders (in this case, a general ability factor [g] that has substantial loadings across all three major ability factors [Verbal, Spatial, and Math]). With an estimation of the factors underlying the ability tests, factor loadings of the knowledge scales are estimated with Dwyer's (1937) extension procedure.[4] The hierarchical factor solutions and extended factor loadings for the knowledge scales are shown in Table 19.3 for the older group.

The Dwyer extension results show that, after accounting for a general ability factor (g), little common variance remained between the Math or Spatial Ability factors and knowledge scales. Art, electronics, and tools/shop had salient loadings on the Spatial Ability factor, and only art had a salient loading (negative) on the Math Ability factor. By contrast, many of the knowledge scales showed substantial positive loadings on the first-order Verbal Ability factor (which is the closest that traditional ability assessment methods come to assessing intelligence as knowledge in adults), as predicted by the PPIK theory. By and large, the largest loadings on the Verbal Ability factor come from knowledge scales in arts and literature and to a somewhat lesser extent history and western/American civilization and social sciences and law/business. Biology and physics knowledge scales had substantial positive loadings on the Verbal Ability factor, even taking note of the fact that all common ability variance is first accounted for in the g factor loadings. Finally, the second-order g factor was significantly and positively associated with all of the knowledge scale scores.

In summary, factor solutions for the older participants and the respective extension analyses indicated that an underlying Verbal Ability factor showed substantial common variance with many of the knowledge scales, even in addition to the variance in common between verbal ability and g. By contrast, math and spatial abilities (which figure prominently in traditional measures of intelligence) appear to have substantially less common variance with knowledge in the domains under consideration, once their common variance associated with general intelligence is partialed out. As such, the PPIK-inspired hypotheses are supported. That is, verbal and crystallized abilities are more highly associated with what adults "know" across a wide variety of topics, in contrast to the communality between abilities that are more

---

[4]Dwyer's (1937) extension analysis procedure allows extending a factor solution to determine correlations between "new" variables (in this case, the Knowledge Scale scores) and the previously determined factor solution (the ability factors), given knowledge of the correlations between these "new" variables and the "old" variables used to derive the factor solution. Using extension analysis to determine the loadings of the new variables on the predetermined factor solution allows one to derive the original factors independently of the variables hypothesized to relate to them and avoids the psychometric problems inherent in factor scores.

TABLE 19.3   Orthogonalized Hierarchical Factor Analysis Solution for Ability Tests, With Loadings of Knowledge Scales on Ability Factors by Dwyer Extension Procedure, for the Older Sample

Ability area and measure	g	Verbal	Spatial	Math
Verbal ability				
Verbal Analogies	.659	.595	.005	.157
Controlled Associations	.363	.450	−.023	.056
Extended Range Vocabulary	.393	.676	.021	−.024
Spatial ability				
Paper Folding	.434	.030	.517	.001
Verbal Test of Spatial	.598	.027	.481	.108
Spatial Orientation	.367	−.082	.519	.002
Math and numerical ability				
Math Knowledge	.612	.098	.170	.228
Problem Solving	.578	.005	.244	.208
Number Series	.638	−.055	.011	.364
Extension analysis: Knowledge scales				
Astronomy	.370	.341	.137	.027
Biology	.455	.431	.238	−.001
Chemistry	.580	.216	.150	.179
Physics	.559	.353	.244	.080
Statistics	.433	.208	.119	.115
Business/management	.283	.357	.182	−.046
Economics	.430	.128	.132	.135
Geography	.421	.139	.190	.100
Law	.377	.295	.213	.013
Psychology	.255	.449	.096	−.055
American government	.468	.290	.132	.100
American history	.381	.418	.078	.033
Western civilization	.333	.507	.037	−.006
American literature	.166	.618	.003	−.120
Art	.203	.550	.378	−.241
Music	.282	.499	−.034	.000
World literature	.235	.634	.074	−.119
Electronics	.432	.178	.346	.025
Technology	.521	.508	.196	.028
Tools/shop	.357	.191	.461	−.071

Note.   Salient loadings are in boldfaced type.

associated with intelligence as process (i.e., spatial and mathematical abilities) and what adults "know."

The ability–knowledge association demonstration is the first step in validating the PPIK theory and putting the theory to use in educational and occupational applications. The next steps for the research are to take into account other trait correlates of individual differences in knowledge and to determine how traits may interact during adult development to determine individual differences in the depth and breadth of knowledge. The remaining analyses reported here represent attempts to further validate the nonability portions of the PPIK theory as well as to further sift the trait universe to concentrate later on the traits that are most likely to determine the paths of adult intellectual development.

Nonability Correlates of Knowledge

Self-Concept and Self-Estimates of Ability

Correlations between self-report measures of self-concept and self-estimates of ability with the knowledge scales are reported in Table 19.4. Consistent with earlier investigations that correlated self-concept scales and abilities, self-report knowledge, and other traits (e.g., see Ackerman, 1997; Ackerman et al., 1995), there is thematic correspondence between self-concept, self-estimates of abilities, and objective data (e.g., objective aptitude measures). In this case, spatial ability and skill self-concept, mechanical ability and skill self-concept, and self-estimates of mechanical knowledge correlated positively and significantly with individual differences in scores on the natural and physical sciences knowledge scales and with the technology and tools/shop scales. Similarly, math self-concept and self-estimates of math ability correlated with natural and physical sciences knowledge.

Verbal self-concept and self-estimates of verbal ability showed substantial positive correlations with many of the knowledge scales and negative correlations with none of the scales. The largest communalities were found for arts and literature, history, and western/American civilization and for social sciences and law/business. As expected, smaller communalities were found for technology and tools, and the natural and physical sciences knowledge categories. Such results are again consistent with the predictions made by the PPIK theory, supporting a broad framework for Gc, both in aptitude and in nonability traits, such as self-concept.

Interests

Table 19.5 shows the correlations between interest theme scores from the UNIACT and knowledge scale scores for the combined participant sample. Correlations between interests and knowledge scales are concordant with the predictions from the PPIK theory (Ackerman, 1996). That is, the domains of knowledge under consideration were generally not associated with individual differences in social, enterprising, or conventional interests but were positively and significantly associated with realistic, investigative, and artistic interests. Salient positive correlations were found between artistic interests and knowledge scales in the arts and literature category (namely American literature, art, music, and world literature). Similarly, realistic interests showed positive correlations with knowledge scales in the technology and tools category (namely electronics, technology, and tools/shop). Finally, investigative interests (which was originally called "intellectual" interests by Holland, 1959), correlated positively and significantly with all of the knowledge scales except for one (statistics), which appeared to be more indicative of flaws in the knowledge test than anything else. Clearly, there is a substantial correspondence between such intellectual interests and actual level of knowledge acquired. The question of where to put the "causal arrow" (i.e., interests → knowledge; knowledge → interests, or some other variable determines both interests and knowledge) continues to be an important issue for future longitudinal research.

TABLE 19.4 Correlations Among Self-Concept, Self-Estimates of Ability, and Knowledge Scale Scores (Whole Sample)

Knowledge scale	Self-concept						Self-estimates of ability				
	Mechanical	Self-management	Verbal	Clerical	Math	Spatial	Verbal	Math	Self-management	Clerical	Mechanical knowledge
Astronomy	.251**	.166*	.110	.146*	.148*	.255**	.139*	.207**	−.080	−.049	.226**
Biology	.233**	.176**	.333**	.194**	.022	.202**	.366**	.130*	.000	.081	.150*
Chemistry	.362**	.076	.066	.058	.363**	.279**	.077	.466**	−.107	−.135*	.210**
Physics	.390**	.133*	.185**	.109	.137*	.193**	.205**	.237**	−.121*	−.062	.304**
Statistics	.109	−.006	.126*	.094	.063	.075	.165**	.140*	−.067	.115	.093
Business/management	.177**	.172**	.310**	.139*	−.075	.071	.400**	−.060	−.008	.107	.123*
Economics	.223**	.121*	.109	.055	.125*	.108	.226**	.174**	−.108	−.093	.151*
Geography	.209**	.066	.182**	.155*	.034	.253**	.254**	.100	−.072	.012	.165*
Law	.200**	.185**	.280**	.173**	−.056	.077	.359**	−.026	−.064	.050	.123*
Psychology	.148*	.212**	.285**	.111	−.059	.111	.302**	−.005	.023	.000	.110
American government	.119	.120*	.256**	.113	.032	.033	.351**	.102	−.089	.025	.094
American history	.256**	.178**	.299**	.135*	−.014	.103	.437**	.037	−.012	.011	.207**
Western civilization	.168**	.123*	.314**	.044	−.021	.125*	.469**	.071	−.047	−.062	.082
American literature	.113	.125*	.405**	.072	−.157**	.048	.495**	−.103	−.010	−.010	.077
Art	.016	.090	.429**	.115	−.155*	.119	.442**	−.175**	−.082	.122	−.001
Music	.130*	.156*	.439**	.232**	−.127*	.089	.439**	−.114	.000	.161*	.084
World literature	.136*	.186**	.453**	.145*	−.152*	.101	.515**	−.090	.013	.058	.061
Electronics	.395**	.234**	.183**	.199**	.040	.292**	.196**	.107	−.047	−.006	.287**
Technology	.329**	.187**	.279**	.198**	.068	.258**	.311**	.180**	−.055	.043	.253**
Tools/shop	.463**	.086	.049	.140*	.075	.251**	.060	.141*	−.137*	−.020	.423**

Note. The maximum sample size for the combined younger and older groups was 278. Salient correlations are in boldface.
*$p < .05$. **$p < .01$, two-tailed.

TABLE 19.5 Correlations Between Interests (From UNIACT) and Knowledge Scale Scores (Whole Sample)

Knowledge scale	UNIACT Interest scale					
	Realistic	Investigative	Artistic	Social	Enterprising	Conventional
Astronomy	.142*	.215***	.117	−.124	−.073	−.014
Biology	.173***	.388***	.199***	−.011	−.178**	−.133*
Chemistry	.160***	.299***	−.039	−.053	−.166***	−.049
Physics	.250***	.292***	.113	−.054	−.107	−.020
Statistics	.052	.103	.122	.007	.025	.001
Business/management	.188**	.276***	.211**	−.053	−.024	−.008
Economics	.134*	.178**	.071	−.107	.031	.051
Geography	.155*	.232***	.211**	−.068	−.093	−.042
Law	.190**	.198***	.187***	−.144*	−.020	.050
Psychology	.120*	.288***	.240***	.103	−.017	−.035
American government	.089	.189***	.197***	−.112	−.043	−.037
American history	.165*	.243***	.271***	−.086	−.023	−.059
Western civilization	.104	.285***	.255***	.001	−.042	−.102
American literature	.149*	.320***	.332***	−.024	−.082	−.131*
Art	.113	.297***	.417***	−.060	−.105	−.186**
Music	.180**	.299***	.366***	−.047	−.144*	−.096
World literature	.157***	.349***	.373***	−.026	−.092	−.098
Electronics	.319***	.360***	.149*	−.108	−.153*	.011
Technology	.292***	.388***	.209***	−.086	−.131*	−.018
Tools/shop	.384***	.283***	.043	−.099	−.124*	.039

Note. The maximum sample size was 278 for the combined younger and older groups. Salient correlations are in boldface. UNIACT = Unisex Edition of the ACT Interest Inventory (ACT = American College Testing).
*$p < .05$. **$p < .01$, two-tailed.

Personality and Motivation

The personality and motivational trait correlations with knowledge scale scores, shown in Table 19.6, provide general confirmation of predictions. That is, neuroticism and agreeableness did not correlate significantly with knowledge scales. TIE, and to some degree openness, did correlate highly and significantly with knowledge scales, especially in arts and literature domains. Interestingly, conscientiousness failed to correlate significantly with any of the knowledge scales, providing additional support for the notion that this particular Big Five personality factor is more about "plodding" kinds of behaviors than "dedicated" kinds of behaviors (e.g., see the clerical/conventional trait complex in Ackerman & Heggestad, 1997). The correlations between extraversion and knowledge scale scores were uniformly large and significantly negative, indicating that higher levels of extraversion were associated with lower scores on the knowledge tests.

The only scale of motivational traits to consistently correlate with the knowledge scales was Competitiveness, and that measure correlated negatively with arts and literature knowledge, technology and tools knowledge as well as with business/management knowledge. Such results are concordant with recent theorizing about adult motivation traits and assessment procedures (Kanfer & Heggestad, 1997) that have suggested that the extant measures are missing substantial sources of individual-differences variance in motivation.

Some Preliminary Conclusions

Among both the younger and older adult samples, g and verbal ability (even after g was partialed from this ability) were positively and consistently related to individual differences on the 20 knowledge scales. No consistent pattern of correlations between spatial and math abilities were found, once general intelligence was partialed from these abilities. The verbal tests associated with traditional assessment of Gc are most highly predictive of standing on the knowledge scales. However, it is important to note that verbal ability does not account for all of the knowledge scale performance — indeed, many knowledge scales only weakly loaded on an independent Verbal Ability factor (e.g., scales from the technology and tools domain, and the natural and physical sciences domain). It is thus important to note this asymmetry from these results. That is, at least qualitatively, the results demonstrate that knowledge is something more than verbal abilities (or Gc as traditionally measured).

Vocational interests are very much in line with predictions from Ackerman's (1996) PPIK theory and from the review of interest–intelligence associations (Ackerman, 1997; Ackerman & Heggestad, 1997). That is, realistic, investigative, and artistic interests were positively associated with knowledge scale scores across a wide variety of scales (with predictable correspondences, such as artistic interests and art or music knowledge, and realistic interests and electronics and tools/shop knowledge). Interests in social, enterprising, and conventional domains were largely uncorrelated with performance on the knowledge scales.

The personality traits of openness and TIE were substantially positively correlated with many knowledge scales, especially in the arts and literature domains. By contrast, competitiveness was negatively associated with several knowledge scales. Also,

TABLE 19.6 Correlations Between Personality and Motivational Traits (NEO-FFI, TIE, and WOFO) and Knowledge Scale Scores (Whole Sample)

Knowledge scale	Personality and motivational scales								
	Neuroticism	Extraversion	Openness	Agreeableness	Conscientiousness	TIE	Work	Mastery	Competitiveness
Astronomy	0.37	-.288**	.214**	-.109	-.081	.241**	.035	.088	.063
Biology	-.051	-.296**	.275**	.014	.044	.371**	.154*	.054	-.025
Chemistry	-.039	-.247**	.108	.014	-.021	.157**	.048	.028	.048
Physics	-.063	-.275**	.218**	-.035	-.002	.278**	.100	.038	-.065
Statistics	.007	-.167**	.121	-.071	-.030	.199**	.062	.064	.062
Business/ management	-.044	-.246**	.306**	.088	.101	.364**	.132*	-.018	-.267**
Economics	-.032	-.300**	.170**	-.037	-.002	.252**	.053	.039	.008
Geography	.010	-.261**	.285**	.017	-.101	.325**	-.025	.033	-.078
Law	-.044	-.292**	.242**	.024	.089	.337**	.132*	.061	-.146*
Psychology	-.000	-.235**	.294**	.101	.047	.347**	.211**	.004	-.098
American government	-.007	-.361**	.253**	.004	-.045	.334**	-.023	-.085	-.104
American history	-.027	-.324**	.343**	.045	-.015	.447**	-.007	.015	-.156*
Western civilization	-.042	-.267**	.358**	.058	-.120	.425**	-.015	.003	-.048
American literature	.013	-.314**	.460**	.041	-.049	.486**	-.002	-.017	-.257**
Art	-.017	-.222**	.453**	.070	-.006	.459**	.019	.084	-.237**
Music	.016	-.298**	.404**	.065	.053	.416**	.024	.036	-.214**
World literature	-.013	-.290**	.511**	.107	-.032	.556**	.005	.042	-.268**
Electronics	-.126	-.210**	.284**	.087	.103	.340**	.196**	.147*	-.156*
Technology	-.079	-.302**	.372**	.081	.047	.422**	.133*	.058	-.169*
Tools/shop	-.108	-.228**	.186**	.014	-.078	.205**	.070	.009	-.148*

Note. The maximum sample size was 278 for the combined younger and older groups. Salient correlations are in boldfaced type. NEO-FFI = NEO Five-Factor Inventory; TIE = typical intellectual engagement; WOFO = Work and Family Orientation Questionnaire.
*$p < .05$. **$p < .01$, two-tailed.

somewhat surprisingly, extraversion was significantly negatively correlated with performance on nearly all of the knowledge scales.

In general, these results are consistent with the PPIK approach to adult intellect that represents the foundation for this program of research. Most of all, though, these results argue for a more integrated view of adult intellect than that provided by traditionally separate perspectives offered by single-domain researches (e.g., processes, traits, or content). The many communalities found among predictor variables and individual differences in knowledge support an approach that has the following fundamental tenets (which, of course, are subject to empirical verification):

1. Whether through genetic or environmental causes (or their interactions), individual differences in basic information-processing capabilities provide a "starting point" for human intellect.
2. Early in development, through positive and negative cultural and educational experiences, individuals develop a set of coherent interests, personality, and abilities.
3. As common educational and cultural experiences are replaced during adolescence and beyond by unique or occupationally or avocationally distinct experiences, individual differences in knowledge structures develop, both in breadth and depth.
4. What an adult knows is determined initially by individual differences in basic information-processing abilities and later by investment of intellectual capital (in terms of time and effort), in concert with a relatively small set of key interest, personality, and self-concept traits.
5. By the time an individual is an adult (especially through middle age), what the individual is capable of, in terms of day-to-day interactions with the world at large, is expected to be more dependent on the adult's knowledge and less dependent on individual differences in information-processing speed and accuracy.

REFERENCES

Ackerman, P. L. (1984). *A theoretical and empirical investigation of individual differences in learning: A synthesis of cognitive ability and information processing perspectives.* Unpublished doctoral dissertation, University of Illinois, Urbana.

Ackerman, P. L. (1986). Individual differences in information processing: An investigation of intellectual abilities and task performance during practice. *Intelligence, 10,* 101–139.

Ackerman, P. L. (1988). Determinants of individual differences during skill acquisition: Cognitive abilities and information processing. *Journal of Experimental Psychology: General, 117,* 288–318.

Ackerman, P. L. (1990). A correlational analysis of skill specificity: Learning, abilities, and individual differences. *Journal of Experimental Psychology: Learning, Memory, and Cognition, 16,* 883–901.

Ackerman, P. L. (1992). Predicting individual differences in complex skill acquisition: Dynamics of ability determinants. *Journal of Applied Psychology, 77,* 598–614.

Ackerman, P. L. (1994). Intelligence, attention, and learning: Maximal and typical performance. In D. K. Detterman (Ed.), *Current topics in human intelligence: Vol. 4. Theories of intelligence* (pp. 1–27). Norwood, NJ: Ablex.

Ackerman, P. L. (1996). A theory of adult intellectual development: Process, personality, interests, and knowledge. *Intelligence, 22,* 229–259.

Ackerman, P. L. (1997). Personality, self-concept, interests, and intelligence: Which construct doesn't fit? *Journal of Personality, 65,* 171–204.

Ackerman, P. L., & Goff, M. (1994). Typical intellectual engagement and personality: Reply to Rocklin (1994). *Journal of Educational Psychology, 86,* 150–153.

Ackerman, P. L., & Heggestad, E. D. (1997). Intelligence, personality, and interests: Evidence for overlapping traits. *Psychological Bulletin, 121,* 219–245.

Ackerman, P. L., & Kanfer, R. (1993). Integrating laboratory and field study for improving selection: Development of a battery for predicting air traffic controller success. *Journal of Applied Psychology, 78,* 413–432.

Ackerman, P. L., Kanfer, R., & Goff, M. (1995). Cognitive and noncognitive determinants and consequences of complex skill acquisition. *Journal of Experimental Psychology: Applied, 1,* 270–304.

Ackerman, P. L., & Rolfhus, E. R. (1998a). *Knowledge structures and adult intellectual development* (College Board Research Rep. No. 98-3). New York: College Board.

Ackerman, P. L., & Rolfhus, E. R. (1998b). *Knowledge structures and ability, personality, and interests: A cross-sectional comparison of younger and middle-aged adults.* Manuscript under review.

Alexander, P. A., Kulikowich, J. M., & Schulze, S. K. (1994). The influence of topic knowledge, domain knowledge, and interest on the comprehension of scientific exposition. *Learning and Individual Differences, 6,* 379–397.

Baldwin, R. S., Peleg-Bruckner, Z., & McClintock, A. H. (1985). Effects of topic interest and prior knowledge on reading comprehension. *Reading Research Quarterly, 20,* 497–504.

Baltes, P. B., & Schaie, K. W. (1976). On the plasticity of intelligence in adulthood and old age: Where Horn and Donaldson fail. *American Psychologist, 31,* 720–725.

Carroll, J. B. (1993). *Human cognitive abilities: A survey of factor-analytic studies.* New York: Cambridge University Press.

Cattell, R. B. (1943). The measurement of adult intelligence. *Psychological Bulletin, 40,* 153–193.

Cattell, R. B. (1957). *Personality and motivation structure and measurement.* Yonkers-on-Hudson, NY: World Book.

Cattell, R. B. (1987). *Abilities: Their structure, growth and action.* Amsterdam: North-Holland. (Original work published 1971)

Charness, N. (1987). Component processes in bridge bidding and novel problem-solving tasks. *Canadian Journal of Psychology, 41,* 223–243.

Chase, W. G., & Ericsson, K. A. (1981). Skilled memory. In J. R. Anderson (Ed.), *Cognitive skills and their acquisition* (pp. 141–189). Hillsdale, NJ: Erlbaum.

Chase, W. G., & Simon, H. A. (1973). Perception in chess. *Cognitive Psychology, 4,* 55–81.

Chi, M. T. H., Glaser, R., & Rees, E. (1982). Expertise in problem solving. *Advances in the Psychology of Human Intelligence, 1,* 7–76.

Detterman, D. K., & Andrist, C. G. (1990). Effect of instructions on elementary cognitive tasks sensitive to individual differences. *American Journal of Psychology, 103,* 367–390.

Dwyer, P. S. (1937). The determination of the factor loadings of a given test from the known factor loadings of other tests. *Psychometrika, 2,* 173–178.

Goff, M., & Ackerman, P. L. (1992). Personality–intelligence relations: Assessing typical intellectual engagement. *Journal of Educational Psychology, 84,* 537–552.

Hebb, D. O. (1942). The effect of early and late brain injury upon test scores, and the nature of normal adult intelligence. *Proceedings of the American Philosophical Society, 85,* 275–292.

Hebb, D. O. (1949). *The organization of behavior: A neuropsychological theory.* New York: Wiley.

Holahan, C. K., & Sears, R. with Cronbach, L. J. (1995). *The gifted group in later maturity.* Stanford, CA: Stanford University Press.

Holland, J. L. (1959). A theory of vocational choice. *Journal of Counseling Psychology, 6,* 35–45.

Holland, J. L. (1973). *Making vocational choices: A theory of careers.* Englewood Cliffs, NJ: Prentice Hall.

Horn, J. L. (1965). *Fluid and crystallized intelligence: A factor analytic study of the structure among primary mental abilities.* (University Microfilms No. 65–7113).

Horn, J. L. (1968). Organization of abilities and the development of intelligence. *Psychological Review, 75,* 242–259.

Horn, J. L., & Cattell, R. B. (1966). Refinement and test of the theory of fluid and crystallized general intelligences. *Journal of Educational Psychology, 57,* 253–270.

Horn, J. L., & Donaldson, G. (1976). On the myth of intellectual decline in adulthood. *American Psychologist, 31,* 486–498.

Humphreys, L. G., & Taber, T. (1973). Postdiction study of the Graduate Record Examination and eight semesters of college grades. *Journal of Educational Measurement, 10,* 179–184.

Hunter, J. E. (1983). A causal analysis of cognitive ability, job knowledge, job performance, and super-

459

visor ratings. In F. Landy, S. Zedeck, & J. Cleveland (Eds.), *Performance measurement and theory* (pp. 257–266). Hillsdale, NJ: Erlbaum.

Kanfer, R., & Heggestad, E. (1997). Motivational traits and skills: A person-centered approach to work motivation. In L. L. Cummings & B. M. Staw (Eds.), *Research in organizational behavior* (Vol. 19, pp. 1–57). JAI Press, Greenwich, CT.

Lowman, R. L., Williams, R. E., & Leeman, G. E. (1985). The structure and relationship of college women's primary abilities and vocational interests. *Journal of Vocational Behavior, 27,* 298–315.

MacLeod, C. M. (1991). Half a century of research on the Stoop effect: An integrative review. *Psychological Bulletin, 109,* 163–203.

Rocklin, T. (1994). The relationship between typical intellectual engagement and openness: A comment on Goff and Ackerman (1992). *Journal of Educational Psychology, 86,* 145–149.

Rogers, W. A., Fisk, A. D., & Hertzog, C. (1994). Do ability–performance relationships differentiate age and practice effects in visual search? *Journal of Experimental Psychology: Learning, Perception and Cognition, 20,* 710–738.

Rolfhus, E. L. (1998). *Assessing individual differences in knowledge: Knowledge structures and traits.* Unpublished doctoral dissertation, University of Minnesota, Twin Cities.

Rolfhus, E. L., & Ackerman, P. L. (1996). Self-report knowledge: At the crossroads of ability, interest, and personality. *Journal of Educational Psychology, 88,* 174–188.

Rolfhus, E. L., & Ackerman, P. L. (1998). *Assessing the student's knowledge: Test development and communalities with abilities, personality, and interests.* Manuscript under review.

Salthouse, T. A. (1996). The processing-speed theory of adult age differences in cognition. *Psychological Review, 103,* 403–428.

Schaie, K. W. (1970). A reinterpretation of age related changes in cognitive structure and functioning. In L. R. Goulet & P. B. Baltes (Eds.), *Life-span developmental psychology* (pp. 423–466). New York: Academic Press.

Schaie, K. W. (1974). Transitions in gerontology: From lab to life. *American Psychologist, 29,* 802–807.

Schmid, J., & Leiman, J. M. (1957). The development of hierarchical factor solutions. *Psychometrika, 22,* 53–61.

Schmidt, F. L., & Hunter, J. E. (1993). Tacit knowledge, practical intelligence, general mental ability, and job knowledge. *Current Directions in Psychological Science, 2,* 8–9.

Signorella, M. L., & Jamison, W. (1986). Masculinity, femininity, androgyny and cognitive performance: A meta-analysis. *Psychological Bulletin, 100,* 207–238.

Snow, R. E. (1989). Aptitude–treatment interaction as a framework for research on individual differences in learning. In P. L. Ackerman, R. J. Sternberg, & R. Glaser (Eds.), *Learning and individual differences: Advances in theory and research* (pp. 13–59). New York: Freeman.

Staudinger, U., & Baltes, P. (1994). Psychology of wisdom. In R. J. Sternberg (Ed.), *Encyclopedia of human intelligence* (Vol. 2, pp. 1143–1152). New York: Macmillan.

Stauffer, J. M., Ree, M. J., & Carretta, T. R. (1996). Cognitive-components tests are not much more than *g*: An extension of Kyllonen's analysis. *Journal of General Psychology, 123,* 193–205.

Sternberg, R. J. (1977). *Intelligence, information processing, and analogical reasoning: The componential analysis of human abilities.* Hillsdale, NJ: Erlbaum.

Sternberg, R. J. (1985a). *Beyond IQ: A triarchic theory of human intelligence.* Cambridge, England: Cambridge University Press.

Sternberg, R. J. (Ed.). (1985b). *Human abilities: An information-processing approach.* New York: Freeman.

Sternberg, R. J., & Berg, C. A. (1987). What are theories of adult intellectual development theories of? In C. Schooler & K. W. Schaie (Eds.), *Cognitive functioning and social structure over the life course* (pp. 3–23). Norwood, NJ: Ablex.

Stroop, J. R. (1935). Studies of interference in serial verbal reactions. *Journal of Experimental Psychology, 18,* 643–662.

Whipple, G. M. (1922). Intelligence tests in colleges and universities. *The twenty-first yearbook of the National Society for the Study of Education* (Chap. 10, pp. 253–270).

Willingham, W. W. (1974). Predicting success in graduate education. *Science, 183,* 273–278.

Discussion

Discussion following Ackerman's paper started with inquiries about the relationship between typical intellectual engagement and need for cognition. Subsequent discussion concerned the difference between Ackerman's approach to knowledge as intelligence and other approaches, such as the study of wisdom.

Dr. Stanovich: Before we became aware of your typical intellectual engagement scale, we did a little work with need for cognition. I was wondering if you could either tell us how need for cognition relates to TIE.

Dr. Ackerman: I'm afraid I don't know the answer to that. I don't know where need for cognition fits to anything. The work that I've seen is confused about where a need for cognition fits in the nomological space.

Dr. Pisoni: Could you explain what that is, the need for cognition?

Dr. Stanovich: Well, it seemed to have some overlap with typical intellectual engagement. The need to stay engaged in mental activities. It bears similarities in the sense that it deals with typical performance rather than maximal performance.

Dr. Ackerman: But it's not as academic and culturally oriented as the typical intellectual engagement scale is. And I would guess need for a cognition fits a little closer to personality measures than to intelligence measures, but I don't have the specific data on it.

Dr. Deary: You've shown some fields in which older people do better. Can I mention another one where we always assume they did? That is in wisdom. Paul Baltes's group (Staudinger & Baltes, 1994), as you know, spent some years trying to operationalize and validate the measures of wisdom. One of the surprises is, except for those individuals who were nominated as being very wise and probably often turn out to be people like Nobel Prize winners, the average older person doesn't

461

seem to be all that wise in their studies. Do you want to comment on that with respect to your orientation?

Dr. Ackerman: If I wanted to be evaluative, where Baltes et al. went wrong (at least as far as my own theory is concerned) is that wisdom is considered as processing new information. They gave people scenarios, and they say "figure out the right answer." So it still involves probably a fair amount of fluid intelligence in conceptualizing the problem and dealing with it. What Baltes et al. didn't do was to take an individual who is, say, an accountant, and say here's an accounting problem, show us your wisdom about accounting. What he did was he said here's a general life question or here's a novel question. And what I'm saying is, as the artificial intelligence people have said, general problem solvers are not how people do things in the real world. It's mostly knowledge driven. That means you can't ask everybody the same question. You have to be able to tap that which individuals know, and a carpenter is going to know a lot that's different from a physicist.

Dr. Deary: The other aspect of their measure of wisdom is that you seem to get a lot of points for being indecisive. The more you can prevaricate about the question, the wiser you're supposed to be.

Dr. Ackerman: That is, it is similar to Guilford's divergent production, right? For example, any idea you come up with, for the use of a brick counts as a positive mark for creativity.

Dr. Gustafsson: I was reminded by some Swedish work where Anette Andersson, who is a graduate student of mine, has analyzed the grades from the Swedish comprehensive school, which are awarded when the kids leave at the age of 16. There are 17 different subject matter areas, and there is a strong general factor, which probably to a large extent is a halo effect. But when the general factor is taken out, we can see that there are four or five dimensions which define different profiles, and the profiles seem to be very much patterned along knowledge domain areas and seem to be highly predictive of lines of study in upper secondary school and at universities. So my question, or my comment, is that the profiling of competence may start early. You seem to be looking at the adult age. But perhaps it will be worthwhile to try to locate this in younger age groups as well?

Dr. Ackerman: I think that's right. And there is a lot to be said for earlier development during adolescence. What I am trying to do is to developmentally separate a general curriculum from differential curricula. In this country, children proceed through sixth grade or seventh grade before they start getting electives and can take different courses. So yes, I think especially in a place where are students are put into "tracks" (which is less frequent in this country) into vocational schooling or university or academic preparation schooling. That provides for a lot more individual differences in knowledge that are developed, and I think it would provide a wonderful place to assess this longitudinally.

Dr. Wagner: Where did your older sample come from?

Dr. Ackerman: The general broader university community. The University of Minnesota has this huge night and extension class program, and students come in from all over the Twin Cities and sign up. And we paid them a lot of money.

Dr. Wagner: I just wondered if maybe there were going to be some differences in knowledge, and the typical intellectual engagement might be differences in the population where people are kind of hanging around the university when they're 30 to 40.

Dr. Ackerman: That is absolutely right. And in the future, we hope to be able to sample more broadly. However, we didn't have the funding to go beyond the university community, and that's certainly a limitation of this study.

Author Index

Numbers in italics refer to listings in reference sections.

463

Subject Index

About the Editors

Phillip L. Ackerman, PhD, is Professor of Psychology at the Georgia Institute of Technology. He is a Fellow of the American Psychological Association, the American Psychological Society, and the Human Factors and Ergonomics Society. From 1987 to 1990 he held the McKnight-Land Grant Professorship at the University of Minnesota. He is an editorial board member of *Intelligence: A Multidisciplinary Journal, Human Performance* and *Learning and Individual Differences: A Multidisciplinary Journal in Education.* He has coedited two books on learning and individual differences. In 1992, he was the recipient of the American Psychological Association's Distinguished Scientific Award for Early Career Contribution to Psychology (in the field of Applied Research/Psychometrics). His current research concerns ability determinants of skill acquisition, personality–interest–ability relations, and adult intellectual development.

Patrick C. Kyllonen, PhD, is Senior Scientist in the Manpower and Personnel Research Division (Human Resources directorate) of the U.S. Air Force Research Laboratory and Director of the Learning Abilities Measurement Program (LAMP). He is a Fellow of the American Psychological Association and a recipient of the American Psychological Association Division 15 Outstanding Early Contribution Award, the Air Force Human Resources Laboratory's Scientific Achievement Award, the Air Force Science and Technology Achievement Award, and the Air Force's Basic Research Award (honorable mention). He serves on the editorial boards of the journals *Intelligence: A Multidisciplinary Journal, Human Factors* and the *Spanish Journal of Psychology.* His research interests center around the topic of individual differences and cognition and recently have focused on time estimation, psychomotor abilities, mood and personality as they affect learning and performance, and knowledge assessment.

Richard D. Roberts, PhD, is a National Research Council Fellow at the Human

Resources Directorate, U.S. Air Force Research Laboratory, Brooks Air Force Base, Texas. He is the coauthor of a forthcoming book on mental speed and cognitive ability. His research interests concern development of a taxonomic model of mental processing speed and investigations of less well understood domains of individual differences (e.g., emotional intelligence, tactile and olfactory abilities, circadian rhythms, and confidence ratings).

BF 318 .L3853 1999 C.1

Learning and individual
  differences

DATE DUE	
APR 1 5 1999	
9/12/04 ILL	
MAR 09 2006	
GAYLORD	PRINTED IN U.S.A.